Afoot & Afield

Los Angeles County

259 Spectacular Outings in Southern California

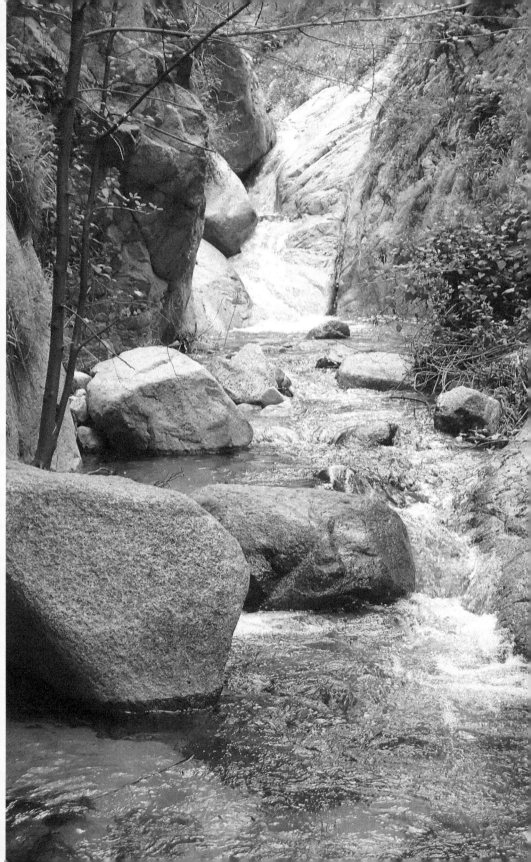

Afoot & Afield

Los Angeles County

259 Spectacular Outings in Southern California

FOURTH EDITION

Jerry Schad and David Harris

WILDERNESS PRESS ... *on the trail since 1967*

IN MEMORY OF JERRY SCHAD, 1949–2011

Afoot & Afield Los Angeles County: 259 Spectacular Outings in Southern California

Copyright © 1991, 2000, 2010 by Jerry Schad
Copyright © 2020 by David Harris

Published by Wilderness Press
Distributed by Publishers Group West
Fourth edition, first printing

Editor: Ritchey Halphen
Photos: David Harris, except where noted
Maps: David Harris and Scott McGrew
Cover design: Scott McGrew
Text design: Andreas Schüller, with updates by Annie Long
Proofreader: Emily C. Beaumont
Indexer: Joanne Sprott/Potomac Indexing

LCCN: 2019021676; ISBN: 978-1-64359-041-7; ISBN: 978-0-89997-870-3 (e-book)

Published by: **𝍏 WILDERNESS PRESS**
An imprint of AdventureKEEN
2204 First Ave. S., Ste. 102
Birmingham, AL 35233
800-443-7227; FAX 205-326-1012

Visit wildernesspress.com for a complete listing of our books and for ordering information. Contact us at info@wildernesspress.com, facebook.com/wildernesspress1967, or twitter.com/wilderness1967 with questions or comments. To find out more about who we are and what we're doing, visit blog.wildernesspress.com.

Cover photos: (Front cover, clockwise from top) Wildflowers in bloom at Point Dume, Malibu (see Trip 1.1, page 25), Luc Mena/Shutterstock; evening light at Vasquez Rocks Natural Area (see Trip 12.6, page 184), Jon Bilous/Alamy Stock Photo; hiker and dog on the Zuma Ridge Trail, Malibu (see Trip 8.2, page 102), Debra Behr/Alamy Stock Photo. (Back cover) Rocky Peak summit (see Trip 5.3, page 58), David Harris

Frontispiece: First Water welcomes travelers on the Old Mount Wilson Trail (see Trip 24.8, page 324); photo: David Harris

Safety Notice Although Wilderness Press and the authors have made every attempt to ensure that the information in this book is accurate at press time, they are not responsible for any loss, damage, injury, or inconvenience that may occur to anyone while using this book. You are responsible for your own safety and health while in the wilderness. The fact that a trail is described in this book does not mean that it will be safe for you. Be aware that trail conditions can change from day to day. Always check local conditions, and know your own limitations.

Acknowledgments

I am grateful to many people for their help with this project.

Many reviewers have helped improve this book. They include the following: Christy Araujo, Tim Hayden, and James Valdez, California State Parks; David Baumgartner, Restoration Legacy Crew; Jane Baumgartner, Fisheries Resource Volunteer Corps and San Gabriel Canyon Gateway Center; Melanie Beck, National Park Service; Jessica Boudevin and Morgan Robson, Catalina Conservancy; Christopher Brennen; Russell Brown and Adam Dedeaux, Griffith Park; Tom Chester; Bryan Conant, Los Padres Forest Association; Andrea Gullo, Puente Hills Habitat Preservation Authority; Anna Huber, Conejo Open Space Conservation Agency; Kyle Kuns; Louise Olfarnes, Palos Verdes Peninsula Land Conservancy; Deveron Shudic, Glendale Community Services & Parks; Dash Stolarz, Mountains Recreation and Conservation Authority; Bob Spears; Ben White, San Gabriel Mountains Trailbuilders; Richard Wismer, Mount Baldy Visitor Center; and Helen Wong, Eaton Canyon Natural Area.

I am also grateful to Werner Zorman and Elizabeth Thomas, who woke up in the wee hours for countless Thursday Morning Hiking Club expeditions, and to my sons, Abraham, Samuel, and Benjamin, who helped me evaluate many of the kid-friendly hikes.

Finally, I would like to thank the team at Wilderness Press for making this book come together: Ritchey Halphen, who did a marvelous job of editing and managing the project; Annie Long, who perfected the design, and Monica Ahlman, who executed her vision; Emily Beaumont, who carefully proofread the pages; and indexer Joanne Sprott.

—*David Harris*
Upland, California
September 2019

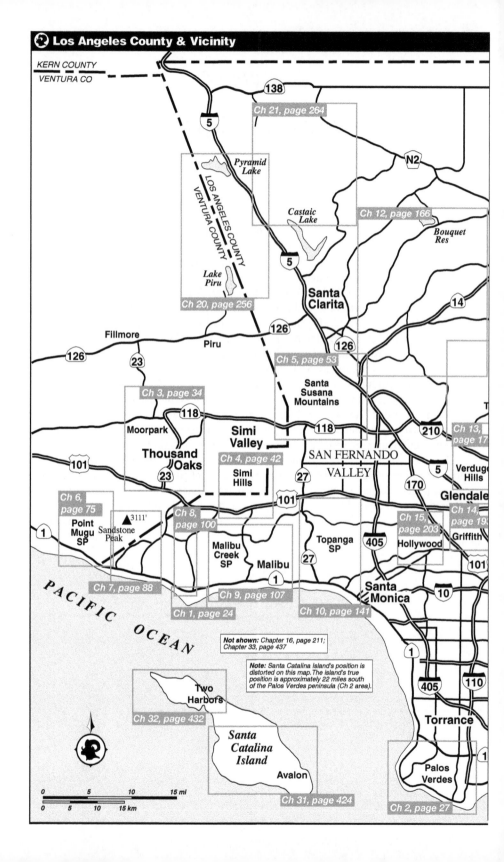

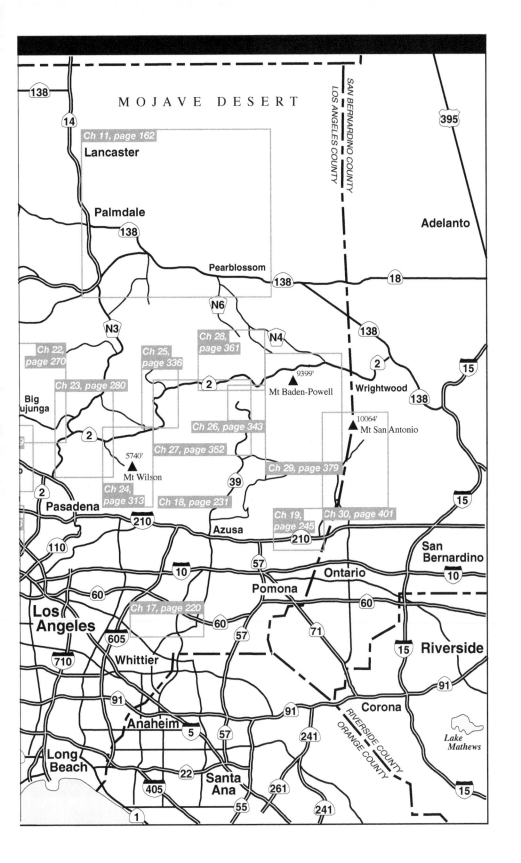

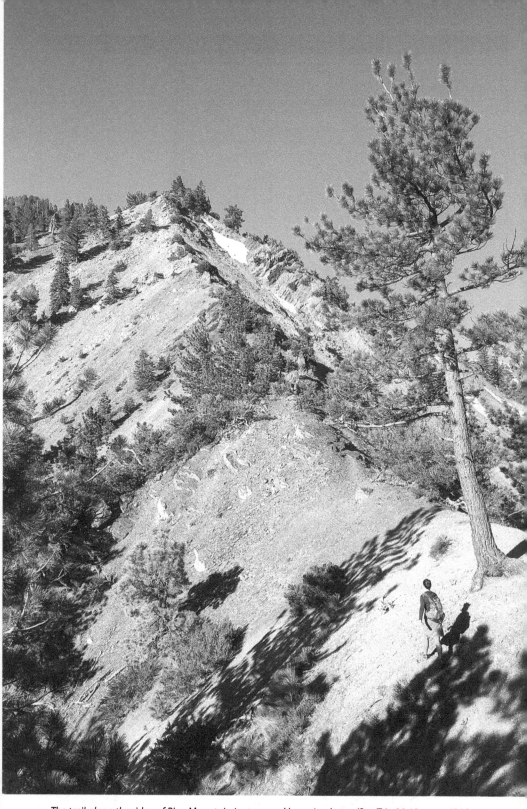

The trail along the ridge of Pine Mountain is steep and loose in places. (See Trip 30.13, page 420.)
Photo: Werner Zorman

Contents

Preface

Pummeled by great heavings of the earth's crust, desiccated by drought, torn by flood, tortured by fire, and pestered by the threat of human intervention, Los Angeles's wild spaces are nonetheless not the wastelands they may appear to be when viewed through a brown veil of smog or haze. In fact, if you take the time to venture almost anywhere beyond the sprawling metropolitan borders, you'll discover that nature is not only alive out there, it's often triumphant.

While doing field research for this book, I (Jerry) have clambered over sandstone boulders the size of trucks, cooled off in the spray of frothing waterfalls, and trekked down a Wild and Scenic River. In the high country of the San Gabriel Mountains, I stood in stunned silence as a herd of two dozen bighorn sheep scooted across a rocky pass just below me. From a chaparral-clad slope above Glendale, I witnessed the strange juxtaposition of a deer's silhouette against the Oz-like towers of downtown L.A.

With friends I've admired sea stars in crystalline tide pools on the Malibu coast, scuffed through powdery snow in the San Gabriels, and inhaled the nectar-rich air of the Mojave Desert in bloom. From the Angeles Crest, we've spotted white sails in Santa Monica Bay and watched the sun sink toward a blue horizon dimpled by four offshore islands. Alone at dawn on the mile-high rim of the L.A. Basin, I've watched the glare of a million lights succumb to the pink twilight.

In all of my field trips for this book, totaling more than 1,000 miles of walking, never have I needed to venture more than 20 air-miles from the fringe of Los Angeles or its populous satellite cities. Yet once on the trail, I've seldom felt the weight of the teeming millions all around me; indeed in a few places I've walked all day without seeing another person.

This wide-ranging guide covers an equally wide-ranging county: a kingdom in itself, with elements of coast, foothill, mountain, and desert rolled into a 4,083-square-mile space. Remove the urbanized coastal plain and the semideveloped western Mojave from the county's area, and you're still left with nearly 2,000 square miles of wild or lightly developed land.

Most of L.A. County's publicly accessible open spaces lie north and west of the heavily populated coastal plain. **Angeles National Forest,** encompassing most of the San Gabriel Mountains, sprawls across 652,000 acres (1,019 square miles), about one-quarter of the county's land area. In spite of Southern California's dry climate, the Angeles Forest supports about 240 miles of perennial streams and in some areas a forest cover resembling parts of the high Sierra Nevada. About 600 miles of trail—including a segment of the Pacific Crest National Scenic Trail—connect high and low points within the forest, linking such disparate locations as the L.A. Basin and the Mojave Desert. In 2014, President Barack Obama designated 364,177 acres of the range as **San Gabriel Mountains National Monument,** but little new funding or other changes have yet followed.

Tucked into the southwestern corner of the county and spilling over into Ventura County are the **Santa Monica Mountains.** This coastal range includes a patchwork of private and public lands, the latter under the jurisdiction of the National Park Service (**Santa Monica**

Mountains National Recreation Area) and various state and local agencies. The pace of park-land acquisition in the Santa Monicas has quickened in recent years, and the trail network is continually expanding

Close to the heart of the county's urban core are scattered islands of open space: the **Santa Susana** and **Verdugo Mountains,** bordering the San Fernando Valley; the **Puente Hills,** in the San Gabriel Valley; and, of course, venerable **Griffith Park.**

Rounding out the list of better places to explore in the county are some more-or-less natural stretches of Pacific coastline, the rim of the western Mojave Desert, and **Santa Catalina Island.**

Every trip in this book was hiked by each of the authors at least once, and every effort has been made to ensure that the information herein is current as of the day of publication. Road access and trailheads do change, however. New acreage is being acquired for public use, and the near future will doubtless see the construction of more trails.

—Jerry Schad

I am honored to follow in Jerry Schad's footsteps and keep his book current and vibrant. For the fourth edition, I rehiked nearly every trail in this book, with the exception of a few that are still closed due to fire damage. The field work involved more than 1,500 miles of walking and 20,000 miles of driving over two-and-a-half years. I have added 66 new trips and removed 15 trips, mostly because of access issues; a handful of others were either just uninteresting or wiped out by wildfire.

Updates and future editions of this book are planned, so please keep me apprised of recent developments and/or changes by writing me in care of Wilderness Press, or email me at info@wildernesspress.com. Your comments are appreciated.

—David Harris

Goat Rocks at Malibu Creek State Park is near the Lookout Loop. (See Trip 9.8, page 119.)

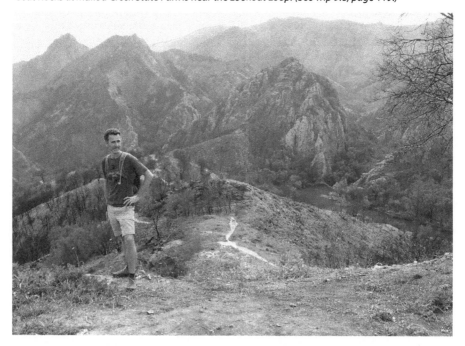

Overview of Hikes

HIKE NUMBER	HIKE	DISTANCE (miles)	ELEVATION GAIN (feet)	TRAIL TYPE	BACKPACKING	MOUNTAIN BIKING	EQUESTRIANS	DOGS	KIDS
Chapter 1: MALIBU COAST									
1.1	Point Dume to Paradise Cove	2.9	200	point-to-point					🚸
Chapter 2: PALOS VERDES PENINSULA									
2.1	Top of the Peninsula	1.8	300	out-and-back				🐕	🚸
2.2	Malaga Cove to Bluff Cove	1.9	200	loop					🚸
2.3	Bluff Cove to Point Vicente	6	200	point-to-point					
2.4	White Point to Cabrillo Beach	3.4	200	point-to-point					🚸
Chapter 3: THOUSAND OAKS & MOORPARK									
3.1	Happy Camp Canyon	10.5	1,500	loop		🚲			
3.2	Paradise Falls	2.7	500	loop				🐕	🚸
3.3	Los Padres Loop	4.1	700	loop		🚲		🐕	🚸
3.4	Los Robles Trail	11	2,000	out-and-back				🐕	
3.5	Lake Eleanor Open Space	2.6	600	out-and-back				🐕	🚸
Chapter 4: SIMI HILLS									
4.1	Sage Ranch	2.1	400	loop		🚲		🐕	🚸
4.2	Castle Peak	1.2	650	out-and-back				🐕	
4.3	Lasky Mesa	3.7	500	loop		🚲	🐎	🐕	🚸
4.4	Victory to Las Virgenes	3.0	100	point-to-point		🚲	🐎	🐕	🚸
4.5	Upper Las Virgenes Canyon	5.4	300	out-and-back		🚲	🐎	🐕	🚸
4.6	Cheeseboro Canyon	6.5	850	loop				🐕	
4.7	China Flat Loop	9	2,100	loop				🐕	
Chapter 5: SANTA SUSANA MOUNTAINS									
5.1	Hummingbird Trail	3.5	1,150	out-and-back				🐕	🚸
5.2	Chumash Loop	9	2,000	loop		🚲		🐕	
5.3	Rocky Peak	5.5	1,400	out-and-back		🚲		🐕	
5.4	Corriganville Park	1.3	100	loop					🚸
5.5	Old Stagecoach Road	2.7	700	out-and-back					🚸

TRAIL TYPE LEGEND: ↻ = loop ↗ = out-and-back ⟋ = point-to-point

OVERVIEW OF HIKES *(continued)*

HIKE NUMBER	HIKE	DISTANCE (miles)	ELEVATION GAIN (feet)	TRAIL TYPE	BACKPACKING	MOUNTAIN BIKING	EQUESTRIANS	DOGS	KIDS
Chapter 5: SANTA SUSANA MOUNTAINS *(continued)*									
5.6	Devil Canyon	2.4+	450+	↗				🐕	🧍
5.7	Oat Mountain	4.8	1,400	↗		🚲		🐕	
5.8	Porter Ranch Loop	8	1,000	↻			🐎	🐕	
5.9	Bee Canyon	2.2	200	↗				🐕	🧍
5.10	Mission Point	4.7	1,450	↻				🐕	
5.11	Rice Canyon	2.5	350	↗				🐕	🧍
5.12	East Canyon Loop	7	1,300	↻		🚲	🐎	🐕	
5.13	Don Mullally Loop	5	1,100	↻		🚲		🐕	
5.14	Pico Canyon	7	1,200	↗		🚲		🐕	
Chapter 6: POINT MUGU									
6.1	Mugu Peak	2.0	1,250	↗					
6.2	La Jolla Falls	1.8	250	↗					🧍
6.3	La Jolla Valley Loop	11	1,950	↻	🥾				
6.4	Overlook Loop	2.8	500	↻					🧍
6.5	Serrano & Big Sycamore Loop	10	1,200	↻					
6.6	Sycamore Canyon Waterfall	3.2	500	↗					🧍
6.7	Old Boney Loop	11	2,000	↻					
6.8	Satwiwa Loop via Wendy Trail	2.4	400	↻				🐕	🧍
Chapter 7: ARROYO SEQUIT & SANDSTONE PEAK									
7.1	Leo Carrillo Ocean Vista	2.0	600	↻					🧍
7.2	Leo Carrillo Traverse	5.5	1,600	↗					
7.3	Nicholas Pond	1.2	100	↗					🧍
7.4	The Grotto	2.6	500	↗				🐕	🧍
7.5	Sandstone Peak	6	1,700	↻				🐕	
7.6	Arroyo Sequit Park	2.0	400	↻				🐕	🧍
7.7	Charmlee Wilderness Park	2.4	400	↻			🐎	🐕	🧍
Chapter 8: ZUMA CANYON									
8.1	Lower Zuma Canyon	2.8	100	↗				🐕	🧍
8.2	Zuma Canyon & Zuma Ridge Loop	8	1,700	↻				🐕	
8.3	Newton Canyon	0.8	150	↗				🐕	🧍
8.4	Rocky Oaks	1.0	150	↻		🚲	🐎	🐕	🧍
Chapter 9: MALIBU CREEK									
9.1	Escondido Canyon	3.4	500	↗				🐕	
9.2	Lower Solstice Canyon	2.4	350	↗				🐕	🧍

TRAIL TYPE LEGEND: ↻ = loop   ↗ = out-and-back   ↗ = point-to-point

OVERVIEW OF HIKES (continued)

HIKE NUMBER	HIKE	DISTANCE (miles)	ELEVATION GAIN (feet)	TRAIL TYPE	BACKPACKING	MOUNTAIN BIKING	EQUESTRIANS	DOGS	KIDS
Chapter 9: MALIBU CREEK (continued)									
9.3	Rising Sun & Sostomo Loop	7	1,900	↻				✓	
9.4	Corral Canyon	2.2	500	↻				✓	✓
9.5	Peter Strauss Trail	1.3	200	↻				✓	✓
9.6	Paramount Ranch	1–3	300	↻			✓	✓	✓
9.7	Ladyface Mountain	2.0	1,200	↗				✓	
9.8	Lookout Loop	3.8	700	↻					✓
9.9	Century Lake	3.0	250	↗		✓			✓
9.10	Lost Cabin Trail	6	700	↗					
9.11	Bulldog & Backbone Loop	14	3,000	↻		✓			
9.12	Phantom Loop	7	1,200	↻			✓		
9.13	Upper Las Virgenes View Trail	4.6	900	↗		✓	✓	✓	
9.14	New Millennium Loop	12	2,700	↻		✓		✓	
9.15	King Gillette Ranch Inspiration Point	1.7	250	↻				✓	✓
9.16	Piuma Overlook	0.6	150	↗				✓	✓
9.17	West Ridge of Saddle Peak	3.5	−1,500	↗				✓	✓
9.18	Saddle Peak	3.2	900	↗				✓	
9.19	Red Rock Canyon	4.0	700	↗		✓		✓	✓
9.20	Calabasas Peak	3.6	1,000	↗		✓		✓	
9.21	Topanga Lookout & Stunt High Loop	6.5	1,800	↻				✓	
9.22	Hondo Canyon	3.5	−1,600	↗				✓	
Chapter 10: PACIFIC PALISADES & TOPANGA									
10.1	Eagle Rock Loop	6.5	1,300	↻	✓				✓
10.2	East Backbone Trail	10	1,400	↗					
10.3	Santa Ynez Waterfall	2.5	200	↗					✓
10.4	Topanga Overlook	5	1,200	↗		✓			
10.5	Temescal Canyon	2.8	850	↻					✓
10.6	Rivas Canyon	2.7	600	↗				✓	
10.7	Will Rogers Park	2.0	350	↻		✓		✓	✓
10.8	Rustic Canyon Loop	5.5	1,000	↻					
10.9	Sullivan Canyon	10.5	1,600	↻		✓		✓	
10.10	Viewridge Trail	2.6	400	↻				✓	✓
10.11	Summit Valley	1.6	450	↗				✓	✓
10.12	Woodland Ridge	2.3	600	↗				✓	
10.13	Caballero Canyon	4.5	1,000	↗		✓			
10.14	San Vicente Mountain	1.6	300	↗		✓		✓	✓

OVERVIEW OF HIKES (continued)

HIKE NUMBER	HIKE	DISTANCE (miles)	ELEVATION GAIN (feet)	TRAIL TYPE	BACKPACKING	MOUNTAIN BIKING	EQUESTRIANS	DOGS	KIDS
Chapter 11: ANTELOPE VALLEY									
11.1	Arthur B. Ripley Desert Woodland State Park	1.2	50	↻					🧍
11.2	Antelope Valley California Poppy Reserve	1–4	200+	↻					🧍
11.3	Saddleback Butte	3.8	1,100	↗					
Chapter 12: DESERT GATEWAY									
12.1	Elsmere Canyon Falls	2.6	300	↗				🐾	🧍
12.2	Whitney Canyon	3.4	300	↗		🚲		🐾	🧍
12.3	Placerita Canyon	3.6	400	↗				🐾	🧍
12.4	Manzanita Mountain to Los Pinetos Canyon	7	1,800	↻	🥾			🐾	
12.5	Los Pinetos Waterfall	1.6	350	↗				🐾	🧍
12.6	Vasquez Rocks Natural Area	3.5	300	↗				🐾	🧍
12.7	Sierra Pelona & Mount McDill	12	2,500	↗			🐎	🐾	
12.8	Jupiter Mountain	3.8	1,600	↗				🐾	
Chapter 13: GLENDALE & VERDUGO MOUNTAINS									
13.1	Deukmejian Wilderness Park	2.5	800	↻		🚲		🐾	🧍
13.2	Mount Lukens Southern Approach	10	2,800	↻		🚲		🐾	
13.3	Haines Canyon	3.4	1,000	↗		🚲		🐾	🧍
13.4	La Tuna Loop	9	1,900	↻				🐾	
13.5	Verdugo Peak Traverse	6	1,800	↗				🐾	
13.6	Beaudry Loop	5.5	1,600	↻		🚲		🐾	
13.7	Vital Link Trail	3.2	1,500	↗				🐾	
13.8	West Side Loop	9	2,000	↻				🐾	
13.9	Stough Canyon Loop	3.0	800	↻				🐾	
Chapter 14: GRIFFITH PARK									
14.1	Hollywood Sign via Cahuenga Peak	2.8	1,000	↗				🐾	🧍
14.2	Mulholland Ridge	3.6	1,000	↗				🐾	
14.3	Mount Hollywood	4.7	1,000	↻				🐾	🧍
14.4	Beacon Hill	4.1	800	↻				🐾	🧍
14.5	East Side Loop	6	1,300	↻				🐾	
14.6	Mount Bell	5	1,100	↻				🐾	
Chapter 15: HOLLYWOOD HILLS									
15.1	Franklin Canyon	1.8	400	↻				🐾	🧍
15.2	Coldwater to Fryman Canyon	2.9	500	↗				🐾	🧍
15.3	Wilacre & Coldwater Loop	2.7	500	↻				🐾	🧍
15.4	Trebek Open Space	2.5	400	↗				🐾	🧍
15.5	Runyon Canyon	2.0	500	↻				🐾	🧍

TRAIL TYPE LEGEND: ↻ = loop   = out-and-back   = point-to-point

OVERVIEW OF HIKES (continued)

Hike Number	Hike	Distance (miles)	Elevation Gain (feet)	Trail Type	Backpacking	Mountain Biking	Equestrians	Dogs	Kids
Chapter 16: URBAN PARKS									
16.1	San Rafael Hills	5	900	loop		🚲	🐎	🐕	
16.2	Debs Park	5	1,000	loop				🐕	
16.3	Elysian Park	2.5	300	loop				🐕	👪
16.4	Hahn Park	2.6	350	loop		🚲		🐕	👪
16.5	Baldwin Hills Scenic Overlook	1.2	350	loop					👪
Chapter 17: PUENTE HILLS									
17.1	Sycamore Canyon	2.6	200	point-to-point					👪
17.2	Hellman Wilderness Park	2.5	700	loop				🐕	👪
17.3	West Skyline Loop	4.7	1,100	loop		🚲	🐎	🐕	
17.4	Worsham Canyon Loop	4.2	1,000	loop		🚲	🐎	🐕	
17.5	Arroyo Pescadero Loop	2.8	300	loop			🐎	🐕	👪
17.6	Schabarum Loop	6	1,000	loop		🚲	🐎	🐕	
17.7	Powder Canyon Loop	4.2	700	loop		🚲	🐎	🐕	
17.8	Schabarum–Skyline Trail	16	2,800	point-to-point		🚲	🐎	🐕	
Chapter 18: SAN GABRIEL VALLEY									
18.1	Monrovia Canyon Falls	2.6	600	point-to-point				🐕	👪
18.2	Ben Overturff Trail	7	1,800	loop		🚲	🐎	🐕	
18.3	Fish Canyon Falls	5	800	point-to-point				🐕	👪
18.4	Big Dalton Mystic Loop	3	1,300	loop				🐕	
18.5	Big Dalton Canyon	2.1	500	loop				🐕	👪
18.6	Glendora South Hills Wilderness	2.9	800	loop				🐕	👪
18.7	Walnut Creek	5	350	point-to-point		🚲		🐕	👪
18.8	Bonelli Regional Park	8	800	loop		🚲	🐎	🐕	
Chapter 19: SAN DIMAS–LA VERNE–CLAREMONT HILLS									
19.1	Lower Marshall Canyon	2.5	300	loop		🚲	🐎	🐕	👪
19.2	Middle Marshall Canyon	1.7	300	loop		🚲	🐎	🐕	👪
19.3	Upper Marshall Canyon	4.5	800	loop		🚲	🐎	🐕	👪
19.4	Johnson's Pasture	2.2	400	point-to-point		🚲	🐎	🐕	👪
19.5	Sycamore Canyon	2.3	600	loop				🐕	👪
19.6	Claremont Hills Wilderness Park	5	1,000	loop		🚲	🐎	🐕	👪
19.7	Potato Mountain	4.5	1,200	point-to-point		🚲			
19.8	Thompson Creek Trail	4.5	300	point-to-point		🚲		🐕	👪
Chapter 20: PIRU CREEK									
20.1	Oak Flat Trail	2.8	1,000	point-to-point				🐕	👪
20.2	Pothole–Agua Blanca Loop	20	3,600	loop	🥾			🐕	
20.3	Piru Creek	21	600	point-to-point	🥾			🐕	

OVERVIEW OF HIKES (continued)

HIKE NUMBER	HIKE	DISTANCE (miles)	ELEVATION GAIN (feet)	TRAIL TYPE	BACKPACKING	MOUNTAIN BIKING	EQUESTRIANS	DOGS	KIDS
Chapter 21: LIEBRE MOUNTAIN & FISH CANYON									
21.1	**Liebre Mountain**	10	2,000	↗	🚶			🐾	
21.2	**Fish Canyon Narrows**	10	800	↗	🚶			🐾	
Chapter 22: TUJUNGA CANYONS									
22.1	Yerba Buena Ridge	4.6	1,400	↗	🚶	🚴	🐴	🐾	
22.2	Trail Canyon Falls	4.5	1,000	↗				🐾	
22.3	Condor Peak & Trail Canyon	16	4,300	↗	🚶			🐾	
22.4	Mount Lukens & Grizzly Flats Loop	13	3,400	↻	🚶			🐾	
22.5	Messenger Flats	3.3	800	↻				🐾	🧒
Chapter 23: ARROYO SECO & FRONT RANGE									
23.1	Lower Arroyo Seco	5	300	↗	🚶	🚴	🐴	🐾	🧒
23.2	Down the Arroyo Seco	10	−2,300	↗	🚶	🚴		🐾	
23.3	Switzer Falls	3.8	700	↗	🚶			🐾	🧒
23.4	Royal Gorge	13	1,800	↗	🚶			🐾	
23.5	World of Chaparral Trail	2.8	700	↗				🐾	
23.6	Hoyt Mountain	3.4	1,300	↻				🐾	
23.7	Josephine Peak	8	2,100	↻				🐾	
23.8	Strawberry Peak	7	2,700	↗				🐾	
23.9	Colby Canyon to Big Tujunga	7	1,700	↗	🚶			🐾	
23.10	Mount Lawlor	6	1,300	↗				🐾	
23.11	San Gabriel Peak	3.7	1,400	↗				🐾	
23.12	Mount Lowe	3.2	500	↗				🐾	
23.13	Inspiration Point	6	1,600	↻	🚶			🐾	
23.14	Bear Canyon	8	−2,800	↗	🚶			🐾	
23.15	Millard Canyon Falls	1.4	300	↗				🐾	🧒
23.16	Dawn Mine Loop	6	1,600	↻				🐾	
23.17	Upper Millard Canyon	11	2,700	↻	🚶			🐾	
23.18	Brown Mountain Traverse	12	3,200	↻				🐾	
23.19	Echo Mountain	5.5	1,400	↗				🐾	
23.20	Mount Lowe Railway	11	2,700	↻	🚶			🐾	
Chapter 24: MOUNT WILSON & FRONT RANGE									
24.1	Henninger Flats	5	1,400	↗	🚶	🚴		🐾	🧒
24.2	Mount Wilson Toll Road	9	−4,200	↗	🚶	🚴		🐾	🧒
24.3	Eaton Canyon Falls	3.8	400	↗				🐾	🧒
24.4	Idlehour Descent	12	−5,300	↗	🚶			🐾	
24.5	Valley Forge & DeVore Trails	7	1,700	↗	🚶			🐾	

TRAIL TYPE LEGEND: = loop ↗ = out-and-back   = point-to-point

OVERVIEW OF HIKES (continued)

HIKE NUMBER	HIKE	DISTANCE (miles)	ELEVATION GAIN (feet)	TRAIL TYPE	BACKPACKING	MOUNTAIN BIKING	EQUESTRIANS	DOGS	KIDS
Chapter 24: MOUNT WILSON & FRONT RANGE *(continued)*									
24.6	Bailey Canyon	1.2	300	↗				🐕	🚶
24.7	Jones Peak	6	2,300	↗				🐕	
24.8	Mount Wilson to Sierra Madre	7	−4,800	↗	🚶			🐕	
24.9	Santa Anita Ridge	7	1,300	↗		🚴		🐕	
24.10	Hoegees Loop	5.5	1,300	↻	🚶			🐕	
24.11	Sturtevant Falls	3.4	700	↗				🐕	🚶
24.12	Santa Anita Canyon Loop	8.5	2,200	↻	🚶			🐕	
24.13	Mount Wilson Loop	13.5	4,100	↻	🚶			🐕	
24.14	Angeles Crest to Chantry Flat	12	1,800	↗	🚶			🐕	
Chapter 25: CHARLTON–CHILAO RECREATION AREA									
25.1	Vetter Mountain	3.6	700	↻				🐕	🚶
25.2	Chilao & Charlton Loop	5.5	800	↻		🚴		🐕	🚶
25.3	Mount Hillyer	6	1,100	↻				🐕	🚶
25.4	Pacifico Mountain	10	1,700	↗	🚶			🐕	
Chapter 26: CRYSTAL LAKE RECREATION AREA									
26.1	Lewis Falls	0.8	300	↗				🐕	🚶
26.2	Mount Islip South Ridge	10	2,800	↻	🚶			🐕	
26.3	Crystal Lake Nature Trails	1	Varies					🐕	🚶
26.4	Mount Islip via Windy Gap	7	2,500	↗	🚶			🐕	
26.5	Mount Hawkins Loop	11	3,000	↻	🚶			🐕	
Chapter 27: SAN GABRIEL WILDERNESS									
27.1	Upper Devils Canyon	6	1,600	↗	🚶			🐕	
27.2	Mount Waterman Trail	8	1,400	↗	🚶			🐕	
27.3	Mount Waterman & Twin Peaks	12	4,000	↗	🚶			🐕	
27.4	Smith Mountain	7	1,800	↗				🐕	
27.5	Bear Creek Trail	11	1,100	↗	🚶			🐕	
Chapter 28: HIGH COUNTRY & NORTH SLOPE									
28.1	Winston Peak and Ridge	1.2+	500+	↗				🐕	🚶
28.2	Cooper Canyon Falls	3.2	800	↗	🚶			🐕	🚶
28.3	Burkhart Trail	12	2,000	↗	🚶			🐕	
28.4	Kratka Ridge	1.8	400	↗				🐕	🚶
28.5	Mount Williamson	4.2	1,500	↗	🚶			🐕	
28.6	Pleasant View Ridge	11	4,900	↗	🚶			🐕	
28.7	Sierra Alta Nature Trail	0.2	100	↻				🐕	🚶
28.8	South Fork Trail	5	−2,100	↗				🐕	
28.9	Mount Islip: North Approach	6	1,200	↗	🚶			🐕	🚶
28.10	Devil's Punchbowl Loop Trail	1.0	300	↻				🐕	🚶

OVERVIEW OF HIKES (continued)

HIKE NUMBER	HIKE	DISTANCE (miles)	ELEVATION GAIN (feet)	TRAIL TYPE	BACKPACKING	MOUNTAIN BIKING	EQUESTRIANS	DOGS	KIDS
Chapter 28: HIGH COUNTRY & NORTH SLOPE *(continued)*									
28.11	Devil's Chair	6	1,200	out-and-back	🚶			🐾	
28.12	Lower Punchbowl Canyon	2.5	400	out-and-back	🚶			🐾	🧒
28.13	Holcomb Canyon	4	700	loop	🚶			🐾	
Chapter 29: BIG PINES & SHEEP MOUNTAIN WILDERNESS									
29.1	Shoemaker Canyon Road	5.5	800	out-and-back		🚲		🐾	
29.2	Rattlesnake Peak	9.5	4,200	out-and-back				🐾	
29.3	Cattle Canyon	7.5	700	out-and-back	🚶			🐾	🧒
29.4	Bridge to Nowhere	9.5	1,000	out-and-back	🚶			🐾	
29.5	Iron Mountain	13.5	6,200	out-and-back				🐾	
29.6	Down the East Fork	15.5	−4,800	out-and-back	🚶			🐾	
29.7	Big Horn Mine	3.8	500	out-and-back				🐾	
29.8	Ross Mountain	14	5,500	out-and-back	🚶			🐾	
29.9	Mount Baden-Powell Traverse	8	2,100	out-and-back	🚶			🐾	
29.10	Mount Lewis	0.8	500	out-and-back				🐾	🧒
29.11	Lightning Ridge Nature Trail	0.6	200	loop				🐾	🧒
29.12	Jackson Lake Loop	7	1,300	loop		🚲		🐾	
29.13	Table Mountain Nature Trail	1+	200+	loop				🐾	🧒
29.14	Big Pines Nature Trail	0.5	100	loop				🐾	🧒
29.15	Blue Ridge Trail	5	1,300	out-and-back				🐾	🧒
Chapter 30: SAN ANTONIO CANYON & OLD BALDY									
30.1	Stoddard Peak	6	1,100	out-and-back				🐾	
30.2	Sunset Peak	6	1,200	out-and-back	🚶	🚲		🐾	
30.3	Bear Flat	4.0	1,300	out-and-back				🐾	🧒
30.4	Mount Baldy via Bear Ridge	13	5,800	out-and-back	🚶	🚲		🐾	
30.5	Icehouse Canyon	7	2,600	out-and-back		🚲		🐾	
30.6	Cedar Glen	4.5+	1,300+	out-and-back	🚶			🐾	
30.7	Cucamonga Peak	12	3,800	out-and-back	🚶			🐾	
30.8	Ontario Peak	12	3,600	out-and-back	🚶			🐾	
30.9	The Three Ts	13	5,000	point-to-point	🚶			🐾	
30.10	San Antonio Falls	1.2	200	out-and-back		🚲		🐾	🧒
30.11	Baldy Loop	10.5	3,900	loop	🚶			🐾	
30.12	San Antonio Ridge	16	6,000	point-to-point	🚶			🐾	
30.13	Baldy North Backbone Traverse	11.5	5,100	out-and-back	🚶			🐾	
30.14	Baldy Devil Backbone	6	2,300	out-and-back	🚶			🐾	

TRAIL TYPE LEGEND: ↻ = loop   ↗ = out-and-back   ↗ = point-to-point

HIKE NUMBER	HIKE	DISTANCE (miles)	ELEVATION GAIN (feet)	TRAIL TYPE	BACKPACKING	MOUNTAIN BIKING	EQUESTRIANS	DOGS	KIDS
OVERVIEW OF HIKES *(continued)*									
Chapter 31: **SANTA CATALINA ISLAND: AVALON**									
31.1	East Mountain	10	2,000	↻				🐾	
31.2	Lone Tree Point	6	1,800	↻				🐾	
31.3	Airport Loop Trail	2.3	400	↻				🐾	🧍
31.4	Airport in the Sky to Little Harbor	12	2,000	↻	🥾			🐾	
Chapter 32: **SANTA CATALINA ISLAND: TWO HARBORS**									
32.1	Parsons Landing	14	2,300	↻	🥾			🐾	
32.2	Silver Peak & Starlight Beach	11	3,100	↻				🐾	
32.3	Harbor to Harbor	5.5	1,500	↗	🥾			🐾	
Chapter 33: **LONG-DISTANCE TRAILS**									
33.1	Silver Moccasin Trail	52	14,600	↗	🥾	🚲	🏇	🐾	
33.2	Gabrielino Trail	28	4,900	↗	🥾	🚲		🐾	
33.3	High Desert Loop	41	10,000	↻	🥾			🐾	
33.4	Santa Monica Mountains Backbone Trail	67	13,300	↗	🥾	🚲	🏇	🐾	
33.5	Trans-Catalina Trail	38.5	8,000	↗	🥾			🐾	
33.6	San Gabriel River Trail	38	–700	↗		🚲	🏇	🐾	

Santa Anita Canyon draws throngs of hikers, but you can find seclusion on Santa Anita Ridge (left). Mount Wilson is the high point on the right. (See Trip 24.9, page 326.)

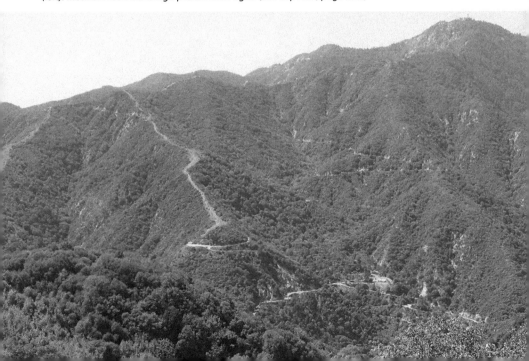

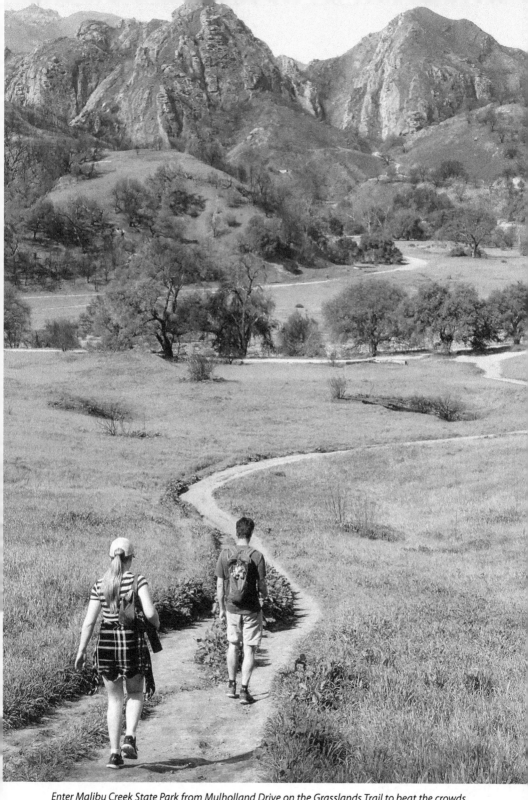

Enter Malibu Creek State Park from Mulholland Drive on the Grasslands Trail to beat the crowds. (See Trips 9.9–9.11, pages 121, 122, and 124.)

Introducing Los Angeles County

L os Angeles County sits astride one of the earth's most significant structural features: the San Andreas Fault. For more than 10 million years, movements along the San Andreas and neighboring faults have shaped the dramatic geology and topography evident throughout the region today. The very complexity of the shape of the land has in turn spawned a variety of localized climates. These varied climates, along with the diverse topography and geology, have resulted in a remarkably diverse array of plant and animal life.

Exploring all of this wonderful variety right in L.A.'s backyard isn't hard to do. Conveniently enough, many of the best hiking opportunities start right on the edge of town—right off the freeway. Other trailheads can be quickly reached by way of lesser roads such as Pacific Coast Highway, Mulholland Highway, and Angeles Crest Highway. Fewer than a dozen of the hikes described in this book involve any kind of dirt-road driving to reach, and every trip (except for those on Santa Catalina Island) lies within a 90-minute drive of downtown L.A., assuming light traffic.

In the next few pages of this book, we'll examine Los Angeles County's several climates, its spectacular geology, and its native plants and animals. In the short sections that follow, you'll find some important notes about safety and appropriate behavior on the trail; some useful tips on how to use this book effectively; and finally some helpful advice on how to choose and time your visits so as to avoid smog, excessive heat, and other discomforts that can detract from an otherwise pleasant outing. After perusing that material, you can dig into the heart of this book: descriptions of more than 250 hiking routes from the coast to the mountains, from sea level to 10,000 feet.

Happy reading—and happy hiking!

Land of Many Climates

A fairly accurate and succinct summary of Los Angeles County's climate might take the form of just two phrases: "warm and sunny" and "winter-wet, summer-dry." In the worldwide range of climates, this pattern can be described as Mediterranean and is typical of less than 3% of the world's landmass.

Actually, a lot of variation exists, a fact readily apparent to anyone traveling almost any direction through the county. Inland, away from the moderating influence of the ocean, temperatures usually climb higher in the day and usually drop lower at night. Also, higher elevations mean cooler temperatures and more rainfall. Because both of these influences are at work in the L.A. area, it's helpful to picture the county as divided into several climate zones, each zone characterized by particular combination of weather characteristics. Informally, let's divide the county into five of these zones.

The **coastal (or maritime fringe) zone** extends only a few miles inland across the coastal slopes of the Santa Monica Mountains, but about 15 miles across the flat, central urban basin of Los Angeles. Moist air from over the cool Pacific waters sweeps into this zone with some regularity during the daytime hours, while at night the marine layer often turns into fog or low overcast. Average Fahrenheit temperatures range from the 60s/40s (daily high/low) in winter to the 70s/60s in summer. Rainfall averages about 12–15 inches annually, except in the Santa Monicas. The higher profile of this coastal range snags extra moisture from rain-bearing winter storms, yielding an additional 10–15 inches.

The **inland valley zone** encompasses such corners of urban L.A. as the San Gabriel and San Fernando Valleys, plus the north slope of the Santa Monica Mountains and the lower foothills of the San Gabriel Mountains. This area, only partially under the influence of moderating sea breezes, experiences more-extreme temperatures, both daily and seasonally: typically from the 60s/30s in winter to the 90s/50s in summer. Precipitation averages about 15 inches annually, somewhat more in the foothills.

Higher lands even more removed from coastal influences are classified as having either **transitional** or **mountain climates.** Both these zones are found in interior mountain ranges and are characterized by somewhat lower average temperatures. The subtle difference between the two involves rainfall. Annual rainfall in the semiarid transition zone, which encompasses the northwest corner of Angeles National Forest and the desert-facing slopes of the San Gabriel Mountains, is typically about 15–20 inches. The mountain climate zone, including most of the Front Range of the San Gabriels (facing the San Gabriel Valley) and the higher country along Angeles Crest Highway, receives upwards of 30 inches—enough to support large areas of coniferous and broadleaf forest. Mount Wilson, in the Front Range, for example, gets about 35 inches of precipitation, including about 4 feet of snow, annually. Average temperatures there range from the 50s/30s in winter to the 80s/50s in summer. Mount Wilson's hilltop position spares it from the effects of cold-air drainage at night, so the day–night thermometer change is rather small. Not so for the canyon bottoms, especially in winter, when temperatures can plummet more than 40°F as the sun sinks out of sight.

In the High Country of the San Gabriel Mountains, enough snow falls and remains on the ground during the winter to permit skiing for about four months a year in a few areas. Several small but thriving winter-sports facilities exist here. Still higher, Mount San Antonio (10,064') lies very near timberline, where the climate verges on alpine.

North of the San Gabriels, 50 or more miles inland, lies the county's driest climate zone, the **High Desert,** which encompasses the westernmost Mojave Desert, aka the Antelope Valley. This area is almost completely cut off from the moderating influence of the ocean, and it experiences a relatively extreme continental type of climate. Temperatures typically range from 50s/20s in winter to 90s/60s in summer. The coastal mountains serve as a barrier to rain-bearing clouds moving inland, so annual precipitation amounts to only about 7 inches—somewhat more at the western tip of the valley near Interstate 5, and somewhat less at the county's northeast corner near Edwards Air Force Base.

The precipitation figures mentioned above, which are long-term averages, should be taken with a grain of salt—the last 35 years or so have seen a drying trend locally and throughout much of the Western states. (For evidence of this, examine any freshly cut tree stump in the local mountains, and note that the tree rings are crowded together toward the outside edge.) We are in the beginning stages of a long-term drought.

Also, it's worth noting that average statistics tell only part of the story. Hot spells, for example, descend upon the county with some regularity, especially in the fall when searing Santa Ana winds come roaring down through the mountain passes toward the coast. This condition occurs when dry air moves southwest from a high-pressure area in the interior US out toward Southern California. Flowing across low gaps in the mountains (notably Cajon Pass on the east flank of the San Gabriels, and Soledad Pass south of Palmdale), this air sometimes reaches the coastline or even Santa Catalina Island. As the air moves

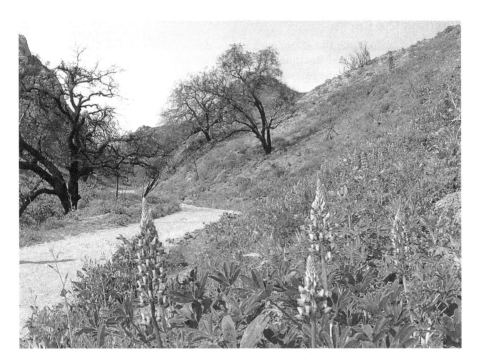

Lupine sprouts along the Century Lake Trail months after the 2018 Woolsey Fire. (See Trip 9.9, page 121.)

downward, it compresses and warms about 5°F for every 1,000 feet of descent. At Malibu or Santa Monica, daytime highs can soar to 90°F–100°F, rivaling the hottest temperatures recorded nationwide that day. High in the mountains, Santa Anas are much cooler, but they can assume gale and even hurricane force. Mount Wilson has experienced more than a hour of steady winds in the range of 80–90 mph.

Santa Ana winds spread wildfires easily. Early Santa Anas (October and November) often coincide with the tail end of months of summer drought. Most wildfires in L.A. County are quickly controlled, but the combination of hot winds, dry chaparral, and flammable hillside homes has set the stage time and time again for disasters of monstrous magnitude, including the Fire of 1924 and the 2009 Station Fire. Climate change is a contributing factor in the largest and most damaging fires that have plagued the state in recent years.

In a similar way, the generally bland average statistics for rainfall fail to reveal the normal situation—which is, metaphorically, feast or famine. A string of drought years can be followed by one or two very wet ones. In wet years much of the moisture received comes in the form of rather short but intense winter storms. A case in point is a monumental downpour recorded in January 1942 at Hoegees Camp in the Front Range of the San Gabriels: more than 26 inches of rain fell in a 24-hour period. On another occasion in the San Gabriels, a rain gauge collected 1 inch in 1 minute. When dumped on steep slopes denuded of vegetation after a fire, such intense rainfall sends debris flows—torrents of water, rocks, and soil with a consistency of wet aggregate concrete—down through the canyons.

Despite nature's occasional temper tantrums, more than 9 times out of 10 your outings in Los Angeles County are likely to coincide with dry weather and temperatures in a moderate register for at least part of the day. Few other areas around the country, and probably no other great city in the world, can offer such good odds.

Reading the Rocks

A good way to approach the subject of L.A. County's geology is to think about the geomorphology, or shape and structure, of the landscape. Of California's many geomorphic provinces, the county claims parts of three: the **Los Angeles Basin,** the **Transverse Ranges,** and the **Mojave Desert.** The bulk of the county's urban area dominates the Basin province, while the mostly undeveloped San Gabriel Mountains and semideveloped Santa Monica Mountains (the two ranges containing most of the hikes in this guide) belong to the Transverse Ranges. Because only a few of the trips in this guide border on the Mojave Desert, it is not discussed in any detail here.

The Los Angeles Basin province extends from the base of the San Gabriel and Santa Monica Mountains in the north to the Santa Ana Mountains and San Joaquin Hills of Orange County on the south. It's a huge, deeply folded basin filled to a depth of up to 6 miles by some volcanic material and land-deposited sediments, but mostly by sediments of marine origin—sand and mud deposited on the ocean bottom from 80 million years ago to as recently as 1 million years ago.

Then, after uplift during the past 1–2 million years, the surface of the basin accumulated a layer of terrestrial sediment shed from the surrounding hills and mountains. The basin, in fact, would still be filling with sediment today were it not for the installation of flood-control barriers in the mountains, dams to catch debris at the mouths of the canyons, and more than 2,000 miles of storm drains and concrete-lined flood channels that carry flood waters to the sea. (Amazingly, some of the sediment cleaned out from behind the flood-control dams is trucked back up into the mountains; there's no room for it down in the city!)

The Transverse Ranges province encompasses in Los Angeles County the Santa Monica and San Gabriel mountains, plus the mini-ranges of Liebre Mountain, Sawmill Mountain, and Sierra Pelona lying northwest of the San Gabriels. Outside L.A. County, the province takes in part of the coastal ranges of Santa Barbara and Ventura County, and the San Bernardino and Little San Bernardino Mountains. As indicated by the name *Transverse,* these east–west trending mountains stand crosswise to the usual northwest–southeast grain of California's other major mountain groups: the Coast Ranges, Sierra Nevada, and Peninsular Ranges. This kink in the alignment of California's mountains is mirrored by a similar east–west jog in the San Andreas Fault, which defines the north edge of the San Gabriel Mountains.

The San Andreas Fault, of course, represents the boundary between two of the earth's major tectonic plates—the largely oceanic Pacific Plate and the largely continental North American Plate. For at least 10 million years, lands on the west side of the boundary have been sliding (often lurching) northwest relative to lands on the east side. Currently the average rate of movement is about 2 inches per year—enough, if it continues, to put Los Angeles abreast of San Francisco about 10 million years from now.

A growing body of evidence now suggests that the movements along the San Andreas Fault do not simply involve one plate slipping past another; they also produce compression, which accelerates and possibly controls the process of mountain building along the Central and Southern California coast. In the area of the kink, centered on the San Gabriel Mountains, the compression forces are greatest. In this view, the San Gabriels are being squeezed horizontally about a tenth of an inch each year, and being thrust upward at least as fast. This means that Mount San Antonio is rising by more than a mile per million years even as it's eroding away almost as fast. At the same time, the Los Angeles Basin, which is underlain by folded and crumpled structures under its blanket of sediment, may be losing an average of a quarter acre per year due to compression.

The kink in the San Andreas Fault, and therefore in the alignment of the coastal mountains, might be explained by the fact that the part of the North American Plate over Nevada

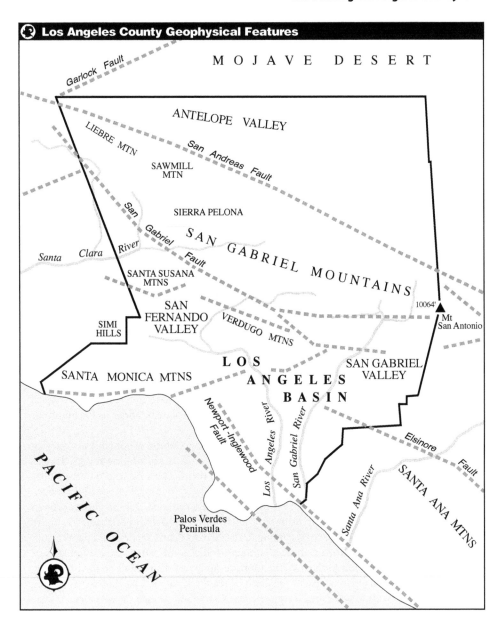

Los Angeles County Geophysical Features

MOJAVE DESERT

Garlock Fault

ANTELOPE VALLEY

LIEBRE MTN

San Andreas Fault

SAWMILL MTN

SIERRA PELONA

San Gabriel River

SAN GABRIEL MOUNTAINS

Santa Clara River

Fault

SANTA SUSANA MTNS

10064' Mt San Antonio

SIMI HILLS

SAN FERNANDO VALLEY

VERDUGO MTNS

SANTA MONICA MTNS

LOS ANGELES BASIN

SAN GABRIEL VALLEY

Newport-Inglewood Fault

Los Angeles River

San Gabriel River

Elsinore Fault

Santa Ana River

SANTA ANA MTNS

PACIFIC OCEAN

Palos Verdes Peninsula

and Utah is stretching and spreading outward because it is thin and is closer to the earth's mantle there. The western Mojave Desert, which rides on the western edge of the North American Plate, may be jamming against the plate boundary, producing the kink.

Regardless of what has pushed them to their present heights, the mountains of the Transverse Range are just a few million years old, relatively young as upthrust units. This is not true of the ages of most of the rocks that compose them. The oldest rock found exposed in the Santa Monica Mountains—Santa Monica Slate—checks out at about 150 million years. Some rocks in the San Gabriels are representative of the oldest found on the Pacific Coast: more than 600 million years of age.

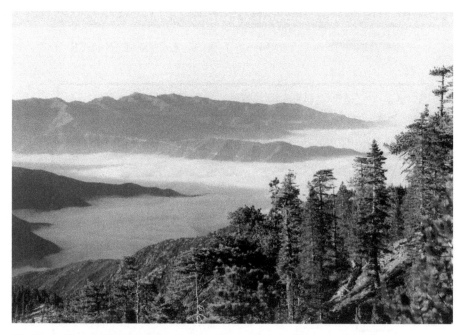

The forested San Gabriel Mountains rise above the marine layer blanketing the valley.

The geological history of the San Gabriels, which have been called the most complicated mountain range in North America, may never be fully deciphered. As one expert put it, "The San Gabes look like a flake kicked around on plate boundaries for hundreds of millions of years."

Caught in the tectonic frenzy of the moment, the San Gabriel Mountains are surging upward as fast as any mountain range on Earth. They are also disintegrating at a spectacular rate. Although they consist mainly of durable granitic rocks, much like those in the sturdy Sierra Nevada, the San Gabriel rocks have been through a tectonic meat grinder. Like mountains made of soft material, the tops of the San Gabriels are rounded. But the slopes are often appallingly steep and unstable. An average of 7 tons of material disappears from each acre of the front face each year, most of it coming to rest behind debris barriers and dams below.

As you hike through the San Gabriel Mountains, and also the Santa Monicas (which to a lesser degree suffer erosion problems), the ultimate futility of dam-building, road-building, and even trail-building in many places will become readily apparent. Like sandcastles waiting for the next ocean tide, the man-made improvements and even the natural vegetation clinging to mountain slopes wait for advancing tides of fire, flood, and earthquake to sweep them away.

Native Gardens

As mentioned earlier, Los Angeles County's varied climate, topography, and geology have set the stage for a remarkable diversity of plants. There's a second reason too: Los Angeles County, and coastal Southern California for that matter, lies between two major groups of flora: a southern group, represented by drought-tolerant plants characteristic of northern Mexico, and a northern group, represented by moisture-loving plants typical of the Sierra Nevada and California's north coastal ranges. As the climate fluctuated, seesawing from cool and wet to warm and dry over the past million years or so, species from both groups invaded the present-day county borders. Once established, many of these species remained in protected niches even as the climate turned unfavorable for them. Some survived unchanged; others evolved into unique forms. Some are present today only in very specific habitats. If you invest the time to learn the common plants, you'll eventually be rewarded by seeing old friends each time you visit the mountains.

Several common, widely distributed trees—gray pine, limber pine, big-leaf maple, valley oak, and California buckeye—reach their southernmost limits on the Pacific coast in or near L.A. County. California walnut and big-cone Douglas-fir, the former a foothill-dwelling tree and the latter an inhabitant of the higher mountains, have more-restricted ranges centered approximately on the L.A. Basin. The Joshua tree, the trademark of the Mojave Desert, reaches its westernmost limit near the 5 Freeway (I-5) in northern L.A. County, and is widely distributed in the Antelope Valley and along the northern base of the San Gabriels.

The bulk of Los Angeles County's undeveloped and naturally vegetated land can be grouped into several general classes, which botanists often call plant communities or plant associations. (In a broader sense, these are biological communities, because they include animals as well as plants.) Several of the major plant communities in the county are briefly described, in the order you would encounter them on a journey from the coast, up into the San Gabriel High Country, and then down to the desert.

The **sage-scrub (or coastal sage-scrub) community** lies mostly below 2,000 feet elevation, on south-facing slopes in the Santa Monica Mountains, the Simi Hills, the Santa Susana Mountains, and on some of the lower, hotter slopes of the San Gabriel Mountains. The dominant plants are small shrubs, typically California sagebrush, black sage, white sage, and California buckwheat. Two larger shrubs often present are laurel sumac and lemonade berry, which, like poison oak, are members of the sumac family. In some areas along the coast, prickly-pear cactus thrives within this community. Interspersed among the somewhat pliable and loosely distributed shrubs is a variety of grasses and wildflowers, green and colorful during the rainy season, but dry and withered during the summer and early fall drought. Much of the sage-scrub vegetation is "summer-deciduous"—dormant and dead-looking during the warmer half of the year, lush green and aromatic during the cool, wet half.

The **chaparral community** is commonly found between 1,000 and 5,000 feet elevation just about anywhere there's a slope that hasn't burned recently. Were it not for roads, firebreaks, and other interruptions, the chaparral would run in wide unbroken swaths along the flanks of most of the county's mountains. At low elevations, chaparral—which requires more moisture than sage-scrub—tends to stick to slopes protected from the full glare of the sun. At higher elevations, which get more rainfall, chaparral takes over the south slopes, while oaks and conifers thrive on slopes receiving less sun. The dominant chaparral plants include chamise, scrub oak, manzanita, toyon, mountain mahogany, and various forms of ceanothus (wild lilac). Whipple yuccas, known for their spectacular candle-shaped blooms, often frequent the chaparral zones. The chaparral plants are tough and intricately branched evergreen shrubs with deep root systems that help the plants survive during the long, hot summers. Chaparral is sometimes referred to as elfin forest—a good description of a mature stand. Without benefit of a trail, travel through mature chaparral, which is often 15 feet high and incredibly dense all the way up from the ground, is almost impossible.

The **coniferous forest,** which has two phases in Los Angeles County, takes over roughly above 4,000 feet elevation, at least in areas with sufficient rainfall. The yellow-pine phase includes conifers such as big-cone Douglas-fir, ponderosa pine, Jeffrey pine, sugar pine, incense cedar, and white fir, and forms tall, open forest. These species are often intermixed with live oaks, California bay (bay laurel), and scattered chaparral shrubs such as manzanita and mountain mahogany. Higher than about 8,000 feet, in the lodgepole-pine phase, lodgepole pine, white fir, and limber pine are the indicator trees. These trees, somewhat shorter and more weather-beaten than those below, exist in small, sometimes dense stands, interspersed with such shrubs as chinquapin, snowbrush, and manzanita.

Pinyon–juniper woodland is found in narrow zones bordering the Antelope Valley and along the semiarid Soledad Canyon area southwest of Palmdale, elevation roughly 3,000–5,000 feet. Here are found a couple of rather stunted conifers—the one-leafed pinyon pine and the California juniper. Usually these trees do not predominate but are mixed with typical chaparral shrubs.

Joshua tree woodland, found in scattered locales along the north base of the San Gabriel Mountains, and more abundantly on rocky hills poking up from the Antelope Valley floor, is dominated by an outsize member of the yucca family—the Joshua tree. (L.A. County's best spot to view them is **Saddleback Butte State Park,** east of Lancaster; see Trip 11.3, page 165.)

Aside from this coast-to-desert cross-section of plant communities, there are others of more restricted range:

Southern oak woodland, widely distributed in coastal and inland valleys and on some of the mountains near Antelope Valley's western tip, consists of dense to open groves of live oak, valley oak (near the coast), black oak (near the desert), and California walnut trees. Scattered conifers such as Coulter pine, gray pine, and big-cone Douglas-fir intermix with the oaks in some areas.

Riparian (streamside) woodland, one of the rarest (in terms of the land it covers) communities, thrives at lower and middle elevations, where water is always present on or close to the surface. Massive live oaks, sycamores, alders, big-leaf maples and cottonwoods, and a screen of water-hugging willows are the hallmarks of riparian woodland. Not only is this kind of environment essential for the continued survival of many kinds of birds, animals, and fish, it's also very appealing to the senses. Riparian woodland is somewhat reminiscent of Eastern forests, with a palpable sense of dampness year-round. Much of this habitat in Southern California has been destroyed or is threatened by continued urbanization and attendant development of water resources or flood-control measures.

Other communities found in snippets along the coast or far afield in the Mojave Desert include rocky shore, coastal strand, coastal salt marsh, freshwater marsh, grassland, sagebrush scrub, creosote-bush scrub, and alkali sink. In many places in the foothills and mountains of the county, you will also find planted trees introduced from other parts of the world. Eucalyptus, pepper, and other exotic trees are often on the sites of many old ranches, while many roadsides, especially in the Angeles National Forest, have been planted with drought-resistant cypress trees and nonnative pines.

Some nonurbanized areas of the county are natural grasslands given over to agriculture and grazing. In areas characterized by heavy grazing, one finds grassy flats and bald slopes—sometimes called potreros (pastures)—supporting mostly nonnative vegetation like wild oats, filaree, fennel, mustard, and thistle. Many noxious invasive plants grow in disturbed areas, including castor bean, tobacco bush, thistle, mustard, and scotch broom.

Early-to-mid spring is the best time to appreciate the cornucopia of Los Angeles County's plant life. Many of the showiest species—spring wildflowers, for example—brighten the sage-scrub and chaparral zones at that time, and other plants exhibit fresh new growth. Peak periods for wildflowers vary according to elevation, slope, and proximity to coastal fogs. Generally, April is the best month. Common mountain wildflowers include lupine, penstemon, paintbrush, and purple nightshade. Common chaparral species include monkey flower, phacelia, California fuchsia, wild cucumber, and poppies.

One of the county's best wildflower spots is **Antelope Valley California Poppy Reserve,** a small state park west of Lancaster (Trip 11.2, page 164). Parched and uninspiring 10 or 11 months of the year, it comes alive (in years of average rainfall or better) with carpets of orange poppies around April. These desert-dwelling members of a species that is more at home in the valleys and hills of Central California evidently invaded the Antelope Valley through low-elevation passes to the west.

Creatures Great and Small

One's first sighting of a mountain lion, a bighorn sheep, an eagle, or any other seldom-seen form of wildlife is always memorable. Because of the diversity and generally broad extent of its habitats, and the inaccessibility of many of its wilderness areas, Los Angeles County plays host to a healthy population of indigenous creatures. If you're willing to stretch your legs a bit and spend some time in areas favored by wild animals, you'll eventually be rewarded with some kind of close visual contact.

The most numerous large creature in the county is the **mule deer,** with a population of at least several thousand. Deer are abundant in areas of mixed forest and scattered chaparral up in the higher mountains, and also close to the coast in the Santa Monica Mountains. Deer like to have a protective screen of vegetation near them at all times, along with a good supply of tasty leaves to munch on, so you won't often see them in wide-open spaces.

The **mountain lion,** once hunted to near-extinction in California, has made a substantial comeback. In Los Angeles County, perhaps two dozen lions roam the San Gabriel Mountains, and about a dozen more roam the Santa Monica Mountains. They're secretive but wide-ranging creatures, so you're much more likely to spot the tracks of this cat than meet one face to face. Still, several serious attacks and two fatalities involving mountain lions

*Antelope Valley California Poppy Reserve puts on a great show after a wet winter.
(See Trip 11.2, page 164.)*

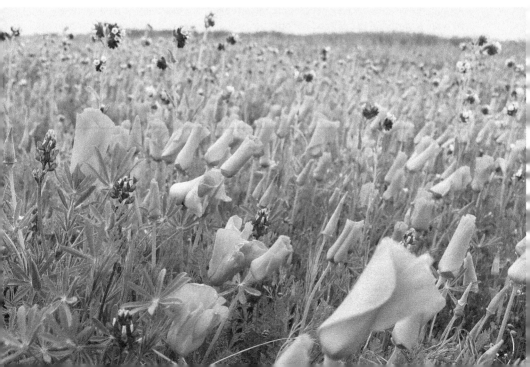

have occurred in California in the last three decades, so caution is warranted (learn more about this in the next section, "Health, Safety, and Courtesy").

Bobcats, which pose no danger unless cornered and harassed, are encountered on occasion in L.A.'s wild spaces, scampering through the canyons of the Santa Monicas or zipping across the Angeles Crest Highway at night.

A number of **black bears**—some of them so-called problem bears deported from Yosemite, others apparently the result of gradual migration south from the Sierra Nevada—inhabit the deeper canyons of the San Gabriels. They can be a nuisance at the both the developed campgrounds and the trail camps of Angeles National Forest.

Coyotes are universally abundant, adapting to just about any habitat with ease. At the foot of the mountains, where the urban–wildland interface is often a matter of a backyard fence or the curb of a cul-de-sac, coyotes make regular forays into the suburbs to snatch small pets or obtain water and food left unattended.

The county's most interesting (and surprisingly abundant) large mammal is the **bighorn sheep.** Several hundred of these agile animals maintain a tough existence on the steep slopes and rocky crags of the San Gabriel Mountains. Unlike mule deer, the bighorn prefer lightly vegetated, rugged terrain, on which they are capable of escaping almost any predator. They also shun contact with humans, although it's not unusual to spot them quite near such popular High Country summits as Mount Williamson and Mount Baden-Powell. The sheep are superbly adapted to surviving on meager supplies of water and coarse vegetation, conditions that characterize the San Gabriel and Sheep Mountain wilderness areas, which were set aside partly for their benefit.

The county's mammals also include gray foxes; raccoons; and various rabbits, squirrels, wood rats, and mice. Amphibians include tree frogs, salamanders, and pond turtles. Many streams supporting populations of rainbow trout exist in the San Gabriels. Some are artificially stocked to meet the demand of fishermen; others are natural fisheries where catch-and-release is the only method allowed. The tiny, unarmored three-spine stickleback, an endangered species, inhabits streams in Soledad and Bouquet Canyons.

Among the commonly seen reptiles are **rattlesnakes,** discussed in the next section.

Bird life is varied in the county, not only because of the coast-to-desert range of habitats but also because the county lies along the Pacific Flyway route of spring–fall migration and also serves some overwintering birds.

Los Angeles County is also an ancestral home of several other creatures symbolic of wild America. The **California condor,** a large vulture with a wingspan of up to 9 feet, was commonly seen over the San Gabriel and Santa Monica Mountains in the 19th century. By the 1980s the condor population statewide had declined so precipitously that the remaining few condors were captured, taken to zoos, and bred in captivity with the eventual goal of returning their offspring to the wild. This last-ditch strategy worked: now there are hundreds of California condors, some housed in zoos and many others released into the wild areas of Arizona, central and Southern California, and Baja California. **Peregrine falcons** are another comeback success story. These birds, which can achieve speeds of 200 miles per hour when diving for prey, have established nests on L.A. skyscrapers, as well as on secluded cliffs in Southern California's mountains.

Hunted and trapped with vigor until the late 19th century, grizzly bears were once the terror of the San Gabriel Mountains; thankfully for hikers, they won't return. Also gone are the pronghorn antelope that once wintered in the Antelope Valley. Unaccustomed to barriers in their natural open habitat, the pronghorn would not cross or jump over even the most trivial obstacles. Fences and railroads built across Mojave Desert migration routes sealed their fate—death by starvation.

Health, Safety, and Courtesy

Good preparation is always important for any kind of recreational pursuit, and hiking Southern California's backcountry is no exception. Although most of our local environments are usually not hostile or dangerous to life and limb, there are some pitfalls that you should consider.

Preparation and Equipment

An obvious safety requirement is being in good health. Some degree of physical conditioning is always desirable, even for the trips in this book designated as easy or moderate. The more challenging trips, rated moderately strenuous to very strenuous, require stamina and occasionally some technical expertise. Fast walking, running, bicycling, swimming, in-line skating, aerobic dancing, or any similar exercise that develops both the leg muscles and the aerobic capacity of the whole body are recommended as preparatory exercise.

For long trips over rough, cross-country terrain (there are several of these in this book) there is no really adequate way to prepare other than practicing the activity itself. Start with easy- or moderate-length cross-country trips first to accustom the leg muscles to the peculiar stresses involved in walking over uneven terrain and scrambling over boulders, and to acquire a good sense of balance. Sturdy hiking boots are recommended for such travel.

Several of the hiking trips in this book reach elevations of 7,000 feet or more—altitudes at which sea-level folks may notice a big difference in their rate of breathing and their energy. A few hours or a day spent at altitude before exercising will help almost anyone acclimate, but that's often impractical for short day trips. Still, you might consider spending a night at Buckhorn Campground (6,450') or Crystal Lake Campground (5,800') before taking a hike along the Angeles Crest, or at Manker Flats Campground (6,000') before tackling Old Baldy.

Altitude sickness strikes some victims at elevations as low as 8,000 feet. If you become dizzy or nauseated, or you suffer from congested lungs or a severe headache, the antidote may be as simple as descending a couple of thousand feet.

Your choice of equipment and supplies on the longer hikes in this book can be critically important. The essentials you should carry with you at all times in the backcountry are the things that would allow you to survive, in a reasonably comfortable manner, one or two unscheduled nights out. It's important to note that no one ever plans these nights! No one plans to get lost, injured, stuck, or pinned down by the weather. Always do a what-if analysis for a worst-case scenario, and plan accordingly. These essential items are your safety net; keep them with you on day hikes, and take them with you in a small day pack if you leave your backpack and camping equipment behind at a campsite.

Chief among the essential items is **warm clothing.** Inland Los Angeles County is characterized by wide swings in day and night temperatures. In mountain valleys, for example, a midday temperature in the 70s or 80s can be followed by a subfreezing night. Layer your clothing: it's better to take along two or more middleweight outer garments than to rely on a single heavy or bulky jacket to keep you comfortable at all times. Add to this a cap, gloves, and a waterproof or water-resistant shell (a large trash bag will do in a pinch), and you'll be quite prepared for all but the most severe weather experienced in Southern California.

In hot, sunny weather, **sun-shielding clothing** is another essential. This would normally include a sun hat and a light-colored, long-sleeve top.

Water and food are next in importance. Most streams and even some springs in the mountains have been shown to contain unacceptably high levels of bacteria or other contaminants. Even though some of the remote watersheds are probably pristine, it's wise to treat by filtering or chemical methods any water obtained outside of developed camp or picnic sites. Unless the day is very warm or your trip is a long one, it's usually easiest to carry (preferably in sturdy plastic bottles) all the water you'll need. Don't underestimate your water needs: during a full day's hike in 80°F temperatures, you may require as much as a gallon of water. Food is needed to stave off hunger and keep energy stores up, but it's not as essential as water in a survival situation.

Down the list further, but still essential, are a **map and compass** (or a GPS unit or app and the knowledge of its use); **flashlight; fire-starting devices** (examples: waterproof matches or lighter and candle); and **first aid kit.**

Items that aren't always essential, but potentially very useful and convenient, are sunglasses, pocketknife, whistle (or other signaling device), sunscreen, and toilet paper. A cell phone may be of use in an emergency, but be aware that it may fail to work for one reason or another, run out of charge, or you could easily be out of range of an antenna relay in just about any remote location. Consider buying a satellite locator beacon if you visit remote areas.

The essential items mentioned above should be carried by every member of a hiking party, because individuals or splinter groups may end up separating from the party for one reason or another. If you plan to hike solo in the backcountry, being well equipped is very important. If you hike alone, be sure to check in with a park ranger or leave your itinerary with a responsible person. In that way, if you do get stuck, help will probably come to the right place—eventually.

Special Hazards

Other than getting lost or pinned down by a sudden storm, the four most common hazards found in the L.A. County backcountry are **steep, unstable terrain; icy terrain; rattlesnakes;** and **poison oak.**

Exploring some parts of the San Gabriel Mountains—even by way of the trails—involves travel over structurally weak rock on steep slopes. The erosive effects of flowing water, of wedging by roots and by ice, and of brush fires tend to pulverize such rock even further. Slips on such terrain usually lead to sliding down a hillside some distance. If you explore cross-country, always be on the lookout for dangerous run-outs, such as cliffs, below you. The side walls of many canyons in the San Gabriels may look like nice places to practice rock-climbing moves, but this misconception has contributed to many deaths over the years.

Statistically, mishaps associated with snow and ice have caused the greatest number of fatalities in the San Gabriel Mountains. This is not because the San Gabriels are somehow inherently more dangerous than other ranges. Rather, it's because inexperienced lowlanders, never picturing their backyard mountains as true wilderness areas, are attracted here by the novelty of snow and the easy access by way of snowplowed highways. Icy chutes and slopes capable of avalanching can easily trap such visitors unaware. Winter travel in the more gentle areas of the high country can be accomplished on snowshoes or skis; but the steeper slopes require technical skills and equipment such as an ice ax and crampons, just as in any other high mountain range.

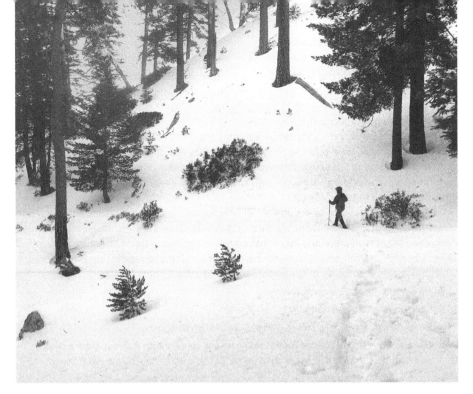

A winter wonderland in Icehouse Canyon (see Trip 30.5, page 409)   Photo: Werner Zorman

Rattlesnakes are fairly common in most parts of Los Angeles County below about 7,000 feet. Seldom seen in either cold or very hot weather, they favor temperatures in the 75°F- to 90°F range—mostly spring–fall in the lower areas and summer in the higher mountains. Most rattlesnakes are as interested in avoiding contact with you as you are with them. The more hazardous areas include rocky canyon bottoms with running streams. Watch carefully where you put your feet, and especially your hands, during the warmer months. In brushy or rocky areas where sight distance is short, tread with heavy footfalls, or use a stick to bang against rocks or bushes. Rattlesnakes will pick up the vibrations through their skin and will usually buzz (unmistakably) before you get too close for comfort.

Poison oak grows profusely along many of the county's canyons below 5,000 feet. It's often found in the form of a bush or vine on the banks of streams, where it prefers semi-shady habitats; quite often it's seen beside or encroaching on well-used trails. Every California hiker should learn to recognize its distinctive three-leafed structure and avoid contact with skin or clothing. Because poison oak loses its leaves during the winter (and sometimes during summer and fall droughts) but still retains some of the toxic oil in its stems, it can be extra-hazardous at that time because it is harder to identify and avoid. Midweight pants, like blue jeans, and a long-sleeve shirt will serve as a fair barrier against the toxic oil of the poison oak plant. Do, of course, remove these clothes as soon as the hike is over, and make sure they are washed carefully afterward. If you come in contact with poison oak, rinse off the oil with cold water. If you get a rash, various creams and antihistamines may help.

Here are a few more tips:

Ticks can sometimes be a scourge of overgrown trails in the sage-scrub and chaparral country, particularly during the first warm spells of the year, when they climb to the tips of shrub branches and lie in wait for warm-blooded hosts. If you can't avoid brushing against vegetation along the trail, be sure to check yourself for ticks frequently. Upon finding a host, a tick will usually crawl upward in search of a protected spot, where it will try to attach itself. If you can be aware of the slightest irritations on your body, you'll usually intercept ticks long before they attempt to bite. Wearing long pants, long sleeves, and insect repellent helps ward off ticks. Ticks can carry Lyme disease, so consult your doctor promptly if you have a rash, fever, headache, or fatigue following a tick bite.

For decades, encounters with mountain lions (cougars) were almost never reported in Southern California. This began to change in the 1990s, due, in part certainly, to an increase in cougar population, a decrease in cougar habitat (especially in areas where suburban and rural housing development is increasing), and abnormal geographic displacement of deer, a prime source of food for cougars.

Several incidents involving cougars stalking or menacing campers, hikers, and mountain bikers have occurred throughout Southern California since 1994. In the worst such incident, a woman was attacked and killed by a cougar while hiking near Cuyamaca Peak in San Diego County. The following precautions are urged for all persons entering cougar country, which may include virtually every nonurban Los Angeles County locale:

- Hike with one or more companions.
- Keep children close at hand.
- Never run from a cougar. This may trigger an instinct to attack.
- Make yourself large, face the animal, maintain eye contact with it, shout, blow a whistle, and do not act fearful. Do anything to convince the animal that you are not its prey.

Despite the recent interest in and the increased use of hiking trails in Los Angeles County, there is paradoxically less money (especially in Angeles National Forest) for building and maintaining them. Most of that work is left to volunteer crews nowadays. In the chaparral areas, trails can become overgrown quickly, so that travel along them can become

Scarcely a mile from the freeway, you can get away from it all in the Santa Susana Mountains. (See Trip 5.11, page 69.)

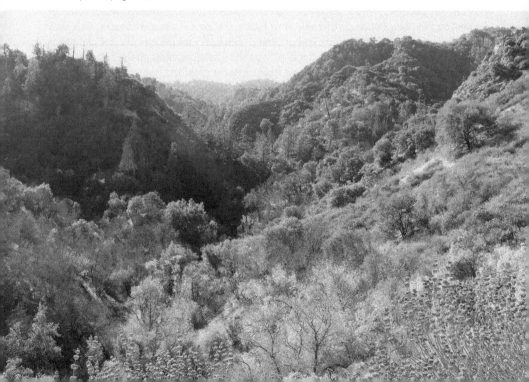

an exercise in bushwhacking. Traveling certain trailless canyon bottoms and ridgelines also involves some bushwhacking. Blue jeans (in spite of their reputation as being worthless in cold, wet conditions) are very good at protecting your legs when you're dodging or pushing through dry chaparral.

Camping and Permits

Overnight camping in roadside campgrounds is not always a restful experience. Off-season camping (late fall through early spring) offers relief from crowds but not from chilly night-time weather. Campgrounds in Angeles National Forest are less well supervised than those in the Santa Monica Mountains, and therefore sometimes attract a noisy crowd. In my experience, facilities with a campground host promise a better clientele, and a better night's sleep.

The nice advantage of a developed campground is that you can always build a campfire, unless the facility itself is closed or there is a total fire ban in the forest. On the national-forest trails, campfires are allowed most of the year in the stoves provided at trail camps or on ground cleared to bare mineral soil to a 5-foot radius (campfire builders must also carry a shovel to bury the embers). Fire permits, valid for the length of a fire season, must be obtained from the U.S. Forest Service (USFS) for the use of any campfire or flame device (camp stoves, gas lanterns) on the trail. Be aware that any jurisdiction—national forest, state, county, city, or private—may declare fire closures in which all access is prohibited during critical fire conditions. Call first if you're in doubt.

Angeles National Forest allows remote, primitive-style camping: under this policy, you're not restricted to staying at a developed campground or designated trail camp. For sanitation reasons, you are required to locate your primitive camp at least 200 feet from the trail and the nearest source of water. And, of course, you must observe the fire regulations stated earlier. Contact the USFS to confirm these rules if you intend to do any remote camping.

Most federally managed wilderness areas around the state require special wilderness permits for entry. At present, however, permits are not required for **San Gabriel Wilderness** or **Pleasant View Wilderness,** or for **Sheep Mountain Wilderness** except at the East Fork Station gateway, where free self-issue wilderness permits are available. **Cucamonga Wilderness** in San Bernardino County (represented in one hike in this book) also requires a free self-issue permit, available at ranger stations or the Icehouse Canyon Trailhead.

Other Regulations

This book contains much trail information of interest to **mountain bikers.** Mountain biking regulations, however, vary according to jurisdiction. Currently, bikes are allowed on all Angeles National Forest roads and trails except the Pacific Crest Trail and trails within wilderness areas. Elsewhere, bikes are usually permitted on fire roads, but not on singletrack trails. Mountain bikers should yield the right-of-way to both hikers and equestrians.

Deer-hunting season in Angeles National Forest occurs during midautumn. Although conflicts between hunters and hikers are rare, you may want to confine your explorations at that time to the state, county, and city parks, where hunting is prohibited.

Once allowed over a wide area of the mountains, **target shooting** is now legally restricted to a small number of private shooting ranges and designated shooting areas in Angeles National Forest. Some illegal shooting continues to take place in canyons just off some of the mountain highways. Try to report this kind of activity to the sheriff or a ranger. Shooting in the lawful pursuit of game is easy to distinguish from automatic-weapon fire in non-designated areas.

For Your Protection

There is always some risk in leaving a vehicle in an unattended area. Automobile vandalism, burglary, and theft are small but distinct possibilities. Report all theft and vandalism of personal property to the county sheriff, and report vandalism of public property to the appropriate park or forest agency.

Obviously, it's unwise to leave valuable property in an automobile. To prevent theft of the car, you can disable your car's ignition system or use a locking device on the steering wheel. Many of the routes in this book are written up as one-way, point-to-point trips requiring either a car shuttle (leaving cars at both ends) or an arrangement by which someone drops you off and later picks you up. Choose the latter method if you're concerned about security.

Trail Courtesy

Whenever you travel in the natural areas of the county, you take on a burden of responsibility to keep the backcountry as you found it. Aside from commonsense prohibitions against littering, vandalism, and illegal fires, there are some less obvious guidelines every hiker should be aware of. We'll mention a few:

Never cut trail switchbacks. This practice breaks down the trail tread and hastens erosion. Improve designated trails by removing branches, rocks, or other debris if you can. Springtime growth can quite rapidly obscure pathways in the chaparral country, and funding for trail maintenance is often scarce, so try to do your part by joining a volunteer trail crew or by performing your own small maintenance tasks while walking the trails. Report any damage to trails or other facilities to the appropriate ranger office.

When backpacking, be a **Leave No Trace** camper: leave your campsite as you found it, or leave it in an even more natural condition.

Collecting specimens of minerals, plants, animals, and historical objects without special permit is prohibited in state and county parks. This means common things, too, such as pine cones, wildflowers, and lizards. These should be left for all visitors to enjoy. Some limited collecting of items like pine cones may be allowed on the national forest lands—check first.

We've covered most of the general regulations associated with the use of the public lands in Los Angeles County. But you, as a visitor, are responsible for knowing any additional rules as well. The capsulized summary for each hike described in this book includes a reference to the agency responsible for the area you'll be visiting. Addresses and phone numbers for those agencies appear in Appendix D.

Where and When to Go

Clearly, two of the most detrimental aspects of living in most parts of Los Angeles are air pollution and traffic congestion. Air pollution affects, to a greater or lesser degree, all of the trips in this book, and traffic congestion affects (at least at certain times) how quickly you can escape the city and be on your merry way down the trail. In this section we'll look into some of the strategies you can use to sidestep these difficulties and also take advantage of optimum conditions of weather and visibility.

Beating the traffic isn't too difficult once you're out of the urban core. On weekdays, the flow of automobiles is mostly inward toward congested parts of the city during the morning, and outward during the afternoon and evening. Driving out of town early on weekend mornings is a breeze, but getting back into town later in the afternoon can be a bit of a problem.

Nearly all the trails of Los Angeles County are refreshingly underutilized on weekdays. Sometimes you can walk for hours without seeing another traveler. Fair-weather weekends

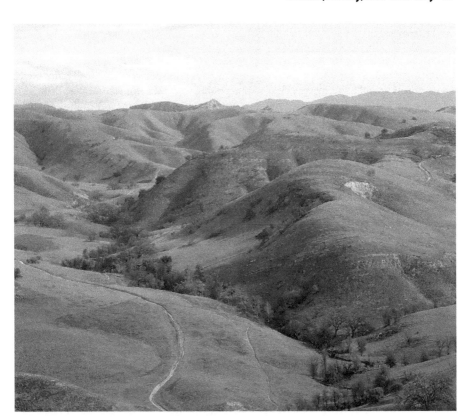

The Simi Hills wear an emerald mantle after winter rains. (See Chapter 4.)

bring large numbers of people to a relatively small number of popular trailheads, while other trailheads have plenty of room for parking. Chantry Flat and Sunset Ridge (Millard Canyon), both easily accessible from San Gabriel Valley communities, have outside gates that can and do close to incoming traffic whenever the parking situation gets intolerable. The moral of all this is: hike on weekdays when you can, or on weekends as long as you get an early start.

There's a strong belief, even among most Southern Californians, that summer equals the hiking season. This prejudice probably comes from the fact that so many Southland residents have emigrated from other areas where this may be true. Actually, summer is the worst season to visit most of the wild lands of Los Angeles County. Summer–early fall is a time of drought, when much of the chaparral and scrub vegetation blanketing the mountain slopes turns drab and crispy, and the land bakes under a near-vertical sun. Summer hikes can be rewarding, however, if the trip is short and you get an early-morning start.

Summer—early summer especially—is fine for areas above 6,000–7,000 feet. Some of the highest elevations in the San Gabriel Mountains don't experience much of a summer at all, the snows of winter disappearing in July or not long before the first subfreezing nights of September or October. Summer is also a perfectly good time to visit the beaches, and the lower slopes and canyons of the Santa Monica Mountains that benefit from the coastal breezes.

Late fall brings autumn color to the oak woodlands and wet canyons of the county. The leaves of the valley oak, black oak, and walnut turn a crispy yellow in the valleys and on the hillsides. Big-leaf maples, cottonwoods, willows, and sycamores contribute similar hues to canyon bottoms spotted with red-leafed poison oak vines. This is a time when the marine layer over the coastline and basin often lies low (at least in the morning) while the air above can be extraordinarily clean and dry.

Instead of suffering through days-long episodes of bad weather in winter, we Southern Californians usually experience a string of sunny days interspersed with short, rainy spells. Some storms are followed by very clear weather along with cold winds from the north. This is when you should seize the moment: hop in the car, and head for a trail in the nearby foothills or mountains leading to some prominent high point. The views will often stretch from snow-covered peaks to the island-dotted Pacific Ocean.

Spring comes on gradually, each week a little warmer (with a heat wave or two tossed in) and a little hazier. The marine layer is thicker now, but superb views are still possible from mile-high summits in the San Gabriels such as Mount Lowe and Strawberry Peak. Sunrises can be dramatic up there, with much of the surrounding lowland enveloped in a bank of low clouds. Annual wildflowers seem to pop up everywhere, wild lilacs paint the hillsides white and blue, and the scents of sage and nectar float on the air. When the marine layer is very deep, fogs bearing light drizzle may envelop the canyons of the Santa Monicas and San Gabriels, like the mists of Sherwood Forest. The High Country is often snowbound through May, although it may be possible to approach some of the passes and high points by way of southern routes.

In any season, the infamous Los Angeles smog can seriously affect your enjoyment of wild areas. At worst, the eye-smarting, lung-irritating air can turn an otherwise pristine watershed into one that looks like a hellish abyss. Strict emissions controls implemented over the past five decades have resulted in dramatic improvements in air quality.

Often, that's not very hard. Prevailing ocean breezes keep the western Santa Monica Mountains fairly clean most of the year. The High Country and northern slopes of the San Gabriels are more affected by marine air moving up the Santa Clara River valley than by dirty air blown in from the city. For example, Charlton–Chilao Recreation Area, just 10 airline miles from the edge of the L.A. Basin, gets an average of only about 40 slightly smoggy days a year.

Air pollution often and seriously affects such L.A. Basin–bordering areas as Griffith Park, the Verdugo Mountains, the Santa Susana Mountains, the Puente Hills, and the Front Range of the San Gabriels. But there are clear spells as well. Much of the smog originating in the L.A. Basin is photochemically produced (sunlight reacting on automobile exhaust gases), so morning air tends to be cleaner than afternoon air. Weekends are a little cleaner than weekdays, because traffic volumes are somewhat reduced.

When the weather is stable, and a strong temperature inversion (warmer air overlying cooler air) exists, the smog-bearing marine layer stays close to the ground until about midday. By afternoon local sea breezes are transporting it east to Riverside and San Bernardino Counties, and up the Front Range canyons and slopes.

Less commonly, regional winds kick the smog north or northeast into the Antelope Valley, west along the Malibu coast to Oxnard and Ventura, or south as far as San Diego. Sometimes smog covers the whole county as a gauzy curtain, but more often it lies quite close to the ground in a localized area, leaving upwind areas with clear, blue skies.

Using This Book

Whether you wish to use this book as a reference tool or as a guide to be read cover to cover, you should take a few minutes to read this section. Herein we explain the meaning of the capsulized information that appears before each trip description, and we also describe the way in which trips are grouped together geographically.

One way to expedite the process of finding a suitable trip, especially if you're unfamiliar with hiking opportunities in Los Angeles County, is to turn to "Best Hikes" (page 464). This is a cross-reference of the most highly recommended hikes described in this book.

Each of the 259 hiking trips belongs to one of 33 geographic regions, which are organized as chapters in this book. Each chapter has its own introductory text and map. The San Gabriel Mountains and Santa Monica Mountains account for the largest share of hikes, but many interesting trips can be found along the coastline, in the desert, in the Los Angeles Basin, and on Santa Catalina Island. The overview map (see "Los Angeles County & Vicinity," pages vi–vii) shows the coverage of each chapter map, and "Contents" (page ix) shows the page numbers for each region, chapter, and trip.

The introductory text for each area includes any general information about the area's history, geology, plants, and wildlife not included in the trip descriptions.

Important information about possible restrictions or special requirements (wilderness permits, for example) appears here, too, and you should review this material before starting on a hike in a particular chapter. In particular, you should be aware that many trips on Angeles National Forest land require that you post a **National Forest Adventure Pass** on your parked car. See page 21 for more information.

Each chapter also contains a sketch map of the locations and routes of all hikes in the area covered by that chapter. The numbers in the squares on those maps correspond to trip numbers in the text. These boxed numbers refer to the start and end points of out-and-back and loop trips. The point-to-point trips have two boxed numbers, which indicate separate start and end points. For some hikes, the corresponding chapter map alone is complete enough and fully adequate for navigation; for other hikes, more detailed topographical or other maps are recommended. A legend for the maps appears on page 20.

Capsulized Information

The following is an explanation of key at-a-glance information that appears at the beginning of each trip description. If you're simply browsing this book, these summaries alone can be used as a tool to eliminate from consideration hikes that are either too difficult, or perhaps too trivial, for your abilities.

DISTANCE

An estimate of total distance is provided. Out-and-back trips show the sum of the distances of the out and back segments; some trips have alternative paths that change the distance. Your mileage may vary.

Map Legend

Freeway	══════	County line	─── ─ ── ─
Major paved road	───────	Stream or canyon with tributaries	
Minor paved road	─────		
Dirt road	▪▪▪▪▪▪▪▪▪▪▪	Body of water	
Trail	------------	Start/end point of single trip	**6**
Cross-country route	··················	Start point of a range of trips	**7–9**
Parking lot	**P**	Point of interest	■
Trailhead	**T**	Peak	▲
Ranger station/ visitor center		Gate	•—•
Picnic area			
Campground		North arrow	

Distances measured with an odometer or GPS are generally reported to the nearest tenth of a mile. Beware, however, that two different GPS units will yield slightly different mileages, even when carried by the same person at the same time. Total trip distance is generally rounded to the nearest mile for longer trips.

After the trail distance, we've noted whether the trip, as described, is a loop, an out-and-back route, or a point-to-point trip requiring a car shuttle. There is some flexibility, of course, in the way in which a hiker can actually follow the trip.

HIKING TIME

This figure is for the average hiker and includes only the time spent in motion. It does not include time spent for rest stops, lunch, etc. Fast walkers can complete the routes in perhaps 30% less time, and slower hikers may take 50% longer. We assume the hiker is traveling with a light day pack. Hikers carrying heavy packs could easily take twice as long, especially if they are traveling under adverse weather conditions. Remember, too, that the progress made by a group as a whole is limited by the pace of the slowest member(s).

ELEVATION GAIN/LOSS

These are an estimate of the sum of all the vertical gain segments and the sum of all the vertical loss segments along the total length of the route (includes both ways for out-and-back trips). This is often considerably more than the net difference in elevation between the high and low points of the hike. You can reduce the elevation gain for some one-way trips by hiking in the downhill rather than uphill direction.

DIFFICULTY

This overall rating takes into account the length of the trip and the nature of the terrain. The following are general definitions of the five categories:

- *Easy:* Suitable for every member of the family
- *Moderate:* Suitable for all physically fit people
- *Moderately Strenuous:* Long length, substantial elevation gain, and/or difficult terrain; suitable for experienced hikers only
- *Strenuous:* Full day's hike (or overnight backpack) over a long and often difficult route; suitable only for experienced hikers in excellent physical condition
- *Very Strenuous:* Long and rugged route in extremely remote area; suitable only for experienced hikers/climbers in top physical condition

Each higher level represents more or less a doubling of the difficulty. On average, moderate trips are twice as hard as easy trips, moderately strenuous trips are twice as hard as moderate trips, and so on.

TRAIL USE

All trips are open to hikers. We've also noted whether trips are well suited for dogs, equestrians, mountain bikers, families with kids, or backpackers.

BEST TIMES

This is the seasonal range that the authors have estimated as best for each trail. Nearly all of the short trips in this book are suitable year-round. Some of the longer trips in the warmer, interior areas are simply too hot during the summer season. Hikes at high altitude can become inaccessible during the winter because of road closures, or they may be dangerous because of snow and ice. Generally, however, the range of months indicates when the hike is most rewarding.

AGENCY

Lists the entity that manages the area in which the hike is located. Agency contact data is listed in Appendix D (page 469).

PERMITS

Only a few wilderness areas in Los Angeles County require permits for entry. Some popular areas have quotas that fill up long in advance on summer weekends, so plan ahead.

Many popular trailheads in Angeles National require parked cars to display a **National Forest Adventure Pass.** These passes cost $5 for a day or $30 for a year. You may also use an **America the Beautiful Pass,** which covers admission to national parks and most other federal lands.

In the 2014 *Fragosa et al. v. U.S. Forest Service* decision, the California Central District Court ruled that people who do not use facilities and services such as restrooms, picnic tables, and trash cans cannot be required to buy a pass to park in or enter a national forest. The USFS has agreed to designate free parking close to developed trailheads, but signage is still in flux.

National Forest Wilderness Permits are different from Adventure Passes. The latter cost money and are required to park your car at developed sites; Wilderness permits are free, subject to quota limits, and required for entering many wilderness areas. For more information on both, visit www.fs.fed.us/visit/passes-permits.

Anyone 16 years of age or older must possess and wear a **California Sport Fishing License** while angling. Licenses, good for one calendar year, can be purchased from the California Department of Fish and Wildlife or from authorized agents. See wildlife.ca.gov/licensing /fishing for more information.

Access fees listed in this edition were accurate at press time but are subject to change, so check the resources in Appendix D (page 469) for the latest information.

SUPPLEMENTAL MAPS

For trips in this book, maps are categorized as *optional, recommended,* or *required.* If you already know an area well, you may be able to do without a recommended map. Required maps, however, are essential for successful navigation.

Where available, this book recommends **Tom Harrison** or *National Geographic* **Trails Illustrated** maps or other specialty commercial maps. These are regularly updated and cover more trails for less money than the aging U.S. Geological Survey (USGS) 7.5-minute-series topographic maps. Tom Harrison maps tend to be the most accurate. In addition, many parks and open-space areas in L.A. Count provide excellent hiking maps to visitors at entrances and trailheads at minimal or no cost—when these maps are freely available online, they are mentioned here. When free or commercial maps are unavailable, the USGS map is listed, but be aware that not all trails are shown on these older maps.

Most of these supplemental maps can be purchased from local outdoor-equipment stores, ranger stations, and rei.com, as well as directly from the publishers. See Appendix E (page 472) for more information.

DIRECTIONS

Whenever driving directions are given for trips in the rural or remote areas of Los Angeles County, certain reference points along numbered highways may be keyed to the roadside mile markers posted at frequent intervals. County highways often have small, paddle-shaped signs with mileage figures on them. State highways have reflective paddles stenciled with numbers like "29.54." The mileage signs may appear at half-mile intervals, 1-mile intervals, or at irregular intervals. When the driving directions stipulate a turn at, say, mile 39.7, this doesn't necessarily mean there's a marker at that exact spot. Rather, it would typically indicate a spot 0.3 mile from a milepost labeled 40.0. In general, highway mileage increases northward for north–south highways and increases eastward for east–west highways.

ELECTRONIC SUPPLEMENTS

The free **eTrails** app for iOS complements this book. It contains high-quality maps and waypoints for these trips, as well as for the Pacific Crest Trail and several other books; it also helps automate driving from your present position to the trailheads. Download eTrails from the Mac App Store; in the app, go to the menu tab, select "AALA4e" as the book, and then pick the hike(s) that interests you.

The GPS tracks and waypoints for most of the trips in this book can also be downloaded directly from eTrails.net.

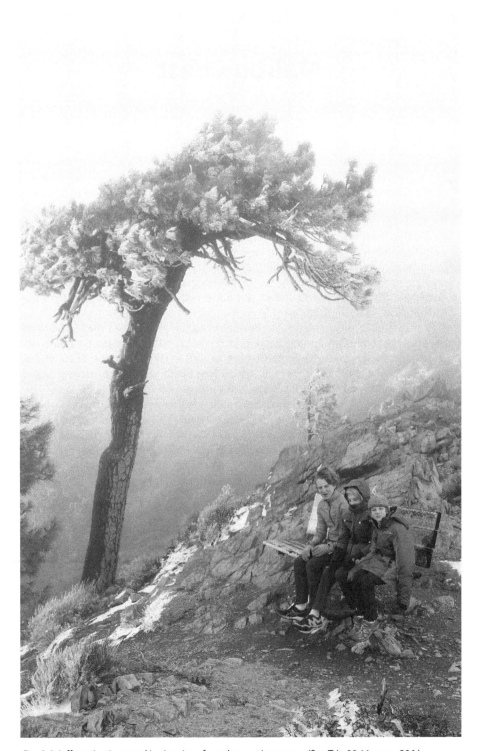

Brrr! *A Jeffrey pine is coated in rime ice after a late-spring storm. (See Trip 29.11, page 396.)*

chapter 1

Malibu Coast

Fabled Malibu stretches 25 miles from the edge of the Los Angeles Basin at Santa Monica upcoast toward the Ventura County line. This odd, ribbonlike community—the home of many of L.A.'s rich and famous—doggedly follows the course of the narrow, curvy Pacific Coast Highway, itself confined to a precariously unstable coastal terrace at the foot of the Santa Monica Mountains. Parts of Malibu consist of unbroken rows of townhouses perilously jammed between the highway and the surf. Just back of the coastal strip, stilted houses have gained airy footholds on precipitous slopes overlooking the coast. Periodic wildfires sweeping over the mountains and the erosive battering of the ocean waves have done little to discourage urban-style growth. But a rising antigrowth sentiment among residents may well accomplish what nature has failed to do.

If you like strolling on crowded public beaches, or ogling fancy houses, the Malibu coastline has plenty of both. Quieter stretches of coastline, removed from the sight of houses and the roar of traffic, are a little harder to find but are well worth seeking out. These include (in the middle section of Malibu) Malibu Lagoon State Beach, which has a saltwater lagoon favored by migrating birds, a surfing beach, and a pier, as well as Malibu Bluffs Park.

If you're an avid hiker, though, you'll head a little farther west to a stretch of coastline wrapping around the flat-topped headlands of Point Dume. This southward-pointing promontory, jutting into the Pacific Ocean some 20 miles west of Santa Monica, is a widely visible landmark. Just east of the point itself, an unbroken cliff wall shelters a secluded beach from the sights and sounds of the civilized world. On this beach, you can forget about whatever else may lie just over the cliff rim; your world is simply one of crashing surf, tangy salt spray, pearly sand, and fascinating tide pools.

Sea star and sand-coated anemones hang out in Dume Cove tide pools.

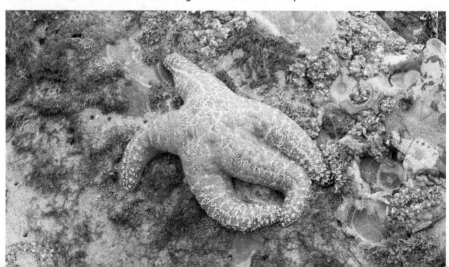

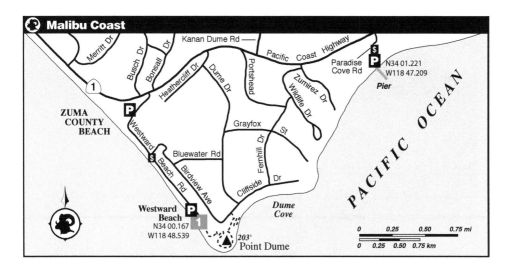

Malibu Coast

Kanan Dume Rd

Merritt Dr
Busch Dr
Bonsall Dr
Heathercliff Dr
Dume Dr
Portshead
Pacific Coast Highway
Zumirez Dr
Wildlife Dr

Paradise Cove Rd
N34 01.221
W118 47.209
Pier

ZUMA COUNTY BEACH

Westward Beach Rd

Grayfox

Fernhill Dr

St

Bluewater Rd

Birdview Ave

Cliffside

Dr

PACIFIC OCEAN

Westward Beach
N34 00.167
W118 48.539

Dume Cove

203'
Point Dume

0   0.25   0.50   0.75 mi
0   0.25   0.50 0.75 km

---

trip 1.1   **Point Dume to Paradise Cove**

Distance	6 miles (out-and-back) or 3 miles (one-way)
Hiking Time	3 hours
Elevation Gain	400'/200'
Difficulty	Moderate
Trail Use	Good for kids
Best Times	Year-round (low tide recommended)
Agency	National Park Service
Optional Map	Tom Harrison *Zuma–Trancas Canyon* or Trails Illustrated *Santa Monica Mountains National Recreation Area (253)*

DIRECTIONS From Santa Monica drive west (up the coast) on Pacific Coast Highway (Highway 1) about 25 miles to Westward Beach Road (0.4 mile west of mile marker 001 LA 54.5). Turn south and follow Westward Beach Road to its end, where there is a spacious pay parking lot. Alternatively, park free on the roadside before you reach the pay station, and then stroll 0.7 mile southeast along the beach to Point Dume.

To make this a one-way trip, park your getaway car or bike on the shoulder of the highway near the intersection with Paradise Cove Road, 2 miles east of Westward Beach Road. You can also park at the private resort of Paradise Cove, but expect a hefty parking fee unless you patronize the restaurant.

A pleasant walk anytime the tide is low, this trip is doubly rewarding when the tide dips as low as –2 feet. The rocky coastline below the cliffs of Point Dume harbors a mind-boggling array of marine plant and animal life, much of it under water most of the time. That includes, based on what I (Jerry) have seen myself: limpets, periwinkles, chitons, tube snails, sandcastle worms, sculpins, mussels, shore and hermit crabs, green and aggregate anemones, three kinds of barnacles, and two kinds of sea stars. Extreme low tides occur during the afternoon two or three times each month from October through March. Consult tide tables to find out exactly when. Captain George Vancouver named Point Dume in 1793 in misspelled honor of Padre Francisco Dumetz of Mission San Buenaventura.

From the parking lot at Westward Beach, you have two choices. The shorter, much easier route profiled here (and the only practical alternative during all but extremely low tides) is the trail slanting left up the cliff. Stay right at a junction onto a path hugging the top of the cliffs. On top you'll come to an area popular for sighting gray whales during their

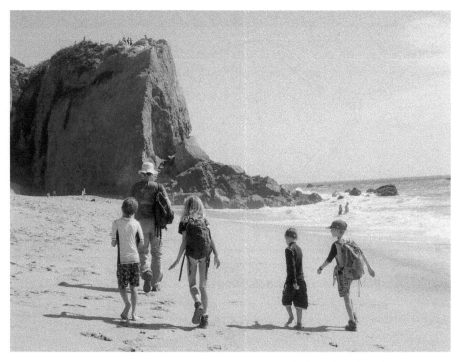

A family walks along Westward Beach toward Point Dume as rock climbers belay from the summit.

southward migration in winter. You'll also discover a state historic monument. Point Dume was christened by the British naval commander George Vancouver, who sailed by in 1793. As you stand on Point Dume's apex, note the marked contrast between the lighter sedimentary rock exposed on the cliff faces both east and west, and the darker volcanic rock just below. Like the armored bow of an ice-breaker, this unusually tough mass of volcanic rock has thus far resisted the onslaught of the ocean swells. You may see (and smell) a colony of sea lions on the rocks below. After you descend from the high point, some metal stairs will take you down to crescent-shaped Dume Cove.

The alternative route is for skilled climbers only—it's definitely not appropriate for small children. During the lowest or low tides, you can edge around the point itself, making your way by hand-and-toe climbing in a couple of spots over huge, angular shards of volcanic rock along the base of the cliffs. The tide pools here and also to the east along Dume Cove's shoreline harbor some of the best displays of intertidal marine life in Southern California. This visual feast will remain for others to enjoy if you refrain from taking or disturbing in any way the organisms that live there (this hike is part of Point Dume Natural Preserve, where all features are protected). Be aware that exploring the lower intertidal zones can be hazardous. Be very cautious when traveling over slippery rocks, and always be aware of the incoming swells. Don't let a rogue wave catch you by surprise.

The going is easy once you're on Dume Cove's ribbon of sand. When you reach the northeast end of Dume Cove, swing left around a lesser point and continue another mile over a somewhat wider beach. You can travel as far as Paradise Cove, the site of an elegant beachside restaurant and private pier, 2.9 miles from your starting point.

If you left a getaway vehicle at Paradise Cove Road, you'll find it by walking up the Paradise Cove Road for 0.3 mile to the highway. Otherwise, return the way you came.

chapter 2

Palos Verdes Peninsula

Forged by local uplift of the seafloor roughly 2 million years ago, Palos Verdes lay surrounded by the ocean for hundreds of thousands of years. Today the vast sheet of alluvium filling the L.A. Basin connects Palos Verdes to the mainland—yet in a figurative sense Palos Verdes has never really lost its identity as an island.

When the South Bay cities of Torrance and Long Beach are cloaked by fog or brown haze, the adjoining cities of Palos Verdes Estates and Rancho Palos Verdes often stand head and shoulders above the murk. Sometimes you can stand on top, enjoying views of far-off Santa Catalina Island and Old Baldy but failing to make out L.A. Harbor just a few miles away.

Palos Verdes is a distinct economic and cultural island as well. Rimmed by oil refineries, gritty industrial neighborhoods, and wall-to-wall people, the peninsula itself is dominated almost exclusively by opulent ranch-style homes and sprawling, lavishly landscaped estates. The contrast is startling.

Fortunately, Palos Verdes offers miles of near-pristine coastline and big patches of hillside open space within Palos Verdes Nature Preserve for explorers on foot to enjoy. Start with Trip 2.1, below, for an easy overview of the area and later graduate to one of the tougher scrambles (Trips 2.2–2.4) along the base of the coastal cliffs. Contact the Palos Verdes Peninsula Land Conservancy (pvplc.org) for information about other open spaces in the area.

trip 2.1   ## Top of the Peninsula

see map on next page

Distance	1.8 miles (out-and-back)
Hiking Time	1 hour
Elevation Gain	300'
Difficulty	Easy
Trail Use	Dogs allowed, good for kids
Best Times	Year-round
Agency	City of Rancho Palos Verdes Department of Recreation, Parks, and Open Space
Optional Maps	USGS 7.5' *Torrance, San Pedro*

DIRECTIONS From Highway 1 in Torrance, drive south on Crenshaw Boulevard, one of L.A.'s longest and busiest thoroughfares, all the way to its southern end. Park on the shoulder before the dead-end of the road (observing parking restrictions).

At Del Cerro Park, on top of the Palos Verdes Peninsula, you need only climb a small, grassy hill to take in one of L.A.'s truly great ocean views. With a little bit more ambition, you can hoof it less than a mile to an even more panoramic view spot. Ideally, you could be here when a chilly north wind (which usually follows the passage of major winter storms) cleanses the Southland of polluted air. But don't neglect the early spring. During

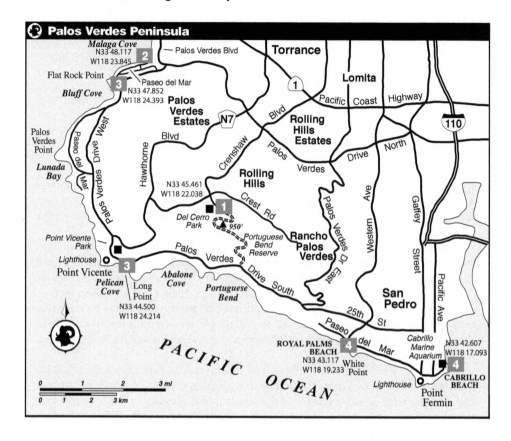

Palos Verdes Peninsula

March and April the sages, native wildflowers, and weedy grasses magically transform the normally drab-colored hillsides into tapestries of velvet green. Even with hazy skies, however, the view seems ethereal.

This trip lies within the 399-acre Portuguese Bend Reserve, established in 2005 as part of the Palos Verdes Nature Preserve. The place-name derives from Portuguese whalers who hunted along this bend in the coastline in the 1870s.

At Crenshaw's dead end, step around the steel gate and follow Burma Road, the dirt fire road beyond, into Portuguese Bend Reserve. Soon you're in a rare patch of open space surrounded by, but largely removed from, the curving avenues and palatial estates of Rancho Palos Verdes. Since the mid-1950s, when more than 100 houses were destroyed or seriously damaged by landslides in the Portuguese Bend area, most of the steep area above the Bend has remained off-limits to development.

At 0.6 mile stay on the main road as the Peacock Flats and Ishibashi Trails fork off. Continue a curving descent until you reach a flat area about 0.3 mile farther. Leave the road there and take the Eagle's Nest Trail to the top of a 950-foot knoll, dotted with planted pines, on the left. Atop this serene little overlook, you'll enjoy a 150° view of the ocean, with Santa Catalina Island sprawling at center stage in the south. If the air is very clear, try to spot San Nicolas Island, some 70 miles away to the southwest.

The knoll you're standing on is a remnant of one of the 13 marine terraces that have made the Palos Verdes hills a textbook example familiar to geology students. The terraces, rising like rounded and broken stairs from sea level to 1,300 feet, are the result of wave erosion modified by uplift and fluctuating sea levels during the past 2 million years. From this spot (despite the effects of decades of grading and construction on some of the adjacent ridges) you will probably recognize at least seven of the terraces in the topography around you.

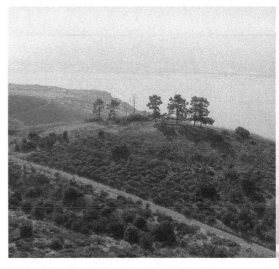

VARIATION

With some extra time, you can explore the spiderweb of trails that lace the hills located between Del Cerro Park and Palos Verdes Drive South. Following the paths downhill will eventually get you to the Ishibashi Farm Trailhead near Palos Verdes Drive in 2–2.5 miles. For a change of scenery, turn right on Palos Verdes Drive, and then walk past the South Bay Archery Club to the signed Sacred Cove Trail to Inspiration Point. A spur called the Bow and Arrow Trail drops to the

The Pacific Ocean lies beyond the Eagle's Nest Viewpoint in Portuguese Bend Reserve.

east side of Inspiration Point, where you can explore tide pools and visit a sea cave at the end of the point, roughly 3 miles. Another branch of the Sacred Cove Trail departs the road a bit farther west and leads you down to the shore in the beautiful cove. Slightly farther west, the Smugglers Trail brings you out to Portuguese Point and to the Olmsted Trail into Abalone Cove. If the 1,200-foot climb back to Del Cerro Park looks daunting, you can hail a ride-sharing service back up instead.

---

trip 2.2   Malaga Cove to Bluff Cove

Distance	1.9 miles (loop)
Hiking Time	1.5 hours
Elevation Gain	200'
Difficulty	Moderate
Trail Use	Good for kids
Best Times	Year-round (low tide recommended)
Agency	City of Palos Verdes Estates
Optional Map	USGS 7.5' *Redondo Beach*

see map opposite

DIRECTIONS From the 110 Freeway, exit west on the Pacific Coast Highway (Highway 1). In 0.6 mile turn left on Normandie. Then, in 0.5 mile, veer right onto Palos Verdes Drive North. Follow this scenic winding road for 6.7 miles; then keep left onto Palos Verdes Drive West. In 0.2 mile turn right onto Via Almar. In 0.6 mile turn right again onto Via Arroyo and, in 0.1 mile, turn right yet again onto Paseo del Mar, where you will find a large parking area in front of Malaga Cove Intermediate School.

If dancing across wave-rounded boulders is your cup of tea, you'll enjoy this moderately difficult rock-hop in the Palos Verdes Estates Shoreline Preserve, along the northernmost edge of the Palos Verdes Peninsula. With near-vertical cliffs on one side and foamy surf on the other, you'll truly feel that you're treading the edge of the continent. Shoes or boots with good ankle support are recommended to deal with the uneven terrain.

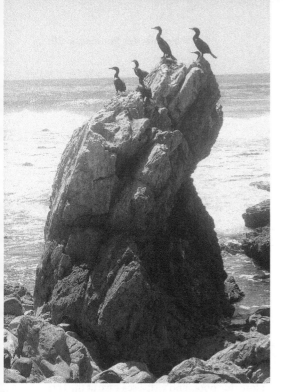

Walk to the east end of the parking lot, where you'll find a trail just beyond a gazebo overlooking the Pacific. Follow the trail down to Malaga Cove. This hike leads left (southwest) along the rocks beneath the sea cliffs. If the tide looks too high or the surf is excessive, consider diverting right instead and taking a stroll along Torrance Beach.

Otherwise, pick a path over the sedimentary rocks. Surfers flock to the cove to test their skills on the waves. Look carefully for small sea anemones, snails, and hermit crabs in the tide pools. In 0.3 mile watch (and sniff) for a natural mineral spring emerging from rocks near the ocean's edge. Continuing along the rocks, watch for rusted metal debris from an unknown wreck.

After a slow mile you arrive at Flat Rock Point, another popular area for tide pooling when the tide is low. Wide, curving Bluff Cove lies just ahead. Your goal is to reach Paseo del Mar above. An

Cormorants claim this rock along the Palos Verdes coastline.

extremely steep and potentially hazardous trail leads straight up from Flat Rock Point. A safer choice is to continue along the cove to find a graded path on the left. In either event, once you reach Paseo del Mar, turn left and walk half a mile back to your vehicle, enjoying the elaborately landscaped mansions along the way.

trip 2.3 Bluff Cove to Point Vicente

see map on p. 28

Distance	6 miles (one-way)
Hiking Time	4 hours
Elevation Gain	200'
Difficulty	Strenuous
Best Times	Year-round (low tide recommended)
Agencies	Cities of Palos Verdes Estates and Rancho Palos Verdes
Optional Map	USGS 7.5' *Redondo Beach*

DIRECTIONS This trip requires a car or bike shuttle or ride-sharing service. If you plan a shuttle, leave your getaway vehicle at Pelican Cove Park on Palos Verdes Drive South, 0.8 mile south of Hawthorne Boulevard (accessible only from the eastbound lane).

To reach the northern trailhead, go east on Palos Verdes Drive until you can make a U-turn; then drive west and north on Palos Verdes Drive for 5.8 miles. Turn left onto Via del Puente, then immediately left again onto Via Almar. In 0.4 mile turn right on Via Arroyo, then left onto Paseo Del Mar. Continue 0.7 mile to park on the street by the Flat Rock Point Trail, a dirt road/trail descending to Bluff Cove.

This long trek down Palos Verdes' wild west side visits crescent-shaped Lunada Bay, plus a half-dozen mini-coves, and traverses the wave-torn base of the sea cliffs below Point Vicente. Time your hike so that low tide occurs when you're below the lighthouse at

Point Vicente, which is one of the tighter spots along the coastline. If you're out during the late morning or noon hour on a sunny day, you may want to reverse the route from that described here in order to avoid facing the sun the whole way. Shoes or boots with good ankle support are recommended to deal with the uneven terrain, but do realize that exposure to salt water may shorten their life. The loose rocks demand constant concentration, making the hike substantially more demanding than the distance might suggest.

On the Flat Rock Point Trail, you descend quickly to Bluff Cove. Onward to Lunada Bay, the going is easy—as long as you stay close to the base of the cliffs. Often there are occasions where you can walk out farther to tide pools that are well exposed during tides of –1 foot or lower. These moderately rich pools contain green anemones, crabs, and sometimes purple sea urchins—but probably not too many of the more interesting creatures such as sea stars.

At around 2 miles, short of Palos Verdes Point (aka Rocky Point) you'll come upon the dismembered remains of the Greek freighter *Dominator,* which ran aground in 1961. Rusting pieces of the ship now litter a stretch of coastline nearly a half mile long.

Once around the point, the beautiful, semicircular Lunada Bay lies before you. The beige-tinted sedimentary cliffs encircling the bay are of Monterey shale, a thinly bedded and easily eroded formation that composes about 90% of the exposed rock on the Palos Verdes Peninsula. The formation consists of former seafloor rich in diatoms, the skeletons of microscopic single-celled plants that float about in the ocean. A steep trail leads up the cliff at Lunada Bay to connect with Paseo del Mar. The first two of the half dozen indentations pocking the coastline beyond Lunada Bay also have steep paths going up to Paseo del Mar. Keep this in mind if you want to bail out and avoid the more rugged and rocky shoreline ahead.

Rock-hopping becomes de rigueur in the last mile before Point Vicente. Some hand and foot work will get you over the piles of broken rocks just below the whale-watching overlook and lighthouse. A short way ahead, you'll come to a steep path slanting up the cliff to the Point Vicente Fishing Access parking lot at the end of the traverse. The point was named by Captain George Vancouver in 1790 for Friar Vicente of Mission Buenaventura and the spelling was changed by the Pacific Geographical Society in 1933.

Before or after your hike, consider visiting nearby Point Vicente Lighthouse. Open daily, the park features an interpretive center, which includes a nice relief map of the peninsula and offers great views of the winter-migrating gray whales from the brink of the sea cliffs.

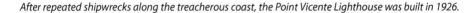

After repeated shipwrecks along the treacherous coast, the Point Vicente Lighthouse was built in 1926.

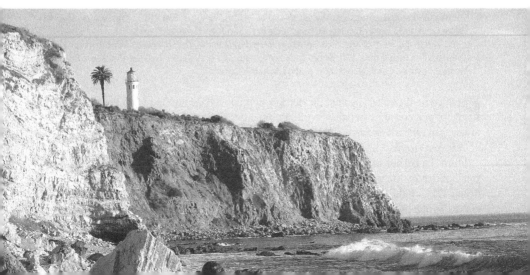

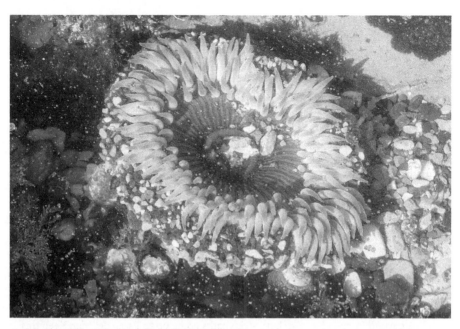

Sea anemone in a Palos Verdes tide pool (see Trip 2.3)

trip 2.4   **White Point to Cabrillo Beach**

see map on p. 28

Distance	3.4 miles (one-way)
Hiking Time	2 hours
Elevation Gain	200'
Difficulty	Moderate
Trail Use	Good for kids
Best Times	Year-round (low tide recommended)
Agency	Los Angeles County Department of Beaches & Harbors
Optional Map	USGS 7.5' *San Pedro*

DIRECTIONS This trip requires a 3-mile car shuttle or ride share. Place a vehicle at the end of the trip at Cabrillo Marine Aquarium. Near the south end of Pacific Avenue in San Pedro, turn east on Stephen White Drive, then right on Oliver Vickery Circle Way, and then right again on Shoshonean Road.

To reach the start of the hike by White Point/Royal Palms Beach, drive back north on Pacific Avenue; then turn left on 19th Street. In 1.3 miles turn left on Western Avenue. Proceed 0.8 mile on Western to its end at Paseo del Mar, and park on the street.

Pressed hard and fast against the densely populated community of San Pedro, the rocky ribbon of coastline between White Point and Cabrillo Beach looks out over a 20-mile, watery gap separating Santa Catalina Island from the mainland. On clear winter days, the island seems to float like a dusky shadow over the sparkling surf.

From the corner of Western and Paseo del Mar, follow a clifftop path southeast. Soon you'll arrive at the entry kiosk on the road leading down to White Point/Royal Palms Beach. (You could also park on Paseo del Mar near the kiosk or pay a fee and drive down to park by the beach.) Walk down the road to the beach. At low tide, you'll find tide pools full of sea anemones and crabs.

Cabrillo Beach commemorates Juan Rodríguez Cabrillo, who in 1542–43 became the first European to explore the coastline of present-day California. Point Fermin was named in 1793 by Captain George Vancouver in honor of Father Fermín Francisco de Lasuén, who founded nine Spanish missions in California.

Walk east past White Point, making your way over tilted slabs of sedimentary rock and small boulders. Here and on the bluffs above lie the skimpy remains of early-20th-century resorts and spas that capitulated to the 1933 Long Beach earthquake and decades of pounding surf. The checkered history of this stretch of coastline is interpreted in a display at the Cabrillo Marine Aquarium, which lies at the end of this hike.

At about 1.5 miles, before the shoreline terrace you're following narrows to practically nothing at Point Fermin, you'll reach metal steps going up the bluff. This is your safe ticket to getting past Point Fermin. (If the tide is extremely low and the surf is relatively calm—conditions that are most likely to occur on only a few afternoons during the fall—expert scramblers can try to edge around the point itself and reach the sand of Cabrillo Beach beyond.) Point Fermin's cliff faces, though not the highest on the peninsula, present the wildest scene in the area. When I (Jerry) scooted over them during a tide of –1 foot, dozens of sleek black cormorants perched on tiny niches above observed my every move.

At the top of the metal stairs, a path leads to the west end of Point Fermin Park, a grassy strip popular among joggers and strollers. Keep heading east along the edge of the cliffs, passing the antique Point Fermin Lighthouse, built in 1874 with materials shipped around Cape Horn. Farther east, the 1929 Sunken City landslide blocks your way. The mysterious-sounding area has been gated and closed to the public since 1987 because at least 18 deaths have occurred at the unstable cliffs.

Turn inland one block to reach Shepard Street; then follow it east to Pacific Avenue, and continue straight ahead on Bluff Place down to Cabrillo Beach. Here you can enjoy the only true beach for miles in either direction and pay a visit to the aquarium, which features some excellent marine and historical exhibits. If you want to stretch your legs further, try walking out to sea atop the San Pedro breakwater, one of several artificial barriers protecting the Los Angeles–Long Beach harbor complex from ocean swells.

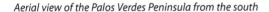

Aerial view of the Palos Verdes Peninsula from the south

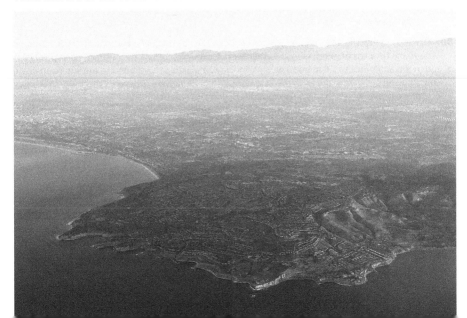

chapter 3

Thousand Oaks & Moorpark

Interior Ventura County is dominated by long, parallel ridges associated with the Transverse Ranges. Shallow, often wide valleys lie between those ridges. Housing developments have spread far and wide over some of the valleys and hillsides here, but much open land remains.

Historical uses such as agriculture, cattle grazing, and oil production are fading in Ventura County, whereas habitat preservation and recreational opportunities are in greater demand. That is why key parcels of this spacious landscape are bit by bit being transferred into public ownership. One goal is to create a Rim of the Valley natural area—a connected patchwork of open spaces stretching around the San Fernando Valley from Ventura County to Glendale.

While the parks described in this chapter are not within Los Angeles County itself, they are located nearby and are easily accessible to San Fernando Valley residents—hence their inclusion here.

trip 3.1   Happy Camp Canyon

Distance	10.5 miles (loop)
Hiking Time	5 hours
Elevation Gain	1,500'
Difficulty	Moderately strenuous
Trail Use	Suitable for mountain biking
Best Times	October–June
Agencies	Mountains Recreation & Conservation Authority, Santa Monica Mountains Conservancy
Optional Map	USGS 7.5' *Simi*

DIRECTIONS Follow the 118 Freeway west from Simi Valley or the 23 Freeway north from Thousand Oaks to the New Los Angeles Avenue exit. Go west 1 mile to Moorpark Avenue (signed Highway 23), turn right, and proceed 2.6 miles to where Highway 23 makes a sharp bend to the left. Keep going straight here, but then make an immediate right turn on Broadway. Proceed a short way to the east end of Broadway, where there's a spacious dirt parking lot and trailhead.

Happy Camp Canyon nuzzles in a crease between the long, rounded ridge called Big Mountain, just north of Simi Valley, and Oak Ridge, a taller parallel ridge to the north. These ridges and plenty more, like the Santa Monica Mountains, are caterpillar-like parallel segments of the Transverse Ranges, which stretch from Santa Barbara County in the west to San Bernardino County to the east.

Oil-bearing shales predominate in this region, evidenced by various oil wells and dirt roads built to access them scattered across the surrounding hillsides. On your ramble through the lower and middle parts of the canyon, keep an eye out for bright red stones, sometimes exhibiting a glassy texture, some right under you feet and others visible in outcrops. These rocks were formed by the slow combustion of organic material trapped in layers of shale.

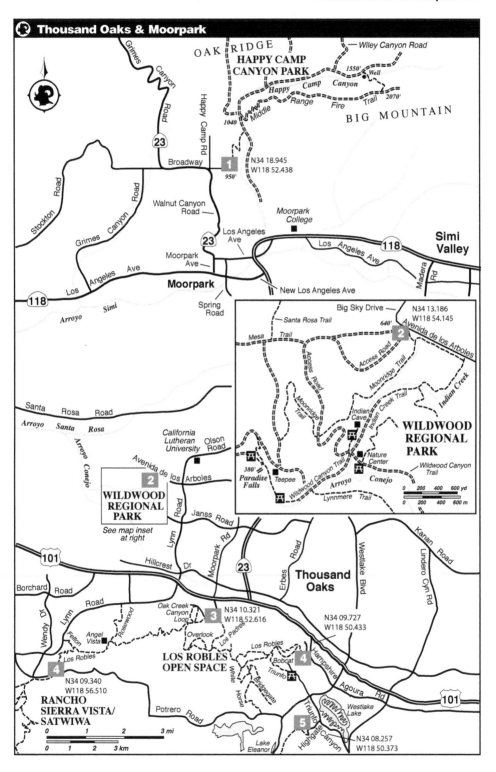

Thousand Oaks & Moorpark

Happy Camp Canyon itself remains quite pristine. Several groups of Chumash Indians called this place home in past centuries; later it became a part of an immense cattle ranch founded by a pioneer Simi Valley family. Purchased as a future state park in the late 1960s, it was later traded to Ventura County for use as a regional park. Today, save for a few dirt roads and a smattering of artifacts from the days of cattle ranching, the 3,000-acre canyon park serves as prime natural habitat for native plants and animals, and a restful retreat for hikers seeking to escape from the sights and sounds of city and suburban life.

From the trailhead, follow the path heading north and east along gentle, grassy slopes down onto the wide floor of Happy Camp Canyon. As you look down on a golf course at the canyon's mouth, note the terraced aspect of the landscape on both sides. These are fluvial (streamside) terraces—sedimentary deposits from earlier flows of Happy Camp Canyon's creek.

Pass two minor side trails on the left (leading up to a maze of equestrian trails on the hill) and then another two on the right. At 1.0 mile you join the dirt Happy Camp Canyon Fire Road in the bottom of the canyon. Turn left and 0.2 mile later you pass through a gate marking the start of the "wilderness" section of Happy Camp Canyon Park. At a fork just beyond, stay left (north) into the main canyon.

By 2.0 miles the canyon floor has become narrow, you've turned decidedly east, and you are strolling through beautiful coast live-oak woods (plus native sycamore and walnut trees), which continue intermittently up the canyon in the next 3 miles. A little stream flows in the bottom of the canyon during, and for some weeks or months after, the winter rains. You're climbing at a gentle rate of about 200 feet of elevation gain per mile. You pass the ascending Wiley Canyon Road on the left at 4.1 miles, and at 4.7 miles you reach the site of an old well and pump. Large oak trees shade a cluster of picnic tables for a convenient lunch stop. Continue following the graded dirt road about 300 yards past the well. The road ends, but a bulldozed track, eroded and very steep at first, curls 0.7 mile up the south slope of Happy Camp Canyon then joins Middle Range Fire Trail on the crest of Big Mountain. If you are coming in the other direction, the easy-to-miss junction is marked by a cairn on a saddle. Use that ridge-running fire trail to return to lower Happy Camp Canyon at a point just above the gate marking the wilderness-area boundary.

trip 3.2   Paradise Falls

Distance	2.7 miles (loop)
Hiking Time	2 hours
Elevation Gain	500'
Difficulty	Moderate
Trail Use	Dogs allowed, good for kids
Best Times	Year-round
Agency	Conejo Recreation & Park District
Optional Map	USGS 7.5' *Newbury Park*

see map on p. 35

DIRECTIONS From Highway 101 at Exit 45 in Thousand Oaks, take Lynn Road north 2.5 miles to Avenida de los Arboles. Turn left and follow Avenida de los Arboles 1 mile west. At this point traffic goes sharply right on Big Sky Drive—you make a U-turn and park on the right at Wildwood Park's principal trailhead, open 8 a.m.–5 p.m.

Wildwood Park in Thousand Oaks is Ventura County's most scenic suburban park. The scenery here has been imprinted in the minds of many in the over-60 age group: the area was once an outdoor set for Hollywood movies as well TV's *Gunsmoke*, *The Rifleman*, and *Wagon Train*. The short but steep hike—down and then up—described here takes you to Wildwood Park's scenic gem: the Arroyo Conejo gorge and Paradise Falls. The lovingly maintained park offers drinking fountains, picnic tables, interpretive signs, and shady rest spots along this fine loop.

Three trails radiate from the Avenida de los Arboles trailhead. Two of them are wide, relatively bland dirt roads. The third trail—the one that you want, the narrow and scenic Moonridge Trail—descends sharply from the east side of the parking area (that is, the left side of the parking area as you drove into Wildwood Park). Immediately after you start on the trail, come to a T-intersection amid oak woods. Turn right, remaining on the Moonridge Trail.

The trail descends a sunny slope covered with aromatic sage-scrub vegetation. Beware of the prickly pear cactus flanking the trail. There's a brief passage across a shady ravine using wooden steps and a plank bridge. At 0.5 mile you cross over a dirt road and continue on the narrow Moonridge Trail.

Ahead, the trail curls around a deep ravine, edging into the crumbly sedimentary rock. At 0.9 mile you join another dirt road and use it to descend toward a large wooden tepee structure on a knoll just below. Make a right at the tepee, descending farther into the Arroyo Conejo gorge. As you descend, watch for the narrow side trail on the left that will take you straight down to Paradise Falls—a beautiful, 30-foot-high cascade that makes its presence known by sound before sight. Keep an eye out for poison oak, especially on the far side of the creek.

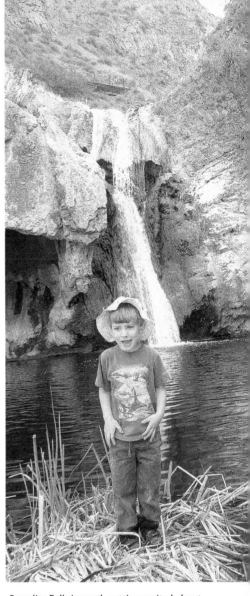

Paradise Falls is worth getting excited about.

After you've admired the falls, continue by climbing back up the slope in the direction you came and taking the fenced, cliff-hanging trail around the left (east) side of the falls. Beyond that fenced stretch, the narrow trail descends a little and sidles up alongside the creek, where large coast live oaks spread their shade.

Soon you'll find yourself continuing on a path of dirt-road width. Stay with that path until you reach a major crossroads. It's worth a 0.1 mile detour straight ahead to the walk-through Indian Cave. Then, returning to the junction, cross the bridge. The small Wildwood Nature Center is just around the bend to the right, and your return route up along Indian Canyon is to the left.

On the Indian Creek Trail, you pay your debt to gravity by ascending nearly 300 feet in about 0.7 mile. The beautifully tangled array of live oak and sycamore limbs along this trail keeps your mind off the climb. At one point, you can look down into a deep ravine where an inaccessible mini-waterfall and pool lie practically hidden. When you finally reach Avenida de los Arboles, turn left and return a short distance to the trailhead parking lot.

VARIATION

An extensive network of trails radiates in all directions from Wildwood Park. Regular visitors will want to download the *Wildwood Park Trail Map* to aid exploration: tinyurl.com /wildwoodtrailmap.

---

trip 3.3 Los Padres Loop

Distance	4.1 miles (loop)
Hiking Time	2 hours
Elevation Gain	700'
Difficulty	Moderate
Trail Use	Suitable for mountain biking, dogs allowed, good for kids
Best Times	Year-round
Agency	Conejo Open Space Conservation Agency
Recommended Map	*Los Robles Trail Map* (free online from Conejo Open Space Conservation Agency) or Trails Illustrated *Santa Monica Mountains National Recreation Area (253)*

see map on p. 35

DIRECTIONS From Highway 101 at Exit 44 in Thousand Oaks, take Moorpark Road south. In 0.3 mile turn left on Los Padres Drive. Proceed 0.1 mile to the signed trailhead on the right and park on the road.

The Scenic Loop Trail along the Los Padres Trail visits oaks, grassland, and chaparral.

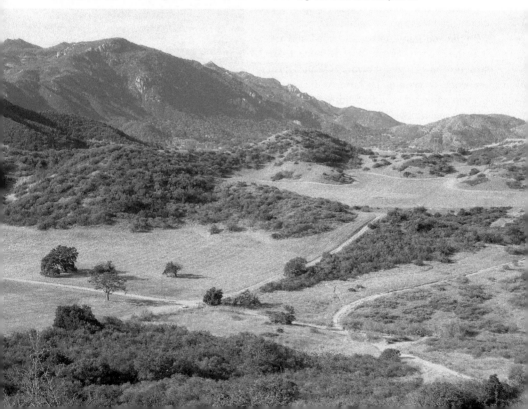

The hills in the Conejo Open Space are laced with an intricate network of trails. This appealing loop is just the right length for a moderate workout and thus draws throngs of hikers, dog walkers, and mountain bikers.

Pass through a gate at the trailhead and follow the Los Padres Trail through a beautiful glen of coast live oaks. In 0.5 mile turn right onto a fire road. In another 0.5 mile reach a junction with the Los Robles Trail near a gated ranch.

To take in a good view, turn left and walk 0.2 mile east on the Los Robles Trail. Turn left onto a decomposing paved road and follow it 0.1 mile to Hill 1450. Then return to the Los Robles Trail.

Continue west on Los Robles for 0.1 mile to a junction with the Scenic Loop Trail on the right. This trail rejoins Los Robles in 0.5 mile. You could take either one, but the Scenic Loop follows a low ridge with views and hence is, you guessed it, more scenic.

When the two trails rejoin, descend southwest through tall chaparral to a picnic bench; then turn north and continue to a junction of fire roads in 1.0 mile. Stay right and go 0.4 mile to the Los Robles Trailhead at the end of Moorpark Road. Then follow Moorpark 0.3 mile back to Los Padres Drive where you began the trip.

trip 3.4 Los Robles Trail

Distance	11 miles (one-way)
Hiking Time	5 hours
Elevation Gain	2,000'
Difficulty	Strenuous
Trail Use	Dogs allowed
Best Times	Year-round
Agency	Conejo Open Space Conservation Agency
Recommended Map	Los Robles Trail Map (free online from Conejo Open Space Conservation Agency) or Trails Illustrated Santa Monica Mountains National Recreation Area (253)

see map on p. 35

DIRECTIONS This one-way trip involves a 9-mile shuttle. If you aren't returning using a ride-sharing service, leave one vehicle at the west end (Potrero Road) trailhead in Newbury Park. From the 101 Freeway, take Exit 45 for Lynn Road. Follow Lynn southwest for 3.9 miles; then turn left on to Wendy Drive. In 0.6 mile turn left onto Potrero Road. Proceed 0.5 mile to the trailhead parking on the left.

To reach the east end, return to the 101 and go east; then take Exit 41 for southbound Hampshire Road. In 0.3 mile turn right on Foothill Drive. In 0.1 mile park on the street where Foothill turns sharply right.

Since 1977, the City of Thousand Oaks and the Conejo Recreation and Park District have done an admirable job acquiring and protecting open space overlooking town. The crowning accomplishment of this effort is the Los Robles Trail, running the skyline from Westlake Village to Newbury Park by way of a series of nature preserves. Many spur trails connect to neighborhoods so you can visit this trail in segments (see Trip 3.3 for one of the best), or you can go the whole distance for a strenuous workout. The western terminus of the trail is on Potrero Road. Three branches exist on the east end; this trip begins on the Foothill Drive trailhead to make the longest continuous path.

The trail is a portion of the Juan Bautista de Anza National Historic Trail. In 1775–76, de Anza led 240 Spanish settlers and 1,000 head of stock 1,200 miles from the Tubac Presidio in New Spain (now Mexico) to a new settlement at the San Francisco Bay. His route through the Conejo Valley more closely tracks the 101 Freeway, but the historic trail takes the more scenic ridgeline route.

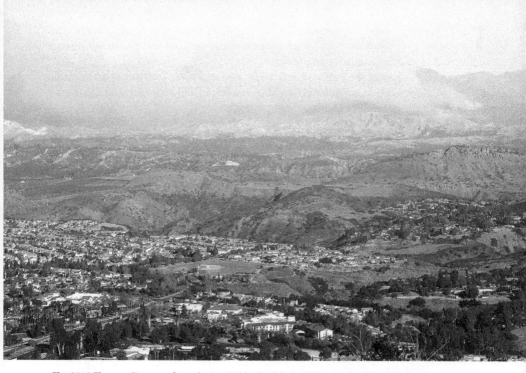
The 2017 Thomas Fire, seen from the Los Robles Trail, burned the parched Ventura County mountains.

Follow the unsigned Los Robles Trail from Foothill Road that climbs 0.1 mile to a T-junction with a fire road. Turn right. At a bend in 0.3 mile, meet gated Fairview Avenue on the right and the narrow Bobcat Trail on the left. Stay on the fire road or take the Bobcat Trail, which is slightly longer but has better views. Both rejoin at a saddle in 0.6 mile.

Continuing west for 0.3 mile and watching for various narrow social trails that have developed, pass a trail on the left descending the canyon to Triunfo Community Park. In another 1.2 miles, pass the White Horse Canyon Trail on the left that descends to the Fox-field Stables on Potrero Road (no hiker parking). Our Los Robles Trail continues west for 0.9 mile, passing spurs up two hills, to meet the Los Padres Trail on the right.

In 0.1 mile reach a junction with the Scenic Loop Trail on the right. Take either path; the Scenic Loop climbs to the ridge and has better views over Thousand Oaks but is slightly longer, rejoining Los Robles in 0.4 mile.

The next narrow stretch of trail is particularly scenic, curving down into a canyon. In 1.0 mile turn left at a junction. In another 0.1 mile, the Spring Canyon Trail stays right, while Los Robles narrows and makes another scenic climb. Pass a spur to a vista point in 1.6 miles. Cross a private road in 0.9 mile. In another 0.5 mile, the Rosewood Trail veers right. It's worth making a 0.2-mile detour here to Angel Vista, the best viewpoint along the trail.

Our path now descends and squeezes through an easement in a neighborhood of mansions. In 1.2 miles pass a spur on the right leading to the Felton Street trailhead. In 1.1 miles cross a paved road. In 0.1 mile the Los Robles Trail ends at a large lot on Potrero Road.

VARIATION

For an even longer hike, a trail crosses Potrero Road and leads on to Rancho Sierra Vista and Point Mugu State Park.

trip 3.5   Lake Eleanor Open Space

Distance	2.6 miles (out-and-back)
Hiking Time	1.5 hours
Elevation Gain	600'
Difficulty	Easy
Trail Use	Dogs allowed, good for kids
Best Times	Year-round
Agency	Conejo Open Space Conservation Agency
Optional Map	USGS 7.5' *Thousand Oaks*

see map on p. 35

DIRECTIONS From the 101 Freeway, take Exit 40 for southbound Westlake Boulevard. In 1 mile turn left onto Triunfo Canyon Road. In 0.6 mile turn right onto Highgate Road. Proceed 0.5 mile and park on the street at the end near 2123 Highgate Road.

The 529-acre Lake Eleanor Open Space is named for a small reservoir dammed in 1889. The lake and surrounding ridges were acquired in 1986 by the Conejo Open Space Conservation Agency, and a scenic trail runs along the ridge west of the lake. Spring wildflowers can be gorgeous here. (Note that the lake itself is closed to public use.)

Walk past the gate up the paved (but closed) road, and within 50 yards look for an unmarked trail departing on the right side. Stay on the main trail as you pass spurs descending to other neighborhoods. The trail climbs to a high point with views of the Las Virgenes Reservoir and Westlake Lake, then veers left. As you continue southwest along the ridgeline, you'll encounter three forks. At each, you can go left to bypass a hill, or right to climb over the top. The first hill is definitely worth climbing for its excellent views down to Lake Eleanor in a gorge below the volcanic cliffs of Lake Eleanor Sentinel. The trail ends abruptly at Denver Springs Drive. Although you could walk back on streets, it is faster and more scenic to return the way you came.

Lake Eleanor is a nesting site for hawks and great blue herons.

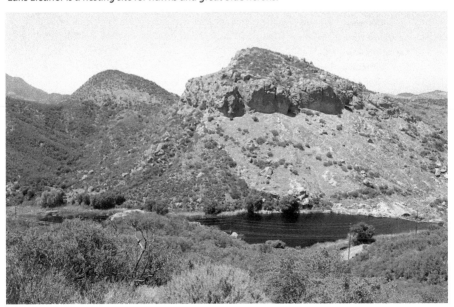

chapter 4

Simi Hills

U p until the 1970s the pastoral grazing lands of the Simi Hills were remote from the city. Today, spillover growth along the Ventura Freeway from the San Fernando Valley to Thousand Oaks has made substantial inroads. On the brighter side, more than 16,000 acres have been acquired and protected by the National Park Service and other agencies, from the Victory Trailhead in West Hills all the way to Thousand Oaks. This has assured protection for most of the area's valley-oak savanna habitat, established a permanently protected link in the north–south wildlife migration corridor, and created a recreational resource for millions of people who live in the greater Los Angeles area.

In 2003, a big parcel of land on the west rim of the San Fernando Valley—the Ahmanson Ranch—was purchased with the help of state bond money and additional grants. The acquisition of this parcel, now titled the Upper Las Virgenes Canyon Open Space Preserve, ensures that an uninterrupted block of natural landscape can remain in between the San Fernando Valley and the city of Thousand Oaks.

The 2018 Woolsey Fire started near the Santa Susana Field Laboratory and, driven by intense Santa Ana winds, burned across most of the Simi Hills and much of the Santa Monica Mountains. The grasslands and oak woodlands of the Simi Hills have endured many fires in the past and will eventually recover.

trip 4.1 Sage Ranch

see map opposite

Distance	2.1 miles (loop)
Hiking Time	1 hour
Elevation Gain	400'
Difficulty	Easy
Trail Use	Suitable for mountain biking, dogs allowed, good for kids
Best Times	October–June
Agencies	Mountains Recreation & Conservation Authority, Santa Monica Mountains Conservancy
Optional Map	Tom Harrison *Cheeseboro–Palo Comado Canyons*
Fees/Permits	$5 parking fee

DIRECTIONS From the 101 Freeway in Calabasas, take Exit 29 for northbound Valley Circle Boulevard. In 5.7 miles turn left onto Woolsey Canyon Road. Follow it 2.5 miles to a T-junction by the entrance to the Santa Susana Field Laboratory. Turn right, go 0.2 mile, and then turn left into Sage Ranch. Continue 0.2 mile up the paved road to a parking area.

T he 635-acre Sage Ranch owes its name not to the predominant sage-scrub vegetation growing there, but rather to the former owner of the ranch, one Orrin Sage Sr., who

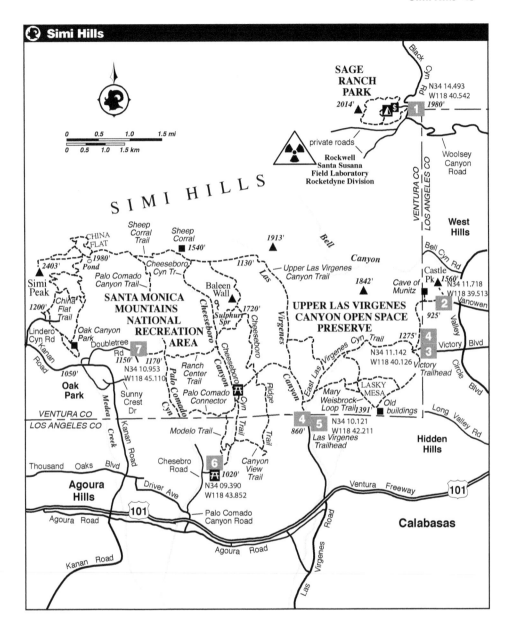

SAGE
RANCH
PARK
2014'

N34 14.493
W118 40.542
1980' 1

private roads

Rockwell
Santa Susana
Field Laboratory
Rocketdyne Division

Woolsey
Canyon
Road

West
Hills

S I M I   H I L L S

Sheep
Corral
Trail

Sheep
Corral

CHINA
FLAT
1980'
Pond

1540'

1913'

Bell

Canyon

Castle
Pk *1560'*
N34 11.718
W118 39.513
Yanowen

2403'

1130'

Upper Las Virgenes
Canyon Trail

Las

Cheeseboro
Cyn Tr

1842'

Cave of
Munitz

Palo Comado
Canyon Trail

Baleen
Wall

2

Simi
Peak

1200'

China
Flat

1720'

Cheeseboro

UPPER LAS VIRGENES
CANYON OPEN SPACE
PRESERVE

925'

SANTA MONICA
MOUNTAINS
NATIONAL
RECREATION
AREA

Sulphur
Spr

Las Virgenes

East Las Virgenes Cyn Trail

1275'

4

N34 11.142
W118 40.126

Victory

Blvd

Trail

Lindero
Cyn Rd

Oak Canyon
Park

Victory
Trailhead

3

Doubletree
Rd

7

1150' *1170'*

N34 10.953
W118 45.110

Ranch
Center
Trail

Cheeseboro Canyon

Cheeseboro Cyn Trail

LASKY
MESA

Circle

Blvd

Kanan Road

1050'

Oak
Park

Sunny
Crest
Dr

Palo Comado Connector

Ridge Trail

Mary
Weisbrock
Loop Trail

1391'

Old
buildings

Long Valley Rd

VENTURA CO
LOS ANGELES CO

Medea Creek

Palo Comado Cyn

Modelo Trail

Canyon Trail

4 5

860'

N34 10.121
W118 42.211

Las Virgenes
Trailhead

Hidden
Hills

Thousand   Oaks   Blvd

Agoura
Hills

Kanan Road

Chesebro
Road

6

1020'

N34 09.390
W118 43.852

Canyon
View
Trail

Ventura   Freeway

101

101

Driver Ave

Agoura   Road

Palo Comado
Canyon Road

Calabasas

Kanan   Road

Agoura   Road

Las Virgenes

Virgenes Road

grazed cattle here for a time and planted orange and avocado orchards on a portion of the
property in 1981. Previous to Sage's ranching, dozens of Hollywood westerns were filmed
here. Purchased by the state in 1990, this pocket-size patch of publicly owned open space
has become a model park for recreational activities such as hiking, bird-watching, and
nature study, as well as a critical wildlife corridor. A 10-site campground within the park is
available by reservation to organized groups only.

Tilted sandstone outcrops and boulders punctuate the landscape hereabouts, the result of uplift of Cretaceous marine sedimentary rock. This rock originated from layers of sandy muck deposited near the ocean shore some 70 million years ago. Framed by these sometimes dramatic outcrops, the hiker's view on a clear day extends broadly toward Simi Valley and the Santa Susana Mountains in the north, San Fernando Valley in the east, and the Santa Monica Mountains in the south. You can see Sage Ranch at its very best in early spring, a time when wildflower fragrances, mixed with the scent of orange blossoms, suffuse the air.

The closer-at-hand view to the south and west includes some worn-out-looking former Rocketdyne Santa Susana Field Laboratory aerospace test facilities. The facility was the site of 30,000 rocket engine tests that spilled toxic rocket fuel into the ground. In 1959, an experimental nuclear reactor partially melted down and released radioactive gas over Southern California, but the disaster was kept secret until 1989. To this day, children in the area experience elevated cancer rates. Boeing now owns most of the Rocketdyne facility and continues to resist completing the incredibly expensive cleanup. Parts of the field lab burned in the 2018 Woolsey Fire, but Sage Ranch narrowly escaped. Although Sage Ranch is operated as a park open to the public, you should use your own judgment about whether you feel comfortable this close to a toxic- and nuclear-waste site.

The single loop trail (with minor spurs) going around the property follows graded and ungraded roads, passing near dramatic rock formations known as Turtle Rock and Sandstone Ridge, and skirting a maintained grove of orange trees. Start counterclockwise by walking north from the parking lot through a gate. At the time of this writing, part of the loop trail is closed for cleanup of an old shooting range, and you'll be detoured onto a gorgeous path through the center of the park that emerges at the campground.

Explore the oaks and tilted sandstone outcrops in Sage Ranch.

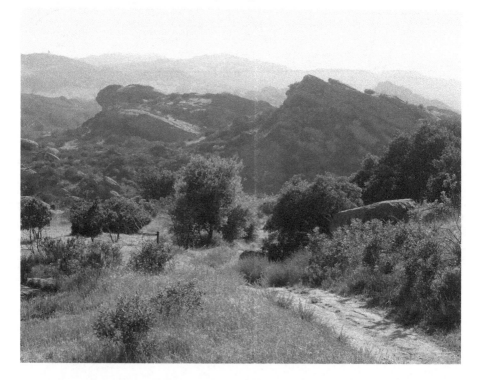

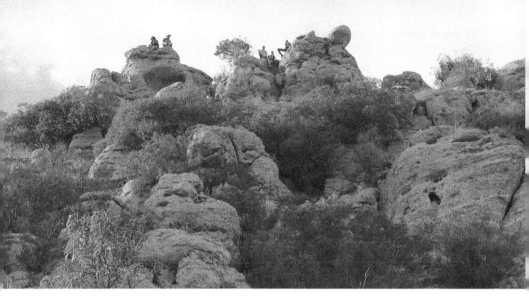

Scramble up the rocks to enjoy great views on Castle Peak.

see map on p. 43

trip 4.2 Castle Peak

Distance	1.2 miles (out-and-back)
Hiking Time	1 hour
Elevation Gain	650'
Difficulty	Moderate
Trail Use	Dogs allowed
Best Times	Year-round
Agency	Los Angeles Department of Recreation and Parks
Optional Map	Tom Harrison *Cheeseboro–Palo Comado Canyons*

DIRECTIONS From the 101 Freeway, take Exit 29 for northbound Valley Circle Boulevard. In 2.9 miles turn left on Vanowen Street. Go 0.1 mile and park along the street at El Escorpión Park.

Topped by craggy blocks of white conglomerate rock, Castle Peak (1,699') affords what is probably the most expansive view of the San Fernando Valley's west side. From the top, a sea of ground-hugging subdivisions is seen lapping at the foot of the mountain and stretching toward a vaporous horizon. In the middle distance, a bevy of skyscrapers at Warner Center rises up starkly, symbolizing the valley's evolution toward a presumably more vertical type of metropolitan environment in the future. Castle Peak burned in the 2018 Woolsey Fire, but the trailhead remains open.

To the Chumash Indians living in the Simi Hills centuries ago, Castle Peak was known as Huan, a gigantic monument used to keep track of repetitive celestial and earthly cycles. Every year during the winter solstice, Huan's pointed afternoon shadow swept across a Chumash village located near the mouth of Bell Canyon. Even today, there's a sense of timeless drama on Huan's summit as you watch (on a crystal-clear December or January afternoon especially) the shadows of the Simi Hills stretch across the urban plain.

Although Castle Peak's summit can be reached from all sides, the shortest and most direct route is from El Escorpión Park just below the southeast slope. Follow an old dirt road going west into a broad, valley-oak-dotted canyon. Soon you will spot, on the right, a steeply inclined path heading straight up toward Castle Peak's craggy summit. Some scrambling gets you to the highest outcrop.

Hawks and ravens patrol the air spaces above (and often below) you as you survey the landscape. If you wish, you can follow the trailless ridgeline east to Peak 1639 for a better view of the rolling Simi Hills to the west.

VARIATION

Just up the canyon from Castle Peak is an unusual formation called the Cave of Munits. You can visit the cave by continuing 0.5 mile west up the canyon to a Santa Monica Mountains Conservancy Zone sign, then turning right and following a well-used trail to the cave entrance, which, from a distance, resembles a vertical gash in the rock. Scramble up a ramp into the conglomerate cave; small children will need assistance. The skylit cathedral-like interior was a sacred site for the Chumash. Adventurous scramblers can find a window exit leading to a balcony, from which one could gain the ridgeline and follow it east to Castle Peak. According to legend, the cave is named for a shaman who lived here and who was executed after killing a chief's son.

---

trip 4.3   Lasky Mesa

see map on p. 43

Distance	3.7 miles (loop)
Hiking Time	2 hours
Elevation Gain	500'
Difficulty	Moderate
Trail Use	Suitable for mountain biking, equestrians, dogs allowed, good for kids
Best Times	October–May
Agencies	Mountains Recreation & Conservation Authority, Santa Monica Mountains Conservancy
Optional Map	Tom Harrison *Cheeseboro–Palo Comado Canyons* or Trails Illustrated *Santa Monica Mountains National Recreation Area (253)*
Fees/Permits	$3 parking fee at Victory Trailhead

DIRECTIONS From the 101 Freeway in Calabasas, take Exit 29 for northbound Valley Circle Boulevard. Go 2.1 miles; then turn left on Victory Boulevard, and proceed 0.7 mile to the trailhead at the west end. Park free on the street or for a fee in the lot beyond the gate. The trails are open during daylight hours.

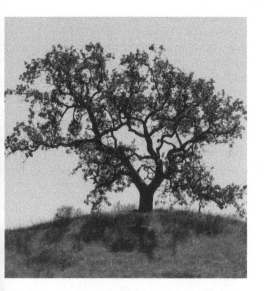

Lasky Mesa, an elevated, treeless plain located in the southeast corner of Upper Las Virgenes Canyon Open Space Preserve, offers sweeping vistas in any direction you care to look. That view is most impressively open on sparkling clear winter days—yet nothing beats being here in early spring in a year of average or better rainfall. That's when the whole area can acquire an almost impossibly vivid emerald-green sheen.

The route described here keeps you entirely on old dirt roads, which today are essentially maintained as wide multiuse trails. This area has a maze of unsigned social trails, so try to

Las Virgenes Canyon Open Space Preserve is renowned for its valley oaks.

stay on the widest and most heavily used paths. From the Victory Trailhead, follow the broad fire road southwest, descending 0.1 mile to a junction where you make a sharp left onto the Joe Behar Trail, briefly reversing your path (your return route lies on the right). You then wind uphill past valley oaks that are clinging to the grassy slopes. Look back at the ostentatious mansions crammed up against the park boundary.

Before long the climb moderates and spacious Lasky Mesa lies ahead. Meadowlarks and redwing blackbirds sing, accompanied by the droning hum of distant traffic on Highway 101, unseen from this vantage point. At 1.2 miles stay left where a segment of the Mary Weisbrock Loop Trail intersects on the right. Behar and Weisbrock were both leaders in the effort to preserve this area from becoming yet another huge subdivision.

At 1.5 miles you swing by some old ranch buildings that were used in the movie and television industries. Starting in 1914, motion picture pioneer Jesse Lasky set his big scenes in the surrounding landscape. Movies such as *Gone with the Wind* and *The Charge of the Light Brigade* were partially filmed here, as was the TV series *Petticoat Junction*. The Ahmanson Land Company made plans in 1986 to build an enormous community atop the mesa, sparking a 17-year land-use fight that ended when the Santa Monica Mountains Conservancy acquired the property for $135 million, the largest public-land acquisition in county history.

Bypass the ranch buildings and swing to the right (north), remaining on the Mary Weisbrock Loop Trail. Continue north, ignoring other old ranch roads. At 1.9 miles keep straight where the north segment of the loop trail comes in from the right.

Now you begin a delightful descent down off the mesa, past fine specimens of coast live oak, and later through willow trees. Turn right at the major junction (2.6 miles) and head east, uphill, on the East Las Virgenes Canyon Trail, which will take you back toward your starting point.

trip 4.4   Victory to Las Virgenes

see map on p. 43

Distance	3.0 miles (one-way)
Hiking Time	1.5 hours
Elevation Gain/Loss	100'/400'
Difficulty	Moderate
Trail Use	Suitable for mountain biking, equestrians, dogs allowed, good for kids
Best Times	Year-round
Agencies	Mountains Recreation & Conservation Authority, Santa Monica Mountains Conservancy
Optional Map	Tom Harrison *Cheeseboro–Palo Comado Canyons* or Trails Illustrated *Santa Monica Mountains National Recreation Area (253)*
Fees/Permits	$3 parking fee at Victory Trailhead

DIRECTIONS This trip requires a 9-mile car shuttle or trip with a ride-sharing service. Leave a getaway vehicle at the Las Virgenes Trailhead: From the 101 Freeway in Calabasas, take Exit 32 for northbound Las Virgenes Road. Go 1.4 miles and park at the end of the road.

To reach the other end at the Victory Trailhead, return to the eastbound 101 Freeway and take Exit 29 for northbound Valley Circle Boulevard. Go 2.1 miles; then turn left on Victory Boulevard and proceed 0.7 mile to the trailhead at the west end. Park for free on the street, or for a fee in the lot beyond the gate. The trails are open during daylight hours.

This one-way traverse across the Upper Las Virgenes Canyon Open Space Preserve—easy for just about anyone when traveled in the east-to-west, downhill direction as suggested here—can be pleasantly accomplished anytime the weather is not excessively hot. You start

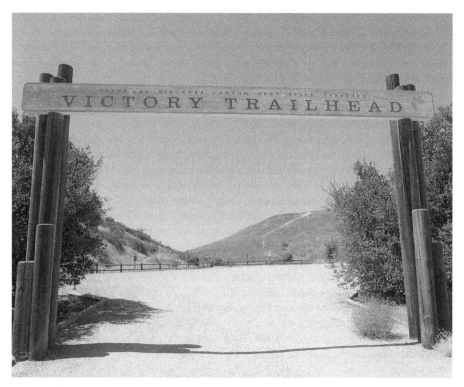

The Victory Trailhead marks the west end of 25-mile Victory Boulevard, a major San Fernando Valley thoroughfare named in honor of soldiers returning from World War I.

in a saddle at the head of the upper east branch of Las Virgenes Canyon (the site of the Victory Trailhead) and finish at the northern terminus of Las Virgenes Road (Las Virgenes Trailhead). For an afternoon hike, consider reversing the direction so as to avoid having sun glare in your eyes the entire way. Las Virgenes is an abbreviation of the 1802 Spanish land grant Nuestra Señora la Reina de las Virgenes ("Our Lady Queen of the Virgins").

From the Victory Trailhead, follow the broad dirt road leading left (southwest). Beware of a maze of social trails in this area; try to stay on the widest and most heavily used path. Descend 0.1 mile to a trail junction and veer right. You're on the East Las Virgenes Canyon Trail, which twists and turns a bit as it swoops into a shallow tributary of Las Virgenes Canyon. You're also on the signed Juan Bautista de Anza National Historical Trail, which rather closely traces the famed overland route of the 1775–76 Spanish expedition. On that expedition, some 30 families traveled from southern Arizona into California. Most settled in the San Francisco Bay Area.

On your gradually descending route, stay on the East Las Virgenes Canyon Trail as other trails intersect on the left and the right. Enjoy the spacious vistas of wide-open grassland, highlighted here and there by valley and live oaks, willows, and sycamores. The scene is most impressive when the sun angle is low, as in early morning or late afternoon.

After traveling for a total of 2.5 miles, you arrive at the "confluence" of Las Virgenes Canyon's east and main branches; some of the oaks here burned in the 2018 Woolsey Fire. Turn left here on the Upper Las Virgenes Canyon Trail, and complete the remaining short distance over to the Las Virgenes Trailhead.

trip 4.5 Upper Las Virgenes Canyon

Distance	5.4 miles (out-and-back)
Hiking Time	2.5 hours
Elevation Gain	300'
Difficulty	Moderate
Trail Use	Suitable for mountain biking, equestrians, dogs allowed, good for kids
Best Times	October–June
Agencies	Mountains Recreation & Conservation Authority, Santa Monica Mountains Conservancy
Optional Map	Tom Harrison *Cheeseboro–Palo Comado Canyons* or Trails Illustrated *Santa Monica Mountains National Recreation Area (253)*

see map on p. 43

DIRECTIONS From the 101 Freeway in Calabasas, take Exit 32 for northbound Las Virgenes Road. Go 1.4 miles and park at the end of the road. The trailhead is open during daylight hours.

Upper Las Virgenes Canyon is one of those places where you can make the sight and sound of a huge metropolitan area simply disappear after a short drive from a major freeway and only a few minutes' walk. The area even seems removed from the flight paths of major aircraft. Portions of the canyon burned in the 2018 Woolsey Fire, but the walk remains worthwhile.

The out-and-back jaunt into the upper canyon is great for kids, too. What creatures might they discover? Cottontail rabbits, for sure. A frog perhaps, or (as we did) a scorpion. If the kids get tired, you can turn back anytime. Expect to encounter two or three foot-wetting and possibly muddy stream crossings in the early part of the hike.

From the trailhead, simply head north on the main trail (an old dirt road), which imperceptibly gains elevation in the canyon's initially wide flood plain. In a couple of places ahead, narrow side trails higher on the canyon slope exist, but they may be too heavily overgrown by vegetation to follow. There are enough oaks, sycamores, and willows around to keep much of the trail decently shaded, even during the middle of the day.

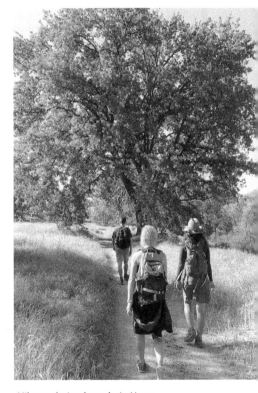

Hikers admire the oaks in Upper Las Virgenes Canyon.

After about 2.5 miles the ascent into the upper canyon quickens, and you go sharply up and sharply down twice. Afterward, you bend right and transit a gallery of overarching coast live oak limbs. The trail then executes a hairpin turn and starts to climb out of the canyon at a point below Peak 1913. You've come 2.7 miles from the start, and this is a good place to turn back—for this casual hike at least. If your goal is to connect to the extensive trail systems lacing through Cheeseboro and Palo Comado Canyons to the west, then by all means press on.

trip 4.6	**Cheeseboro Canyon**

Distance	6.5 miles (loop)
Hiking Time	3 hours
Elevation Gain	850'
Difficulty	Moderate
Trail Use	Dogs allowed
Best Times	November–May
Agency	National Park Service
Optional Map	Tom Harrison *Cheeseboro–Palo Comado Canyons* or Trails Illustrated *Santa Monica Mountains National Recreation Area (253)*

see map on p. 43

DIRECTIONS From the 101 Freeway in Agoura Hills, take Exit 35 for northbound Chesebro Road (spelling is correct). Go 0.1 mile and then turn right onto signed Chesebro Road. Drive 0.7 mile north to Cheeseboro Canyon's entrance and trailhead on the right.

Instantly a hit when it first opened to the public in the late 1980s, Cheeseboro Canyon now draws a host of hikers, mountain bikers, equestrians, and even some wheelchair explorers to its network of old roads and newer trails. Friendly rangers patrol the roads and trails on horseback, eager to tell anyone willing to lend an ear about the park's natural features and wildlife (deer and coyotes especially). This area was singed by the 2018 Woolsey Fire, but the National Park Service reopened it within a month.

For a good overview of the entire area, follow the 6.5-mile route described here, which goes up the canyon floor and back along the east ridge. Two optional, worthwhile side trips could add more miles—if you're up to it. If you're traveling on a mountain bike, be aware that they are allowed only on the wide trails designated for such use, not for the entire trip described here.

Starting from the trailhead, the wide Cheeseboro Canyon Trail goes east and then bends north up the wide, nearly flat canyon floor, while the Modelo Trail slants left and curves up along the canyon's rounded west wall. At 1.6 miles, near the Palo Comado Connector trail joining from the west, you come upon a pleasant trailside picnic area. Stay on the main, wide trail going north along the Cheeseboro Canyon bottom, passing statuesque valley oaks, which are deciduous, and gnarled coast live oaks, which retain their smaller cup-shaped leaves year-round.

After 2.5 miles, turn right onto the steep, narrow Baleen Wall Trail—be aware that no mountain bikes are allowed on the ascending stretch ahead—and then begin climbing the grass- and sage-covered east canyon wall. (From this junction you could make an out-and-back side trip: by keeping straight on the main trail, you would pass some sulfurous-smelling seeps and later emerge in an open valley dotted with sandstone boulders. An old sheep corral made of wire lies in the upper reaches of Cheeseboro Canyon, 2 miles from the Baleen Wall turnoff.)

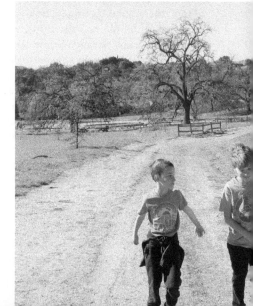

Oaks and broad hiking trails make Cheeseboro Canyon a popular destination.

After some huffing and puffing up the Baleen Wall Trail, you come to a power-line access road roughly following the east ridgeline. (Here you could begin a second side trip by going north along the road 0.5 mile to the lip of the Baleen Wall, a whitish sedimentary outcrop, for an impressive view of the upper canyon.)

To continue on the main route, walk south on the power-line access road, the Cheeseboro Ridge Trail, past a large water tank and down to a trail junction. Turn right and continue descending toward the picnic area you passed earlier. From there, retrace your steps down the Cheeseboro Canyon Trail back to the trailhead.

trip 4.7   China Flat Loop

see map on p. 43

Distance	9 miles (loop)
Hiking Time	5.5 hours
Elevation Gain	2,100'
Difficulty	Moderately strenuous
Trail Use	Dogs allowed
Best Times	November–May
Agency	National Park Service
Optional Map	Tom Harrison *Cheeseboro–Palo Comado Canyons* or Trails Illustrated *Santa Monica Mountains National Recreation Area (253)*

DIRECTIONS From Highway 101 in Agoura Hills, take Exit 36 for northbound Kanan Road and drive north 2.2 miles to Sunnycrest Drive. Turn right and continue 0.8 mile to a wide gated trail entrance on the right signed Public Recreation Trail. At this point, the street's name changes to Doubletree Road. Abundant curbside parking is available. Note that several similar trails branch off Sunnycrest, so be sure you've gone the right distance.

This rambling loop route includes a little of everything: a long ascent up pristine Palo Comado Canyon, a visit to a reflecting pool (well, an old stock pond) at China Flat, broad views of the surrounding suburbs from Simi Peak, a passage through Oak Canyon Park, and a concluding stretch on suburban streets. Although the route as described here is customized for hikers, mountain bikers can at least appreciate the stretch through Palo Comado Canyon and into China Flat. Only extreme mountain bikers will enjoy the steep climb to the summit of Simi Peak and the rocky descent of the China Flat Trail.

From the trailhead, pass through a gate and take a broad fire road east through grassland. Pass an unsigned service road, over a rise, and descend into broad Palo Comado Canyon, 0.5 mile. Turn left on the dirt road going left, up the canyon, and enjoy a pleasant stroll amid stately sycamores and gnarled live oaks. Unlike Cheeseboro Canyon to the east, Palo Comado is pleasantly free from the visual annoyance of power lines. Wildlife is plentiful hereabouts but often circumspect. Deer, bobcats, coyotes, rabbits, owls, and various birds of prey can be spotted here, especially in the early morning.

Stay on the main Palo Comado fire road as you pass an unsigned and unmaintained singletrack on the right climbing to the Sheep Corral Trail. At around 1.5 miles, the dirt road begins a vigorous and sometimes crooked ascent. Looking behind you, you gaze upon a lovely tapestry of canyon-bottom woods and slopes adorned with dense patches of chaparral and sandstone outcrops.

Pass the signed Sheep Corral Trail on the right at 2.2 miles, and climb more gently over a summit at 3.1 miles and proceed another 0.2 mile downhill to the edge of oak-dotted China Flat. Pass a trail on the left beside an old corral and water tank. Shortly thereafter,

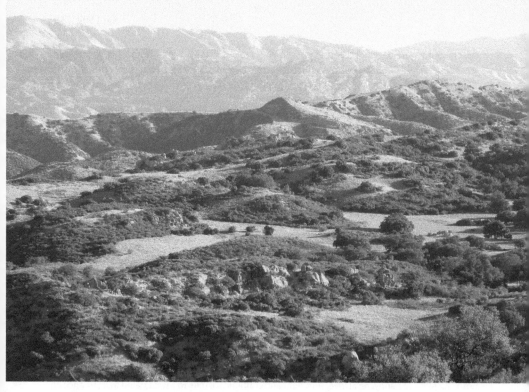

Looking north from the Simi Peak Trail over China Flat

the signed China Flat Trail veers right—stay left on a narrower trail. Look to the left for an old stock pond forming a small reflecting pool when it brims with water during and after the rainy season.

Continue west through China Flat for 0.2 mile to yet another junction with the China Flat Trail just before a lovely grove of coast live oaks. The way back to suburbia stays left, but our trip goes right for an enjoyable excursion to Simi Peak, 0.8 mile away by trail. Descend to cross a wash; then stay left to follow the Simi Peak Trail west. Eventually pass a branch on the right looping back to Oak Flat, but continue west and then curl up the steep, rocky north slope of Simi Peak. South and west from the jagged summit, your gaze takes in the broad sweep of the Santa Monica Mountains and scattered patches of cityscape embedded in the rolling landscape below.

After visiting the peak, return to China Flat and turn right on the China Flat Trail. You duck under the canopy of oaks, climb for a few minutes and pass over a saddle (5.8 miles), before joining an abandoned and highly eroded dirt road. There are many unsigned paths that all eventually reach Oak Canyon Park. For the most direct route, stay on the main ridge descending south.

At the bottom of the road, stay right to pass a maintenance yard and then cross a paved road into well-manicured Oak Canyon Community Park, where you'll find a drinking fountain, restrooms, and picnic grounds (7.3 miles). Follow a paved path to the lowermost playground; then walk down through the trees, and ford Medea Creek to reach a wide dirt path on the far side. Turn left and follow this path down along the creek to the southern end of the park, where you emerge on Kanan Road (7.7 miles).

Now only 1.2 miles remain—entirely on sidewalks. Turn left onto Hollytree Drive and left again onto Doubletree Road to get back to your starting point by the shortest route.

chapter 5

Santa Susana Mountains

Barren and austere when viewed by midday light, but soft and pillowy under the sun's slanting rays, the Santa Susana Mountains, rising from the northeast corner of the San Fernando Valley, have long been recognized as an important reservoir of open space. Conservation organizations have spearheaded the effort to acquire from private interests bits and pieces of what will hopefully become a broad tapestry of protected land for wildlife habitat and low-impact recreation.

Overlooking the valley from the east end of the range is 672-acre O'Melveny Park, the second biggest (after Griffith Park) city park in Los Angeles. Noted for its picture-perfect picnic grounds with white fences and towering eucalyptus trees, the park also challenges hikers with several miles of steep, backcountry fire roads and primitive trails.

Behind (north of) O'Melveny Park, on slopes facing the Santa Clarita Valley, lie some 6,000 acres of attractively wooded ridges and canyons that are a part of the Santa Clarita Woodlands Park and various parks and preserves acquired or managed by the Santa Monica Mountains Conservancy. Four trips in this chapter explore this surprisingly beautiful patch of open space.

Farther west, hikers can enjoy a network of riding and hiking paths in suburban Porter Ranch, ascend the south slope of Oat Mountain, probe the narrow confines of Devil Canyon, trace an old stagecoach trail that preceded the 20th-century roads through Santa Susana Pass, and climb view-rich Rocky Peak. Worth mentioning (but not included as a trip in this chapter) is Stony Point in Chatsworth, a spectacular but graffiti-scarred pile of sandstone boulders popular among rock-climbing enthusiasts and scramblers of all ages.

The 14 trips in this chapter give a taste of what is currently available for hikers in the Santa Susanas. The presently existing parks and open spaces in this area are but a part of a visionary Rim of the Valley natural area that will include, it is hoped, a trail stretching 100 miles around the north rim of the San Fernando Valley—from Ventura County to Glendale. Los Angeles County has released a Santa Susana Mountains Trails Master Plan that will likely lead to significant expansion of the trail network in this area.

continued on page 56

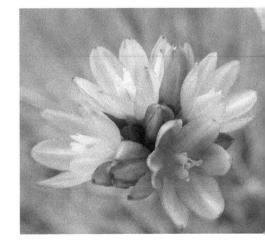

Blue dicks (Dichelostemma capitatum, also known as wild hyacinth or brodiaea) bloom early in the spring throughout the lower mountains of Los Angeles County.

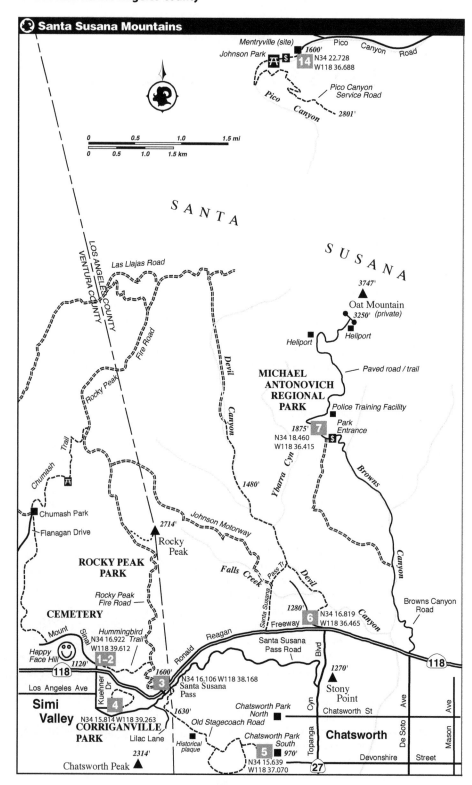

Santa Susana Mountains

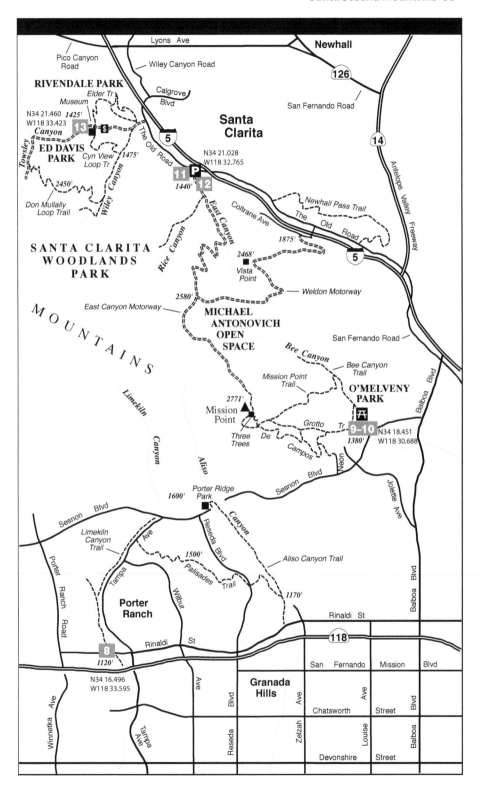

continued from page 53

trip 5.1   Hummingbird Trail

Distance	3.5 miles (out-and-back)
Hiking Time	3 hours
Elevation Gain	1,150'
Difficulty	Moderately strenuous
Trail Use	Dogs allowed, good for kids
Best Times	October–May
Agency	Santa Monica Mountains Conservancy
Optional Map	USGS 7.5' *Simi Valley East*

see map on p. 54

DIRECTIONS From the 118 Freeway in Simi Valley, take Exit 30 for Kuehner Drive. Go north 0.3 mile and park on the right side of Kuehner near the trailhead sign, taking care to observe parking restrictions.

The Hummingbird Trail starts at the extreme northeast corner of Simi Valley and deviously ascends boulder-studded slopes to the crest of a long ridge leading north to Rocky Peak. This out-and-back jaunt is perfect for early-morning exercise, when the trail lies mostly in shadow. Hikers and runners use it, as well as some intrepid mountain bikers who may risk life and limb on a couple of the steeper, more slippery pitches.

From the signed trailhead outside the private Hummingbird Nest Ranch, follow the Hummingbird Trail down to the bottom of a ravine called Hummingbird Creek. The trail repeatedly braids and rejoins; you will have to choose a path. After veering south to reach a point close to the freeway embankment, the trail switches back and starts to dart upward, trending east via many zigs and zags, sometimes over barren rock. At one point, it ascends a slab next to a cliff; between the slab and cliff is an interesting slot to explore. The steep climb continues more or less unabated until near the end, where the trail straightens, heads straightforwardly east, and finally reaches the Rocky Peak Fire Road at a point 0.8 mile

The Hummingbird Trail zigzags through sandstone outcrops near Rocky Peak.

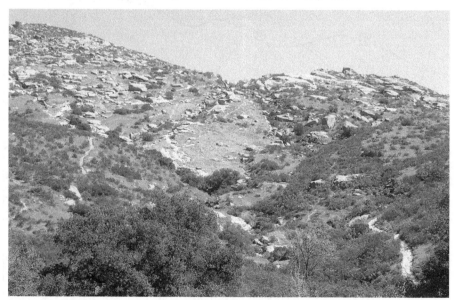

north of the fire road's origination point alongside the 118 Freeway at Santa Susana Pass. Take in the view from a bench and return the way you came.

Along the way up and the way back down you're seldom out of earshot of traffic on the neighboring freeway. Yet there are consistently panoramic views to enjoy whenever you want to take a break. If you have a camera, it's fun to pose your hiking companion atop any number of rounded boulders alongside the trail, with a background, perhaps, of the geometric patterns of subdivisions on the flat Simi Valley floor.

trip 5.2   Chumash Loop

Distance	9 miles (loop)
Hiking Time	3 hours
Elevation Gain	2,000'
Difficulty	Strenuous
Trail Use	Suitable for mountain biking, dogs allowed
Best Times	October–May
Agency	Santa Monica Mountains Conservancy
Optional Map	USGS 7.5' *Simi Valley East*

see map on p. 54

DIRECTIONS From the 118 Freeway in Simi Valley, take Exit 30 for Kuehner Drive. Go north 0.3 mile and park on the right side of Kuehner near the trailhead sign, taking care to observe parking restrictions.

This fun and invigorating loop explores the blocky sandstone country around Rocky Peak. It ascends the Chumash Trail, then follows the Rocky Peak Road until you can loop back on the Hummingbird Trail. The area is very popular with mountain bikers, but much skill is necessary to negotiate the trails, especially the steep and rocky Hummingbird Trail.

The trail is named for the Chumash, an American Indian people who lived along the coastal region of California from Malibu to Morro Bay. (*Chumash* may mean "bead maker" or "seashell people.") Tens of thousands of Chumash lived in over 150 villages before the arrival of the Spanish. The Chumash were enslaved by the missionaries and decimated by European diseases. The genocide accelerated under Mexican and United States rule as Indians were murdered and systematically forced out of their land. By the start of the 20th century, the Chumash numbered only about 200, and their territory was reduced to

Eroded sandstone windows line the Rocky Peak Fire Road.

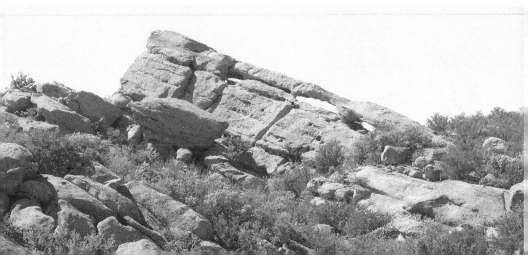

a 127-acre reservation near Santa Ynez. The last native speaker of the Chumash language died in 1965.

Make a clockwise loop to get the dull section out of the way and end with the best. From the Hummingbird Trailhead, walk south down Kuehner Drive; then make a right on Mount Sinai Drive, where you can follow a fenced path alongside the road. Pass a subdivision below Happy Face Hill, and continue to an unmarked trail just beyond the Mount Sinai cemetery entrance in 0.8 mile. Follow this trail up to a hilltop; then continue north along a path that soon parallels Flanagan Drive. Beware of many side trails branching off in this area. Pass Chumash Park and find the signed Chumash Trail at the north end of Flanagan Drive (1.6 miles).

You now leave civilization behind and head north. Immediately pass an unsigned trail on the left leading to a subdivision, and begin a steady climb through the sage scrub. The thick-leaf yerba santa attracts bees to its purple blossoms in the spring. At 3.0 miles step off the trail to a bench where you can catch your breath and enjoy sweeping views over the valley. Continue up to meet the Rocky Peak Fire Road at 4.2 miles.

Make a right and follow the fire road over the shoulder of Rocky Peak. At 5.4 miles pass a spur on the left leading toward the summit (see the next trip for this optional detour). Staying on the main road, descend through a basin and step down again to the signed Hummingbird Trail at 7.1 miles. Turn right and pick a path down this braiding trail past sandstone outcrops (see Trip 5.1, page 56). After you ford a seasonal creekbed at the bottom, stay right and follow the main trail back to your vehicle.

trip 5.3	**Rocky Peak**

Distance	5.5 miles (out-and-back)
Hiking Time	3 hours
Elevation Gain	1,400'
Difficulty	Moderately strenuous
Trail Use	Suitable for mountain biking, dogs allowed
Best Times	October–May
Agencies	Mountains Recreation & Conservation Authority, Santa Monica Mountains Conservancy
Optional Map	USGS 7.5' *Simi Valley East*

see map on p. 54

A feathered visitor enjoys the view from the Rocky Peak summit.

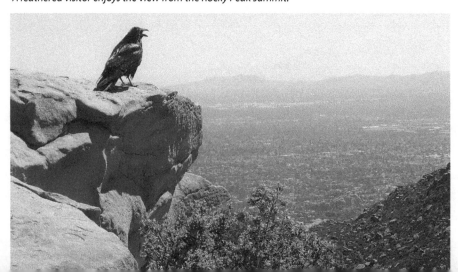

DIRECTIONS From the westbound 118 Freeway, take Exit 32 for Rocky Peak Road. Park in the small dirt lot on the right (north) side of the off-ramp, taking care to observe parking restrictions. From the eastbound 118, take Exit 30 for southbound Kuehner Drive. In about 1.2 miles, Kuehner Drive curves east and becomes Santa Susana Pass Road. In another 1.7 miles, turn left on Rocky Peak Road and go 0.1 mile over the freeway bridge to reach the trailhead parking area above. Overflow parking is available south of the bridge just before the turnoff.

In 1990 the Santa Monica Mountains Conservancy entered negotiations with entertainer Bob Hope to purchase Rocky Peak Park—a 4,369-acre parcel of land overlooking the Simi and San Fernando Valleys. Today, the entire spread, long locked up in private ownership and more recently threatened by creeping suburbia, welcomes hikers and bikers who can start their trip, conveniently enough, at the end of a freeway off-ramp.

A look at a topographic map of the area reveals a loopy pattern of closely spaced contour lines, indicative of terrain topped by immense boulder piles. The sandstone that underlies this area dates from the Cretaceous period more than 65 million years ago. Relatively recent uplift, weathering, and erosion has carved this rock into impressively huge and intricate structures at the surface.

Your steep ascent from the trailhead begins immediately on the Rocky Peak Fire Road. At 0.8 mile note the junction of the Hummingbird Trail (see Trip 5.1, page 56) on the left. Keep climbing. At about 1.5 miles, your relentless ascent is temporarily reversed by a brief drop into a little flat where, on the right, you can find shade and rest under a lone live-oak tree.

After passing larger and more impressively convoluted outcrops of sandstone, the fire road tops out on a prominent ridgeline (2.4 miles). There an older, disused road joins on the right, leading circuitously toward Rocky Peak. In 0.2 mile the path peters out at a summit with excellent views that will satisfy most visitors. Purists will want to continue 0.1 mile to the true high point, but this involves a faint trail that passes east of two more bumps on the ridge to avoid a tricky boulder scramble.

The 2,714-foot Rocky Peak summit defines a waypoint on the boundary between Los Angeles and Ventura Counties. The view from the top at best encompasses large parts of these two counties, plus the Pacific Ocean—partly obscured by the undulating Santa Monica Mountains.

trip 5.4	**Corriganville Park**

Distance	1.3 miles (loop)
Hiking Time	1 hour
Elevation Gain	100'
Difficulty	Easy
Trail Use	Good for kids
Best Times	October–June
Agency	Rancho Simi Recreation and Park District
Maps	None

see map on p. 54

DIRECTIONS From the 118 Freeway in Simi Valley, take Exit 30 for southbound Kuehner Drive. In 1.3 miles turn left on Smith Road. In 0.4 mile turn left again into the Corriganville Park parking lot.

What could be more appropriate for Los Angeles County than hiking around a semi-abandoned film lot? Corriganville Park is named for Ray "Crash" Corrigan, who acquired the land in 1937 and built movie and television sets here. Corrigan was a well-known actor and stunt man, best known for playing the gorilla in *Tarzan and His Mate* and

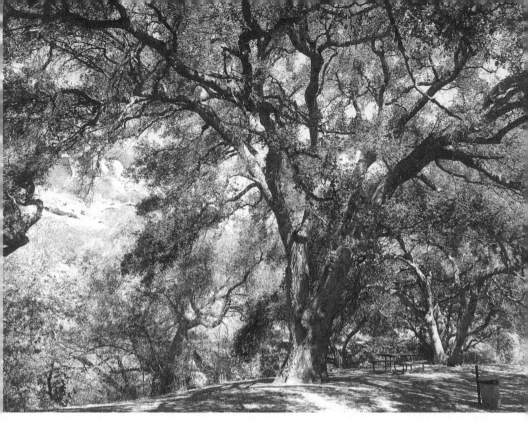

Beware of Robin Hood's Merry Men when picnicking in the Sherwood Forest.

for starring in low-budget Westerns. Corrigan operated the ranch as an amusement park on weekends from 1949 to 1965, drawing up to 20,000 people a day for the Western-themed entertainment. Bob Hope acquired the property in 1965, but the land and structures burned in 1970 and 1979. The City of Simi Valley purchased the 190-acre park in 1988 for public use. Now you can walk a short loop around Corriganville and listen for the ghosts of heroes and outlaws roaming the rocks and woods.

To make a counterclockwise loop, begin by walking to the far east end of the parking lot, where you'll find the signed Interpretive Trail circling the massive sandstone ridge in the middle of the park. The poorly marked trail has many forks, so try to stay on the heavily used paths.

You begin by following the often-dry Arroyo Simi on a broad path shaded by imposing coast live oaks. One of the oak groves, known as Sherwood Forest, was a set for the 1950s *Robin Hood* TV series. You can stop at a picnic bench to soak up the memories. You'll soon reach Robin Hood Lake, now an empty concrete pool. Look for windows beneath the bridge where underwater scenes were filmed.

At the northeast corner of the park, you'll enter Camp Rotary, operated by the Rotary Club for youth groups. Veer left at the large picnic shelter and cross Simi Arroyo; then pass an amphitheater. The old roadbed is cut into the sandstone bedrock as it climbs to a low saddle. From the saddle, you can go right or left around a rocky hill before reaching an open area that was once the site of *Fort Apache*, where John Ford directed the so-named 1948 film starring John Wayne and Henry Fonda. Nearby is the site of Vendetta Village, where Howard Hughes produced his less-successful film *Vendetta* in 1950. You'll soon complete the loop and emerge at the parking area.

trip 5.5 **Old Stagecoach Road**

Distance	2.7 miles (out-and-back)
Hiking Time	1.5 hours
Elevation Gain	700'
Difficulty	Moderate
Trail Use	Good for kids
Best Times	Year-round
Agencies	California State Parks, Los Angeles Department of Recreation and Parks
Optional Maps	USGS 7.5' *Oat Mountain, Simi Valley East*

see map on p. 54

DIRECTIONS From the 118 Freeway in Chatsworth, take Exit 34 for southbound Topanga Canyon Boulevard. In 1.5 miles turn right on Devonshire Street, and go 0.5 mile to its end at Chatsworth Park South. Continue through the park, which is open weekdays 9 a.m.–10 p.m. and weekends 9 a.m.– 5 p.m., to the large lot near the community center at the end of the road.

Clear-air vistas of the San Fernando Valley and surrounding mountain ranges are as spectacular as they come when seen from the Old Stagecoach Road above Chatsworth. The boulder-stacked hillsides rising from the valley seem strongly reminiscent of the golden backdrops seen in old Western movies and television shows, because they really did play a background role in many of those productions.

The area traversed by the Old Stagecoach Road has been incorporated into the 670-acre Santa Susana Pass State Historic Park. The pass has been, and continues to be, a key link in a major coastal transportation corridor connecting Northern and Southern California. The Spanish Army Captain Gaspar de Portolá passed this way in 1769, blazing a trail from San Diego to Monterey Bay. The route later became a part of El Camino Real (King's Highway), which linked the Spanish system of presidios, pueblos, and missions along California's coast and coastal–inland valleys. Today, railroad tracks and the Simi Valley Freeway traverse the Santa Susana Pass slightly north of where an earlier, devilishly steep road called the Devil's Slide, was built to accommodate stagecoaches. Surprisingly, this long-abandoned stage route can be traced today on foot. The trails are presently poorly marked and the directions might change by the time you visit.

At Chatsworth Park South, head west through the grassy picnic grounds. At the west end, cross the fenced Old Stagecoach Equestrian Trail, jog right a few steps, and find a trail leading west into a canyon and then up the hillside. Soon reach paved Powerhouse

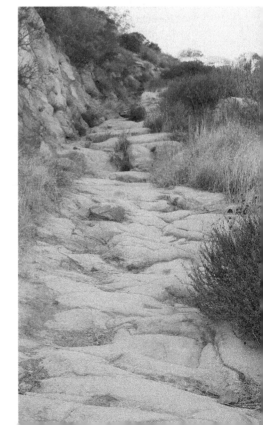

The Old Stagecoach Road was carved from solid rock up the Devil's Slide.

Road, where you turn right and go 80 yards, then leave it for the unsigned rocky Chatsworth Wagon trail, climbing to your left.

If you've managed to stay on route through this maze, the rest is easy. You'll soon reach a bend in the signed Old Stagecoach Road. Turn right and follow it all the way to the top. Veer right at the next two signed junctions to stay on your trail. Pass the unsigned Hill Palmer Trail on the right dropping into a ravine.

You're now on a well-preserved section of Devil's Slide, a key link in the 1860–1890 coastal stage road linking Los Angeles and San Francisco. A tiled historical plaque, installed in 1939 by the Native Daughters of the Golden West, commemorates the road. As you walk up the hard sandstone bed, notice the carefully hewn drainage chutes on both sides. Watch for grooves cut in the sandstone by iron-banded wagon wheels as horse teams struggled up the formidable grade. Pass unsigned trails on the right to a rocky viewpoint (a great place to watch trains coming through the tunnel), and left to a small dam where rainwater was captured for the horses. The grade eventually relaxes and you soon reach the Devil's Slide summit (1,630'), where you cross the L.A.–Ventura County line and reach a trailhead sign on Lilac Lane in an area of scattered residences. North, behind a hill, is today's Santa Susana Pass, threaded by the Simi Valley Freeway and the older Santa Susana Pass Road. Some 600 feet below you is the 1.4-mile-long Santa Susana railroad tunnel, whose east entrance can be seen back near Chatsworth Park South.

---

trip 5.6 Devil Canyon

Distance	2.4–9 miles (out-and-back)
Hiking Time	1–5 hours
Elevation Gain	450'–1,000'
Difficulty	Easy–Moderate
Trail Use	Dogs allowed, good for kids
Best Times	October–June
Agency	Santa Monica Mountains Conservancy
Optional Map	USGS 7.5' *Oat Mountain*

see map on p. 54

DIRECTIONS From the 118 Freeway in Chatsworth, take Exit 34 for Topanga Canyon Boulevard. Turn north and immediately go west on Poema Place. In 0.3 mile park on the side of the street near the entrance to the 11500 unit of the Summerset Village apartment complex.

A surprisingly cool and pleasant retreat just back of the hot, dry northwest corner of the San Fernando Valley, Devil Canyon sports abundant growths of live oak and willow and a small, intermittent stream. Fire and flood have long since removed almost all traces of an old auto road in the canyon; in its place hikers have beaten down a narrow trail. Come here in the early spring to enjoy the wildflowers and blooming ceanothus on the hillsides, or in winter (wear an old pair of shoes) if you don't mind tramping through lots of good, clean mud.

You can adjust the length of this hike to your choosing. The junglelike lower segment of Devil Canyon is most dramatic. If you are seeking a workout, you can continue all the way to Brown Mountain Road at the head of the canyon.

Walk into the apartment complex parking area and make your first right turn by unit 11504. Pass through a gate at the end of the parking spur, and walk down the stairs. Turn left and join an old dirt road that soon deposits you by the creek bed on the canyon floor. Follow the willow-lined creek bed upstream; don't be tempted out onto side paths. The at-first uninspiring scenery improves greatly as you swing around a couple of sharp bends

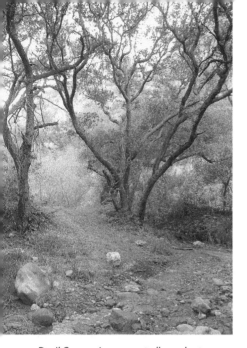

Devil Canyon is unexpectedly verdant and refreshing.

and lose sight of wall-to-wall condos on the bluff above. Scattered riparian vegetation accompanies you for most of the way as you work your way up along the canyon bottom; beware of poison oak. The wind and water-carved sandstone canyon walls, a part of the same formation exposed at Stony Point and Santa Susana Pass, originated from sediments laid down in a marine environment roughly 80 million years ago. Shallow caves can be found in Devil Canyon's tributaries, especially Falls Creek, if you don't mind doing a little bushwhacking.

At 1.2 miles reach an unmarked trail that leads steeply out the left side of the canyon. This is the Santa Susana Pass Trail, which continues 1.0 mile to the gated Indian Springs community on Iverson Road. Those seeking a short trip could turn around here.

At 2 miles watch for a spur trail on the right into Ybarra Canyon, by a grove of oaks. The main path becomes better defined and the canyon walls recede. Higher in the canyon, you will encounter more oaks, meadows, and sage scrub. At 4.6 miles your trail ends at a T-junction with the Brown Mountain Road.

VARIATION

For an 11-mile hike with a 2-mile car, bike, or ride sharing shuttle, you can turn left on Brown Mountain Road and go 0.4 mile to a ridgetop junction. Las Llatas Road continues straight, but you turn left onto Rocky Peak Motorway. Follow the rolling ridge all the way back to the Rocky Peak parking area (see Trip 5.3, page 58), passing many side roads and interesting rock formations along the way.

---

trip 5.7   Oat Mountain

Distance	4.8 miles (out-and-back)
Hiking Time	2.5 hours
Elevation Gain	1,400'
Difficulty	Moderately strenuous
Trail Use	Suitable for mountain biking, dogs allowed
Best Times	October–May
Agencies	Mountains Recreation & Conservation Authority, Santa Monica Mountains Conservancy
Optional Map	USGS 7.5' *Oat Mountain*
Fees/Permits	$5 parking fee at Antonovich Regional Park

see map on p. 54

DIRECTIONS From the 118 Freeway in Chatsworth, take Exit 35 for northbound De Soto Avenue; the northern extension of De Soto is called Browns Canyon Road. Follow this narrow, twisty road 3.3 miles around some outlying houses, up along the Browns Canyon stream, and finally up a steep hill to the main Antonovich Park entrance, where you must deposit a fee in the iron ranger. There's a lower parking lot on the left, but continue 0.4 mile to a large upper lot just shy of where the road is blocked to public traffic.

A rambling patch of open space with a long-winded name, Michael D. Antonovich Regional Park at Joughin Ranch spreads over a south-facing slope, culminating in a 3,747-foot summit called Oat Mountain, the high point of the Santa Susana Mountains. On this trip, you drive about halfway up the mountain (as measured from the San Fernando Valley floor) and travel on foot most of the remaining distance to Oat Mountain, whose summit lies on private property. The entrance fee for this forlorn park is shocking; the park has no facilities whatsoever, and the only trail is the paved service road up the mountain. The mountaintop is adorned with a Doppler weather radar and many communications antennas and is off-limits to the public. However, on a clear day, the ever more spacious view gets ever more stupendous; on a hazy or smoggy day you won't like either the impaired view or the dirty air moving in and out of your lungs.

After parking in the upper lot—as far as you can drive on Browns Canyon Road—trudge on, uphill and sometimes steeply so, continuing on the same paved road. By 0.6 mile into the hike, you're passing the decommissioned LA-88 Nike Missile air defense base, where nuclear-tipped Hercules missiles were first deployed to deter Soviet bombers. Little remains after the 2008 Sesnon Fire. The base was repurposed as an L.A. Police Department SWAT training site but now appears to be mostly used by vandals. The sharp increase in elevation gain so far has yielded a significantly wider panorama of the vast, flat, and densely populated San Fernando Valley below. Above the base, the close-at-hand landscape assumes a more impressive character, with wild grasses—mostly wild oats, after which the peak above was named—bending in a supple fashion in the zephyrs of springtime, or chafing in the dry breezes of the other seasons.

At 1.1 miles you traverse a cattle grate and temporarily enter a parcel where cattle graze contentedly. Soon, after crossing a second grate, you're back in Antonovich parkland, where the ascent quickens. The valley view to the south now assumes a pseudo-aerial character,

Watch for scallop fossils in the rocks where a 50-million-year-old seabed was pushed up to form the Santa Susana Mountains.

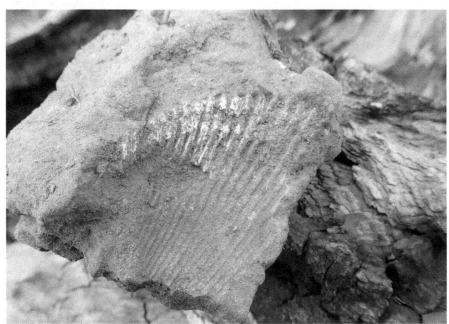

and the green or golden (depending on the season) slopes seem to roll sensuously upward, downward, and sideways.

At 2.0 miles, alongside a heliport (a large flat spot for firefighting helicopters to land), you start to get a view to the north, which consists of miles of ridges sparsely dotted with valley oaks and an occasional rocker pump struggling to extract the very last drop of crude oil remaining in the permeable strata far below.

Keep going another half mile to a second heliport, this one on the right, which offers perhaps the most comprehensive vista so far. Unfortunately, because the road is gated just beyond, hikers must turn around here. After contemplating the scene and taking a deep pull from your water bottle, it's time to return. Use the same route—a possibly knee-jarring experience at times.

---

trip 5.8   **Porter Ranch Loop**

Distance	8 miles (loop)
Hiking Time	4 hours
Elevation Gain	1,000'
Difficulty	Moderately strenuous
Trail Use	Equestrians, dogs allowed
Best Times	October–May
Agency	Los Angeles Department of Recreation and Parks
Optional Map	USGS 7.5' *Oat Mountain*

see map on p. 54

DIRECTIONS From the 118 Freeway in Northridge, take Exit 37 for Tampa Avenue. Go north for one block, turn left on Rinaldi Street, go 0.2 mile, and find a place to park where Rinaldi crosses Limekiln Canyon Park.

The open spaces and trails lacing the well-to-do Porter Ranch subdivision could serve as a nice model for community development anywhere in the Southland. Of course, it could also be argued that the world would be better off without the square miles of new housing developments here and elsewhere along the rim of the San Fernando Valley. But at least local residents—and the public at large—have the opportunity to wander the remaining vestiges of two riparian canyons and a cliff-rimmed hillside blanketed with aromatic sage. Suitable for horses as well as hikers, this trip is best taken on a cool day. A look at this chapter's map (or any street map of the area) reveals ways to abbreviate the trip if you don't want to go the full 8 miles.

George Porter and partners acquired 57,000 acres in 1874 that are now known as Porter Ranch. Porter was the first major citrus grower in the San Fernando Valley, and he later subdivided his ranch. The region became popular for horse ranches and movie studios, and portions of *E.T. the Extra-Terrestrial* were filmed here. Porter Ranch is now the site of upscale gated communities.

From Rinaldi Street, pick up the equestrian trail going north through the landscaped linear park along Limekiln Canyon's trickling creek, which the trail repeatedly fords. Stay on the main path at numerous forks, some of which go up to neighborhoods and others down to the creek. In 2.0 miles arrive at Sesnon Boulevard, near the mouth of the Aliso Canyon Natural Gas Storage Field.

Oil was discovered in this canyon in 1938. As it was pumped out, a huge hollow was left in the underground rock formations. When the oil was depleted, the field was repurposed for natural gas storage, and now the Southern California Gas Company holds up to 86

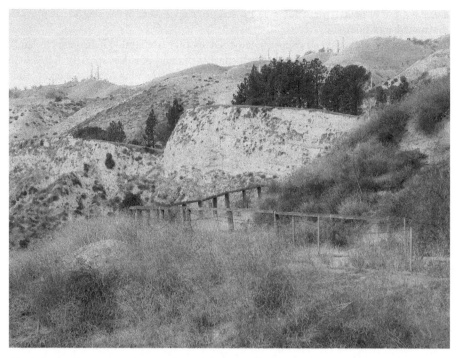

The Palisades Trail escapes the sprawling subdivisions of Porter Ranch.

billion cubic feet of gas at the site, the second largest in the United States. The gas company reported a leak in one of the wells in October 2015. Over the next three months, roughly 100,000 tons of natural gas escaped, smelling like rotten eggs, causing nosebleeds, and forcing over 11,000 residents and two schools to relocate. Seven attempts to plug the leak failed, the last creating a 25-foot-deep crater, before SoCal Gas was able to drill a relief well and fill the leaking shaft from below.

Turn right and follow the sidewalk of Sesnon Boulevard 0.6 mile to its dead end on the edge of steep-sided Aliso Canyon. Walk around the pipe gate on the left and down into Aliso Canyon. Follow the unsigned Aliso Canyon Trail south along the canyon floor, passing various spurs branching to neighborhoods, until you reach a junction at the confluence of Aliso Canyon and a tributary to the west in 1.3 miles. Turn right onto the unsigned Palisades Trail, which doubles back up a ravine, climbs a slope, passes some houses, and reaches Reseda Boulevard. Cross Reseda, continue uphill on the west sidewalk for about 0.3 mile, and then veer off on the wide trail, bordered by a wooden fence, descending left along a sage-covered slope with panoramic views.

Soon you start contouring along the base of some craggy sedimentary bluffs—the so-called palisades. You're well above the valley floor here, so the view takes in thousands of rooftops in the foreground and the purple Santa Monica Mountains rising above the valley haze in the south.

At 6.5 miles the Palisades Trail goes over a saddle and then drops to Tampa Avenue. Pick up the Limekiln Canyon Trail on the far side, and then return to your car, retracing your earlier steps.

see
map on
p. 54

trip 5.9   Bee Canyon

Distance	2.2 miles (out-and-back)
Hiking Time	1.5 hours
Elevation Gain	200'
Difficulty	Moderate
Trail Use	Dogs allowed, good for kids
Best Times	Year-round
Agency	Los Angeles Department of Recreation and Parks
Optional Map	USGS 7.5' *Oat Mountain*

DIRECTIONS From the 118 Freeway in Granada Hills, take Exit 40A for Balboa Boulevard. Drive north 2.3 miles to Sesnon Boulevard. Go left (west) and continue 0.6 mile to the parking lot for O'Melveny Park on the right.

O'Melveny Park's Bee Canyon is a terrific place for exploring with little ones. Presided over by sky-scraping cliffs and shaded by a veritable jungle of young willow saplings, this is natural L.A.'s answer to Disneyland's Adventureland. During most of the year water seeps, or flows, down the canyon's silty bottom, so you'd better wear old shoes if you intend to probe the canyon's upper, nearly trailless reaches. The park is named for Henry O'Melveny, who founded a law firm in 1885 that has grown to become the noted O'Melveny & Meyers LLP. O'Melveny was a founding member of the California State Parks Commission. The family acquired a ranch here in 1941, and it was converted into a city park in 1973. At 627 acres, O'Melveny Park is the second largest park in Los Angeles.

From the park's entrance, follow the paved trail uphill through the tree-shaded picnic grounds. After the path turns to dirt and becomes the O'Melveny Trail, simply follow the path of least resistance into the hills, straight up the V-shaped gorge ahead, which is Bee Canyon. On the left (southwest) side of the canyon, live oak and California walnut trees stand as battered but proud survivors of fire and flood. On the right, barren sedimentary cliffs soar 500 feet. Movements along the Santa Susana thrust fault, which cuts east–west across the Santa Susanas, have helped produce this towering feature. In the wetter times of

Dramatic Bee Canyon is a short stroll from O'Melveny Park.

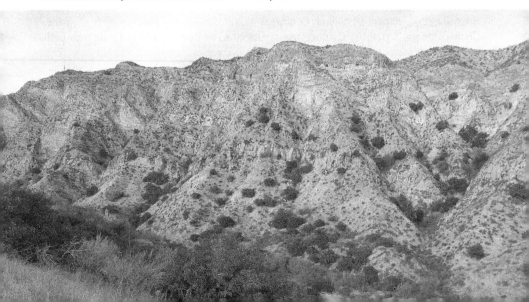

year water seeps out of cracks in the layered rock above and dribbles down several of the steep gullies. (*Note:* The cliffs are unstable and thus unsuitable for climbing.)

At 0.5 mile beyond the picnic area, the main trail bends left to climb the canyon's south wall. A less-traveled trail continues ahead through willow thickets, becoming more and more obscure the farther you venture. Soon you're scrambling over eroded banks and tree roots and squishing through mud puddles. By the time the going gets really rough, you'll be at or near the north boundary of the park—a good turnaround point.

trip 5.10   Mission Point

Distance	4.7 miles (loop)	
Hiking Time	3 hours	see map on p. 54
Elevation Gain	1,450'	
Difficulty	Moderately strenuous	
Trail Use	Dogs allowed	
Best Times	November–May	
Agency	Los Angeles Department of Recreation and Parks	
Optional Map	USGS 7.5' *Oat Mountain*	

DIRECTIONS From the 118 Freeway in Granada Hills, take Exit 40A for Balboa Boulevard. Drive north 23 miles to Sesnon Boulevard. Go left (west) and continue 0.6 mile to the parking lot for O'Melveny Park on the right.

Two centuries ago the treeless bump called Mission Point (2,771') overlooked an arid valley dotted with Indian villages. One century ago, the same vantage point would have revealed an early housing boom amid the citrus groves on the valley floor. Today (whenever the smog chances to clear away) the 150° view of the San Fernando Valley takes in a seemingly endless grid of rectilinear streets and avenues, plus all the visible infrastructure of a city-within-a-city of more than 1.5 million people.

From the park's entrance, a paved trail leads through an orchard and picnic grounds, while a dirt road to the left goes to the dirt equestrian parking area. Walk through the equestrian parking and pick up a fenced equestrian trail that parallels the paved road. In 0.2 mile turn left onto the signed Grotto Trail, which darts up a narrow, almost barren ridge dividing two parallel ravines. California walnut trees dot the bottoms of these ravines. Chances are good you'll spot a deer or a coyote, or a roadrunner flitting across your path.

Numerous social trails veer off the Grotto Trail. Try to stay on the main path as it climbs steeply to a four-way junction. Go right and then, in 0.1 mile, turn left on a wider trail (you'll follow the other fork on your descent), and continue your climb to the high point. Nearing the summit you'll pass a knoll topped by a cluster of three live-oak trees. This tiny oak copse makes a fine picnic spot with a good view to boot.

A small stone monument atop Mission Point's shadeless summit (1.9 miles into the hike) memorializes physician Mario De Campos, a lover of the local mountains. Down in the valley 3 miles southeast, you'll spot the newer Los Angeles Reservoir as well as the dry bed of its predecessor, the Van Norman Reservoir, whose dam very nearly failed during the 1971 Sylmar earthquake. To the west, carved into the dry south slopes of the Santa Susanas, are old oil wells and a tangle of cliff-hanging roads built to serve them.

For a look at the much more agreeable and verdant north slopes of the Santa Susanas, walk farther north about 0.3 mile to where the road begins its descent into the Santa Clarita Woodlands area. There you can get a glimpse of canyon country dotted with live oak, valley

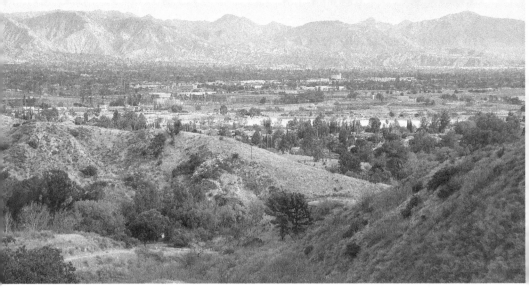

Looking back toward O'Melvany Park from the Grotto Trail

oak, walnut, and big-cone Douglas-fir trees. Why the big difference in vegetation? It's simply the slope aspect, whereby the south-facing slopes bake in year-round sun, while the north-facing slopes experience far more shade and less evaporation of moisture.

On your return to the O'Melveny Park entrance, descend below Mission Point using the path you followed uphill. At the aforementioned junction, turn left onto the unsigned but wide O'Melveny Trail, which will take you down, sometimes steeply, into Bee Canyon. Once you reach the canyon floor, turn downstream and hike the remaining short distance out to the picnic area and your starting point.

VARIATION

You can also reach Mission Point via the less-crowded Dr. Mario A. De Campos Trail up the Sulphur Springs Fire Road starting at the north end of Neon Way. The trail joins the regular route at the three trees. Up-and-back is 5.0 miles with 1,300 feet of elevation gain.

---

trip 5.11   ## Rice Canyon

Distance	2.5 miles (out-and-back)
Hiking Time	1.5 hours
Elevation Gain	350'
Difficulty	Easy
Trail Use	Dogs allowed, good for kids
Best Times	Year-round
Agencies	Mountains Recreation & Conservation Authority, Santa Monica Mountains Conservancy
Optional Map	USGS 7.5' *Oat Mountain*
Fees/Permits	$5 parking fee at East Canyon Trailhead

see map on p. 54

DIRECTIONS From the 5 Freeway in Santa Clarita, take Exit 166 for westbound Calgrove Boulevard. Calgrove becomes The Old Road and veers south. Continue 1.1 miles to the East Canyon Trailhead, on the right. Park on the shoulder of the road for free or in the trailhead lot for a fee.

A pleasant little retreat in almost any season, Rice Canyon hides amid the foothills of the Santa Susana Mountains, just outside the busy suburban community of Santa

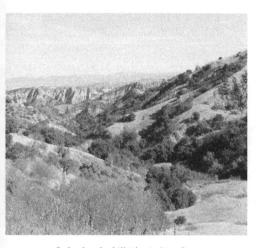

Oaks dot the hillsides in Rice Canyon.

Clarita. Even on the sunniest days, you can find dark pools of shade here, and much cooler temperatures.

From the trailhead, you start with an uninteresting 0.3-mile hike south on an old ranch road to an old water trough and other evidence of former cattle ranching. Look on the right side of the road for the narrow trail going into Rice Canyon, where it is noted that mountain bikes are prohibited. This nearly 1-mile-long trail is enchanting for kids and adults alike—a veritable fairyland complete with a limpid brook and a shade-giving assortment of trees, predominantly coast live oak, but also scrub, canyon, and valley oak and sycamore, willow, and cottonwood.

In the upper part of Rice Canyon, the trail begins to rise sharply along the slope to the right. After climbing sharply for a few minutes, you get a nice view south of steep slopes plunging sheer from the crest of the Santa Susana Mountains. Here and there, higher in elevation, you'll spot big-cone Douglas-fir trees. The trail soon becomes indistinct, so turn around when you've seen enough.

trip 5.12   East Canyon Loop

see map on p. 54

Distance	7 miles (loop)
Hiking Time	3.5 hours
Elevation Gain	1,300'
Difficulty	Moderately strenuous
Trail Use	Suitable for mountain biking, equestrians, dogs allowed
Best Times	October–May
Agencies	Mountains Recreation & Conservation Authority, Santa Monica Mountains Conservancy
Optional Map	USGS 7.5' *Oat Mountain*
Fees/Permits	$5 parking fee at East Canyon Trailhead

DIRECTIONS From the 5 Freeway in Santa Clarita, take Exit 166 for westbound Calgrove Boulevard. Calgrove becomes The Old Road and veers south. Continue 1.1 miles to the East Canyon trailhead on the right. Park on the shoulder of the road for free or in the trailhead lot for a fee.

Verdant East Canyon tucks into steep, north-facing slopes just below the crest of the Santa Susana Mountains. The canyon receives an average of about 20 inches of rainfall annually—just enough, in an environment sheltered from the sun's south-slanting rays, to support an islandlike array of scraggly big-cone Douglas-fir trees. This evergreen species tends to thrive higher up in the nearby San Gabriel Mountains, but in this area some specimens can be found at elevations as low as 2,000 feet. The route is tucked between the Sunshine Canyon Landfill and the Oak Tree Gun Club. Your tranquility may be interrupted by the beeping of heavy machinery and the report of gunfire, but you can be thankful that East Canyon was preserved in its natural form.

Except for some steep pitches here and there, the looping route into East Canyon described here is perfect for mountain biking. You'll see plenty of cyclists on the route, which consists of a combination of paved and dirt roads. The trail is much less crowded than the nearby Towsley Canyon.

From the trailhead, head southeast (on foot or bike) on The Old Road, first under the traffic lanes of the 5 Freeway and then parallel to the freeway; this is the defunct US 99 over Newhall Pass, which has since been replaced by the modern freeway. Stay on The Old Road's shoulder so as to keep away from the fast-moving automotive traffic that still exists here. After a probably tedious (on foot, at least) 1.6 miles you reach Weldon Canyon Road, which crosses the 5 Freeway on a narrow overpass. Make a right at Coltrane Avenue on the far side of that overpass and continue 0.1 mile to Weldon Motorway (a fire road) on the left. The fire road's initial ascent is excruciating, but the uphill grade soon moderates.

The scenery turns gorgeous as you climb, especially during the early morning on many a day, when the entire San Fernando Valley lies unseen beneath a marine-layer blanket of clouds. Watch for toyon, California walnut trees, and especially coast live oak. To the east, the rounded summits of the San Gabriel Mountains rise into a sapphire sky, sometimes flecked with cirrus clouds. Near at hand, note the coast live oaks and a small number of big-cone Douglas-firs dotting the slopes.

At 2.3 miles look for a dead-end road on the left; stay right and proceed along a narrow ridge with dramatic drop-offs on both sides. At 3.1 miles (elevation 2,468') there's a rest stop with a shade ramada overlooking the East Canyon drainage to the north and east.

Continue following the same narrow ridge—essentially the south rim of East Canyon—until you reach a junction of fire roads at 4.6 miles. A left turn here could take you to Mission Point and O'Melveny Park (see Trip 5.8, page 65). You go right, however, and begin the long and sometimes steep descent into East Canyon. Note more fine specimens of big-cone Douglas-firs along the way, their wandlike limbs reaching wide.

By 6 miles you arrive alongside East Canyon's trickling stream and enter a strip of gorgeous riparian–oak woodland. Your starting point along The Old Road is a short mile ahead.

The East Canyon Loop is notable for its oak woodlands.

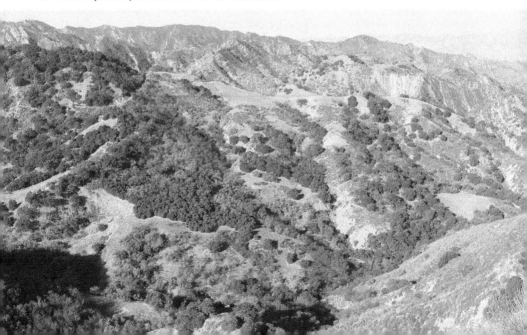

trip 5.13   **Don Mullally Loop**

Distance	5 miles (loop)
Hiking Time	3 hours
Elevation Gain	1,100'
Difficulty	Moderately strenuous
Trail Use	Suitable for mountain biking, dogs allowed
Best Times	October–June
Agencies	Mountains Recreation & Conservation Authority, Santa Monica Mountains Conservancy
Optional Map	USGS 7.5' *Oat Mountain*

see map on p. 54

DIRECTIONS From the 5 Freeway in Santa Clarita, take Exit 166 for westbound Calgrove Boulevard. Calgrove becomes The Old Road and veers south. Continue 0.2 mile to Ed Davis Park on the right, and park at a large free lot just outside the gate.

Santa Clarita Woodlands Park, north of the arid San Fernando Valley and just east of Santa Clarita's dry hills and valleys, encompasses a surprising assortment of strange geologic features and several amazingly lush canyons and north-facing hillsides. For 120 years, Chevron Corporation (formerly Standard Oil of California) owned this land, using it for oil production and limited grazing. The area was slated to become a huge landfill but was preserved as a park thanks to activists led for three decades by naturalist and teacher Don Mullally; state senator Ed Davis championed the land acquisition. In 1995, more than 3,000 acres of this land was transferred to the Santa Monica Mountains Conservancy. With subsequent additions of open space, the protected area now includes about 6,000 acres. Here, as elsewhere on the metropolitan fringe of Los Angeles, it's hard to believe such near-pristine and sublime landscapes can exist so close to a population of millions.

The popular Don Mullally Trail (renamed from the Towsley View Loop in 2014), partly on old roads and partly on singletracks trail, visits narrow canyon bottoms and sunny ridges, all the while exposing you to an ever-changing array of habitats: riparian woodland, oak and walnut woodlands, coastal sage scrub, chaparral, and grassland.

From the parking area, walk west on a paved road for 0.5 mile to an upper pay parking lot near a picnic area and Towsley Lodge (which can be rented for special events). The Elder Trail on the right branches back to where you began, leading 1 mile through Rivendale Park through a zone that burned in the June 2016 Sage Fire.

Our trail passes a chain gate and continues west on the gravel service road going up the wide floodplain of Towsley Canyon. The scenery improves dramatically as you reach, at 0.9 mile, the portals of The Narrows, a slotlike cleft worn through layers of sandstone and conglomerate tilted nearly vertical. The Santa Susana Mountains were built through geologic uplift along thrust faults—a process dramatically demonstrated during the catastrophic 1994 Northridge quake, an event that actually caused the Santa Susanas to rise a foot or more. With all the compression going on, both underground and at the surface, it is not surprising to see a variety of folds (synclines and anticlines) in the rocks exposed here and elsewhere in the Santa Clarita Woodlands.

After a brief passage through The Narrows, you encounter a split in the road. Stay left on the main path. After another 200 yards, stay left again, and begin climbing the canyon slope to the left on what is called the Towsley View Loop Trail. It quickly evolves into a narrow, or singletrack, trail (easy to negotiate on foot, tougher on a mountain bike) that steadily ascends on switchbacks through sage scrub and later through some gorgeous, almost pure stands of California walnut. Watch for a naturally occurring oil seep with gobs of tar. Well

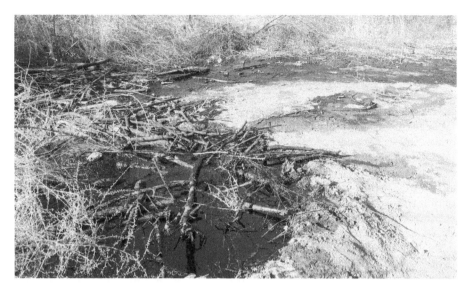

A natural tar seep along the Don Mullally Trail hints at the oil once extracted here.

before any oil was extracted for commercial purposes here, the Tataviam Indians of the area used the asphalt for medicinal applications and to seal their basketry. Higher still the tree canopy thins, with scattered oaks and pungent bay laurel clinging to the hillsides. There you catch sight of the hills and valleys of Santa Clarita to the north and east, which are increasingly being overrun with cookie-cutter subdivisions.

After reaching a high point of 2,450 feet, the trail begins to pitch downward, executing a circuitous and sometimes steep descent down drier slopes into the shady depths of Wiley Canyon. Joining a dirt road there (4.0 miles), you turn left and head north, making your way easily down the canyon and passing another tar pit.

At 4.7 miles pass the Canyon View Loop Trail, on the left. You could take this crooked path up over a ridge and back down to the main road, but your easiest option is to continue along the dirt road to your starting point.

---

trip 5.14 **Pico Canyon**

see map on p. 54

Distance	7 miles (out-and-back)
Hiking Time	3.5 hours
Elevation Gain	1,200'
Difficulty	Moderately strenuous
Trail Use	Suitable for mountain biking, dogs allowed
Best Times	October–May
Agencies	Mountains Recreation & Conservation Authority, Santa Monica Mountains Conservancy
Optional Maps	USGS 7.5' *Newhall, Oat Mountain*
Fees/Permits	$5 parking fee at Mentryville trailhead

DIRECTIONS From I-5 in Santa Clarita, take Exit 167 for Pico Canyon Road, and drive west 2.5 miles to the gated entrance to Santa Clarita Woodlands Park (open daily, sunrise–sunset). Park outside for free, or continue 0.4 mile farther to the large pay parking lot/trailhead at the historic site of Mentryville.

Pico Canyon cuts deeply into the northern Santa Susana Mountains, a few miles south of Six Flags Magic Mountain amusement park. The canyon is considered the birthplace of the oil industry in California (ignoring the small-scale use of oil tar as a caulking agent by early Native Americans and missionaries). All of the wells in the canyon are capped today, and the surrounding property has become a part of the publicly accessible Santa Clarita Woodlands Park.

Historic Mentryville is today a gentrified ghost town. A number of structures in this former oil boom town remain intact: an 1890s barn and chicken coop, the 1898 home of oil driller Charles Alexander Mentry, and the Felton schoolhouse built in 1885 to serve more than 100 families residing in the canyon at that time.

From Mentryville, either by foot or by mountain bike, you may travel up the canyon as little as 0.7 mile to the rest stop known as Johnson Park, or as many as 3.5 miles to a canyon-rim perch offering a panoramic view of the entire Santa Clarita region. The former option is fine for an easy stroll anytime; the latter option involves significant effort and elevation gain, whether you go by foot or bike.

As you proceed uphill on the paved road into Pico Canyon from Mentryville, you'll be right alongside the canyon's sluggishly flowing creek. Enjoy the green ribbon of riparian vegetation and trees—mostly live oaks, cottonwood, walnut, and arroyo willows. Natural tar still seeps into the stream, and it isn't unusual to catch a pungent whiff of it on the passing breeze.

At Johnson Park, a former oil-company picnic site with picnic benches and restrooms, don't mistake the wooden oil derrick you'll see there for a historic artifact; it's in fact an accurate replica of an early-20th-century oil rig.

At 1.5 miles up the canyon from Mentryville, two historical plaques indicate the site of the Pico Canyon Oil Field Well Number 4, which was not only California's first commercially successful oil well, but also the longest continuously operating oil well in the world (1876–1990) at the time of its closure. Its yield of 150 barrels of oil per day was modest compared to modern oil wells.

Just beyond, the Pico Canyon service road bends sharply left, turns to dirt, and rises very steeply onto the brushy slope of the canyon, where the view expands to include the looping coaster tracks at Magic Mountain. After many twists and turns, 3.5 miles into the hike, the road ends at a flat spot some 1,200 feet higher than your starting point. Look for a rusty old sign indicating a defunct Union Oil well. Intrepid hikers have forged a sketchy path along the ridgeline connecting this point to the Towsley Canyon unit of the Santa Clarita Woodlands Park, which lies southeast of here. Your easy option, to be sure, is to return along the same route.

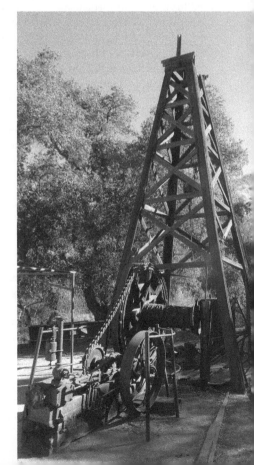

Replica oil rig at Johnson Park

chapter 6

Point Mugu

Mugu, a corruption of the Chumash word *muwu,* meaning "beach," lends its name to a rocky promontory jutting into the ocean, a bald peak towering behind it, and one of the larger state parks in California: 16,000-acre Point Mugu State Park.

Geographically speaking, the Point Mugu area is the last gasp of the Santa Monica Mountains up the coast from Los Angeles. Geologists, however, say that the underpinnings of these mountains really extend as far west as the Channel Islands off Santa Barbara. The intervening low area, occupied by the flat, silty Oxnard Plain and part of the continental shelf offshore, is a structurally huge syncline, or downfold of crustal rocks. Paleontological evidence has shown that for a long period ending 1 or 2 million years ago the islands were linked to the mainland by an isthmus. This ancient feature is named the Cabrillo Peninsula, after the 16th-century explorer Juan Rodríguez Cabrillo, who was buried on the western-most island, San Miguel.

Point Mugu State Park lies entirely outside Los Angeles County's boundary, but because it's an integral and important part of the Santa Monica Mountains National Recreation Area, it merits a chapter in this book. The recreational opportunities here are superb. Almost half of the park's area comprises the Boney Mountain State Wilderness: remote, wild, and open to hikers and equestrians only.

The two principal park entrances—both off Pacific Coast Highway—are Big Sycamore Canyon and the Ray Miller Trailhead at La Jolla Canyon. Big Sycamore Canyon, in particular, is one of the favored areas on the California coast for overwintering Monarch butterflies.

The author hikes in La Jolla Valley with the Boney Mountains in the background.

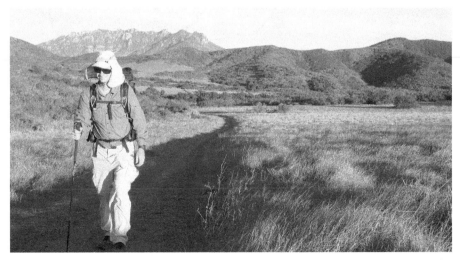

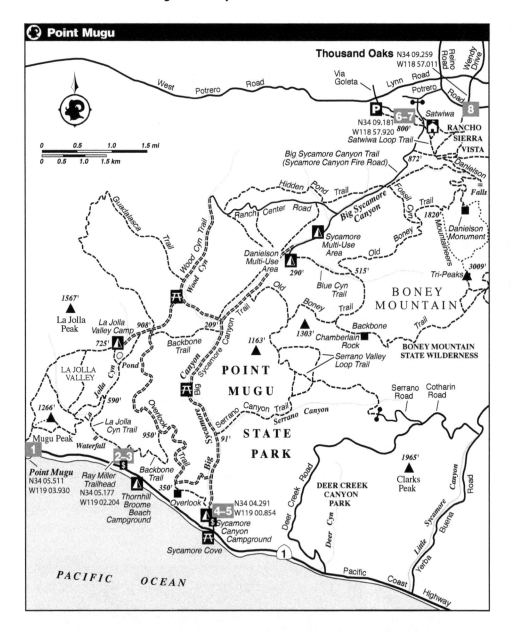

Abutting the north end of the park, next to suburban Newbury Park, is the Rancho Sierra Vista/Satwiwa natural area and cultural park, managed by the National Park Service. In addition to serving as a northern trailhead for the state park (easily accessible from the Ventura Freeway), Rancho Sierra Vista features the Satwiwa Native American Indian Culture Center, where park rangers or Native American hosts offer interpretive programs on the weekends.

With about 100 miles of trails lacing the Point Mugu area, it's possible to devise more than a dozen loop trips significantly different from one another. Six routes are included in this chapter, on trails ranging from paved service roads and graded fire roads to primitive pathways suitable for hikers only. These specific routes are not available for use by mountain bicyclists because they include portions of singletrack trail, which (for the purposes of state park rules) are reserved for hikers and equestrians.

Camping opportunities in the Point Mugu area are plentiful. There are developed campgrounds at Thornhill Broome Beach and Sycamore Canyon (hot showers at the latter). Backpackers can pitch a tent at La Jolla Valley Walk-in Camp, a 2.5-mile hike by the shortest route. Organizations can reserve group-camping facilities at the Danielson and Sycamore Multi-Use Areas.

The 2013 Springs Fire burned 24,000 acres, including 86% of Point Mugu State Park. The fire started along the 101 Freeway in Camarillo. The chaparral recovered quickly, but many of the graceful oaks and sycamores will take decades to regrow. The 2018 Woolsey Fire burned the eastern rim of the park, including much of what the Springs Fire missed along the Chamberlain Trail.

---

trip 6.1   Mugu Peak

Distance	2.0 miles (out-and-back)
Hiking Time	1.5 hours
Elevation Gain	1,250'
Difficulty	Moderate
Best Times	October–June
Agency	California State Parks
Optional Map	Tom Harrison *Point Mugu State Park*

see map opposite

DIRECTIONS From Santa Monica, drive west (up the coast) on Pacific Coast Highway for 36 miles to the large but unsigned Chumash Trailhead parking area on the right (0.4 mile west of mile marker 001 VEN 7.5). This lot is 1.8 miles west of Thornhill Broome State Beach and directly opposite a Navy shooting range.

The steep and sun-baked Chumash Trail up 1,266-foot Mugu Peak at the far west end of Point Mugu State Park draws a steady stream of hikers because it offers a short but intense workout with great ocean views and avoids the substantial parking fees charged elsewhere in the state park. Go on a cool day or be prepared for a sweat-fest.

Lemonade berry, buckwheat, cactus, and other drought-tolerant plants cling to the hillside along the shadeless trail. From March to May, you may see a blooming treelike sunflower called giant coreopsis. You may also hear gunfire, shelling, or explosions from the nearby Point Mugu Naval Air Station or see warplanes dispatched to practice blowing up targets far off shore at San Nicholas Island. After 0.6 mile and 800 feet of climbing, you reach a saddle northwest of Mugu Peak.

To reach the peak, you can jog left and then pick up a very steep use trail going straight up the ridge of the peak. Point Mugu State Park rangers hope to replace this trail with a better one soon. At the summit, you're rewarded by

An American flag flies atop Mugu Peak not far from the naval air station.

a flagpole and great views of the ocean, La Jolla Valley, and the Sandstone Peak area. Return the way you came, taking care on the steep trail.

VARIATION

A better trail descends the southeast ridge of Mugu Peak. You can go down this path and circle back to the saddle at the top of the Chumash Trail. This variation is a mile longer than the direct route.

---

trip 6.2 La Jolla Falls

Distance	1.8 miles (out-and-back)
Hiking Time	1 hour
Elevation Gain	250'
Difficulty	Easy
Trail Use	Good for kids
Best Times	December–June
Agency	California State Parks
Optional Map	Tom Harrison *Point Mugu State Park* or Trails Illustrated *Santa Monica Mountains National Recreation Area (253)*
Fees/Permits	$12 day-use fee

see map on p. 76

NOTES The La Jolla Canyon Trail washed out during storms after the 2013 Springs Fire and remains closed and hazardous at this time of writing, with an anticipated reopening in 2020. When it does reopen, the trail will be rerouted and you will take a spur trail to see the falls. Contact Point Mugu State Park (310-457-8143, parks.ca.gov/pointmugu) for updates.

DIRECTIONS Point Mugu State Park lies some 34 miles west of Santa Monica via Pacific Coast Highway (Highway 1). At mile 001 VEN 5.9, immediately west of Thornhill Broome Beach Campground, turn north onto a poorly marked road and follow it to the end for the Ray Miller Trailhead parking area. If you haven't registered for overnight camping, you'll need to pay your day-use fee here.

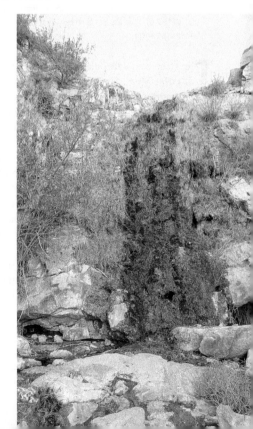

The modest 15-foot-tall cascade in La Jolla Canyon is a pleasant destination for an introductory exploration of Point Mugu State Park. Just be sure to come after recent rains have been sufficient to enliven the flow of water through the canyon.

From the Ray Miller Trailhead, follow the wide La Jolla Canyon Trail north. Your route initially follows a dirt road used to haul stone for the construction of Pacific Coast Highway in the 1920s. After about 0.7 mile, the trail

La Jolla Falls is only a trickle except after recent rains.

passes the quarry site and starts climbing. With a small amount of huffing and puffing, you arrive at the falls. Willows and a native species of walnut tree grace the canyon hereabouts. They're handy if you're looking for some shade.

Beyond the falls, the trail continues sharply uphill toward La Jolla Valley (see next trip)— but you simply turn back at this point, assuming your only destination is the falls.

trip 6.3 La Jolla Valley Loop

Distance	11 miles (loop)
Hiking Time	5.5 hours
Elevation Gain	1,950'
Difficulty	Moderately strenuous
Trail Use	Suitable for backpacking
Best Times	October–June
Agency	California State Parks
Optional Map	Tom Harrison *Point Mugu State Park*
Fees/Permits	$12 day-use fee

see map on p. 76

NOTES The La Jolla Canyon Trail washed out during storms after the 2013 Springs Fire and remains closed and hazardous at this time of writing, with an anticipated reopening in 2020. Contact Point Mugu State Park (310-457-8143, parks.ca.gov/pointmugu) for updates. Until then, you can exit on the Chumash Trail with a 1.8-mile walk, bike, or car shuttle to close the loop.

DIRECTIONS Point Mugu State Park lies some 34 miles west of Santa Monica via Pacific Coast Highway (Highway 1). At mile 001 VEN 5.9, immediately west of the Thornhill Broome Beach Campground, turn north onto a poorly marked road and follow it to the end for the Ray Miller Trailhead parking area. If you haven't registered for overnight camping, pay your day-use fee here.

Lazily curving up the rumpled slopes of the western Santa Monica Mountains, the Ray Miller Trail takes in sweeping views of the Point Mugu coastline and the distant Channel Islands. This is the westernmost link in the Backbone Trail, which skims along the crest of the Santa Monicas for some 67 miles. The Ray Miller Trail offers a well-graded and scenic approach to the rounded ridge that divides the two largest canyons in Point Mugu State Park: La Jolla and Big Sycamore Canyons. The trail was named after California's first official State Park Campground Host, who served here from 1979 until his death in 1989.

The Ray Miller Trail is just the start of the big loop we're suggesting here: a comprehensive trek through the western quadrant of Point Mugu State Park. If this is too big a chunk to bite off for a single day, there are shortcuts, as this chapter's map suggests. You could also extend your trip by staying overnight at La Jolla Valley Walk-in Camp. For that, you must register with a park ranger across the highway at Thornhill Broome Beach Campground.

Start hiking at the Ray Miller Trailhead. Two trails diverge from the parking lot there. The wide one going up along the dry canyon bottom ahead is the La Jolla Canyon Trail—your return route. To begin, take the narrower Ray Miller (aka Backbone) Trail to your right. It doggedly climbs 2.4 miles to a junction with the Overlook Trail, a wide fire road. This is the major ascent along the loop—better to get it over with at the beginning. Ever-widening views of the ocean and fine springtime wildflower displays keep your mind off the effort.

Turn left when you reach the Overlook Trail, and wend your way around several bumps on the undulating ridge. Enjoy the terrific views of Boney Mountain's eroded volcanic core to the east and La Jolla Valley's grassy fields to the west. You arrive at a saddle (4.5 miles

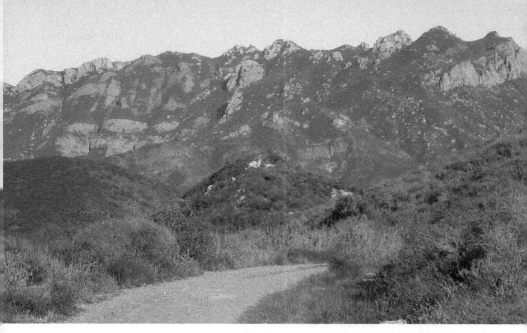

The volcanic crags of the Boney Mountains offer a dramatic backdrop to the La Jolla Valley.

from the start), where five trails diverge. Take the trail to the left (west) that descends into the green- or flaxen-colored (depending on the season) La Jolla Valley.

The valley is managed by the state park as a natural preserve to protect the native bunch-grasses that flourish there. Because so much of California's coast ranges have been biologically disturbed by grazing for more than a century, opportunistic, nonnative grasses have taken over just about everywhere. The authentic California tallgrass prairie in parts of the La Jolla Valley is a notable exception.

The La Jolla Valley Walk-in Camp just ahead has an outhouse and oak-shaded picnic tables, but it no longer has piped water. Just south of here, beside a trail leading directly back to the Ray Miller Trailhead, you'll find a tule-fringed pond, seasonally dry in some years. Look for chocolate lilies on the slopes around it.

From the camp, continue west in the direction of a military radar installation on Laguna Peak. Stay right where marked trails diverge to the left, tracing the perimeter of the La Jolla Valley grassland, and rising sharply on the Chumash Trail to a saddle (7 miles) on the northwest shoulder of the Mugu Peak ridge. At that saddle you'll have a great view of the Pacific Ocean. The popping noises you may hear below are from a military shooting range, near Pacific Coast Highway. Up the coast lies the Point Mugu Naval Air Station.

Beyond the saddle, Chumash Trail descends sharply to Pacific Coast Highway. You veer left on the Mugu Peak Trail, and contour south and east around the south flank of Mugu Peak. (Alternatively, a use trail on the left just before the saddle shortcuts directly to the peak). You arrive (8 miles) at another saddle just east of Mugu's 1,266-foot summit. Five minutes of climbing on a steep path puts you on top, where there's a dizzying view of the east-to-west-oriented coastline. You can look down upon The Great Sand Dune (coastal dunes) and Pacific Coast Highway, where it barely squeezes past some coastal bluffs. On warm days there's a desertlike feel to this rocky and sparsely vegetated mountain, oddly juxtaposed with the sights and sounds of the surf below.

Return to the saddle east of the peak and continue descending to a junction in a wooded recess of La Jolla Canyon. Turn right, proceed east along a hillside, and then hook up with the La Jolla Canyon Trail, where you turn right.

In an exciting stretch down through a rock-walled section of La Jolla Canyon, you'll see magnificent springtime displays of giant coreopsis. This plant is quite common in the Channel Islands but is found only in scattered coastal locales from far western Los Angeles County to San Luis Obispo County. Some coreopsis plants have forked stems towering as high as 10 feet, head and shoulders above the surrounding scrub. The massed, yellow, daisy-like flowers are an unforgettable sight in March and April.

Descending toward the canyon's mouth, you'll pass a little grove of native walnut trees and the small, seasonal La Jolla Canyon waterfall. After a final descent, you'll join an old dirt road that leads straightaway to your starting point, the Ray Miller Trailhead.

trip 6.4   Overlook Loop

see map on p. 76

Distance	2.8 miles (loop)
Hiking Time	1.5 hours
Elevation Gain	500'
Difficulty	Easy
Trail Use	Good for kids
Best Times	Year-round
Agency	California State Parks
Optional Map	Tom Harrison *Point Mugu State Park* or Trails Illustrated *Santa Monica Mountains National Recreation Area (253)*
Fees/Permits	$12 day-use fee

DIRECTIONS From Santa Monica, drive west (up the coast) on Pacific Coast Highway for 32 miles to Sycamore Canyon Campground, on the right, in Point Mugu State Park (at mile 001 VEN 4.3, but no mile marker is nearby). There's a day-use parking lot here.

The Overlook above Sycamore Canyon Campground offers an almost straight-down view of white, foamy surf and turquoise-tinted shallows. When the tide and surf conditions are just right, and the water's glassy, you can watch the swells reflect off the shore and head back out to sea, producing an ever-changing interference pattern on the surface of the water.

A view of the Pacific Ocean and Pacific Coast Highway from the Overlook

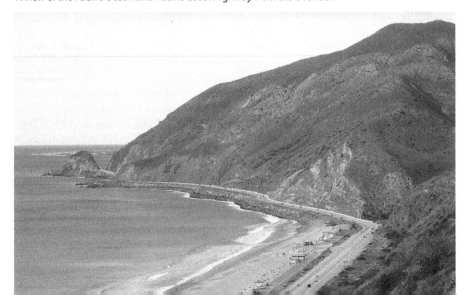

This is an easy loop trip, unlike the much longer one that hikers and mountain bikers often take by linking the entire ridge-running Overlook Trail with trails in Wood and Big Sycamore Canyons. This more leisurely approach will give you time to pay closer attention to the wildflowers and wildlife. Deer frequent these slopes in the early morning and evening. The 2013 Springs Fire incinerated this entire area. Coastal prickly pear cactus survived, and laurel sumac and lemonade berry are among the first shrubs to return.

From the day-use parking lot at Sycamore Canyon Campground, head north up the campground road and past a vehicle gate. Fifty yards past that gate, turn left up the Scenic Trail. You curve up a hillside and arrive after about 15 minutes at a saddle overlooking the ocean. Walk down to a little flat below for a better view. Nestled against the cliff below is a sloping blanket of sand called The Great Sand Dune. Prevailing sea breezes from the west and south keep it in place.

When it's time to go, climb up to join the fire road that curves down the high ridge to the north—the Overlook Trail. Follow its winding course downhill to Big Sycamore Canyon, turn right, and walk back to the campground.

---

trip 6.5   ### Serrano & Big Sycamore Loop

see map on p. 76

Distance	10 miles (loop)
Hiking Time	4.5 hours
Elevation Gain	1,200'
Difficulty	Moderately strenuous
Best Times	October–July
Agency	California State Parks
Optional Map	Tom Harrison *Point Mugu State Park* or Trails Illustrated *Santa Monica Mountains National Recreation Area (253)*
Fees/Permits	$12 day-use fee

DIRECTIONS From Santa Monica, drive west (up the coast) on Pacific Coast Highway for 32 miles to Sycamore Canyon Campground, on the right, in Point Mugu State Park (at mile 001 VEN 4.3, but no mile marker is nearby). There's a day-use parking lot here.

There's something nice about this hike in just about any season. October–December can bring warm, dry winds and fall color—muted yellows and oranges—to the sycamores. During the rainy season, mostly December–March, runoff cascades through the canyon bottoms, and the grasslands come to life. March, April, and May are great for wildflowers—even as the grass bleaches to white and gold. June and July are warm but tolerable under the shade of the spreading oaks in Serrano Canyon, where delicate orange Humboldt lilies sway in the breeze. *Serrano* is a Spanish word for "mountainous" and is an apt word for the region.

Two caveats: bring all the water you'll need and watch out for poison oak, especially in Serrano Canyon. From the day-use parking lot, head north through Sycamore Campground, past the vehicle gate, and up along the wide dirt road (Big Sycamore Canyon Trail) through parklike Big Sycamore Canyon. Proceed to a major fork in the canyon, 1.5 miles from Pacific Coast Highway, and bear right on the Serrano Canyon Trail. After a rather dry, open stretch you enter the steep-walled canyon.

Serrano Canyon is a real treasure—narrow, private, filled with thickets of dark live oaks, pale sycamores, and pungent bay laurels, as well as a green carpet of wild blackberry, ferns, and poison oak. The stream carves its way in a couple of spots through bedrock and gathers in shallow pools. The 2013 Springs Fire burned the lower portion of the canyon and the 2018 Woolsey Fire burned higher on the slopes, but the area remains interesting.

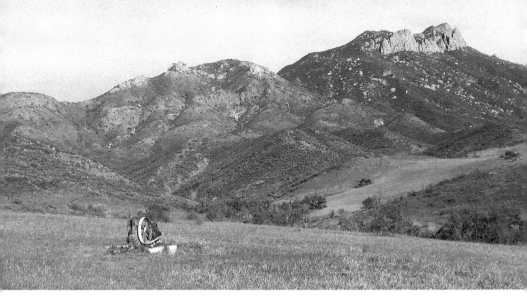

Abandoned farm equipment in the Serrano Valley

At 2.9 miles the Serrano Canyon Trail leaves the canyon, bearing left up a ravine and onto a grassy slope. Stay left at a T-junction marked with a post. The Serrano Valley Loop Trail once curved through the meadow and repeatedly intersected our route, but much has not been restored after the fire as of the time of this writing, and you can simply stay on the clearly defined path until you reach a gap in the ridge above you. At this gap (4.5 miles), you can look down upon a slice of Big Sycamore Canyon. You're now on the far west shoulder of Boney Mountain; eastward the ridge undulates toward its high point at Sandstone Peak. Turn right and follow the trail for another 0.4 mile, up along the ridge and then down a little to meet the Old Boney Trail. Swing left there and go sharply downhill for 1.1 miles to Big Sycamore Canyon Trail.

Four pleasant, easy miles remain in Big Sycamore Canyon. The park's brochure boasts that the canyon is "the finest example of a sycamore savanna in the State Park System." It's true enough. Some of the gangly sycamores soar to heights of about 80 feet. Look for deer, bobcats, and coyotes in the grass and owls and hawks nesting in the trees. If it's fall or early winter, you may see masses of monarch butterflies in some of the trees.

trip 6.6   Sycamore Canyon Waterfall

Distance	3.2 miles (out-and-back)
Hiking Time	2 hours
Elevation Gain	500'
Difficulty	Moderate
Trail Use	Good for kids
Best Times	December–June
Agencies	California State Parks, National Park Service
Optional Map	Tom Harrison *Point Mugu State Park* or Trails Illustrated *Santa Monica Mountains National Recreation Area* (253)

see map on p. 76

DIRECTIONS From Highway 101 in Thousand Oaks, take Exit 45 for Lynn Road. Drive south 5.6 miles on Lynn Road; then turn onto Via Goleta on the left, which leads into Rancho Sierra Vista/Satwiwa. Continue past a gate (open 8 a.m.–sunset) and arrive, after 0.6 mile, at a large trailhead parking area.

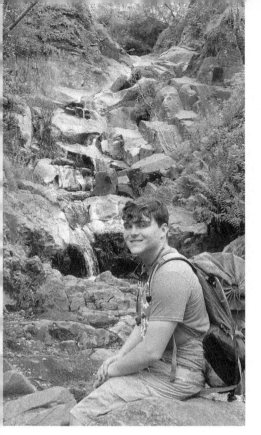

oint Mugu State Park's Big Sycamore Canyon is famous for its miles-long promenade of magnificent California sycamore trees. Higher up and farther inland, hidden in that same drainage, you can find an intimate little waterfall. The falls deliver a melodious whisper most of the year—but try to visit them in the aftermath of recent rainfall, when they play at a larger volume.

From the trailhead, head southeast on an unpaved service road to the paved Big Sycamore Canyon Trail, 0.2 mile away. Jog briefly right, and then veer left on the Satwiwa Loop Trail, bypassing the Satwiwa Native American Culture Center and a Chumash Indian demonstration village (worth a visit on the return leg of your hike). Following signs to the waterfall, aim southeast across a gorgeous meadow, more or less toward the toothy ridgeline called Boney Mountain. You'll pick up Danielson Road, which climbs to a small crest (1.0 mile) and then starts descending into the upper reaches of Big Sycamore Canyon. You're now crossing from Rancho Sierra Vista into Point Mugu State Park.

Sycamore Canyon Falls is a great place to rest for a while.

At the bottom of the grade, your trail swings across the Big Sycamore stream (1.5 miles), and then strikes uphill. Leave the main path and turn left onto the narrow, rough Waterfall Trail. You work your way 0.1 mile upstream to the cascades, which lie in a north-facing grotto almost perpetually shaded from the direct rays of the sun. The falling and flowing water around you is framed by a wild and tangled assortment of oak and sycamore limbs overhead. Given that you've spent only an hour walking in to this spot from the edge of the suburbs, the beauty, serenity, and splendid isolation of the place is a bit hard to believe. Don't get too carried away—rattlesnakes seem to like this cozy corner as well.

---

trip 6.7 **Old Boney Loop**

Distance	11 miles (loop)
Hiking Time	5 hours
Elevation Gain	2,000'
Difficulty	Moderately strenuous
Best Times	November–June
Agencies	California State Parks, National Park Service
Optional Map	Tom Harrison *Point Mugu State Park* or Trails Illustrated *Santa Monica Mountains National Recreation Area* (253)

see map on p. 76

DIRECTIONS From Highway 101 in Thousand Oaks, take Exit 45 for Lynn Road. Drive south 5.6 miles on Lynn Road; then turn onto Via Goleta on the left, which leads into Rancho Sierra Vista/Satwiwa. Continue past a gate (open 8 a.m.–sunset) and arrive, after 0.6 mile, at a large trailhead parking area.

This hike takes you through the heart of the Boney Mountain State Wilderness, which encompasses nearly all the Point Mugu State Park lands east of the Big Sycamore Canyon Trail. As in wilderness areas under federal management (those in the Angeles National Forest and elsewhere), policy here prohibits travel by any mechanical conveyance—even bicycles. Old roads exist from the ranching days, but they are not maintained or improved anymore, except to allow for the passage of hikers and horses.

Boney Mountain, which is the top part of a mass of volcanic rock that solidified roughly 15 million years ago and was later uplifted to its present dominant position, overshadows the area. You'll pass beneath its craggy heights while hiking the Old Boney Trail during the latter part of this trip.

This area is a good place to see spring wildflowers. Hillsides turn golden with masses of California poppies, often interspersed with lupine, morning glory, and desert wishbone bush (with five vivid purple petals and five white stamens). Canyon sunflower, blue dicks, purple nightshade, and fiddlenecks are also plentiful in March, and watchful hikers may identify many other flowers. Spring visitors may find thousands of lizards along the route; side-blotched lizards are especially common and have highly variable coloration but can be recognized by a violet streak just behind the foreleg. Beware of poison oak along the route.

You enter the state park the back way, from Rancho Sierra Vista/Satwiwa. From the trailhead, head southeast on an unpaved service road to the paved Big Sycamore Canyon Trail, 0.2 mile away. Bear right and follow the pavement, passing into Point Mugu State Park and arriving at an 872-foot summit with a bench (0.6 mile). You can now look down on Big Sycamore Canyon and the ribbon of pavement you'll be following for the next 2.8 miles.

Just before the road's end at a ranger residence (3.4 miles), turn left into the Danielson Multi-Use Area, one of two such facilities in the park that cater to organized groups of campers, backpackers, and equestrians. The Danielson facility lies on the grounds of the former Danielson Ranch, which was incorporated into Point Mugu State Park in 1973. There are restrooms and a beautiful, oak-shaded barbecue pit and patio, which is great for a picnic if it's not occupied. Top off your water bottles here with enough to last the rest of the trip.

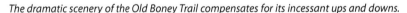

The dramatic scenery of the Old Boney Trail compensates for its incessant ups and downs.

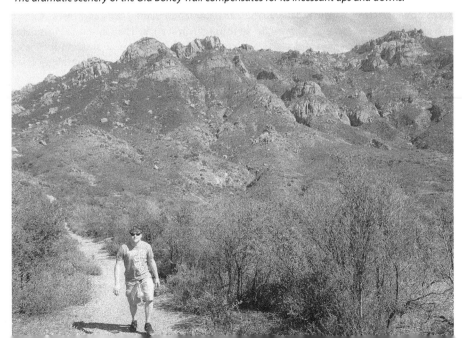

Now the harder part begins. Head east on the Blue Canyon Trail, beneath an oak-and-sycamore canopy, until you reach an intersection with the Old Boney Trail (4.4 miles). Make a sharp left there and trudge uphill through hot, dry chaparral to an open ridge. You'll follow the undulating ridge for a while, under the gaze of Boney Mountain's crags, then climb in earnest to another, higher ridge. You're going against the grain of the land now, and it feels like it. There's a steep descent of about 200 feet and then another climb of about 550 feet to an 1,820-foot summit (7.5 miles). En route you pass the Fossil Trail leading down to Big Sycamore Canyon—stay right. On a clear day all this labor is offset by the tremendous view of the Oxnard Plain, the Channel Islands, the far-off ridges of the Los Padres National Forest, and the discontinuous urban sprawl of Ventura County before you. At the summit, you can take a 0.1-mile spur tunneling through the tall chamise to Hill 1918, with decent views of the surrounding country.

Beyond the 1,820-foot summit, the Old Boney Trail pitches steeply downward, heading toward the uppermost reaches of Big Sycamore Canyon. On the way down, don't miss the side trail on the right, which leads to the Old Cabin Site, consisting of a foundation and a rock chimney. Nearby is a beautiful monument to Richard E. Danielson made of rock and wrought-iron. Danielson and his family donated a part interest in the lands, which were acquired to expand the state park and create the Rancho Sierra Vista/Satwiwa park.

Beyond this point, your trail is known as Danielson Road. By 9 miles you'll be swinging around a hairpin turn that wraps around upper Big Sycamore Canyon's stream. At that turn, a side path (Waterfall Trail; see Trip 6.6, page 83) goes east to some cascades. Don't miss that little detour if the water's flowing decently.

Back on the Old Boney Trail, continue west. Pass several side trails and stay on the main path, eventually crossing a meadow back to the Satwiwa Native American Indian Culture Center, just west of the paved Big Sycamore Canyon Trail and your starting point.

VARIATION

From Hill 1918, you could follow the so-called Mountaineers Route along Boney Mountain's Western Ridge up to the summit of Tri-Peaks (3,009'). Hikers have worn a rough tunnel through the chaparral and up the rocks, but it is slow going because of the steep and rugged terrain. The upper portion burned in the 2018 Woolsey Fire. The summit of Tri-Peaks is a stack of house-size volcanic boulders. You can explore fascinating slots and caves beneath the giant blocks, or make an airy scramble to the highest rock. The Chumash considered Boney Mountain to be a sacred place, a retreat for shamans, and a destination for vision quests. This variation adds 1.5 miles with 1,300 feet of climbing one-way. Consider joining the Backbone Trail or other trails in the area for a longer loop.

| trip 6.8 | **Satwiwa Loop via Wendy Trail** |

Distance	2.4 miles (loop)
Hiking Time	1 hour
Elevation Gain	400'
Difficulty	Easy
Trail Use	Dogs, good for kids
Best Times	October–June
Agency	National Park Service
Optional Map	Tom Harrison *Point Mugu State Park* or Trails Illustrated *Santa Monica Mountains National Recreation Area (253)*

see map on p. 76

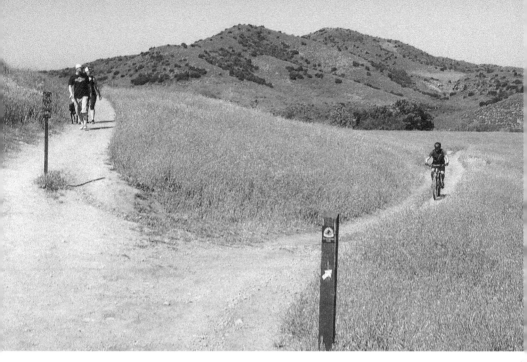

The easygoing Satwiwa Loop draws throngs of springtime visitors.

DIRECTIONS From Highway 101 in Thousand Oaks, take Exit 45 for Lynn Road. Drive south 3.9 miles; then turn left onto Wendy Drive. Wendy Drive ends in 0.6 mile at Potrero Road, where you'll find a large and busy trailhead parking area.

The Rancho Sierra Vista/Satwiwa section of Santa Monica Mountains National Recreation Area features a large meadow noted for spring wildflowers. The area was once a Spanish rancho, and previously was home to the Chumash people, who considered this area sacred. Native peoples have occupied this fertile area for over 10,000 years. This easygoing loop circles the meadow and visits the Satwiwa Native American Indian Culture Center.

Walk through the gate onto the Wendy Trail, which promptly comes to a four-way junction near a seasonal creek. Continue straight across the creek through a grove of oaks. In 0.3 mile turn left onto the Windmill Trail to make a clockwise loop around the valley. Pass the Wendy–Satwiwa Connector on the right; then come to a water tank and old windmill, where you meet the Satwiwa Loop Trail coming up from the meadow. Continue along the edge of the hills, switchbacking up to get views. The chaparral burned in the 2013 Springs Fire. Morning glory vines and purple nightshade are especially plentiful in the new growth. Pass a spur on the left to the Hidden Valley Trail, but descend to meet Danielson Road at 1.2 miles.

Turn right and walk down Danielson briefly to a junction with the Lower Satwiwa Trail (hard right) and Satwiwa Loop Trail (second right). Take the latter trail, which leads across the meadow to the cultural center, where you'll find exhibits and a restroom and drinking fountain (1.6 miles).

When you've seen enough, head east on the Satwiwa Loop Trail for 0.1 mile; then turn left onto a spur that connects to the Wendy Trail, which is a segment of the Juan Bautista de Anza National Historic Trail. Turn right and circle back. At 2.1 miles come to a junction with two parallel paths. For variety, take the left one, which crosses the creek before returning to the junction by the trailhead.

chapter 7

Arroyo Sequit & Sandstone Peak

Toward the western end of the Santa Monica Mountains, the pulse of life slows. Human population is scattered and sparse. People live on little ranches tucked in the canyons, or in modest cottages perched on the hillsides. Some are busy building ostentatious versions of the perfect hilltop dream house, but those are few and far between. Day-trippers and campers come this way to enjoy the ocean, the fresh coastal breezes, and the picturesque, mostly unspoiled backcountry.

The area depicted on this chapter's map, which straddles the Los Angeles–Ventura County line, is dominated by a small stream called Arroyo Sequit. An escarpment stands tall at the northern headwaters of Arroyo Sequit, culminating in a craggy outcrop called Sandstone Peak. At 3,111 feet, it's the highest point in the Santa Monicas. The peak—really an outcrop of volcanic rock that looks like sandstone—is one of several similar-looking summits that make up Boney Mountain, which stretches west into Point Mugu State Park (see the previous chapter).

Much of this area is protected open space, in big chunks of land like Circle X Ranch and Leo Carrillo State Park, and also more modestly sized parcels, like Arroyo Sequit and Charmlee parks. Leo Carrillo State Park (formerly Leo Carrillo State Beach), named after the conservation-minded actor, encompasses a mere 6,000 feet of ocean frontage but 2,000 acres of interior hillsides and canyons.

Readily accessible from either the Ventura Freeway (US 101) to the north or Pacific Coast Highway to the south, the area is a convenient playground for day hikers, campers, and backpackers. Opportunities for camping here (and also in nearby Point Mugu State Park) help make up for the comparative lack of campsites in the eastern Santa Monicas. Leo Carrillo State Park has a campground (with hot showers) along with a hiker-biker annex.

Hiking is generally good year-round immediately next to the coast, where the sea breezes take the heat off the south-facing slopes. Inland, at places like Circle X Ranch, the temperature can climb to 100°F on summer days and drop to well below freezing on calm winter nights.

In addition to hiking, the coastline in and next to Leo Carrillo State Park offers some of the finest beachcombing, surfing, swimming, and sailboarding on the L.A. County coast. At Sequit Point you'll

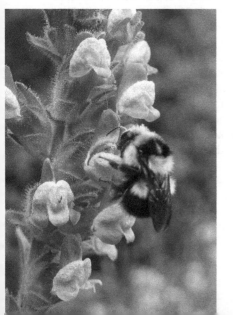

Arroyo Sequit Park (see Trip 7.6, page 97) bursts with spring wildflowers.

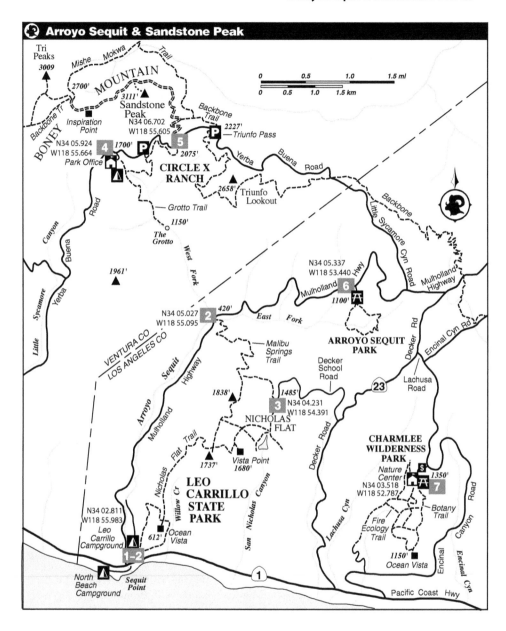

find a jagged stretch of sea bluffs, and rocky pools to explore when the tides are low. Sequit Point is an especially good vantage for spotting gray whales during their winter migrations. Sometimes they can be seen swimming just beyond the surf line.

The trips in this chapter encompass many diverse environments and span 3,000 feet of elevation change—a world in itself that seems quite disconnected from the multimillions of people who live within an hour's drive of the area.

The 2018 Woolsey Fire started near the Santa Susana Field Laboratory and, driven by intense Santa Ana winds, burned across the Santa Monica Mountains all the way to the Pacific. The trails in this chapter were all affected.

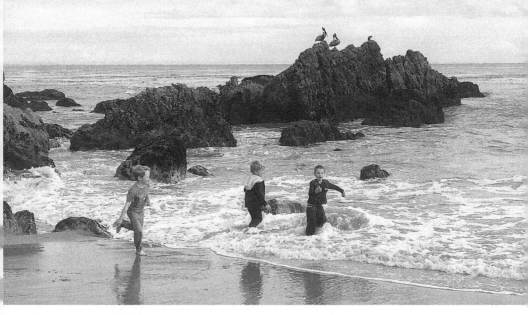

Leo Carrillo State Beach is an excellent place to frolic after hiking nearby.

trip 7.1 Leo Carrillo Ocean Vista

see map on previous page

Distance	2.0 miles (loop)
Hiking Time	1 hour
Elevation Gain	600'
Difficulty	Moderate
Trail Use	Good for kids
Best Times	Year-round
Agency	California State Parks
Optional Map	Tom Harrison *Point Mugu State Park* or Trails Illustrated *Santa Monica Mountains National Recreation Area (253)*
Fees/Permits	$12 day-use fee

DIRECTIONS From Pacific Coast Highway, 27 miles west (up the coast) from Santa Monica near mile 001 LA 62.0, turn north into Leo Carrillo State Park Campground. Day-use parking is available on the left just past the entrance booth; alternatively, look for free parking on the shoulder of the highway outside the campground.

For the modest effort of climbing a 612-foot hill, you can enjoy one of the best ocean views available anywhere in the Santa Monica Mountains. If the morning is fog-free and you're ambitious enough, try to make it to the top in time for sunrise. (The sun rises around 7 a.m. in October, November, and December, so you don't have to lose much sleep, especially if you're camping nearby.) To the sound of booming surf, you can watch the winter sun's golden beams spill over Palos Verdes and glance off the shimmering ocean surface down below. With a pair of binoculars, you might spot whales migrating along the coast. This trip also offers excellent wildflowers in the spring, including prickly lupines, blue dicks, desert wishbone, paintbrush, California poppies, mariposa lilies, morning glories, live-forever, deerweed, and blue and purple sage. Families and surfers enjoy the beach, accessed from the day use parking via an underpass.

Walk back down the park entrance road. Just outside the entrance booth, pick up the signed Camp 13 Trail on the left. Within 0.1 mile come to a signed three-way junction. The

Camp 13 Trail is farthest left, contouring 0.6 mile to the north end of the campground. Our trip uses the other two trails. To make a counterclockwise loop, stay right on the Willow Creek Trail, which slants across a hillside overlooking the highway, then ducks inland along a slope overlooking the V-shaped ravine of Willow Creek. Near the top, you switchback three times and arrive at a four-way junction of trails on a saddle. Turn left and make the short final climb to Ocean Vista.

In addition to the nearby coastline stretching out to Point Dume, you might see the Palos Verdes Peninsula, Santa Catalina Island, and several of the other Channel Islands off Ventura and Santa Barbara. In the north, the toothy crest of Boney Mountain barely peeks over a rounded ridge opposite the Arroyo Sequit. Below, in the west, you'll look down on the sycamore-dotted Leo Carrillo Campground, stretching for almost half a mile along a flat terrace just above Arroyo Sequit's parched bed.

When it's time to go, return to the four-way junction. Take the left branch this time, returning by way of the lower Nicholas Flat Trail.

---

trip 7.2   ## Leo Carrillo Traverse

see map on p. 89

Distance	5.5 miles (one-way)
Hiking Time	3 hours
Elevation Gain/Loss	1,600'/2,000'
Difficulty	Moderately strenuous
Best Times	October–June
Agency	California State Parks
Optional Map	Tom Harrison *Point Mugu State Park* or Trails Illustrated *Santa Monica Mountains National Recreation Area (253)*
Fees/Permits	$12 day-use fee

DIRECTIONS This trip, which requires a shuttle, starts on Mulholland Highway and ends at the entrance to Leo Carrillo State Park Campground. The campground is 27 miles west (up the coast) from Santa Monica on the Pacific Coast Highway (Highway 1) near mile 001 LA 62.0.

Leave one vehicle near the campground entrance—either pay the day-use fee and park at the lot on the left just past the entrance station, or look for parking along Pacific Coast Highway. Then continue west on the PCH and immediately turn right onto Mulholland Highway. Go 3.2 miles north to the signed Malibu Springs Trail on the right. This shuttle can also be done with a bicycle.

This one-way hike goes from the confluence of Arroyo Sequit's East and West Forks to Leo Carrillo State Park Campground—the hard way. Mulholland Highway is the easy way. The trail is lightly maintained and was partially overgrown with mustard and thistle when I visited. Long pants and sleeves are advisable. It has many poorly marked junctions; stay right at all of them. The spring wildflowers are impressive and this is a particularly good trail to spot elusive mariposa lilies.

Keep your eyes open as you hike—this Southern Pacific rattler was coiled just feet from the trail.

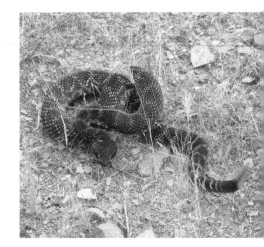

From the Malibu Springs Trailhead on Mulholland Highway, an abandoned bed—now a marked hiking trail—slants up the slope to the south. In essence, you go up and over Arroyo Sequit's east ridge, starting out in oak woodland and chaparral, and ending in coastal sage-scrub vegetation as you approach the ocean. The value of an early-morning start will be apparent as you begin with a bang: 1,400 feet of ascent in 2 miles. On the way up, you swing around several hairpin turns, discovering ever-more-impressive vistas of Boney Mountain and the deep crease in the mountains below it—Arroyo Sequit's West Fork. In the north you'll spot the Triunfo Lookout site, now occupied by a huge, boxy structure serving as a passive reflector for microwave transmissions. Down in the valley to the east are the big, white "ears" of a satellite tracking station.

In 1.8 miles, 200 vertical feet below the top of the ridge, pass a trail that forks left and contours eastward. Take it only if you want to extend your hike by circling around to visit Nicholas Flat. This junction also marks the spot where you leave National Park Service land (Malibu Springs open-space area) and enter Leo Carrillo State Park property.

At an obscure T-junction by Nicholas Flat in another 0.7 mile, jog right and then soon continue south along the Ridge Line Trail. The 1,838-foot summit ahead is the highest point on the brushy ridge, but you'll have better ocean views ahead. Over the next half mile, pass two more trails on the left also leading to Nicholas Flat; then immediately reach a saddle where the Lower Nicholas Flat Trail descends to the right. A firebreak continues south to a 1,737-foot knoll. Detour to the top for the best ocean and coastline view of all; then return to the saddle.

The final bone-jarring descent to Leo Carrillo Campground features almost 1,700 feet of elevation loss in 2.4 miles. A mile from the end, you have a choice: go left down along Willow Creek, or right down the slope overlooking the campground. Both paths are scenic and about equally direct.

trip 7.3 Nicholas Pond

Distance	1.2 miles (out-and-back)
Hiking Time	1 hour
Elevation Gain	100'
Difficulty	Easy
Trail Use	Good for kids
Best Times	Year-round
Agency	California State Parks
Optional Map	Tom Harrison *Point Mugu State Park* or Trails Illustrated *Santa Monica Mountains National Recreation Area (253)*

see map on p. 89

DIRECTIONS From Pacific Coast Highway, at a point 25 miles west of Santa Monica, turn north on Decker Road (Highway 23). Continue 2.5 miles north and turn west on Decker School Road. Proceed 1.7 miles to the road's end, where you'll find the Nicholas Pond Trailhead.

Nicholas Flat harbors a small oasis of live oaks and an old cattle pond backed by picturesque sandstone outcrops. During the spring, the grassy meadows above the pond may put on an eye-popping wildflower show. Because so many plant communities converge in this one area—coastal sage scrub, grassland, chaparral, and oak woodland—Nicholas Flat is a good bet for bird- and wildlife-watching too.

From the trailhead, a pleasant, oak-lined path leads south along a wooded creekbed. Stay on the broad main path as it veers right and crosses a bridge, then turns left again. You will soon arrive at the pond, where a bench flanked by coast live oaks makes an excellent

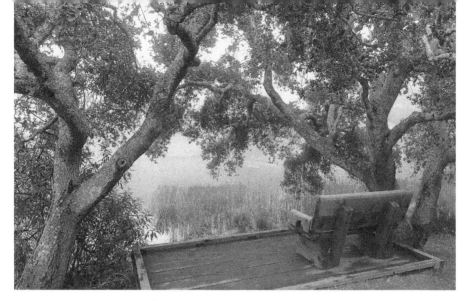

Nicholas Pond is a prime wildlife-watching spot.

place to sit and watch wildlife. In wetter times, the pond brims with water, while in drought years it can turn bone-dry by late summer, with gaping cracks up to 2 feet deep in the adobe mud at the bottom. This is the turnaround point for the short hike.

Numerous lightly maintained trails criss-cross the old ranch land of Nicholas Flat. When I visited, they were partially overgrown with mustard and thistle, but still possible to follow. If you have time to explore, you can make a 3-mile ramble wandering these paths. Amid the oaks you can look for a bedrock metate (grinding slick), where the native Americans of the Chumash tribe milled acorns. Unless you've set up a shuttle, take care not to inadvertently descend to Leo Carrillo State Park or the Malibu Springs Trail, lest you have a strenuous walk back up.

trip 7.4   The Grotto

Distance	2.6 miles (out-and-back)
Hiking Time	1.5 hours
Elevation Gain	500'
Difficulty	Moderate
Trail Use	Dogs allowed, good for kids
Best Times	Year-round
Agency	National Park Service
Optional Map	Tom Harrison *Point Mugu State Park* or Trails Illustrated *Santa Monica Mountains National Recreation Area (253)*

see map on p. 89

DIRECTIONS The Circle X Ranch Ranger Station is located near the western end of the Santa Monica Mountains, a few miles (by crow's flight) south of Thousand Oaks. From the Pacific Coast Highway near mile marker 1 VEN 1.00, turn north onto Yerba Buena Road and proceed 5.4 miles. Or from Highway 101 in Thousand Oaks, take Highway 23 south for 7.2 miles. Turn right (west) on Mulholland Highway; then, in 0.4 mile, turn right again onto Little Sycamore Canyon Road, which soon becomes Yerba Buena Road and reaches the trailhead in 5.5 miles. On either approach, you face a white-knuckle drive on paved but very narrow and curvy roads. You may park at the ranger station or drive 0.1 mile down a dirt road behind the ranger station to signed day-use parking. The trailhead is 0.1 mile farther down at the bottom of the road, beside Circle X Ranch Group Campground (camping by reservation only).

The 1,655-acre Circle X Ranch, formerly run by the Boy Scouts of America but now administered by the National Park Service, is positively riddled with Tom Sawyer–esque hiking paths. The Grotto and Mishe Mokwa Trails (see the next trip for the latter) are among the most interesting in the whole Santa Monica Mountain range.

From the park office, start off on a dirt road leading downhill some 100 yards toward a group campground. Walk through or skirt the campsites, and pick up a trail heading south down along a shady, seasonal creek. Keep heading downhill as you pass, in quick succession, two trails coming in from the left. Very shortly afterward, you cross the creek at a point immediately above a 30-foot ledge that becomes a trickling waterfall in winter and spring. You then go uphill, gaining about 50 feet of elevation, and cross an open meadow

Scrambling at The Grotto is great fun for young hikers.

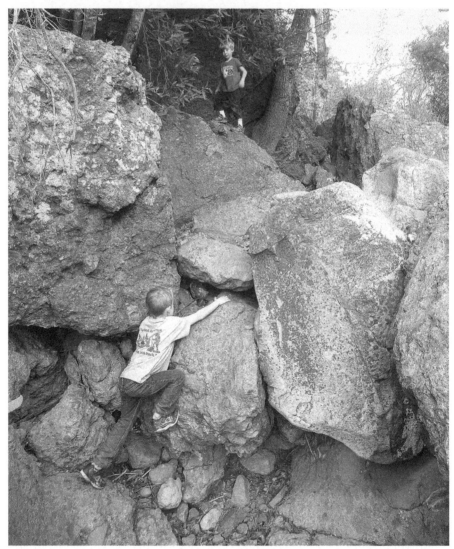

offering fine views of both Boney Mountain above and Arroyo Sequit's West Fork gorge below. Next you begin a steep descent leading to the bottom of the gorge.

When you come upon an old roadbed at the bottom, stay left, cross the creek, and continue downstream on a narrowing trail along the shaded east bank. Curve left when you reach a grove of fantastically twisted live oaks at the confluence of two stream forks. On the edge of this grove, an overflow pipe coming out of a tank discharges tepid spring water. (From this point on, dogs are prohibited on the "trail," which is actually the streambed itself.) Continue another 200 yards down along the now-lively brook to the trail's abrupt end at The Grotto, a narrow, spooky constriction flanked by sheer volcanic-rock walls. If your sense of balance is good and your footwear is appropriate, you can clamber over gray-colored rock ledges and massive boulders that have fallen from the canyon walls—just as thousands of Boy Scouts have done in the past. At one spot you can peer cautiously into a gloomy cavern, where the subterranean stream is more easily heard than seen. Water marks on the boulders above are evidence that this part of the gorge probably supports a two-tier stream in times of flood.

When you've had your fill of adventuring, return by the same route, uphill almost the whole way.

trip 7.5   Sandstone Peak

Distance	6 miles (loop)
Hiking Time	3.5 hours
Elevation Gain	1,700'
Difficulty	Moderately strenuous
Trail Use	Dogs allowed
Best Times	October–June
Agency	National Park Service
Optional Map	Tom Harrison *Point Mugu State Park* or Trails Illustrated *Santa Monica Mountains National Recreation Area (253)*

see map on p. 89

DIRECTIONS From Pacific Coast Highway near mile marker 1 VEN 1.00, turn north onto Yerba Buena Road and proceed 6.4 miles to the Mishe Mokwa/Backbone Trailhead. Or from Highway 101 in Thousand Oaks, take Highway 23 south for 7.2 miles. Turn right (west) on Mulholland Highway; then, in 0.4 mile, turn right again onto Little Sycamore Canyon, which soon becomes Yerba Buena Road and reaches the trailhead in 4.5 miles. On either approach, you face a white-knuckle drive on paved but very narrow and curvy roads.

Sandstone Peak is the quintessential destination for peak baggers in the Santa Monica Mountains. The 3,111-foot summit can be efficiently climbed from the east via the Backbone Trail in a mere 1.5 miles, but the far more scenic way to go is the looping route outlined below. Take a picnic lunch and plan to make a half day of it. Try to come on a crystalline day in late fall or winter to take best advantage of the skyline views. Or, if it's wildflowers you most enjoy, come in April or May, when the native vegetation blooms best at these middle elevations. In addition to blue-flowering stands of ceanothus, the early-to-mid-spring bloom includes monkey flower, nightshade, Chinese houses, wild peony, wild hyacinth, morning glory, and phacelia. Delicate, orangish Humboldt lilies unfold by June. Beware of poison oak growing alongside the trail. Sandstone Peak lies within Circle X Ranch, formerly owned by the Boy Scouts of America and now a federally managed unit of Santa Monica Mountains National Recreation Area.

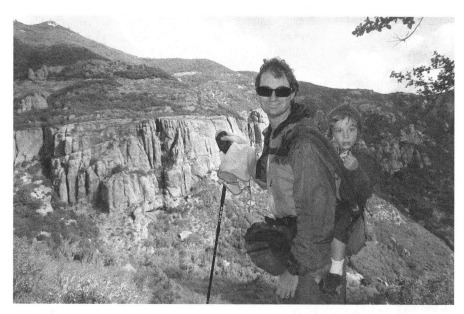

My young son enjoyed riding in an Ergo carrier as we hiked the Mishe Mikwa Trail. In the background, the Echo Cliffs are a popular sport-climbing destination.

From the trailhead, hike past a gate and up a fire road 0.3 mile to where the marked Mishe Mokwa Trail branches right. On this trail, you plunge right away into tough, scratchy chaparral vegetation. The hand-tooled route is delightfully primitive but requires frequent maintenance to keep the chaparral from knitting together across the path. Both your hands and your feet will come into play over the next 40 or 50 minutes as you're forced to scramble a bit over rough-textured outcrops of volcanic rock. You'll make intimate acquaintance with mosses and ferns and several of the more attractive chaparral shrubs: toyon, hollyleaf cherry, manzanita, and red shanks (aka ribbonwood), which is identified by its wispy foliage and perpetually peeling, rust-colored bark. You'll also pass several small bay trees. After about a half hour on the Mishe Mokwa Trail, keep an eye out for an amazing balanced rock that rests precariously on the opposite wall of the canyon that lies just below you.

By 1.7 miles from the start, you'll have worked your way around to the north flank of Sandstone Peak, where you suddenly come upon a couple of picnic tables shaded beneath glorious oaks beside Split Rock, a fractured volcanic boulder with a gap wide enough to walk through (please do so to maintain the Scouts' tradition). An unmaintained trail on the right leads to Balanced Rock—continue on the vestiges of an old dirt road that crosses the aforementioned canyon and turns west (upstream). Pass beneath hefty volcanic outcrops and, at 3.1 miles, come to a signed junction with the Backbone Trail toward Tri-Peaks. Pass water tanks on the right and an unsigned service road leading to them. Shortly thereafter, a sign on the right indicates a side trail to Inspiration Point, which takes you about 50 yards to the top of a rock outcrop. The direction finder there indicates local features as well as distant points such as Mount San Antonio, Santa Catalina Island, and San Clemente Island.

Press on with your ascent. At a point just past two closely spaced hairpin turns in the wide Backbone Trail, make your way up a slippery path to Sandstone Peak's windswept top, the highest point in the Santa Monica Mountains. The plaque on the summit block honors W. Herbert Allen, a longtime benefactor of the Scouts and Circle X Ranch. To the

Scouts this mountain is Mount Allen, although that name has not, so far, been accepted by cartographers. In any event, the peak's real name is misleading. It, along with Boney Mountain and most of the western crest of the Santa Monicas, consists of beige- and rust-colored volcanic rock, not unlike sandstone when seen from a distance.

On a clear day the view is truly amazing from here, with distant mountain ranges, the hazy L.A. Basin, and the island-dimpled surface of the ocean occupying all 360° of the horizon. To complete the loop, return to the Backbone Trail and resume your travel eastward. 1.5 miles of twisting descent will take you back to the trailhead.

VARIATION

You can make an interesting detour to Tri-Peaks by turning right onto the Backbone Trail, then right again onto the Tri-Peaks Trail in a few yards. In 0.3 mile turn right yet again on a spur to Tri-Peaks. The summit of Tri-Peaks is a stack of house-size volcanic boulders. You can explore fascinating slots and caves beneath the giant blocks, or make an airy scramble to the highest rock. This variation adds 1 mile and 400 feet of climbing, round-trip.

---

trip 7.6	**Arroyo Sequit Park**

Distance	2.0 miles (loop)
Hiking Time	1 hour
Elevation Gain	400'
Difficulty	Easy
Trail Use	Dogs allowed, good for kids
Best Times	November–June
Agency	National Park Service
Optional Map	Tom Harrison *Point Mugu State Park* or Trails Illustrated *Santa Monica Mountains National Recreation Area (253)*

see map on p. 89

NOTES This area burned in the 2018 Woolsey Fire and is closed at the time of this writing. Check with the National Park Service (805-370-2301, nps.gov/samo) for updates.

DIRECTIONS From the 101 Freeway, take the Westlake Boulevard (Highway 23) exit in Thousand Oaks. Turn south on Highway 23, and drive 5 miles south to Mulholland Highway, where you turn right. Watch the roadside mileage markers, and drive to mile 5.6 to reach Arroyo Sequit Park, on the left at 34138 Mulholland Highway. Turn left and park in the small lot, which is open daily, 8 a.m.– sunset. This trailhead can also be reached from the south via Pacific Coast Highway by driving 5.6 miles up Mulholland.

Diminutive Arroyo Sequit Park, a 155-acre former ranch that is now a unit of the Santa Monica Mountains National Recreation Area, is a bit hidden in one of the more remote parts of the mountains between Malibu and Thousand Oaks. This patch of land appears drab and dry at least half the year, but winter rains can transform it instantly into an

*Arroyo Sequit Park showcases a tremendous variety of spring wildflowers, including this striking purple sage (*Salvia leucophylla).

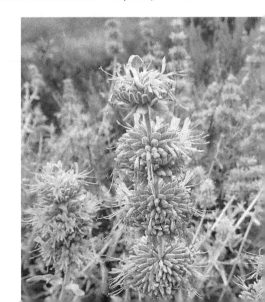

emerald paradise. Bring the kids here for a little hiking, picnicking, wildflower hunting, or bird-watching. It's entirely possible to visit the site on a weekday and see no one else on the trail. The trail is undermaintained and can be brushy at times, so long pants are advisable.

Arroyo Sequit is named for Rancho Topanga Malibu Sequit, a 13,316-acre Spanish land grant made to José Bartolomé Tapia in 1804.

Pass through a gate and walk up the paved access road into the park. In 0.2 mile the road veers left and becomes gravel. Continue 0.2 mile to the signed nature trail on the right. On this trail, you'll circle to the rim of a little canyon (an upper tributary of the stream called Arroyo Sequit), where you can catch an outstanding view of Boney Mountain, the highest promontory in the Santa Monica range, then descend and visit the creek. As you climb back out, you'll reach an odd sign at a T-junction indicating the end of the nature trail. The short spur to the left leads to Bardman Avenue, but this trip turns right and returns to a grassy field by the ranch house. From there, take the paved road back to the trailhead.

trip 7.7   Charmlee Wilderness Park

Distance	2.4 miles (loop)
Hiking Time	1.5 hours
Elevation Gain	400'
Difficulty	Easy
Trail Use	Suitable for mountain biking, equestrians, dogs allowed, good for kids
Best Times	Year-round
Agencies	City of Malibu
Optional Map	Tom Harrison *Point Mugu State Park* or Trails Illustrated *Santa Monica Mountains National Recreation Area (253)*
Fees/Permits	$4 parking fee

see map on p. 89

NOTES Charmlee Wilderness Park burned in the 2018 Woolsey Fire and is closed at the time of this writing. Call 310-456-2489 or check tinyurl.com/charmleewildernesspark for updates.

DIRECTIONS To reach Charmlee Wilderness Park from Santa Monica, drive 25 miles west on Pacific Coast Highway (Highway 1) to a point 0.5 mile west of mile marker 001 LA 59.0. Turn north on Encinal Canyon Road, and proceed 4 miles to the park's well-marked entrance. Gates are open daily, 8 a.m.–sunset. Pay the parking fee at the iron ranger.

Charmlee Wilderness Park, 590 acres of meadow, oak woodland, sage scrub, and chaparral, was first opened to the public in 1981 as a unit of the Los Angeles County park system. Today the City of Malibu administers the park, which lies on that coastal city's western extremity. Never designed to accommodate a large number of visitors, Charmlee's parking lot is often full on the weekends. A spiderweb of trails totaling 8 miles covers the park, making it a great place to ramble with family and friends for the purpose of wildflower spotting in spring, and ocean watching on any clear day. Here's one option to follow on foot.

From the parking lot, walk on pavement to the nature center (if it's open, pick up a guide for the interpretive signposts). Head uphill on a paved road, soon dirt, that bends north up a slope. Make a sharp left turn at the top by a gate, and then follow Potrero Road along the ridge past a hilltop water tank. Boney Mountain, the eroded core of an old volcano, stands prominently on the crest of the Santa Monicas. Curve left at a junction and head east to meet Carmichael Road. From here, consider a short detour left (south) to visit the foundation of an old ranch home in the oaks on a hilltop overlooking the meadow.

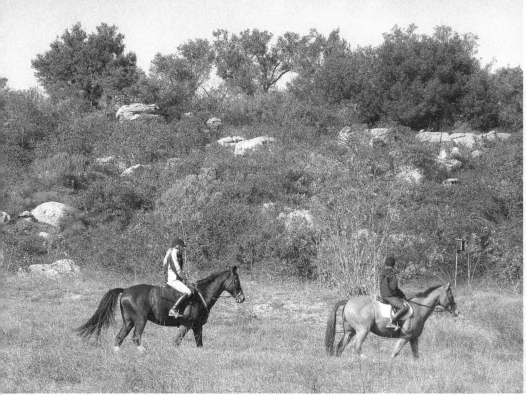

Equestrians enjoyed Charmlee Wilderness Park before the 2018 Woolsey Fire.

Resuming your walk, continue down Potrero Road to the edge of the park's large central meadow, where the road turns left and crosses the meadow. Continue all the way to a dry ridge topped by some old eucalyptus trees and a concrete-lined cistern, both relics of cattle-ranching days. From there descend to the southeast, making a broad switchback. Pass a connector trail on the left, and then make a right onto a short spur leading to the Ocean Vista, which delivers in a big way what its name suggests.

In addition to miles of surf and sand seemingly at your feet, your eyes drink in perhaps a thousand square miles of wind-ruffled ocean. At least six Channel Islands can be identified if the ocean is free of haze. To the west, the small island is Anacapa, with the mountainous Santa Cruz Island looming behind. As your eyes roam left, the low ridge of San Nicholas Island might be glimpsed far out to sea. This island inspired the famous children's book *Island of the Blue Dolphins,* based on the true story of Juana Maria, a Nicoleño Indian girl who survived there alone for 18 years after being stranded when her tribe fled. Closer in, Santa Barbara Island rises from the sea like a broken tooth. Continuing left, look for the low form of San Clemente Island, now a Navy firing range, behind the large Catalina Island. Continuing your panoramic sweep to the left, look for the Palos Verdes hills, the Santa Monica Bay, and Point Dume.

Circle north from Ocean Vista, passing the unsigned connector trail on the left. Watch for a charming oak-shaded glade on the right, where boulders tempt you to stop and sit a bit. Just beyond, pass the East Meadow Cutoff Trail on the left and continue straight on the East Meadow Trail. At the next junction, stay straight onto the Botany Trail and follow it into the woods. The trail ends at a shady picnic area near the parking lot. If it's a spring day and you've kept a tally of wildflowers spotted on the hike, you may be surprised to find that your list includes as many as two dozen or more.

chapter 8

Zuma Canyon

Although it slices only 6 miles inland from the Pacific shoreline near Point Dume, Zuma Canyon harbors one of the deepest gorges in the Santa Monica Mountains. Easily on par with Malibu and Topanga Canyons when it comes to scenic wealth, Zuma Canyon holds the additional distinction of never having suffered the invasion of a major road.

Ongoing acquisitions of open space in Zuma Canyon and neighboring Trancas Canyon to the west by the National Park Service are serving two goals relevant to the desires of hikers. First, there's public access to lower Zuma Canyon—gateway to the most wild and isolated stretch of canyon bottom in the Santa Monicas. Second, the final segment of the Santa Monica Mountains Backbone Trail was completed in 2016 across the uppermost reaches of Zuma and Trancas Canyons (see Trip 33.4, page 449).

The trips in this chapter visit two hiking routes in lower Zuma Canyon; descend toward upper Zuma Canyon, past a couple of waterfalls in Newton Canyon; and ramble through nearby Rocky Oaks Park, a pleasant spot for picnics, wildflower hunting, and bird-watching.

The 2018 Woolsey Fire started near the Santa Susana Field Laboratory and, driven by intense Santa Ana winds, burned across the Santa Monica Mountains all the way to the Pacific. Most of the trails in this chapter were affected.

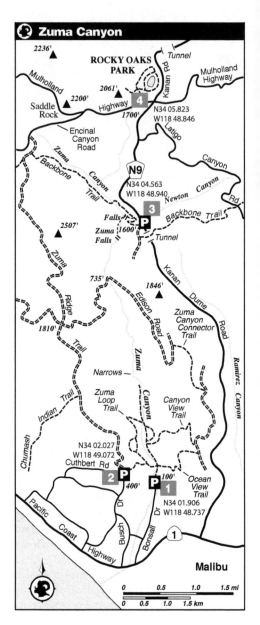

Zuma Canyon

100

trip 8.1   ## Lower Zuma Canyon

Distance	2.8 miles (out-and-back)
Hiking Time	1.5 hours
Elevation Gain	100'
Difficulty	Easy
Trail Use	Dogs allowed, good for kids
Best Times	Year-round
Agency	National Park Service
Optional Map	Tom Harrison *Zuma–Trancas Canyons* or Trails Illustrated *Santa Monica Mountains National Recreation Area (253)*

DIRECTIONS From the intersection of Kanan Dume Road and Pacific Coast Highway at mile marker 001 LA 54.00, go 0.9 mile west on the PCH; then turn north on Bonsall Drive. Follow Bonsall for 1.1 miles to the dirt Zuma Canyon parking lot at its end. There's free day-use parking here.

The wide mouth of Zuma Canyon offers a small network of riding and hiking trails, and plenty of space to wander along the gravelly bed of the canyon's small creek. For starters, try this easy walk.

From the end of Bonsall Drive, walk past a gate and into the sycamore-dotted flood plain ahead. When you reach trails branching left and right after about 0.2 mile, keep straight and follow along the winter-wet, summer-dry creek, crossing it several times in the next mile. You'll pass statuesque sycamores, tall laurel sumac bushes, and scattered wildflowers in season. This is a promising area for spotting wildlife anytime—squirrels, rabbits, and coyotes are commonly seen, deer and bobcats less so.

After about a mile, the canyon walls close in tighter, oaks appear in greater numbers, and you'll notice a small grove of eucalyptus trees across the creek on a little terrace. A short while later, the trail abruptly ends at a pile of sandstone boulders. During the dry months, surface water may get only this far down the canyon. Usually, however, the water trickles or tumbles past here, disappearing at some point downstream into the porous substrate of the canyon floor. Farther travel through the V-shaped canyon ahead is possible only by rock-hopping (see next trip), so this is a good spot to turn around.

VARIATION

On your return, if you want more exercise, you can follow either the Zuma Loop Trail going up along Zuma Canyon's west slope (an extra 0.4 mile and 200' compared with going straight back), or the loop consisting of the Canyon View and Ocean View Trails going high up on the canyon's east slope (an extra 2.3 miles and 800').

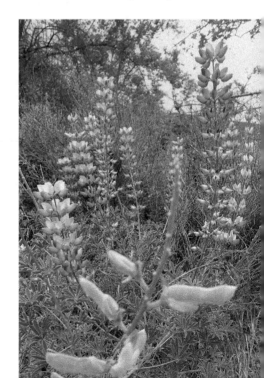

Lupine, a member of the pea family, produces pods after blooming. Some species have edible beans, but others contain toxic alkaloids.

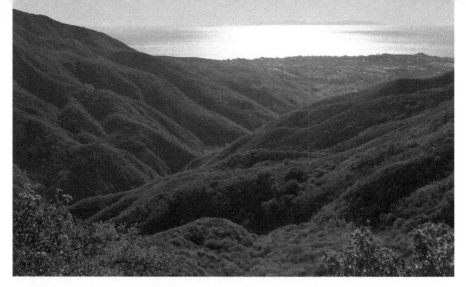

Looking down Zuma Canyon to the Pacific Ocean

trip 8.2 Zuma Canyon & Zuma Ridge Loop

Distance	8 miles (loop)
Hiking Time	6 hours
Elevation Gain	1,700'
Difficulty	Strenuous
Trail Use	Dogs allowed
Best Times	October–June
Agency	National Park Service
Optional Map	Tom Harrison *Zuma–Trancas Canyons* or Trails Illustrated *Santa Monica Mountains National Recreation Area (253)*

see map on p. 100

DIRECTIONS From the intersection of Kanan Dume Road and Pacific Coast Highway at mile marker 001 LA 54.00, go 1.1 miles west on the PCH; then turn north on Busch Drive. Follow Busch 1.4 miles uphill to its end at the dirt Zuma Ridge Trailhead parking area.

Squeezed between walls soaring 1,500 feet or more, the green riparian strip along the bottom of Zuma Canyon's midsection lies undisturbed (save for the crossing of a single dirt road built to provide access to electrical towers). Under cover of junglelike growths of willow, sycamore, oak, and bay, the canyon's small stream cascades over sculpted sandstone boulders and gathers in limpid pools adorned with ferns. These natural treasures yield their secrets begrudgingly, as they should, only to those willing to scramble over boulders, plow through sucking mud and cattails, and thrash through scratchy undergrowth.

Zuma Canyon is passable all the way to the bottom of a 25-foot waterfall just above Newton Canyon. For variety, however, we'll route you part of the way up the canyon and then back on the Edison power-line road and the Zuma Ridge Trail (a fire road). The roads are shadeless, but they offer great vistas of the canyon and the ocean.

Hiking the canyon bottom is least problematic in the fall season before the heavy rains set in. The stream may have shrunk to isolated pools by then, and you'll step mostly on dry rocks with good traction. Winter flooding can render the canyon impassable, but such episodes are rare and short-lived. During spring, the stream flows heartily and there's plenty of greenery and wildflowers; at the same time there's an increased threat of exposure to poison oak (which is found in fair abundance along the banks) and you're more likely to surprise a rattlesnake. Summer days are usually too oppressively warm and humid for such a difficult hike. Whatever the season, take along plenty of water; the water in the canyon is not potable. Expect to get your feet wet, and bring sandals or a change of socks.

From the Busch Drive parking lot, take the Ridge–Canyon Access Trail across the hillside to the east. You lose about 300 feet of elevation as you zigzag down to the flat flood plain at the mouth of Zuma Canyon.

When you reach the bottom in 0.4 mile, bypass the Zuma Loop Trail on the left and go a little farther to the main Zuma Canyon Trail. Turn left there and walk up along Zuma's creek bed for about a mile, passing various trails branching out of the canyon bottom. When the trail ends at a pile of sandstone boulders, you begin a 2-mile stretch of boulder-hopping, 2 or 3 hours' worth depending on the conditions. Other than a few rusting pieces of pipeline from an old dam and irrigation system at the lower end, you may find that the canyon is completely litter-free; please keep it that way.

The great variety of rocks that have been washed down the stream or fallen from the canyon walls says a lot about the geologic complexity of the Santa Monicas. You'll scramble over fine-grained siltstones and sandstones, conglomerates that look like poorly mixed aggregate concrete, and volcanic rocks of the sort that make up Saddle Rock (a local landmark near the head of Zuma Canyon) and the Goat Buttes of Malibu Creek State Park. Some of the larger boulders attain the dimensions of midsize trucks, presenting an obstacle course that must be negotiated by moderate hand-and-foot climbing.

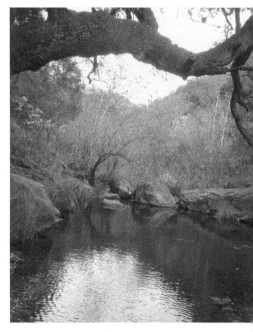

You may wade peaceful pools while hiking up Zuma Creek.

In 1.3 miles you'll pass directly under a set of high-voltage transmission lines—so high that they're hard to spot. These lines, plus the service road built to give access to the towers, represent the major incursion of civilization into Zuma Canyon. If you can ignore them, however, it's easy to imagine what all the large canyons in the Santa Monicas were like only a century ago.

When you finally reach the Edison powerline road, more scrambling and bushwhacking could potentially take you all the way to Kanan Road via Newton Canyon. Going our way, however, you turn left and climb up the twisting service road 2 miles to the top of the west ridge. From there, the Zuma Ridge Trail, a fire road, takes you 2.6 miles back down to the starting point at the end of Busch Drive. On a fine day, you can see all the way to San Jacinto, Santiago Peak, the Palos Verdes Hills, and Catalina, San Clemente, Anacapa, and Santa Cruz Islands.

VARIATION

The Zuma Ridge Trail is a popular exercise route, with a vigorous climb and great ocean views. It's 6 miles one-way to Encinal Canyon Road, although most hikers are satisfied to turn around short of there.

trip 8.3	**Newton Canyon**

see map on p. 100

Distance	0.8 mile (out-and-back)
Hiking Time	1 hour
Elevation Gain	150'
Difficulty	Easy
Trail Use	Dogs allowed, good for kids
Best Times	Year-round
Agency	National Park Service
Optional Map	Tom Harrison *Zuma–Trancas Canyons* or Trails Illustrated *Santa Monica Mountains National Recreation Area (253)*

NOTES Newton Canyon burned in the 2018 Woolsey Fire and is closed at the time of this writing. Check with the National Park Service (805-370-2301 or nps.gov/samo) for updates.

DIRECTIONS You begin at a large trailhead parking area for the Backbone Trail, on the west side of Kanan Dume Road at mile marker 9.62. This is 4.5 miles north of Pacific Coast Highway by way of Kanan Dume Road and 7 miles south of the 101 Freeway by way of Kanan Road and Kanan Dume Road.

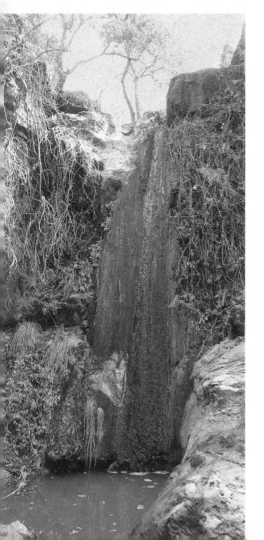

Tucked obscurely into an upper tributary of Zuma called Newton Canyon is a pint-size but charming waterfall accessible by a mere half mile of hiking. Kids will enjoy this little trek. Everyone should be wary of getting too close to the edge of the slippery precipice. Go in the winter or spring after a series of rains, or you may find the falls dry.

Start down the Backbone Trail toward Zuma Ridge Motorway through mature chaparral with an understory of wildflowers and ferns. Make a switchback, and then watch for a use trail on the left shortcutting to the falls. This path is extremely steep, slick, and prone to erosion, so keep going on the main trail and cross Newton Canyon.

Shortly beyond reach a split in the trail. The signed Backbone Trail stays right, but this trip veers left. You quickly come to another fork—take the left path to reach the top of Upper Newton Falls. After you've enjoyed it, return to the fork and then take the other path down to the base of the falls.

VARIATIONS

If you're feeling adventurous, you can extend this hike by following the canyon down to one or two more waterfalls. Lower Newton Falls is a fun rock-hop. You may get wet as you traverse

Don't be surprised to find that Newton Falls is just a trickle on your hike.

sandstone boulders and slabs, and dodge the limbs and branches of oaks, sycamores, and bay laurels. Beware of poison oak, which is hard to recognize in the winter when it loose its leaves. After about 250 yards, you reach the top of Lower Newton Falls, a curtainlike travertine formation about 50 feet high.

If you're feeling even more adventurous, you can continue down to the base of the falls and onto Zuma Falls. A steep, narrow, and potentially dangerous path on the left climbs along the cliffside before plunging down to the base of Lower Newton Falls. Just beyond, you reach the confluence of Newton and Zuma Canyons. Turn left and follow Zuma Canyon, which generally has more water. You will soon have to choose between wading the creek and bushwhacking along the banks. You'll encounter sandstone slabs with lovely cascades before reaching Zuma Falls where a sheet of water flows over an abrupt drop, perhaps the loveliest of the three falls. Going this far and back extends your trip to 2 miles with 300 feet of elevation gain and takes about 2 hours, or possibly more for those who are uncertain of their footing in difficult terrain.

---

trip 8.4   Rocky Oaks

Distance	1.0 mile (loop)
Hiking Time	30 minutes
Elevation Gain	150'
Difficulty	Easy
Trail Use	Suitable for mountain biking, equestrians, dogs allowed, good for kids
Best Times	Year-round
Agency	National Park Service
Optional Map	Tom Harrison *Zuma–Trancas Canyons* or Trails Illustrated *Santa Monica Mountains National Recreation Area (253)*

see map on p. 100

NOTES Rocky Oaks burned in the 2018 Woolsey Fire and is closed at the time of this writing. Check with the National Park Service (805-370-2301 or nps.gov/samo) for updates.

DIRECTIONS From the 101 Freeway in Agoura Hills, take Exit 36 for southbound Kanan Road. Follow Kanan Road 6.3 miles to Mulholland Highway. Turn right (west) on Mulholland, and almost immediately turn right again into Rocky Oaks Park.

Diminutive Rocky Oaks Park is typical of the many small properties that have been purchased or earmarked for future acquisition by the National Park Service in the continuing effort to flesh out Santa Monica Mountains National Recreation Area. The property, a former cattle ranch, was purchased in 1980. Since then it has essentially reverted to a natural state. In the park today, you'll find restrooms, a parking lot, a picnic area, and about 200 acres of wildland consisting of hillsides covered in chaparral and sage scrub, grassy meadows, and (what else?) rocks and oaks. Many of the oaks burned beyond recovery in the Woolsey Fire.

The trails of Rocky Oaks are open 8 a.m.–sunset for multiple uses: hiking, mountain biking, and dog walking. Small kids will perhaps be entertained by the larger-than-life (from their viewpoint) landscape of hills, valleys, and rocky crags. This area was devastated by the Woolsey Fire and will be very different when it reopens.

The Rocky Oaks Loop Trail departs the parking lot at two places. This trip makes a 1-mile clockwise loop, starting at the trailhead in the middle of the lot and ending at the more prominent kiosk at the far end of the lot. From the middle trailhead, cross a seasonal creek, go left, and walk 0.2 mile to a four-way intersection; then continue straight ahead

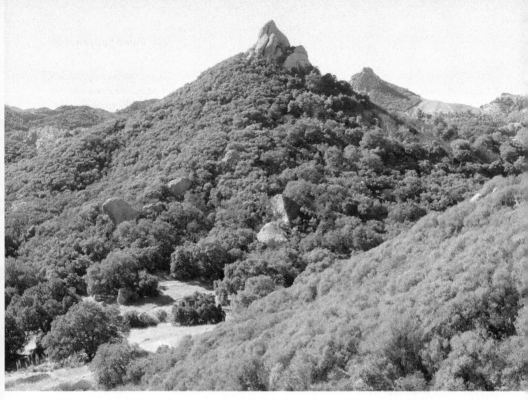

Mitten Mountain rose above the oaks before the Woolsey Fire. Most of the oaks were severely burned.

up a steep slope to reach an overlook at the top of some wood steps. The cattle pond in the valley below may or may not contain water, depending on recent rains. In the opposite direction is Peak 2061 (aka Mitten Mountain), which itself blocks from view the better-known landmark of Saddle Rock. These two crags, as well as the summit you're standing on, consist of the roughly 15-million-year-old Conejo Volcanics rock formation.

The trail continues north, contouring through the tangled growths of chaparral. Dead twigs are accumulating beneath the new growth. In the natural scheme of things, this vegetation sooner or later will burn again, its ashes providing nutrients for the next, almost identical generation of plants. Come to a fence near Kanan Road and abruptly turn back south. To complete the 1-mile loop hike, bear right at the next fork, descend to the meadow below, and make your way past the pond back to the parking lot along any of the maze of trails lacing the area.

chapter 9

Malibu Creek

Nosing its way around an obstacle course of upraised and tilted sandstone, conglomerate, and volcanic rock formations, Malibu Creek clearly has been successful in adapting to the tectonic creaks and groans of Mother Earth. It's the only stream that has managed to cut entirely through the Santa Monica Mountains. Its tentacle-like tributaries reach far west and north, draining parts of the north edge of the Santa Monicas, as well as about one-third of the Simi Hills. Lower Malibu Creek has cut an impressively deep gorge, followed most of the way by the fast, two-lane highway called Malibu Canyon Road.

Hikers and other self-propelled travelers can enjoy 6,000-acre Malibu Creek State Park, which features a quiet stretch of Malibu Creek and picturesque outcrops of sandstone and volcanic rock. Several newer parcels of park and open-space land lie adjacent to the state park, and these are included as well in the 22 trips that belong to this chapter.

In contrast to the area covered in the previous chapter (Topanga), full-blown urbanization is not as much of a factor here. Still, urban-style housing developments have crept into the mountain valleys along Las Virgenes Road and along Mulholland Highway near San Fernando Valley. Timely efforts by park advocates in the 1960s and '70s resulted in the present substantial inventory of park and open-space areas, and these efforts continue today. A quick historical review is helpful in understanding the area's value as parkland and open space.

Bedrock mortars (grinding holes) and other archaeological evidence indicate thousands of years of prehistoric use of the Malibu Creek area, most recently by the coast-dwelling Chumash. These Indians maintained a presence here up to at least the mid-1800s. Some say that Chumash descendants cast the bricks used to build the Sepúlveda Adobe, which stood near Mulholland Highway and Las Virgenes Road from 1863 until it was destroyed in the 2018 Woolsey Fire.

At the turn of the century, a group of wealthy individuals bought property along Malibu Creek and formed the exclusive Crags Country Club. A clubhouse and several private homes were built, but a more lasting effort involved the erection of a dam across a rocky defile on Malibu Creek. The 7-acre lake created by the dam was later named Century Lake by the subsequent owner of the property, 20th Century Fox.

By the mid-1900s, much of Malibu Creek country was a kind of annex for Hollywood movie studios, with sets strategically placed to take advantage of a great variety of exotic backdrops. A vestige of this activity continues today, though most of the sets in Malibu Creek State Park and elsewhere have been removed.

The land owned by 20th Century Fox was purchased by the state in 1974, and adjoining parcels were acquired soon after. In 1976 Malibu Creek State Park was opened to the public. Then, in 1978, Congress established the Santa Monica Mountains National Recreation Area to "preserve and enhance its scenic, natural, and historical setting and its public health value as an airshed for the Southern California metropolitan area while providing for the

continued on page 110

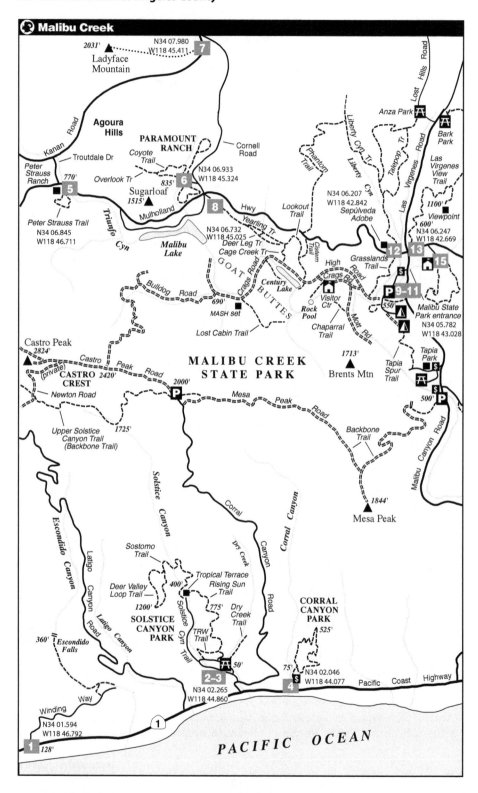

Malibu Creek

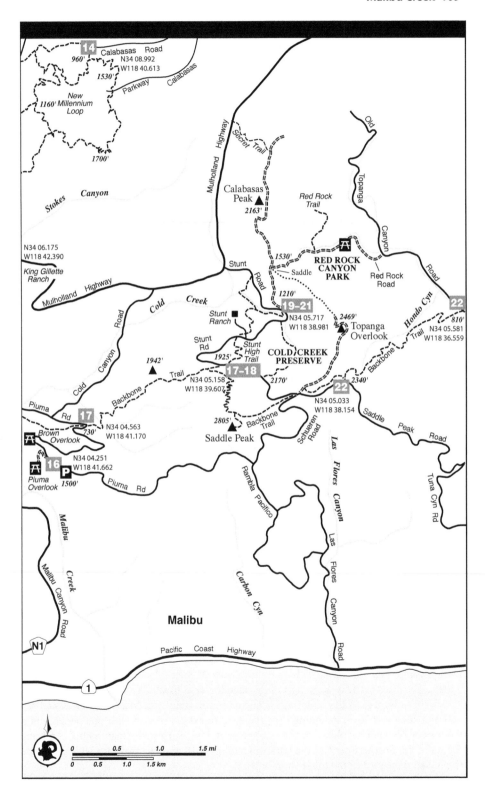

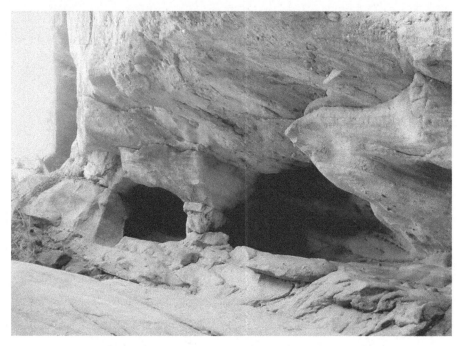

Cavernous sandstone formations resemble eye sockets in Red Rock Canyon. (See Trip 9.19, page 135.)

continued from page 107

recreational and educational needs of the visiting public." To date these goals have been partially realized through the cooperation of several government agencies as well as private landowners. Malibu Creek State Park grew to encompass more than 7,000 acres. All the while, the state-funded Santa Monica Mountains Conservancy, the National Park Service, and private organizations have been busily buying key parcels of land in the Malibu Creek area and beyond for use as open space and parkland. About half of the land shown on our map of the Malibu Creek area is in public ownership so far.

The state park, along with the nearby Paramount Ranch, harbors some of the southernmost valley-oak habitat in California. You can see beautiful specimens of this sprawling, deciduous tree in Liberty Canyon north of Mulholland Highway and along the Nature Trail, located near the state park's main entrance off Las Virgenes Road.

Malibu Creek State Park also has a large, tidy campground with hot showers; it's quiet in the off-season but often full on spring and summer weekends. Even if you live rather close by in the L.A. area, you can stay overnight here and use the campground as a base for early-morning or evening hikes.

The 2018 Woolsey Fire started near the Santa Susana Field Laboratory and, driven by intense Santa Ana winds, burned across the Santa Monica Mountains all the way to the Pacific. The trails in the western part of this chapter were affected but have since reopened.

Also of note, at least five shootings occurred in the vicinity of Malibu Creek State Park between 2016 and 2018, including the June 2018 murder of a man who was sleeping in a tent beside his young children at the campground. Police arrested a man named Anthony Rauda in the northern part of the park in October 2018 and charged him with the crime (he is also suspected in the other shootings).

trip 9.1   Escondido Canyon

Distance	3.4 miles (out-and-back)
Hiking Time	2 hours
Elevation Gain	500'
Difficulty	Moderate
Trail Use	Dogs allowed
Best Times	December–July
Agencies	Mountains Recreation & Conservation Authority, Santa Monica Mountains Conservancy
Optional Map	Tom Harrison *Malibu Creek State Park* or Trails Illustrated *Santa Monica Mountains National Recreation Area (253)*
Fees/Permits	$8 parking fee at Winding Way trailhead

see map on p. 108

DIRECTIONS From a point on Pacific Coast Highway in Malibu at mile marker 1 LA 52.50, 1.7 miles west of Latigo Canyon Road and 1.2 miles east of Kanan Dume Road, turn north on Winding Way and look for a trailhead parking lot immediately on the left.

Escondido ("hidden" in Spanish) Canyon conceals one of the natural treasures of the Santa Monica Mountains: a shimmering waterfall leaping more than 200 feet over a broken cliff. Only during times of rare floods do the falls resemble anything thunderous, but even during an average rainy season the intricate dribblings of water are an inspiration.

On foot, follow the dirt shoulder of Winding Way (a private road that's signed as a public-access trail) for 0.8 mile to a summit, passing palatial houses perched on rounded hilltops and ocean-facing slopes. Continue 0.1 mile past the summit; then follow a narrow trail descending to the left. After another 0.1 mile you cross Escondido Canyon's stream amid oaks, sycamores, and willows. Turn left when you reach the trail on the far side, heading upstream. Stay on the main path, ignoring various narrower spurs. Fine displays of sticky monkey flower adorn the trail in spring and early summer. After the fifth stream crossing, the trail sticks to the east bank and you soon catch a first glimpse of the upper cascades of the multitiered falls dead ahead, its white noise audible over the whisper of the nearby stream.

At the trail's end, a faint sulfurous odor in the air is juxtaposed against the sweet sight of feathery ribbons of water draped across a travertine outcrop, which forms the lowest tier of the falls. Hidden upstream are two more waterfalls, but they're on private property and hikers are unwelcome. Enjoy the soothing ambience of the lowest falls before heading back to the starting point the same way.

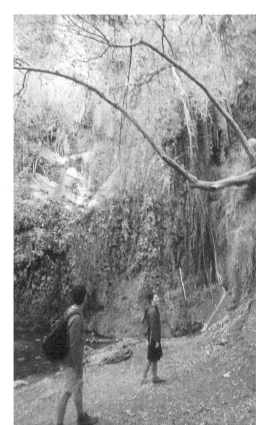

Escondido Falls cascades down a heavily vegetated cliff.

| **trip 9.2** | **Lower Solstice Canyon** |

see map on p. 108

Distance	2.4 miles (out-and-back)
Hiking Time	1.5 hours
Elevation Gain	350'
Difficulty	Easy
Trail Use	Dogs allowed, good for kids
Best Times	Year-round
Agency	National Park Service
Optional Map	Tom Harrison *Malibu Creek State Park* or Trails Illustrated *Santa Monica Mountains National Recreation Area (253)*

DIRECTIONS From Highway 1 in Malibu 0.3 mile west of mile marker 001 LA 50.0, turn north onto Corral Canyon Road. In 0.2 mile turn left into Solstice Canyon Park. There's overflow parking for several cars right at the entrance and a more spacious lot 0.3 mile farther inside at the main trailhead. Park hours are 8 a.m.–sunset.

Easygoing but superbly scenic, Solstice Canyon Trail takes you through the grounds of the former Roberts Ranch, now Solstice Canyon Park, a site administered by the National Park Service. The canyon once hosted a private zoo where giraffes, camels, deer, and exotic birds roamed. At trail's end you come to Tropical Terrace, the site of an architecturally noted grand home that burned in a 1982 wildfire.

Because Solstice Canyon Road is paved, it accommodates road bikes as well as mountain bikes and all travel by foot. Starting at the main trailhead, pass through a gate and continue upstream alongside the canyon's melodious creek. You travel through a fantastic woodland of alder, sycamore, bay, and coast live oak—the latter with trunks up to 18 feet in circumference.

At 1.2 miles you arrive at Tropical Terrace, 90% burned in the 1982 fire. In a setting of palms and giant birds-of-paradise, curved flagstone steps sweep toward the roofless

A striking illustration of the impermanence of human endeavor, Tropical Terrace was wiped out by fire and is being reclaimed by nature.

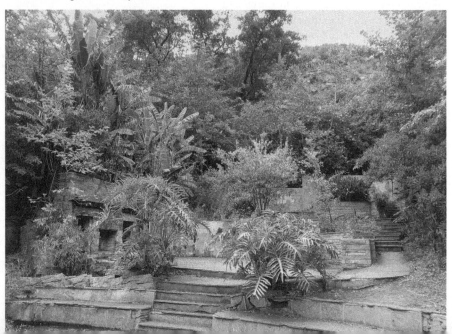

remains of what was for 26 years one of Malibu's grandest homes. Beyond the house, crumbling stone steps and pathways lead to what used to be elaborately decorated rock grottoes, and a waterfall on Solstice Canyon's creek. Large chunks of sandstone have cleaved from the canyon walls, adding to the rubble. For all its perfectly natural setting, Tropical Terrace's destiny was that of a temporary paradise, defenseless against both fire and flood.

When it's time to return, simply go back the way you came. Consider veering onto some of the narrower paths that parallel parts of the paved road.

VARIATION

A beautiful but more strenuous option for a loop hike is to return along the Rising Sun and TRW Loop Trails (see next trip). This adds 400 feet of climbing and 0.7 mile compared with retracing your steps.

VARIATION

If you have a little energy to spare back at the start, take a 0.8-mile (round-trip) side hike up the Dry Creek Trail. An outrageously cantilevered "Darth Vader" house overlooks the Dry Creek ravine, as well as a 150-foot-high precipice that on rare occasions becomes a spectacular waterfall.

---

trip 9.3   **Rising Sun & Sostomo Loop**

Distance	7 miles (loop)
Hiking Time	4 hours
Elevation Gain	1,900'
Difficulty	Moderately strenuous
Trail Use	Dogs allowed
Best Times	October–May
Agency	National Park Service
Optional Map	Tom Harrison *Malibu Creek State Park* or Trails Illustrated *Santa Monica Mountains National Recreation Area (253)*

see map on p. 108

DIRECTIONS From Highway 1 in Malibu 0.3 mile west of mile marker 001 LA 50.0, turn north onto Corral Canyon Road. In 0.2 mile turn left into Solstice Canyon Park. There's overflow parking for several cars right at the entrance and a more spacious lot 0.3 mile farther inside at the main trailhead. Park hours are 8 a.m.–sunset.

This roller coaster–like ramble over the hillsides overlooking lower Solstice Canyon is a nearly complete tour of the entire Solstice Canyon Park. Most of the attractions are in the lower canyon, but the upper portion is worth adding if you are seeking a good workout. It's a sweaty affair if the day is sunny and warm. If you start early enough, however, you can finish in time for lunch under the oaks in the cool, shady canyon bottom.

From the main trailhead, pass through the gate and immediately turn right onto the TRW Loop Trail. After 0.3 mile cross a paved road. Just beyond, make a hard right onto the Rising Sun Trail, which briefly joins the paved road and then continues climbing. There's a fine view of the coastline up near the road; if you arrive by 8:30 a.m. on or near the winter solstice, the risen sun should be gleaming above the Palos Verdes Peninsula, its light scattering into a thousand watery pinpoints on the ocean's surface below.

Resuming your travel on the Rising Sun Trail, you contour above a snaggletoothed outcrop called Lisa's Rock, and then descend sharply to the Tropical Terrace site (1.7 miles). Cross Solstice Canyon's creek, walk down past the ruins of the house, and pick up the Sostomo Trail on the right.

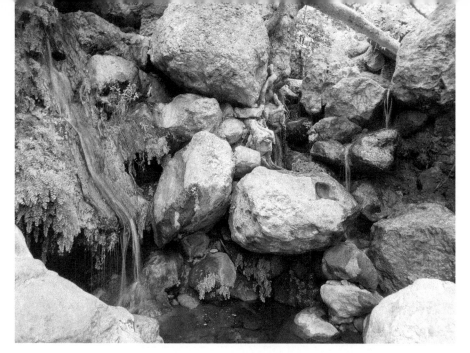

Solstice Falls is tucked away on the creek just above Tropical Terrace.

On the Sostomo Trail, which is an old road to start with, you ascend the west wall of Solstice Canyon, cross the creek (2.0 miles), and then start up the east wall. The trail visits a tiny, burned-out cabin, its forlorn brick chimney bravely poking above the encroaching chaparral. You soon descend and cross the creek again. Going up the west bank you pass another cabin fatality—a roofless stone-and-mortar shell. Looming over the canyon ahead is a spectacular outcrop of sedimentary rock, but our trail route circles south away from it and climbs to a trail junction (3.0 miles). Ahead lies the Deer Valley Loop Trail; go either way around the loop, covering a distance of 1.3 miles. About midway along the loop you reach the shoulder of a ridge at 1,200 feet elevation where you can look down on Point Dume and the coastline. That view is made less dramatic by some high-voltage power lines in the foreground.

To return to the starting point, descend Sostomo Trail back to Tropical Terrace and then take the easiest way back—downhill on the paved Solstice Canyon Road. You can make the walk more interesting by veering onto narrow trails paralleling the road.

---

trip 9.4 **Corral Canyon**

Distance	2.2 miles (loop)
Hiking Time	1.5 hours
Elevation Gain	500'
Difficulty	Moderate
Trail Use	Dogs allowed, good for kids
Best Times	Year-round
Agencies	Mountains Recreation & Conservation Authority, Santa Monica Mountains Conservancy
Optional Map	Tom Harrison *Malibu Creek State Park* or Trails Illustrated *Santa Monica Mountains National Recreation Area (253)*
Fees/Permits	$8 parking fee at Sara Wan Trailhead

see map on p. 108

DIRECTIONS To get to the trailhead, you'll need to be going westbound through Malibu on Pacific Coast Highway (there is no eastbound access to the trailhead). At a point 0.6 mile west of Puerco Canyon Road, 0.4 mile west of mile marker 001 LA 49.5, there's a parking lot on the right at Malibu Seafood restaurant (25623 Pacific Coast Highway); adjacent to this is pay parking at the Sara Wan Corral Canyon Trailhead. Alternatively, you can park on the shoulder of the highway, making sure to observe parking restrictions. LA Metro Bus 534 also stops at the trailhead.

Corral Canyon Park was acquired in the 1990s to protect the undeveloped open space and is now part of the Santa Monica Mountains National Recreation Area. A lazily looping hiking trail traverses the park's grass- and chaparral-covered slopes, inviting your exploration on foot.

Check out the interpretive display at the trailhead and then take off on the trail, which begins by crossing a small area of willow scrub in the often-marshy bottom of Corral Canyon. On the far side, swing left. After 0.1 mile choose the trail to the right, which will take you immediately uphill and counterclockwise on a 2-mile loop. The beautifully graded pathway curls up a grassy hillside swept by fresh Pacific breezes. Hang-gliding humans on parasailing craft can often be seen drifting lazily to and fro along the shoreline, utilizing those same sea breezes.

At 0.8 mile you reach a narrow ridge. A false trail goes right up along the top of that ridge, but you stay left, following a more gently graded trail that continues gaining elevation, going north, parallel to the canyon bottom below. By about 1.1 miles, at an elevation of 550 feet above sea level, there's a sharp switchback. You swing left and initiate a zigzagging descent down into the canyon and then alongside the canyon bottom. Keep an eye on the sky for ravens, hawks, or vultures swooping, soaring, and gliding.

Nearing the end of the hike, you pass a homesite—a cabin burned like so many others in this wildfire-prone region—with its forlorn chimney still standing. Shortly ahead, you come to the aforementioned split in the trail, a short distance shy of the trailhead.

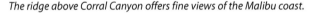

The ridge above Corral Canyon offers fine views of the Malibu coast.

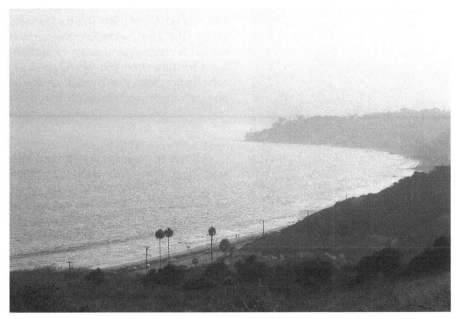

trip 9.5 Peter Strauss Trail

Distance	1.3 miles (loop)
Hiking Time	30 minutes
Elevation Gain	200'
Difficulty	Easy
Trail Use	Dogs allowed, good for kids
Best Times	Year-round
Agency	National Park Service
Optional Map	Tom Harrison *Malibu Creek State Park* or Trails Illustrated *Santa Monica Mountains National Recreation Area (253)*

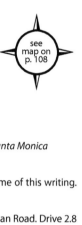

see map on p. 108

NOTES Peter Strauss Ranch burned in the 2018 Woolsey Fire and is closed at the time of this writing. Check with the National Park Service (805-370-2301, nps.gov/samo) for updates.

DIRECTIONS From the 101 Freeway in Agoura Hills, take Exit 36 for southbound Kanan Road. Drive 2.8 miles and turn left on Troutdale Drive. Proceed 0.4 mile south to Mulholland Highway, and turn left. Just ahead, on the right, is the Strauss Ranch parking lot, open 8 a.m.–sunset.

The 65-acre Peter Strauss Ranch, which was owned by actor-producer Peter Strauss before the National Park Service bought the property in 1983, has an interesting past. In the 1930s and '40s this was Lake Enchanto, a popular resort and amusement park, boasting the largest swimming pool west of the Rockies, a terrazzo dance floor, and amusement rides. The upper reaches of Malibu Creek (known here as Triunfo Canyon) were dammed to create the lake itself, a popular draw for boaters and anglers. During the 1960s—long after Lake Enchanto's commercial demise—plans were afoot to develop the property as an elaborate Disneyland-style theme park, but they were never realized.

Today's Lake Enchanto bears only a scant resemblance to the resort it used to be. The dam washed out in 1960 and has not been rebuilt. The great swimming pool remains unfilled. A picturesque stone-and-wood bathhouse remains. Other than guided walks and occasional special events such as dances, plays, art shows, and musical performances held on the grounds, this quiet refuge caters to a relatively small number of hikers, picnickers, and curious folk.

Kids will find plenty to keep them busy here. From spring into early summer, the shallow, sluggish stream is alive with thousands of tadpoles. Careful investigation may reveal crayfish, newts, and pond turtles. Just south of the ranch house, there's a eucalyptus grove overlooking the remains of Lake Enchanto's dam.

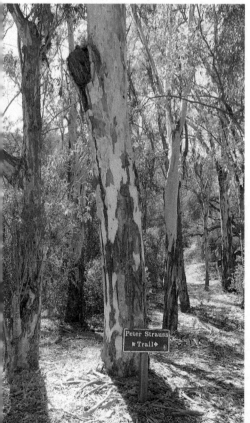

Eucalyptus grove at Peter Strauss Ranch before the Woolsey Fire

To reach the trailhead, walk back onto Mulholland Highway, turn left, and follow the bridge across Malibu Creek; then immediately turn left into the pedestrian entrance to the ranch. Follow the dirt road south for 0.1 mile to the signed start of the Peter Strauss Trail, which makes a loop onto the oak-shaded hillside.

Make a clockwise loop on the trail. Watch for a path on the left leading back across the creek to the parking area. You will soon turn right at an unmarked fork with the Peter Strauss Trail and begin switchbacking up the hill, then briefly traverse and switchback down again.

trip 9.6 Paramount Ranch

see map on p. 108

Distance	1–3 miles (loop)
Hiking Time	30 minutes–1.5 hours
Elevation Gain	Up to 300'
Difficulty	Easy
Trail Use	Equestrians, dogs allowed, good for kids
Best Times	October–June
Agency	National Park Service
Optional Map	Tom Harrison *Malibu Creek State Park* or Trails Illustrated *Santa Monica Mountains National Recreation Area (253)*

DIRECTIONS From the 101 Freeway in Agoura Hills, take Exit 36 for southbound Kanan Road. Drive for 0.5 mile, and turn left on Cornell Way. Immediately ahead, stay right and continue on Cornell Road. Proceed 2 miles south to Paramount Ranch, on the right.

For most of the 20th century, Paramount Ranch served the needs of an entertainment industry always hungry for rustic outdoor scenery. Since 1980, however, the core of this property has been in the hands of the National Park Service (NPS). The park service set

This immense valley oak and the historic Western Town movie set burned in the Woolsey Fire.

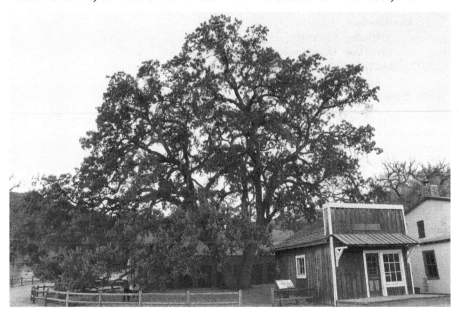

about restoring Western Town, a set where exterior scenes for hundreds of TV Westerns were shot in the 1950s and '60s. Western Town burned to the ground in the 2018 Woolsey Fire, but the park has reopened, and the NPS hopes to rebuild with fire-resistant materials.

Paramount Ranch is a popular spot for guided walks, but you can explore on your own just as easily. A maze of mostly unsigned trails laces the 326-acre property. The oaks were singed in the fire, but many will survive.

The Coyote–Valley Oak Savannah Loop is a 3-mile hike touring the north end of the ranch, including Coyote Canyon and a grassland dotted with valley oaks. From the parking area, walk across the bridge over the creek to Western Town. Look for the signed Coyote Trail behind the old town site. Follow the trail into the canyon; then turn right and climb to a spur leading to a picnic table. The view is blocked by tall chaparral, but you can continue up a use trail a bit farther to look over Western Town. Wildflowers abound in a good year—woolly blue curls, owl's clover, verbena, mallow, and more. Return to the main path and make a clockwise loop around the northern end of the park using the Hacienda, Backdrop, and Bwana Trails. You'll pass many junctions, mostly unsigned, but just aim to stay near the perimeter of the ranch, taking care not to head up the Witches Wood or Paramount Ridge Trails that dead end at the park's western boundary.

The Medea Creek Loop is a 1-mile loop visiting the Western Town Overlook on a hill at the south end of the park. From the parking area, walk south to the poorly marked Medea Creek Trail. To make a counterclockwise loop, stay right at an immediate junction and parallel the creek; then climb up the hillock and take a spur to the overlook at the top. From there, you can look upon the soaring profile of Sugarloaf Peak, which is made of the same stuff as the Goat Buttes: Conejo Volcanics. Continue east and north down through a maze of unsigned trails that all eventually return you to the initial junction.

trip 9.7	**Ladyface Mountain**	

Distance	2.0 miles (out-and-back)
Hiking Time	2 hours
Elevation Gain	1,200'
Difficulty	Moderate
Trail Use	Dogs allowed
Best Times	October–May
Agency	National Park Service
Optional Map	Tom Harrison *Malibu Creek State Park* (trail not shown)

see map on p. 108

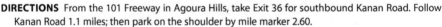

DIRECTIONS From the 101 Freeway in Agoura Hills, take Exit 36 for southbound Kanan Road. Follow Kanan Road 1.1 miles; then park on the shoulder by mile marker 2.60.

From certain vantage points to the east, Ladyface Mountain (2,031') resembles the profile of a woman's head in repose. According to Chumash legend, the woman was watching the sky waiting for her lover's return. A short but steep climbers' trail up the volcanic ridge offers a vigorous workout and great views. Boots with good tread can be helpful on the steep, rocky, and sandy portions of the trail. On an April day in a poor rain year, I (David) noted at least 17 different species of wildflowers along the ridge, with phacelia and sunflowers being particularly common. The ridge was burned to bare earth in the 2018 Woolsey Fire, but the flowers will likely put on an even more impressive show as the area regenerates.

Pick up the trail that begins by your parking area. At an immediate split, stay left and climb steeply to the ridgeline, where you soon stay right to join an old roadbed ascending

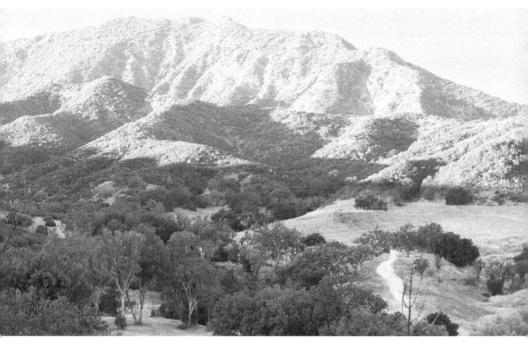

If you squint just right, the ridge might resemble a woman's face staring at the sky.

the ridge. Eventually the road becomes a trail, kept in reasonably good condition by frequent users. At times, you'll have options to stay on the trail or scramble up steeper rocky portions of the ridge. Bypass a rocky false peak on the left (or scramble up it for fun) and continue west to the highest point.

From the summit, you have terrific views of the Santa Monica Mountains to the south, stretching from Sandstone Peak past the Goat Buttes to Saddle Peak. To the north beyond Agoura Hills, you can see the Las Virgenes–Cheeseboro–Palo Comado Canyon area and Rocky Peak. Return the way you came.

trip 9.8   Lookout Loop

Distance	3.8 miles (loop)
Hiking Time	2 hours
Elevation Gain	700'
Difficulty	Moderate
Trail Use	Good for kids
Best Times	November–June
Agency	California State Parks
Optional Map	Tom Harrison *Malibu Creek State Park* or Trails Illustrated *Santa Monica Mountains National Recreation Area (253)*

see map on p. 108

DIRECTIONS From Highway 101 in Calabasas, take Exit 32 for southbound Las Virgenes Road. Drive 3 miles south to Mulholland Highway (traffic light here), turn right, and proceed another 3 miles to the intersection with Cornell Road. Turn left, then left again to reach the spacious trailhead parking lot for the Reagan Ranch.

If it's springtime, you'll want to bring your camera (plus a macro lens or close-up attachment) with you on this hike. After a wet winter, these gentle meadows and oak-dotted hillsides can muster quite a display of wildflowers from March into May or June. Keep an eye out for lupine, larkspur, California poppy, wild pansy, Chinese houses, goldfields, cream cups, wallflower, wild rose, and the ever-present but weedy mustard. You're seldom out of sight or sound of nearby Mulholland Highway, but there's plenty of botanical variety to make the trip an enjoyable one. The 2018 Woolsey Fire swept through this area, but the park quickly reopened and you will be able to watch the process of regrowth.

From the trailhead parking area, walk southeast on paved driveway 0.4 mile to the site of the ranch owned by former president Ronald Reagan before he was elected governor of California in 1966; the buildings burned in the fire. Pick up the signed Yearling Trail, which runs for more than a half mile through a grassy meadow. After 0.1 mile bear right on the Deer Leg Trail (later you'll return to this intersection on the Yearling Trail, the path to the left). The Deer Leg Trail rambles through a strip of oak woodland and then descends to cross tiny Udell Creek. A side path slants left to reconnect with the Yearling Trail, but you stay right on the narrow path that climbs up a brushy slope. In a few minutes, you arrive on top of a ridge overlooking Century Lake and Malibu Creek. In the background, the Goat Buttes soar into a milky blue sky. Strong backlight during most of the day makes this a difficult landscape to capture photographically. Late-afternoon side light, however, does justice to the majesty of the scene.

From the ridgetop, the trail veers north to rejoin the Yearling Trail in the meadow below. Turn right at the bottom, go 0.1 mile east, and go right again on the Cage Creek Trail. After an abrupt 250-foot loss of elevation, you arrive at Crags Road. Turn left, and continue 0.3 mile east past Century Lake to the Lookout Trail on the left. The Lookout Trail swings up a dry ridge to the north, offering more views of the lake and the buttes to the south. You pass the Cistern Trail on the right, which goes to a turnout along Mulholland Highway (an alternative starting point for this hike), and then contour through patches of cool oak woodland and toasty chaparral. Leaving the chaparral, you traverse a grassy saddle and rejoin the Yearling Trail. Follow it back toward the Reagan Ranch and your starting point.

Century Lake Dam blocks the passage between the dramatic Goat Rocks.

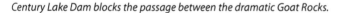

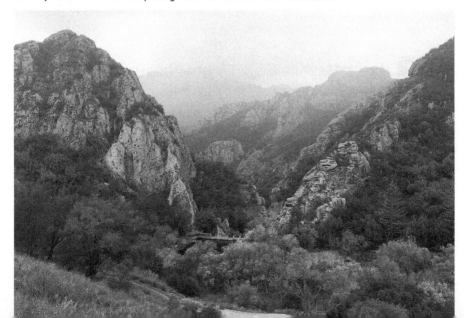

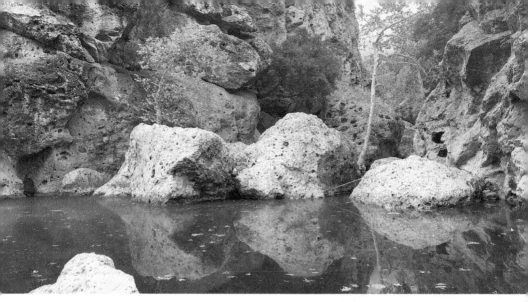

Rock Pool's awesome setting draws rock climbers, cliff jumpers, and bathers—but think twice before submerging your head in these polluted waters.

see map on p. 108

trip 9.9   Century Lake

Distance	3.0 miles (out-and-back)
Hiking Time	1.5 hours
Elevation Gain	250'
Difficulty	Easy
Trail Use	Suitable for mountain biking, good for kids
Best Times	Year-round
Agency	California State Parks
Optional Map	Tom Harrison *Malibu Creek State Park* or Trails Illustrated *Santa Monica Mountains National Recreation Area (253)*
Fees/Permits	$12 day-use fee

DIRECTIONS From Highway 101 in Calabasas, take Exit 32 for southbound Las Virgenes Road. Drive 3 miles south to Mulholland Highway (traffic light here), and continue on Las Virgenes 0.2 mile farther to the Malibu Creek State Park entrance, on the right. Pay the day-use fee and drive 0.4 mile to the hikers' parking lot, open 8 a.m.–10 p.m.

If you only have time to do a single hike at Malibu Creek State Park, this is the one to take. In 3 miles of easy walking you can explore the park's main attractions and also drop by the visitor center (open weekends), which is not accessible by car. Picnic tables are available along the route. The 2018 Woolsey Fire swept through this area, but Malibu Creek State Park quickly reopened, and visitors will be able to watch the process of regrowth.

From the trailhead kiosk just west of the hikers' parking lot, walk west on unpaved Crags Road and immediately make a concrete-ford crossing of Malibu Creek. Youngsters come here to toss in a line for bass, bluegill, and catfish. In 0.3 mile come to an unsigned fork—the High Road stays right, but you veer left down across the creek on Crags Road. In another 0.1 mile, you'll come to a second fork where Mott Road veers left—stay right on Crags Road, heading most directly to the visitor center. (A more interesting, roundabout, and strenuous alternative is to head south on Mott Road, and then follow Chaparral Trail up and over a saddle to reach the visitor center. At that saddle you're rewarded with a great view of the Goat Buttes.)

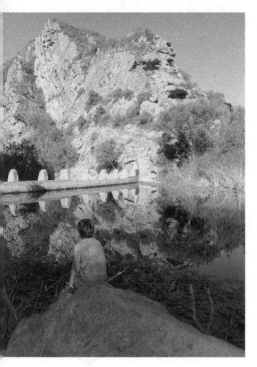

The rock and picnic bench at Century Lake are a good place to watch wildlife or admire the reflection of the crags.

The visitor center is housed in a grand old home once occupied by a member of Crags Country Club and later by the groundskeeper for 20th Century Fox. Even if the center isn't open, you can peruse the interpretive panels set up outside beneath the oaks.

From the visitor center, cross over Malibu Creek on a sturdy bridge and continue up the hill on Crags Road, gaining about 200 feet in elevation. When you reach the crest, look for an unsigned trail descending left. In a minute or two, you'll reach the shady east shoreline of Century Lake, created in 1901 by damming Malibu Creek with a tall concrete structure. Subsequent silting-in has allowed a freshwater marsh to overtake much of what was previously open water. Ducks, coots, and herons frequent the lake, their squallings and callings reverberating off the weathered, honeycombed volcanic cliffs rising from the reservoir's far shore. Redwing blackbirds flit among the cattails and rushes.

When you've had your fill of these engaging sights and sounds, backtrack to the bridge over Malibu Creek. Just before you reach it, though, turn south onto the unsigned Gorge Trail. Pass a picnic area and some pockmarked crags popular with rock climbers, and in a few minutes you'll come upon the Rock Pool, a placid stretch of water framed by volcanic cliffs. This generically wild-looking site has served as a backdrop for outdoor sequences filmed for *Swiss Family Robinson,* the 1930s *Tarzan* movies, and many other productions. Although you're also likely to see young cliff jumpers, beware that cliff jumping here is illegal, the rangers issue citations, the water depth is highly variable, Malibu Search and Rescue responds to accidents here several times a month, and the creek is heavily contaminated with coliform bacteria.

To return to the starting point, simply backtrack to Crags Road, and walk east on it for a scant mile until you reach the main parking lot.

trip 9.10   Lost Cabin Trail

Distance	6 miles (out-and-back)
Hiking Time	3 hours
Elevation Gain	700'
Difficulty	Moderate
Best Times	October–June
Agency	California State Parks
Optional Map	Tom Harrison *Malibu Creek State Park* or Trails Illustrated *Santa Monica Mountains National Recreation Area (253)*
Fees/Permits	$12 day-use fee

see map on p. 108

DIRECTIONS From Highway 101 in Calabasas, take Exit 32 for southbound Las Virgenes Road. Drive 3 miles south to Mulholland Highway (traffic light here), and continue on Las Virgenes 0.2 mile farther to the Malibu Creek State Park entrance, on the right. Pay the day-use fee and drive 0.4 mile to the hikers' parking lot, open 8 a.m.–10 p.m.

It's been said that the number of people on a wilderness trail diminishes in proportion to the square of the distance and the cube of the elevation gain from the nearest road. Perhaps that explains why only about one in every hundred visitors to Malibu Creek State Park bothers to check out the dead-end Lost Cabin Trail. The 2018 Woolsey Fire swept through this area, but Malibu Creek State Park quickly reopened, and visitors will be able to watch the process of regrowth.

In truth, when you reach the end, there's no "there" there: just a trickling brook, a line of willows and oaks, lots of fragrant chaparral on the hillsides, plus the overarching dome of the blue sky. (The cabin, if there ever was one, seems to be truly lost.) This placid scene, however, lies in the heart of the 1,900-acre Kaslow Natural Preserve, the largest of three areas in the park managed for research and low-level public use. The preserve (*Kaslow* means "golden eagle" in the Chumash language) harbors mountain lions, golden eagles, and a rare native plant: the Santa Susana tarweed. (The other natural preserves, incidentally, cover the valley-oak habitat in Liberty Canyon and a small amount of oak-and-chaparral country along Udell Creek, north of Crags Road and south of the Reagan Ranch.)

From the main parking lot, walk west on unpaved Crags Road and immediately make come to a concrete-ford crossing of Malibu Creek. In 0.3 mile come to an unsigned fork—the High Road stays right, but you veer left down across the creek on Crags Road. In another 0.1 mile, you'll come to a second fork where Mott Road veers left—stay right on Crags Road, heading most directly to the visitor center. From the visitor center, cross over Malibu Creek on a sturdy bridge and continue up the hill on Crags Road, gaining about 200 feet in elevation.

The set for the TV classic M*A*S*H *miraculously survived the Woolsey Fire.*

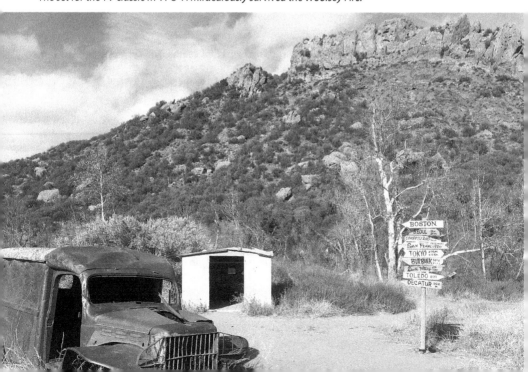

When you start descending, you'll notice on the right the marine-sedimentary Calabasas Formation, consisting of light-colored, easily eroded rocks that are roughly 15 million years old. On the left are the dramatically sheer Goat Buttes, which consist of the erosion-resistant Conejo Volcanics, also about 15 million years old. Ahead on the Lost Cabin Trail, you'll get a look at the south side of those buttes, which features a weird assortment of pockmarked outcrops and boulders.

At 1.7 miles you'll come to a bridge over Malibu Creek. Just ahead, the Forest Trail goes left, providing access to Century Lake's south shore. But this trip follows Crags Road another 0.6 mile, to where an old bulldozed road goes left up along a draw. This is the Lost Cabin Trail, formerly an access road for sites used to film outdoor scenes of the TV series *M*A*S*H*. The main site, dismantled after production on the show's final season was completed in 1982, is marked by a sign along Crags Road. Volunteers have restored the site with a picnic area, a jeep, interpretive signs, and other show memorabilia.

Follow the Lost Cabin Trail, which forks and then rejoins at a divide before descending to its end near the bank of Lost Cabin Creek, a small tributary of Malibu Creek. Downstream, the trickling creek tumbles over a precipice to join Malibu Creek in the gorge between Century Lake and the Rock Pool.

trip 9.11   Bulldog & Backbone Loop

see map on p. 108

Distance	14 miles (loop)
Hiking Time	7 hours
Elevation Gain	3,000'
Difficulty	Strenuous
Trail Use	Suitable for mountain biking
Best Times	November–May
Agency	California State Parks
Optional Map	Tom Harrison *Malibu Creek State Park* or Trails Illustrated *Santa Monica Mountains National Recreation Area (253)*
Fees/Permits	$12 day-use fee

DIRECTIONS From Highway 101 in Calabasas, take Exit 32 for southbound Las Virgenes Road. Drive 3 miles south to Mulholland Highway (traffic light here), and continue on Las Virgenes 0.2 mile farther to the Malibu Creek State Park entrance, on the right. Pay the day-use fee and drive 0.4 mile to the hikers' parking lot, open 8 a.m.–10 p.m.

This is the classic grand tour of Malibu Creek State Park's rugged backcountry. Along the way you'll tramp along the crest of the Santa Monicas, circling high above the park's most conspicuous landmarks. Mountain bikers, who use a slight variation of the route, typically make this a 3- or 4-hour task, but you'd better allow about double that amount of time on foot. There's little shade, so go on a cool day and be prepared with plenty of water (a half gallon or more) and sun protection.

From the main parking lot, walk west on unpaved Crags Road. In 0.3 mile come to an unsigned fork—the High Road stays right, but you veer left down across the creek on Crags Road. In another 0.1 mile, you'll come to a second fork where Mott Road veers left—stay right on Crags Road, heading most directly to the visitor center. From the visitor center, cross over Malibu Creek on a sturdy bridge and continue up the hill on Crags Road, gaining about 200 feet in elevation. Press on past silted-in Century Lake on the left; the Goat Buttes, also on the left; and through the *M*A*S*H* site, where outdoor scenes for the TV series were shot. Birdlife is abundant along this stretch, where the trail parallels Malibu Creek.

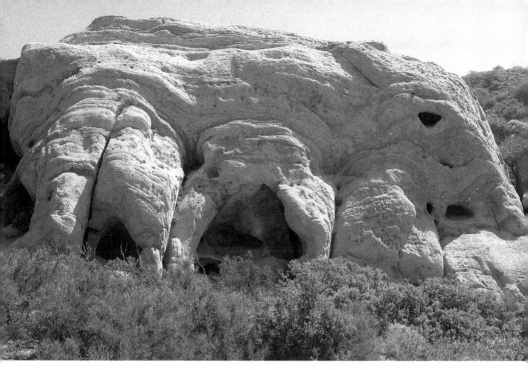

The sandstone caves along Castro Crest were a popular site but have been closed due to vandalism.

After a total of 2.7 miles, bear left on Bulldog Road, aka the Bulldog Motorway, a fire road that also serves as a power-line access road. The road ascends along a small, oak-shaded creek, then rises crookedly along slopes thickly clothed in chaparral. As you climb, you'll pass side roads leading to electrical transmission towers. In a mile stay left at a T and continue up the Bulldog Motorway. The physical effort of negotiating the last steep uphill mile on Bulldog Road is rewarded by ever-expanding views over and beyond the now-shrunken-looking Goat Buttes. Turn left when you top out at Castro Peak Road (Castro Motorway) at 5.8 miles, and start descending east. The Malibu shoreline soon comes into view, with a clear-air vista that includes several of the Channel Islands, Palos Verdes, and the west and south parts of the L.A. Basin. The Castro Crest burned heavily during the 2018 Woolsey Fire.

At the Corral Canyon Road Trailhead parking lot (6.6 miles), stay left on the footpath that goes up a hogback ridge bristling with sandstone pinnacles. (Bikers should stay on the roadways instead of taking the footpath.) Going east along this ridge for 0.5 mile, pass several gargantuan sandstone outcrops—worth climbing if you want to take the time. On the east end of the ridge, you descend to the Mesa Peak Fire Road, which doubles as a segment of the Backbone Trail. More outcrops are worth exploring here, but the famous Corral Canyon cave is posted closed (as of 2017) to recover from extensive graffiti.

After a dull stretch of dirt road, reach a junction at 9.4 miles. The road to Mesa Peak goes right—bear left, staying on the Mesa Peak Fire Road. You now begin a steady descent along the precipitous west wall of Malibu Canyon. Malibu Creek and the curving highway through it come into view occasionally, seemingly straight down. Enjoy the fine views of Saddle Peak ahead and Brents Mountain to the left. At 11.2 miles veer left onto the signed Backbone Trail to bypass the water treatment plant below, and reach the Piuma parking area at 11.8 miles.

The final stretch back to Malibu Canyon Park follows a maze of unsigned trails, and you may prefer to take the road instead. The general idea is to thread your way north, staying east of the Las Virgenes Water Treatment Plant, west of the Tapia Park picnic grounds, east of the Salvation Army Mount Crags Camp, and west of the Camp David Gonzales juvenile-detention facility until you can follow the Tapia Spur Trail over a scruffy ridge to Malibu Creek State Park's group campground. From there, simply walk north out the access road, turn left on the paved road, and head to your car.

VARIATION

You can reach the Corral Canyon Road Trailhead by car from the south, and hike east for up to a mile to explore the sandstone outcrops. Or continue on to Mesa Peak for a 6.5-mile round-trip with 500 feet of elevation gain.

---

trip 9.12 Phantom Loop

see map on p. 108

Distance	7 miles (loop)
Hiking Time	3.5 hours
Elevation Gain	1,200'
Difficulty	Moderate
Trail Use	Equestrians
Best Times	October–June
Agency	California State Parks
Optional Map	Tom Harrison *Malibu Creek State Park* or Trails Illustrated *Santa Monica Mountains National Recreation Area (253)*

DIRECTIONS From Highway 101 in Calabasas, take Exit 32 for southbound Las Virgenes Road. Drive 3 miles south to Mulholland Highway (traffic light here); then turn right and proceed 0.1 mile to park on the shoulder of the road near the signed North Grasslands Trailhead, on the right.

This loop explores the lesser-visited northern end of Malibu Creek State Park by way of Liberty Canyon and the Phantom Trail along a ridgeline before looping back along Malibu Creek. The grassy valley and ridge offer wonderful spring wildflowers and great views to

The Phantom Loop is the best place in the Santa Monica Mountains to admire the majestic valley oak (Quercus lobata).

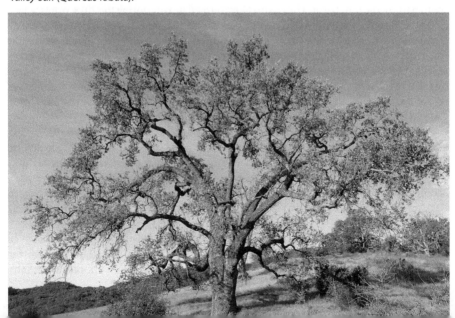

the Goat Buttes. The 2018 Woolsey Fire swept through this area, but Malibu Creek State Park quickly reopened, and visitors will be able to watch the process of regrowth.

Walk north on the North Grasslands Trail past the former site of the Sepúlveda Adobe, a small home built here in 1863 by Don Pedro Alcantra Sepúlveda. Sepúlveda and his wife, Soledad, established a small rancho here and raised 12 children, making a living by selling oak firewood to L.A. residents—a three-day round-trip by wagon along what is now the 101 Freeway. Sadly, the house was destroyed in the 2018 Woolsey Fire.

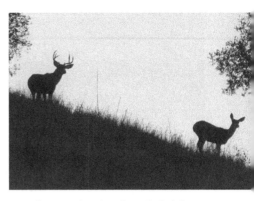

Deer frequent the ridge along the lightly used Talepop Trail (see Variation below).

The trail crosses the meadow and veers right at 0.3 mile onto an old asphalt road that leads to the Edison Crater Substation. The trail resumes on the left at the substation and crosses Liberty Creek on a bridge before meeting the dirt Liberty Canyon Fire Road at 0.8 mile. Turn left and follow the trail through Liberty Canyon Natural Preserve, a 730-acre subunit of Malibu Creek State Park noted for valley oak woodland and savanna. Pass the signed Talepop Trail on the right at 0.9 mile; then pass above a private ranch. At 1.9 miles turn left onto the signed Phantom Trail, which crosses Liberty Creek and reaches a graded gravel ranch road. Turn right on this road, which passes some gorgeous valley oaks; then turn left at a sign where the Phantom Trail resumes (2.2 miles).

Follow the Phantom Trail up a ravine with junglelike oaks, vines, wildflowers, and poison oak. When you reach the ridge at a saddle at 3.0 miles, disregard the unsigned and lightly used Liberty Ridge Trail on the right, and turn left to follow the Phantom Trail along the ridgeline. Stay on the main trail, passing other social paths along the way. Enjoy views of the Goat Buttes before switchbacking down to reach Mulholland Highway at 4.5 mile.

Jog left on the highway; then pick up the signed Cistern Trail on the south side. At a T-junction with the Lookout Trail (4.8 miles), turn left and continue to a trail junction by Century Lake (5.3 miles). It's worth a short detour to explore the north or south side of the lake.

After you've seen the lake, join Crags Road and follow it south and east over a low ridge and down to a four-way junction by Malibu Creek (5.8 miles). In the spring or winter, when there is water on the creek, it's worth a 0.2-mile detour to the right (south) to visit the striking rock pools at the mouth of a narrow canyon flanked by the Goat Buttes. Rock climbers ply their craft on the volcanic crags and boulders.

Returning to the four-way junction, go north and east on the High Road, which parallels Malibu Creek. Look for an unsigned trail at 6.3 miles shortcutting up to meet the Grasslands Trail at a saddle, or, soon after, take the signed Grasslands Trail to the same saddle and onward to reach the trailhead on Mulholland Highway where you began.

VARIATION

The Talepop Loop is 5 miles with 600 feet of elevation gain. Begin the trip as above on the North Grasslands Trail, and then turn right onto the Talepop Trail, which climbs the ridge between Liberty and Las Virgenes Canyons (the trail was named for a Chumash village once situated here). When you meet the Las Virgenes Fire Road at 2.7 miles by a massive valley oak, stay right and follow it south and loop back to the Liberty Canyon Road and North Grassland Trail by the bridge. This hike can also be shortened to 4 miles by starting at Juan Bautista de Anza Park on Lost Hills Road.

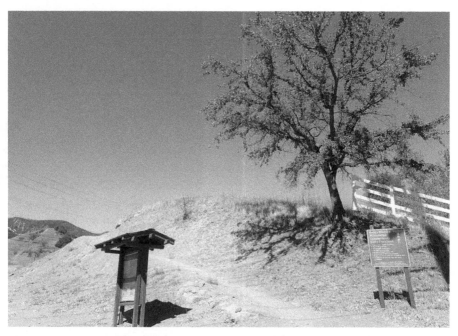

The Las Virgenes View Trail begins at one of the most prominent intersections in the Santa Monica Mountains.

trip 9.13   Upper Las Virgenes View Trail

see map on p. 108

Distance	4.6 miles (out-and-back)
Hiking Time	2 hours
Elevation Gain	900'
Difficulty	Moderate
Trail Use	Suitable for mountain biking, equestrians, dogs allowed
Best Times	October–June
Agencies	Mountains Recreation & Conservation Authority, Santa Monica Mountains Conservancy
Optional Map	Tom Harrison *Malibu Creek State Park* or Trails Illustrated *Santa Monica Mountains National Recreation Area (253)*

DIRECTIONS From Highway 101 in Calabasas, take Exit 32 for southbound Las Virgenes Road. Drive 3 miles south to Mulholland Highway (traffic light here). The small trailhead parking area is on the left, at the northeast corner of the intersection.

The view alluded to in this trail's name is the upper drainage of Las Virgenes Creek, a tributary of Malibu Creek whose tentacles reach north into the Simi Hills west of the San Fernando Valley. The trail climbs through a varied landscape consisting of grassland, chaparral, oak woodland, and a touch of riparian woodland. The overlook at the end of the trail is a worthwhile destination, especially when the air is clean and dry enough to afford distant vistas. Although the trail is popular with mountain bikers, there are a couple of sections cut sharply into a sheer hillside that may prove hazardous to anyone in the saddle.

From the Las Virgenes Road/Mulholland Highway junction, the trail starts by heading crookedly north through weedy grasses, more or less parallel to Las Virgenes Road. After a not-very-promising half mile, the scenery improves greatly as the trail cuts east across a lushly vegetated, north-facing slope, gains elevation, and pulls away from the somewhat noisy sounds of traffic. Before long, you're curling uphill on an oak-dotted ridge and enjoying ever-widening views. At the top of that ridge, the trail turns south, passes a lesser-used spur running the ridge northeast to the New Millennium Loop, and meanders over to an 1,100-foot knoll that serves as an informal viewpoint. There, you can look out over the Las Virgenes Creek floodplain, flanked by sensuously rolling hills, and spot various high points in the Santa Monica Mountains: Saddle Peak, Goat Buttes, Castro Crest, and San Vicente Mountain (with its signature abandoned Nike missile base). Continue to a second knoll for more views. Just beyond, the trail meets a fire road, but return the way you came because the fire road descends to private property with no exit.

trip 9.14 New Millennium Loop

Distance	12 miles (loop)
Hiking Time	6 hours
Elevation Gain	2,700'
Difficulty	Strenuous
Trail Use	Suitable for mountain biking, dogs allowed
Best Times	October–May
Agency	Mountains Recreation & Conservation Authority, Santa Monica Mountains Conservancy
Optional Map	Tom Harrison *Malibu Creek State Park* or Trails Illustrated *Santa Monica Mountains National Recreation Area (253)*

see map on p. 108

NOTES This area burned in the 2018 Woolsey Fire and is closed at the time of this writing. Check with the National Park Service (805-370-2301, nps.gov/samo) for updates.

DIRECTIONS From the 101 Freeway in Calabasas, take Exit 30 for southbound Parkway Calabasas. Make an immediate right onto Calabasas Road, which parallels the highway eastbound. In 0.5 mile stay left (straight) at a funky intersection. In another 0.7 mile, park on the shoulder at mile marker 0.06, just before the end of the road.

The New Millennium Loop circles an extravagant mansion community in the hills of Calabasas. Its ever-changing views encompass oak-dotted grasslands, flowery sage scrub hills, panoramic scenes of the undeveloped mountains, and bird's-eye views of the backyards of the ultra-rich. Mountain bikers prize the singletrack for its variety and challenge.

Beware that two trails depart from the end of Calabasas Road. The Juan Bautista de Anza East Trailhead is at the very end of the road and provides access to the Anza Historic Trail, where the famed Spanish expedition camped on February 22, 1776, en route from south of

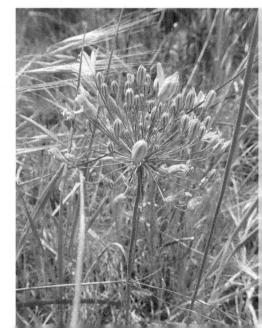

The spectacular golden star flower (Bloomeria crocea) *is always a treat to find.*

Tuscon to San Francisco. However, this trail is a power-line service road mowed through the weeds, scarcely a stone's throw from the noisy 101 Freeway. Our trail starts by mile marker 0.06 at a paved service road blocked by a gate. Walk south on the short service road to where the trail begins, and continue 0.2 mile to a signed junction with the New Millennium Trail.

Turn right and make a counterclockwise loop. The trail climbs through grassy hills studded with valley and coast live oaks. Briefly join an abandoned road cut. At 2.1 miles pass a signed connector on the right leading back down to the Anza Trail. At 4.2 miles pass another signed trail on the right leading 1.2 miles down to the Calabasas Bark Park Trailhead. The vegetation on these south-facing slopes gives way to sage scrub. This area and the Bark Park Trail are great places to look for striking golden stars, which produce a ball of yellow, six-petaled flowers emerging from the top of each stem.

At 5.1 miles come to an unsigned junction. The Las Virgenes View Park Connector Trail on the right follows the ridge southwest 1.4 miles to join the Upper Las Virgenes View Trail (see previous trip), but our loop veers left and gradually descends.

Pass under some hilltop estates, cross another ridge, and then climb the Pyramid Switchbacks to a high point overlooking the massive Oaks Estates (7.3 miles). Built on the site of a former 2,800-acre Warner Bros. film ranch where a Western town was created for *The Oklahoma Kid* in 1939, these castlelike mansions are an iconic symbol of California extravagance. Marketing materials advertise "not one but two 24-hour guard gates," "Hollywood stars of dazzling fame and fortune," homes starting at 10,000 square feet and $10 million, good schools, and the Millennium Loop hiking trail. Ironically, countless oaks must have been cut down to make room for the houses at the Oaks Estates.

The trail descends to cross the Prado Del Grandioso emergency-exit road between two locked gates (8.1 miles), then climbs to the highest point on the loop, with views of lesser mansions and golf courses, before switchbacking down to cross Parkway Calabasas at the

The Too Tight Switchbacks are especially fun for mountain bikers.

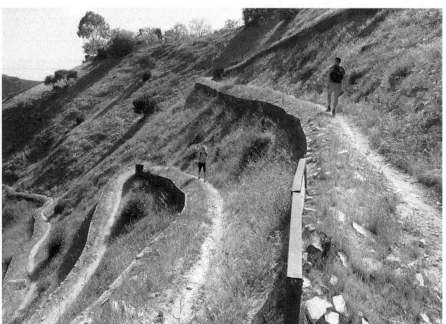

gated entrance of The Oaks at Calabasas (9.3 miles). On the far side, climb back up the Too Tight Switchbacks, held by retaining walls on the steep slope, where even the best cyclists must dismount. Pass a massive water tank at the top (10.0 miles); then descend past oaks, walnut, and grassy fields. Cross a seasonal streambed on a large bridge (11.0 miles); then climb back up and soon meet the Anza connector where the trip began.

trip 9.15   King Gillette Ranch Inspiration Point

see map on p. 108

Distance	1.7 miles (loop)
Hiking Time	1 hour
Elevation Gain	250'
Difficulty	Easy
Trail Use	Dogs allowed, good for kids
Best Times	October–June
Agencies	Mountains Recreation & Conservation Authority, National Park Service, Santa Monica Mountains Conservancy
Optional Map	*King Gillette Ranch* map/brochure or Tom Harrison *Malibu Creek State Park*

DIRECTIONS From Highway 101 in Calabasas, take Exit 32 for southbound Las Virgenes Road. Drive 3 miles south to Mulholland Highway (traffic light here); then turn left, proceed 0.1 mile, and then turn right into King Gillette Ranch, which is now the Interagency Visitor Center for Santa Monica Mountains National Recreation Area. In 0.2 mile turn left into the visitor center parking lot. Free parking is available here for up to 2 hours; if you plan to stay longer, you'll need to continue up the road to the pay lot at the picnic area beside the Gillette mansion.

This short hike takes you through a magnificent grove of coast live oaks up to a knoll called Inspiration Point, from which you can enjoy views west to the imposing rock formations of Malibu Creek State Park and east to towering Saddle Peak. Before you start, stop in the Interagency Visitor Center to get a free trail map—very helpful because none of the trails are presently signed—and enjoy the exhibits.

The mansion on the 588-acre ranch was built in the 1920s for King C. Gillette of razorblade fame. It was later owned by a movie director and a seminary before the National Park Service acquired the land.

King Gillette Ranch is the ideal setting for a picnic beneath the oaks.

From the visitor center, walk southeast across a bridge over Stokes Creek, turn right, and continue to a parking area. Veer right around a building to where the unsigned Gillette Ranch Loop Trail begins as a dirt road climbing the hill. Soon come to a junction. The Ridge Trail continues straight, offering a

1.5-mile longer hike, while two other trails bend left. Take the first left and proceed 80 yards to the hilltop known as Inspiration Point.

Once you've enjoyed the view, return to the junction and take the second left for the Gillette Ranch Loop Trail descending into the oak grove. The trail eventually ends at a dirt road. Turn left and follow the road, which soon becomes paved. Pass under the carport of the Gillette mansion, and find your way back to the point where you began.

trip 9.16	**Piuma Overlook**

Distance	0.6 mile (out-and-back)
Hiking Time	30 minutes
Elevation Gain	150'
Difficulty	Easy
Trail Use	Dogs allowed, good for kids
Best Times	Year-round
Agency	Santa Monica Mountains Conservancy
Optional Map	Tom Harrison *Malibu Creek State Park*

see map on p. 108

DIRECTIONS From Pacific Coast Highway in Malibu near mile marker 001 LA 44.0, turn north on Las Flores Canyon Road. Proceed 3.4 miles to Rambla Pacifico, and turn right. Go 0.6 mile to Piuma Road and turn left. Now head west on Piuma for 3.1 miles, and park on the shoulder near mile marker 3.30. If you reach the David Brown Overlook, you've gone 0.3 mile too far.

In a little patch of open space known as the Malibu Canyon Piuma Ridge, high atop the rim of Malibu Canyon, you can take a short hike to a restful spot with a panoramic view of the Pacific Ocean and the Santa Monica Mountains spilling down toward it.

The easily overlooked trailhead has a chain across an old roadbed and a sign reading SANTA MONICA MOUNTAINS CONSERVANCY ZONE PARKLAND. Follow the roadbed up the brushy slope. After only 0.25 mile, you arrive at a flattish, open area featuring two picnic tables and a virtually unlimited view. Gaze eastward to spot the dramatically tilted sandstone strata on the west flank of Saddle Peak. Look westward into Malibu Creek State Park and spot Brents Mountain and the Goat Buttes within it. Scan the ocean in the south to as far as the transparency of the air will allow. Those bumps out there in various directions are the Channel Islands, the nearest of which is Santa Catalina Island, about 45 miles away.

Piuma Overlook affords great views of Malibu Creek State Park. (Brents Mountain is the peak with the prominent rocky ridge.)

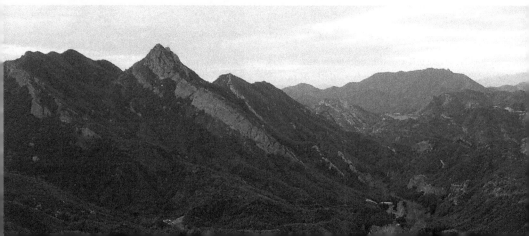

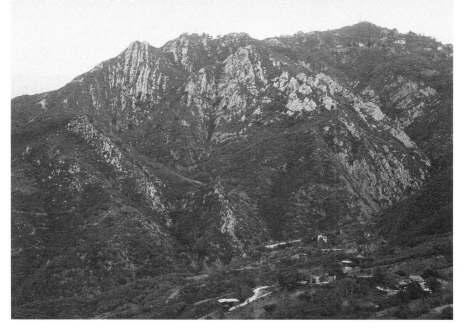

Incredible tectonic forces tilted Saddle Peak's sandstone strata nearly vertical. The peak, viewed here from Piuma Overlook, is a major landmark of the central Santa Monica Mountains.

trip 9.17 **West Ridge of Saddle Peak**

Distance	3.5 miles (one-way)
Hiking Time	1.5 hours
Elevation Gain/Loss	300'/1,500'
Difficulty	Moderate
Trail Use	Dogs allowed, good for kids
Best Times	October–July
Agency	National Park Service
Optional Map	Tom Harrison *Malibu Creek State Park* or Trails Illustrated *Santa Monica Mountains National Recreation Area (253)*

see map on p. 108

DIRECTIONS This one-way trip requires a car shuttle (or retracing your steps). From Highway 101 in Calabasas, take Exit 32 for southbound Las Virgenes Road. Go 3 miles south to Mulholland Highway (traffic light here). Continue south 1.6 mile and turn left on Piuma Road; then proceed 1.2 miles east to a turnout at a hairpin turn at mile marker 1.19, where the Backbone Trail crosses the road—leave a shuttle vehicle here.

   To reach the top trailhead, drive 0.5 mile back down Piuma Road and turn right on Cold Canyon Road. In 2.0 miles turn right (east) on Mulholland Highway. In 0.8 mile turn right on Stunt Road and go 2.9 miles to park on the shoulder by mile marker 2.92.

One of the most scenic sections of the Backbone Trail cuts across the northwest flank of Saddle Peak, accomplishing in 3.5 indirect miles what a bird in flight could traverse in about 1.5 miles. Along its winding, scenic course, the trail passes massive sandstone boulders, slices through tangled thickets of chaparral, penetrates secret copses of live oak and bay laurel, and dips to cross a clear-flowing brook in what is appropriately called Dark Canyon. Easy road access on both ends makes this a good point-to-point hike accomplished by either a car-shuttle or a drop-off-and-pick up arrangement.

   From Stunt Road, start walking southwest on the Backbone connector trail, up through chaparral. Come to a junction in 0.2 mile with the Backbone Trail. Left leads toward Saddle Peak (see next trip), while our route goes right (west).

Wide-open views to the north are interspersed with shady passages across seasonal rivulets descending from Saddle Peak's boulder-studded heights. At 1.2 miles you traverse a grassy meadow astride a small saddle. Northwest of this meadow a 1,942-foot peaklet promises a great view at the expense of a short, leg-scratching climb.

From the saddle you begin a crooked, more-or-less steady descent (1,100 feet in 2 miles) down through mostly chaparral—hot going on a sunny afternoon. A cool and pleasant but brief passage across a north-facing slope precedes a final switchbacking plunge down the steep wall of Dark Canyon. Watch for unmarked use trails, and stay on the main path. There are lots of opportunities to admire Malibu Creek country spread before you—the upthrust Goat Buttes, Brents Mountain, and the green or (depending on the season) gold valleys below. At the bottom, fern-draped Dark Canyon is like a paradise, but the shady passage is a brief one. A final zigzag climb takes you back up into the sunny chaparral, where you come upon Piuma Road.

trip 9.18 Saddle Peak

Distance	3.2 miles (out-and-back)
Hiking Time	2 hours
Elevation Gain	900'
Difficulty	Moderate
Trail Use	Dogs allowed
Best Times	October–July
Agency	California State Parks
Optional Map	Tom Harrison *Malibu Creek State Park* or Trails Illustrated *Santa Monica Mountains National Recreation Area (253)*

see map on p. 108

DIRECTIONS From the 101 Freeway in Calabasas, take Exit 29 for southbound Mulholland Drive. In 0.6 mile turn right onto Valmar Road, which becomes Old Topanga Canyon Road. In 1.2 miles turn right onto Mulholland Highway. In 3.8 miles turn left onto Stunt Road. Go 2.9 miles to the start of a connector trail for the Backbone Trail. The trail originates at a small turnout at mile 2.92.

A hiker plays peekaboo in the shallow sandstone caves on Saddle Peak.

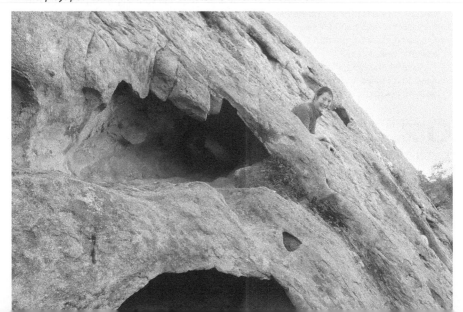

S addle Peak's twin summits—one topped by antennas and fenced off, the other barren but viewful—soar to an elevation of about 2,800 feet. Both preside over a coastline that is only 2.5 miles away. During early morning in spring and early summer, the mountain often stands head and shoulders above a mock ocean of fog that shrouds the coast and sometimes smothers all but the higher ridges of the Santa Monica Mountains. Getting out of bed early to make the trek to the top is worth it to catch the magic of warm sunlight on the pillowy surface of the clouds.

From Stunt Road, start hiking up the Backbone connector trail. Go left in 0.2 mile and proceed uphill though chaparral on a newer stretch of Backbone Trail that at first may seem tedious. By 1.2 miles you reach some blocky sandstone outcrops that lend a spectacular air to the views stretching north—assuming you're not still enveloped in fog. Listen for the whoosh of the wings of cliff swallows as they soar and dive among these crags.

At 1.4 miles turn right (south) on a side trail heading uphill 0.1 mile to a gravel road. Make a left to reach the nearby east (and publicly accessible) summit, or a right to reach the namesake saddle of Saddle Peak.

VARIATION

It's also possible to reach Saddle Peak using the Backbone Trail from Saddle Peak Road. At just 0.8 mile long with 400 feet of elevation gain, this is a shorter but less scenic approach. Using a 1-mile car or bicycle shuttle, you can easily go up one trail and down the other.

---

trip 9.19   **Red Rock Canyon**

Distance	4.0 miles (out-and-back)
Hiking Time	2 hours
Elevation Gain	700'
Difficulty	Moderate
Trail Use	Suitable for mountain biking, dogs allowed, good for kids
Best Times	October–June
Agency	Santa Monica Mountains Conservancy
Optional Map	Trails Illustrated *Santa Monica Mountains National Recreation Area (253)*

see map on p. 108

DIRECTIONS From the 101 Freeway in Calabasas, take Exit 29 for southbound Mulholland Drive. In 0.6 mile turn right onto Valmar Road, which becomes Old Topanga Canyon Road. In 1.2 miles turn right onto Mulholland Highway. In 3.8 miles turn left onto Stunt Road. Go 1.0 mile to a turnout at mile marker 1.00.

S labs of cavernous sandstone and cobbly conglomerate tilted sharply upward in Red Rock Canyon tell a geologic story of deposition by gentle currents and massive floods, later faulting and folding of the resulting sedimentary rock layers, and ongoing weathering and erosion. The beige and purplish-red rock strata contrast nicely with the greens and grays of oaks, sycamores, and chaparral—altogether making the canyon reminiscent of the cinematic Wild West. This description covers the backdoor approach to Red Rock Canyon from its top (west) side, ideal for a weekend stroll or mountain bike ride. In addition, hikers (but not dogs or bikes) may want to try a side trip up the slope north of the canyon using the narrow Red Rock Canyon Trail.

Pick up the gated Calabasas Peak Motorway, which cuts across a hillside to the north. When you reach a junction in a saddle at 0.7 mile, you're at the head of Red Rock Canyon. Turn right on the crooked road descending into the canyon, enjoying the scenery, which becomes more interesting as the canyon becomes narrower and deeper.

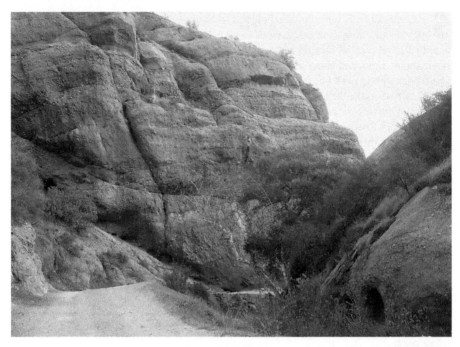

Red Rock Canyon is aptly named for its colorful sandstone.

At 1.5 mile, on the left, the 1-mile-long Red Rock Canyon Trail crosses the canyon's seasonal stream, heads abruptly upward along a ridge, and climbs circuitously to the north rim of the canyon. The side trip is worth it if the weather's clear and cool, otherwise probably not. In another 0.1 mile, an unmarked path on the right leads a few yards to some cavernous sandstone formations well worth exploring. After another 0.3 mile on the canyon road, you come to a picnic site on the grounds of an old Boy Scout camp, which has drinking water. Pass the gate and keep going on the road for 0.2 mile to discover a spectacular little gorge. Return the way you came.

trip 9.20 Calabasas Peak

see map on p. 108

Distance	3.6 miles (out-and-back)
Hiking Time	2 hours
Elevation Gain	1,000'
Difficulty	Moderate
Trail Use	Suitable for mountain biking, dogs allowed
Best Times	October–June
Agency	Santa Monica Mountains Conservancy
Optional Map	Tom Harrison *Malibu Creek State Park* or Trails Illustrated *Santa Monica Mountains National Recreation Area (253)*

DIRECTIONS From the 101 Freeway in Calabasas, take Exit 29 for southbound Mulholland Drive. In 0.6 mile turn right onto Valmar Road, which becomes Old Topanga Canyon Road. In 1.2 miles turn right onto Mulholland Highway. In 3.8 miles turn left onto Stunt Road. Go 1.0 mile to a turnout at mile marker 1.00.

The climb to Calabasas Peak should appeal to both exercise buffs and landscape photographers. The nontrivial gain and loss of elevation make for a great workout, and the geologic formations passed along the way are some of the most photogenic in the Santa Monica Mountains. In any case, an early or a late start is almost always preferred over a midday excursion. The exercise-minded will find the cool morning air most refreshing. Photographers will appreciate the three-dimensional effect of low-angle sunlight on the rock formations and the long shadows slanting across the shaggy mountainsides.

Pick up the gated Calabasas Peak Motorway that cuts across a hillside to the north. Bear left when you reach a road junction at a saddle (0.7 mile), where you get a glimpse of Red Rock Canyon (see previous trip). Continue north, wending your way past a fascinating collection of tilted sandstone slabs and fins.

At 1.6 miles, just beyond a couple of horseshoe curves in the road, you reach the summit ridge, south of the Calabasas Peak summit. Most of Old Topanga Canyon, to the east, is visible below. The road goes on to traverse the peak's east shoulder, so you leave it (and probably your bike, if you have one) and hop onto an easily overlooked firebreak going up toward the 2,163-foot peak itself on your left. A low thicket of chaparral guards the rounded summit.

The foreground view, marred at many points around the compass by the encroaching suburbs, may be a bit disappointing. But on clear days, the long views west toward Castro Crest and east to the San Gabriel Mountains are inspiring all the same.

VARIATION

Calabasas Peak can also be reached from the north via the Calabasas Cold Creek Trail, also known as the Secret Trail. This variation is 4 miles with 900 feet of elevation gain. Start at a signed turnout on Mulholland Highway 0.2 mile south of Dry Canyon Cold Creek Road. Ascend the Secret Trail to the ridgeline; then turn right (south) on the Calabasas Peak Motorway and follow it to the peak.

Like that of nearby Saddle Peak, the sandstone strata on Calabasas Peak has been tilted wildly.

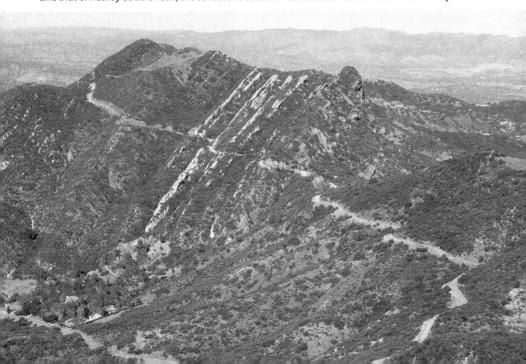

trip 9.21 Topanga Lookout & Stunt High Loop

Distance	6.5 miles (loop)
Hiking Time	3.5 hours
Elevation Gain	1,800'
Difficulty	Moderately strenuous
Trail Use	Dogs allowed
Best Times	October–May
Agency	National Park Service
Optional Map	Trails Illustrated *Santa Monica Mountains National Recreation Area (253)* (trail not fully shown)

see map on p. 108

DIRECTIONS From the 101 Freeway in Calabasas, take Exit 29 for southbound Mulholland Drive. In 0.6 mile turn right onto Valmar Road, which becomes Old Topanga Canyon Road. In 1.2 miles turn right onto Mulholland Highway. In 3.8 miles turn left onto Stunt Road. Go 1.0 mile to a turnout at mile marker 1.00.

This wide-ranging loop follows a climbers' trail up a rocky ridge to the foundation of an old lookout. Save the trip for an exceptionally clear day and you'll be rewarded with vistas that must be seen to be believed.

Pick up the gated Calabasas Peak Motorway that cuts across a hillside to the north. Hike uphill to the saddle at the head of Red Rock Canyon, 0.7 mile from Stunt Road. Take neither the road north to Calabasas Peak nor the road east into Red Rock Canyon below—instead, turn sharply right and climb up a steep bulldozed track. That track soon peters out, but you can continue climbing to a 1,766-foot knoll. There you can see what lies ahead: an undulating, brushy knife-edge ridge buttressed by tilted sandstone slabs and fins. A narrow, but well-beaten trail up along the ridge testifies to its popularity as a mountaineer's route.

Make your way for a painstaking mile up and over or around the sandstone obstacles and through the brush until you reach the terminus of a fire road. Continue on this road for an easygoing 0.4 mile, past a couple of striking columnar rock formations, to the foundation of the long-abandoned Topanga Fire Lookout (2.2 miles). Enjoy the stupefying view, weather permitting. Much of the San Fernando Valley is visible, along with parts of the L.A. Basin and Santa Monica Bay. Downtown L.A.'s office towers point the way toward a low spot on the east horizon—San Gorgonio Pass—flanked by Southern California's highest peaks, San Gorgonio and San Jacinto, both more than 100 miles away.

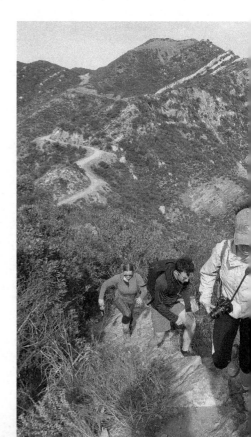

Hikers scramble up the steep ridge toward Topanga Lookout, with Calabasas Peak in the background.

From the lookout site, walk south on the fire road to Saddle Peak Road (3.1 miles), where there's a better view of Santa Monica Bay and Santa Catalina Island. Over at the intersection of paved roads immediately west, bear right on Stunt Road. Walk easily downhill along Stunt Road for a mile, a not-unpleasant task as the road sees only light traffic and affords great views throughout.

At a turnout on the right just beyond another turnout at mile marker 3.00, you'll discover the unsigned top end of the Stunt High Trail. Follow the trail's winding course downhill for 0.8 mile through tall chaparral until you hit Stunt Road again. Turn right and walk 0.1 mile east along Stunt Road's left shoulder to the gated Stunt Ranch entrance road near mile 1.84. The trail resumes at an obscure post at the turnout just before the road. In 0.1 mile the trail crosses the paved Stunt Ranch road. Wind down through chaparral and past a meadow for another 0.4 mile; then pass a trail on the left leading into the Stunt Ranch Preserve, with access by permit only. In another 0.2 mile, reach a T-junction with the Cold Creek Trail, where you turn right. The final, delightfully shaded stretch goes up along the creek and ends at your starting point, the large turnout at mile 1.00 on Stunt Road. As you cross the creek to reach the road, watch for metates, holes in the rock where the Chumash ground acorns.

---

trip 9.22 ## Hondo Canyon

Distance	3.5 miles (one-way)
Hiking Time	2 hours
Elevation Gain/Loss	100'/1,600'
Difficulty	Moderate
Trail Use	Dogs allowed
Best Times	October–June
Agency	Santa Monica Mountains Conservancy
Optional Map	Tom Harrison *Topanga State Park* or Trails Illustrated *Santa Monica Mountains National Recreation Area* (253)

see map on p. 108

DIRECTIONS This one-way trip requires a 13-mile car shuttle (or retracing your steps). From Highway 101, take Exit 27 for southbound Topanga Canyon Road (Highway 27). In 8.1 miles turn right on Old Topanga Canyon Road, and go 0.3 mile to the Backbone Trailhead, at a small turnout near mile marker 5.94—leave a shuttle vehicle here.

To reach the upper trailhead, continue along Old Topanga Canyon Road 5.2 miles; then make a left on Mulholland Highway. In 3.6 miles turn left on Stunt Road. Drive 4.1 miles uphill to the intersection of Saddle Peak Road and Schueren Road. Keep straight there and continue another 0.6 mile east on Saddle Peak Road to reach the trailhead on the left (just beyond mile 0.60 on Saddle Peak Road).

A wonderfully remote segment of the Backbone Trail rises between Old Topanga Canyon Road and Saddle Peak Road, zigzagging along slopes densely clothed in chaparral and oaks, and passing near a number of ephemeral waterfalls in Hondo Canyon that contribute a zenlike atmosphere during the rainy season. Assuming you've set up a car shuttle or planned some similar transportation arrangement, you can have the pleasure of following this easygoing stretch of trail in the downhill (west to east) direction.

You start out in dry chaparral at the top on a short connector trail, quickly making a right turn on the segment of Backbone Trail descending into Hondo Canyon. After a few tedious switchbacks, the trail enters a more thickly wooded area consisting not so much of trees, but rather of a rampant growth of tall chaparral. Watch for occasional burn scars remaining from the October 1993 Malibu fire that ravaged the entire Hondo Canyon drainage.

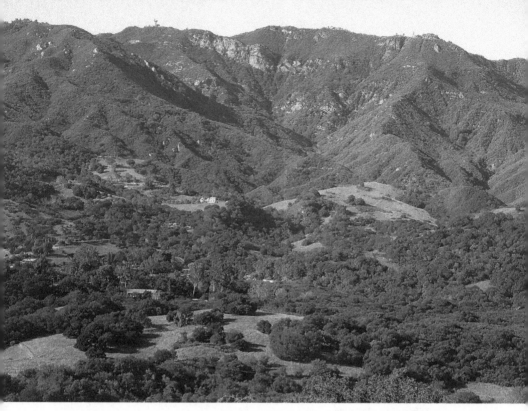

The Santa Monica Mountains Backbone Trail descends through lush Hondo Canyon, here viewed from the Eagle Rock Fire Road.

Many more switchbacks take you inexorably downward along the steep south slope of Hondo Canyon, where you encounter Tolkienesque copses of gnarled live oak and fragrant bay laurel. Nearing the bottom of the canyon at about 2 miles, there's a short side path on the left leading to a point where you can view Hondo Canyon's stream tumbling through a little V-shaped gorge.

Past this point the trail contours to a saddle, veers right, and descends a grassy slope into a separate lesser ravine, whose bottom is beautifully shaded by majestic live oaks. Water flows in this ravine only after a substantial amount of rain has fallen. A few minutes' walk down along the ravine takes you to Old Topanga Canyon's shallow stream and Old Topanga Canyon Road just above it.

chapter 10

Pacific Palisades & Topanga

Topanga: "the place where the mountains meet the sea." That simple and descriptive Gabrielino Indian name aptly applies to the famous canyon and community, and to the big state park sprawling along the canyon's east rim. The ocean is your almost perpetual companion here, if not in sight, at least in the feel of the cool marine air flowing up along the sunny slopes and through the dark, wooded canyons.

Assembled from purchases of public and private lands in the late 1960s and early '70s, Topanga State Park's 11,525 acres—which lie almost entirely within the Los Angeles city limits—rate as one of the world's largest wildlands adjacent to an urban area. The park also serves as a key anchor in the patchwork quilt of public and private lands known as the Santa Monica Mountains National Recreation Area.

Perhaps nowhere else in Southern California is the attack on the integrity of large open spaces so graphically illustrated as right here. The park's ragged boundary necessarily excluded lands earmarked for development in two of the coastal canyons, Santa Ynez and Pulga. Over the past decades, massive grading and construction in and along the walls of these canyons marred the otherwise open vistas. (On the flip side, of course, you need only look east to the Hollywood Hills to imagine how these mountains would probably look decades hence if they lacked any protection at all.)

Topanga State Park's only area developed specifically for drive-in visitors centers around the Trippet Ranch, off Topanga Canyon Boulevard on Entrada Road. The ranch (open during daylight hours) was originally one of the many second-home and resort properties developed in the Topanga Canyon area early in the century. There you'll find a tiny administrative office, a pond, oak-shaded picnic tables, a 1-mile self-guiding nature trail, and trailheads for several of the wide-ranging routes described in this chapter. The trail system is also accessible from several other points on or near the periphery of the park.

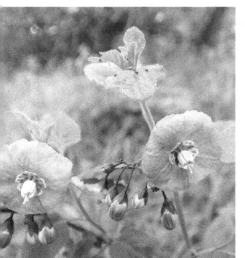

A number of additional hikes outside of the state park proper are included here. This chapter's sketch map includes fire roads and established trails but does not show the dozens of miles of firebreaks and informal paths that thread some of the canyons and going up or along most of the ridges. Some of these seldom-trod pathways have become overgrown; others pass through private lands for which there is no public access.

Purple nightshade (Solanum xanti) is a common but striking chaparral wildflower with a purple flower and bright yellow center.

141

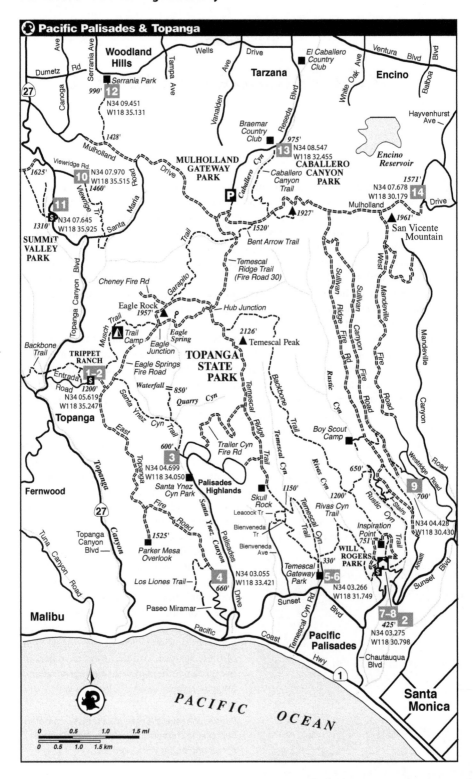

Pacific Palisades & Topanga

trip 10.1 ## Eagle Rock Loop

Distance	6.5 miles (loop)
Hiking Time	3.5 hours
Elevation Gain	1,300'
Difficulty	Moderately strenuous
Trail Use	Suitable for backpacking, good for kids
Best Times	October–June
Agency	California State Parks
Optional Map	Tom Harrison *Topanga State Park* or Trails Illustrated *Santa Monica Mountains National Recreation Area (253)*
Fees/Permits	$10 day-use fee

DIRECTIONS Take Topanga Canyon Boulevard (Highway 27) south from the San Fernando Valley, or north from Pacific Coast Highway. About midway along the highway's twisty 12-mile course from valley to sea, turn east on Entrada Road (signs for Topanga State Park on the highway alert you to this turnoff). Follow winding Entrada Road, carefully observing directional signs for the park, for 1.1 miles to Trippet Ranch, which is the headquarters for Topanga State Park. Pay the day-use fee at the entrance station (open 8 a.m.–sunset), and park in the large lot beyond.

Eagle Rock, the most impressive landmark in all of Topanga State Park, affords hikers an airy perch overlooking the upper watershed of Santa Ynez Canyon and the ocean beyond. Make it your destination for lunch during a lazy day's hike, but do it on a cooler day—there's little shade on the route. This is a figure-eight route, so if you have smaller kids along, you can cut the distance to about 4 miles by avoiding the far loop. Eagle Rock is one of the most popular hikes in the park, so expect plenty of company on a fine day.

From the large parking lot at Trippet Ranch, walk north on a paved drive about 100 yards to where the signed Musch Trail slants to the right across a grassy hillside. You

Imposing Eagle Rock is one of three Southern California outcrops with the same name. (The other two are in northeast Los Angeles and along the Pacific Crest Trail near Warner Springs.)

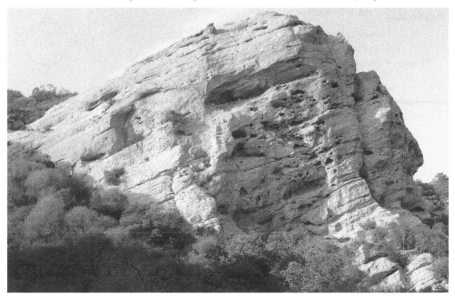

soon plunge into the shade of oak and bay trees. Enjoy the shade—there's not much more ahead. After contouring around a couple of north-flowing ravines, the trail rises to meet a trail campground at the former Musch Ranch (1.0 mile). This camp, and others along the Backbone Trail, serves equestrians and through-hikers. With an advance reservation, you could use it as part of this hike.

Beyond the campground, the trail soon starts climbing through sun-blasted chaparral. After a crooked ascent you reach a ridgetop fire road at Eagle Junction (2.2 miles), from which Eagle Rock looms over the headwaters of Santa Ynez Canyon. This layered sandstone outcrop, pitted with small caves, is an outstanding example of the 15-million-year-old Topanga Canyon Formation. Turn left and follow the fire road up to the gentler north side of Eagle Rock. Walk to the top for the best view.

Back on the fire road, continue east up along a ridgeline and then down to a four-way junction of fire roads at 3.6 miles, called Hub Junction because of its central location in the park. On a side trip south from here you could visit Cathedral Rock and Temescal Peak, but our way goes sharply right on the Backbone Trail (signed EAGLE SPRING FIRE ROAD) leading west under Eagle Rock and back to Eagle Junction. Before you reach the junction, there's a side path on the right to Eagle Spring, where water seasonally trickles out of the sandstone bedrock beneath oaks and sycamores.

When you reach Eagle Junction again (5.0 miles), turn left and return to Trippet Ranch the fast and direct way: Go 1.2 miles down the Eagle Springs Fire Road to the south, and then 0.2 mile northwest on the wide trail leading down to the picnic area and parking lot at Trippet Ranch.

VARIATION

This trip can be extended to 10 miles with 1,600 feet of elevation gain by adding the Garapito and Temescal Ridge/Fire Road 30 Trails between Eagle and Hub Junctions. The Garapito Trail, closed to bikers but popular with trail runners, winds through an elfin forest of chaparral and drops to Garapito Creek before climbing to the fire road.

---

trip 10.2   **East Backbone Trail**

see
map on
p. 142

Distance	10 miles (one-way)
Hiking Time	4.5 hours
Elevation Gain/Loss	1,400'/2,200'
Difficulty	Moderately strenuous
Best Times	October–May
Agency	California State Parks
Optional Map	Tom Harrison *Topanga State Park* or Trails Illustrated *Santa Monica Mountains National Recreation Area (253)*
Fees/Permits	$10 day-use fee at Trippet Ranch, $12 at Will Rogers State Historic Park

DIRECTIONS This one-way trip requires a car shuttle; a ride-sharing service may be more convenient. The state-park parking lots at both ends are open 8 a.m.–sunset, so plan accordingly to avoid getting locked in. Leave one vehicle at the east end at Will Rogers State Historic Park, off Sunset Boulevard 4 miles west of the 405 Freeway. To reach the west end at Trippet Ranch from Will Rogers Park, follow Sunset Boulevard west 3.8 miles to Highway 1, where you turn right and continue west 1.5 miles. Turn right (north) onto Topanga Canyon Road (Highway 27) and go 4.7 miles; then turn right onto Entrada Road. Follow winding Entrada Road, carefully observing directional signs for the park, for 1.1 miles to Trippet Ranch, which is the headquarters for Topanga State Park. Pay the day-use fee at the entrance station, and park in the large lot beyond.

On a cool, clear day, the easternmost section of the Backbone Trail—from Trippet Ranch to Will Rogers State Historic Park—yields dazzling, ever-changing perspectives of the meeting of mountains and sea. A secondary benefit of this one-way trip is that you get to walk downhill most of the time.

From the picnic area at Trippet Ranch, you head southeast on the fire road going up the hill to the Santa Ynez Fire Road (0.2 mile). Turn left at the top and climb to Eagle Junction (1.5 miles). (Purists may prefer to follow the Backbone trail, 0.6 mile longer to this same junction.) Go right there on the Eagle Springs Fire Road, pass under Eagle Rock, climb some more, and arrive at Hub Junction (2.9 miles). Turn right on the Temescal Ridge Trail and walk south, passing a cavernous sandstone outcrop on the left known as Cathedral Rock, to another junction (3.6 miles). The Backbone Trail goes left here on an old fire road. Nearby Temescal Peak, whose summit can be reached

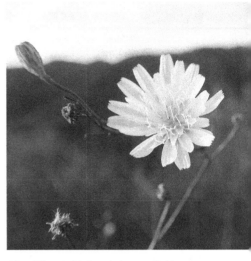

*The cliff aster (*Malacothrix saxatilis*) is a common wildflower in the coastal sage scrub and chaparral communities of the Santa Monica Mountains.*

by way of a short, steep firebreak on its west side, is worth climbing if the visibility is good. This somewhat-undistinguished-looking 2,126-foot bump on the Temescal Ridge holds the distinction of being the highest peak in the Santa Monicas east of Topanga Canyon.

The Backbone Trail (originally the Rogers Trail from here on down to Will Rogers Park) goes east for about a mile, then veers south to loosely follow an undulating ridgeline that always lies west and well above Rustic Canyon and its tributaries. For a couple of miles the upper reaches of Temescal Canyon lie to the west, but then you bear left (southeast) to join the ridge between Rivas and Rustic Canyons. On a flat overlooking the head of Rivas Canyon at 7.3 miles, the Lone Oak provides welcome shade.

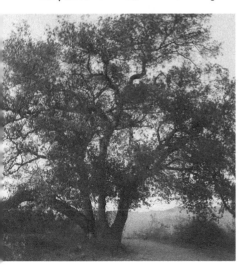

Continue down the footpath and pass a trail coming up from Rustic Canyon (see Trip 10.8, page 152). At 8.6 miles reach a narrow and dramatic section called Chicken Ridge. The Chicken Ridge Bridge spans the narrowest portion. At 9.6 miles come to a junction just above Inspiration Point in Will Rogers Park. Turn right on the wide trail. After 0.3 mile make a left on an unsigned shortcut path (the Lower Betty Rogers Trail) that takes you straight down to the big lawn above Will Rogers's home.

The Lone Oak is a landmark along the East Backbone.

trip 10.3   Santa Ynez Waterfall

Distance	2.5 miles (out-and-back)
Hiking Time	1.5 hours
Elevation Gain	200'
Difficulty	Moderate
Trail Use	Good for kids
Best Times	Year-round
Agency	California State Parks
Optional Map	Tom Harrison *Topanga State Park* or Trails Illustrated *Santa Monica Mountains National Recreation Area (253)*

see map on p. 142

DIRECTIONS From Pacific Coast Highway in Pacific Palisades 0.3 west of mile marker 001 LA 39.0, take Sunset Boulevard north 0.5 mile to Palisades Drive. Follow Palisades north for 2.4 miles; then turn left onto Vereda de la Montura. In 0.1 mile, just before a gated community, find the Santa Ynez Canyon Trailhead on the right—look for a narrow gate that's unlocked during daylight hours. There's abundant free curbside parking.

Twisted live oaks, sycamores, and pungent bay laurel trees highlight the brief trek up the L.A. coast's most easily accessible waterfall-bearing canyon. The goal is an 18-foot cascade tucked into an upper branch of Santa Ynez Canyon. The flow of water in these falls is usually significant from winter through early summer. Both the trail and the falls, however, may be rendered inaccessible if too much rain arrives at one time.

After a short descent from the trailhead, follow the trail going up along Santa Ynez Canyon. Before long, you're dodging stray branches of willow and bay trees, stepping across the soggy creek, and forgetting about the civilized world behind you. The California bay (bay laurel) trees here are commonly found in shady, moist canyons throughout coastal California. Crush one of the dark, elongated leaves and sniff it to get a whiff of the pungent, minty scent. Beware of poison oak, which also grows plentifully in close proximity to the trail.

After 0.6 mile the wide mouth of Quarry Canyon, the site of an old limestone quarry, opens to the right. Stay left and go another 100 yards to a second canyon on the right. The main trail going straight leads to the Trippet Ranch headquarters of Topanga State Park. Take the less-traveled trail right (north) up the second canyon, which is actually the major fork of Santa Ynez Canyon. Beware

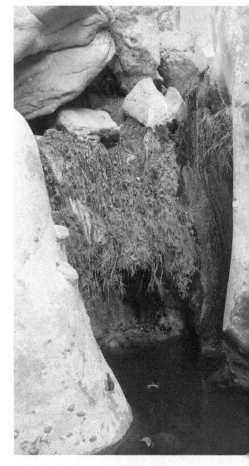

Santa Ynez Waterfall is a beautiful sight even when it's just a trickle.

that this trail is unmaintained. Don't get lured onto deer trails climbing the canyon walls. Many hikers have been trapped and at least two have fallen to their deaths.

After some foot-wetting creek crossings and a slippery scramble over some conglomerate boulders, you arrive at a grotto below the falls. With their orientation subject to deep shadow, the falls are difficult to photograph properly—unless the day is cloudy-bright, in which case the lighting is fine. The cool, damp air here is always refreshing, whether or not the falls are whispering or hissing loudly.

Return the same way. When you return to the junction with the trail to Trippet Ranch, look for the stone chimney of Alphonzo Bell's burned-out hunting cabin (obscured by vegetation near the junction). Bell, a wealthy oil and real estate baron, gave his name to L.A.'s tony Bel-Air district and the communities of Bell and Bell Gardens. Also watch for a sandstone boulder pocked by Indian morteros (mortar holes used centuries ago for the grinding of acorns and other foodstuffs).

VARIATION

The Santa Ynez Canyon Trail continues 1.9 miles from the waterfall junction to Trippet Ranch, allowing a one-way trip of 4 miles/1,000 feet of elevation gain with a car shuttle or a 5-mile out-and-back trip from Trippet Ranch. The trail is posted as unmaintained but was in excellent condition when I visited; its has great spring wildflowers and less poison oak than the main trip.

---

trip 10.4   ## Topanga Overlook

Distance	5 miles (out-and-back)
Hiking Time	2.5 hours
Elevation Gain	1,200'
Difficulty	Moderate
Trail Use	Suitable for mountain biking
Best Times	Year-round
Agency	California State Parks
Optional Map	Tom Harrison *Topanga State Park* or Trails Illustrated *Santa Monica Mountains National Recreation Area (253)*

see map on p. 142

DIRECTIONS From Pacific Coast Highway in Pacific Palisades 0.3 west of mile marker 001 LA 39.0, take Sunset Boulevard north 0.3 mile to Paseo Miramar on the left. Drive up narrow Paseo Miramar 1.3 miles to its end at a vehicle gate with a prominent sign for Topanga State Park; take care not to go astray onto various potentially confusing side roads along the way. Find a place to park back down the road a little way, taking care to observe parking restrictions.

From the perch known as Topanga Overlook, Parker Mesa Overlook, or simply the Overlook, you get a bird's-eye view of surfers off Topanga Beach, the crescent shoreline of Santa Monica Bay, L.A.'s west-side cityscape—and much, much more if the air is really transparent. You can reach the overlook by walking south along Topanga Canyon's east ridge from Trippet Ranch, but we'll describe a shorter and more interesting route from Paseo Miramar, west of Pacific Palisades.

This trip is especially rewarding when done early on certain fall or winter mornings, when tendrils of fog fill the canyons, leaving the mountains to rise above a cottony sea. It's also excellent as a sunset or night hike. For a special treat, do it on any clear, full-moon evening between May and August. In the fading twilight, you'll watch the moon's pumpkinlike disk silently materialize in the east or southeast, hovering over a million glittering lights.

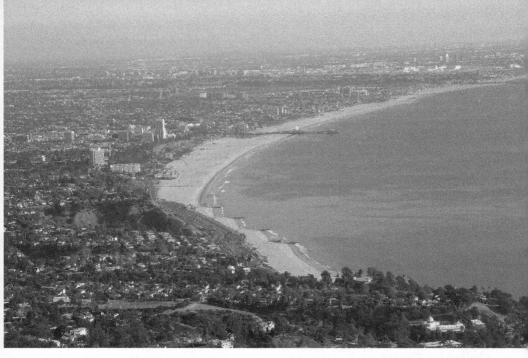

Topanga Overlook offers an unsurpassed view of Santa Monica Bay. It's also a romantic picnic spot.

From the end of Paseo Miramar, walk along the dirt fire road that continues up along a ridge, passing after 0.2 mile a foot trail coming up from Los Liones Drive. Here you have your first outstanding ocean view. Farther ahead you briefly traverse a cool, north-facing slope overlooking Santa Ynez Canyon and neighboring ridges. You arrive at a road junction (2.0 miles) with views of Topanga Canyon to the west. Turn south and walk out along the bald ridge to Topanga Overlook. Down below are Parker and Castellammare mesas, parts of a striking marine-terrace structure that continues east into Pacific Palisades. When it's time to go back, return the way you came.

VARIATION

You can also start this trip from Los Liones Drive, where there is better parking. This adds 1.0 mile and 450 feet of elevation gain.

With a car shuttle, you could make a one-way hike ending at the Trippet Ranch Trailhead. This option is 6 miles with 1,600 feet of elevation gain.

---

trip 10.5 **Temescal Canyon**

Distance	2.8 miles (loop)
Hiking Time	1.5 hours
Elevation Gain	850'
Difficulty	Moderate
Trail Use	Good for kids
Best Times	Year-round
Agencies	Mountains Recreation & Conservation Authority, Santa Monica Mountains Conservancy
Optional Map	Tom Harrison *Topanga State Park* or Trails Illustrated *Santa Monica Mountains National Recreation Area (253)*
Fees/Permits	$10 parking fee at Temescal Gateway Park

see map on p. 142

DIRECTIONS The trail begins at Temescal Gateway Park, on Temescal Canyon Road in Pacific Palisades, 1.0 mile north of Highway 1 and immediately north of Sunset Boulevard. Park here for a fee sunrise–sunset, or look for free curbside parking along Temescal Canyon Road south of Sunset.

A favorite of hikers in West L.A., this short loop includes both wonderful views from high places and a shady passage through riparian and oak woodland.

Using directional signs on the Temescal Gateway Park property, head north up the road past several buildings dating from when the park was a private retreat for the Presbyterian Church. Stay left onto a dirt path and climb to a signed junction where you can pick up the Temescal Ridge Trail on the left. After several twists and turns up the scrubby canyon slope, the trail gains a moderately ascending crest and sticks to it. Pause often so you can turn around and look at the ever-widening view of the coastline curving from Santa Monica Bay to Malibu. Ahead, two short trails, Leacock and Bienveneda, strike off to the left toward a trailhead at the end of Bienveneda Avenue. Ignore those paths and continue a junction (1.3 miles from the start) with the old Temescal Fire Road—signed TEMESCAL RIDGE TRAIL to the north and TEMESCAL CANYON TRAIL to the south. (At this point you have the option of making a side trip north 0.5 mile to a wind-carved, sandstone outcrop known as Skull Rock. The head-shaped rock is best viewed from a distance and requires a bit of imagination to recognize.)

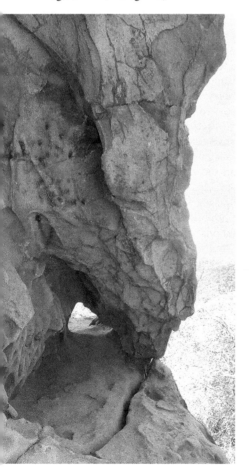

Staying on the loop route, turn right and head downhill on the Temescal Canyon Trail. When you hit the shady canyon bottom (1.7 miles), you'll cross over Temescal Canyon's creek and pick up a smoother section of the old fire road on the far side. Above and below this crossing are small, trickling waterfalls and shallow, limpid pools. Poke around the creek a bit for a look at its typical denizens, water striders and newts.

The final stretch follows the canyon bottom and then contours along a slope to the right of the conference buildings. Lots of live oak, sycamore, willow, and bay trees—their woodsy scents commingling on the ocean breeze—highlight your return.

VARIATION

A signed trail begins just before Bienveneda Avenue enters a gated community. A loop from this trailhead is 3.8 miles with 1,300 feet of elevation gain.

This oddly shaped sandstone outcrop is known as Skull Rock.

trip 10.6   **Rivas Canyon**

Distance	2.7 miles (one-way)
Hiking Time	1.5 hours
Elevation Gain	600'
Difficulty	Moderate
Trail Use	Dogs allowed
Best Times	October–June
Agencies	Mountains Recreation & Conservation Authority, Santa Monica Mountains Conservancy, California State Parks
Optional Map	Tom Harrison *Topanga State Park* or Trails Illustrated *Santa Monica Mountains National Recreation Area (253)*
Fees/Permits	$10 parking fee at Temescal Gateway Park

see map on p. 142

DIRECTIONS This trail leads from Temescal Gateway Park to Will Rogers State Historic Park. If you don't want to retrace your steps or walk back along Sunset Boulevard, it's probably less expensive to call a ride-sharing service for the short trip back than to pay to leave a second vehicle at the Will Rogers parking area.

Temescal Gateway Park is on Temescal Canyon Road in Pacific Palisades, 1.0 mile north of Highway 1 and immediately north of Sunset Boulevard. Park here for a fee sunrise–sunset, or look for free curbside parking along Temescal Canyon Road south of Sunset.

Temescal Canyon and Will Rogers State Historic Park in Pacific Palisades are just two of the many units of parkland and open space that make up the sprawling Santa Monica Mountains National Recreation Area. The Rivas Canyon Trail connects these two park units. This hand-tooled route at times resembles a rabbit run in the brush, so you can be assured of close encounters with the native vegetation. This is exciting and feels like adventurous hiking, but be aware that the encounters may involve poison oak. Be certain you can identify the plant and avoid any physical contact with it.

From any parking lot in Temescal Gateway Park, head north on pavement toward some institutional buildings that make up the former Presbyterian conference grounds, staying right on the paved loop. Take the signed Temescal Rivas Canyon Trail that begins with some steps on the right.

Make your way circuitously up the east wall of Temescal Canyon, gaining a ridgeline after 0.9 mile. You then go up along the ridgeline itself and pass over a crest. You'll enjoy some excellent views along the way, and you can take short unsigned spurs for more views. Descend sharply and crookedly to the

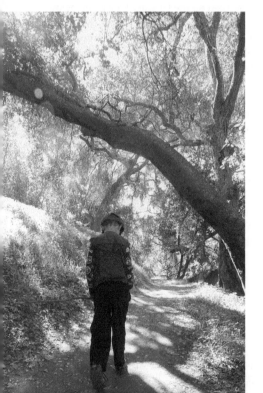

Sun-dappled Rivas Canyon boasts a fine canopy of California live oak.

shady bottom of Rivas Canyon at 1.4 miles. A delightfully gradual downhill promenade ensues, taking you through riparian and oak woodland vegetation. Poison oak is plentiful alongside the trail.

At 2.1 miles reach the end of a paved street by a residential neighborhood—a good turn-around point if you're retracing your steps. Otherwise, the trail resumes across the street on the left and climbs past houses, reaching the main parking lot at Will Rogers State Historic Park at 2.7 miles. (If you're hiking in the opposite direction, the trail starts west just before a small bridge and stairway north of the parking area.)

If you have time, it's worth wandering through the grounds, which includes a polo field and the historic ranch home of famed radio personality and pop philosopher Will Rogers. Or consider extending your hike with a walk up to Inspiration Point (see next trip).

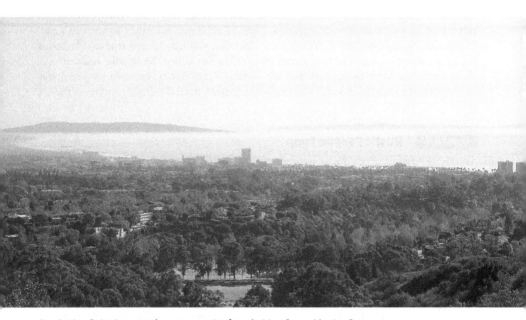

Inspiration Point is a superb vantage point for admiring Santa Monica Bay.

trip 10.7   Will Rogers Park

see map on p. 142

Distance	2.0 miles (loop)
Hiking Time	1 hour
Elevation Gain	350'
Difficulty	Easy
Trail Use	Suitable for mountain biking, dogs allowed, good for kids
Best Times	Year-round
Agency	California State Parks
Optional Map	Tom Harrison *Topanga State Park* or Trails Illustrated *Santa Monica Mountains National Recreation Area (253)*
Fees/Permits	$12 day-use fee

DIRECTIONS From the 405 Freeway, take Sunset Boulevard 4 miles west; then turn right onto the entrance road for Will Rogers State Historic Park. The entrance road curls up a hillside to the park itself, which has abundant parking space. The park is open daily, 8 a.m.–sunset.

Drive up a short mile from the speedway known as Sunset Boulevard toward Will Rogers State Historic Park, and you'll instantly leave the rat race behind. Especially on weekdays or early on weekend mornings, this quiet spot is perfect for getting some exercise and taking advantage of multimillion-dollar views of Santa Monica, West L.A., and downtown.

Newspaperman, radio commentator, movie star, and pop philosopher Will Rogers purchased this 186-acre property in 1922 and lived with his family here from 1928 until his death in 1935. Historic only by Southern California standards, his 31-room mansion is nevertheless interesting to tour.

Our main goal, however, is to reach Inspiration Point, a flat-topped bump on a ridge overlooking the entire spread. Follow the main, wide, riding and hiking trail that makes a 2-mile loop, starting at the north end of the big lawn adjoining the Rogers home. Or use any of several shorter, more direct paths. You may want to obtain a copy of the detailed hikers' map, available at the gift shop in a wing of the home. Printed on the map is one of Will's memorable aphorisms: "If your time is worth anything, travel by air. If not, you might just as well walk."

Relaxing on the benches at the top on a clear day, you can admire true-as-advertised, inspiring vistas stretching east to the front range of the San Gabriel Mountains and southeast to the Santa Ana Mountains. South past the swelling Palos Verdes Peninsula you can sometimes spot Santa Catalina Island, rising in ethereal majesty from the shining surface of the sea.

trip 10.8   Rustic Canyon Loop

see map on p. 142

Distance	5.5 miles (loop)
Hiking Time	3 hours
Elevation Gain	1,000'
Difficulty	Moderately strenuous
Best Times	October–June
Agency	California State Parks
Optional Map	Tom Harrison *Topanga State Park* or Trails Illustrated *Santa Monica Mountains National Recreation Area (253)*
Fees/Permits	$12 day-use fee

DIRECTIONS From the 405 Freeway, take Sunset Boulevard 4 miles west; then turn right onto the entrance road for Will Rogers State Historic Park. The entrance road curls up a hillside to the park itself, which has abundant parking space. The park is open daily, 8 a.m.–sunset.

Rustic Canyon, now almost fully reverted to wilderness condition after nature's one-two punches of fire and flood, was quite lively in the past. Pop philosopher Will Rogers and his associates used it as a retreat back in the 1930s, and it even held the makings of a hideout for Nazi sympathizers later in the 20th century. This is an excellent hike but is unsigned and difficult in places and rangers regularly retrieve lost hikers from this canyon.

The trip begins by climbing to Inspiration Point. Three different trails will all take you here and directions from the Will Rogers country home are difficult to give. The easiest option is to look for the signed trailhead above the parking lot. Cross a small bridge over a gap and follow a fenced trail up the hill. In 100 yards, reach the west branch of the Inspiration Loop Trail. Turn left and follow the trail 0.8 mile to a saddle, where you can turn right and reach the panoramic viewpoint.

Return to the saddle and follow the Santa Monica Mountains Backbone Trail north. As soon as you start climbing the well-defined ridge, you'll realize how appropriate the name *Backbone* is. The trail skips up, over, or around cobbled sandstone "vertebrae" along a stretch

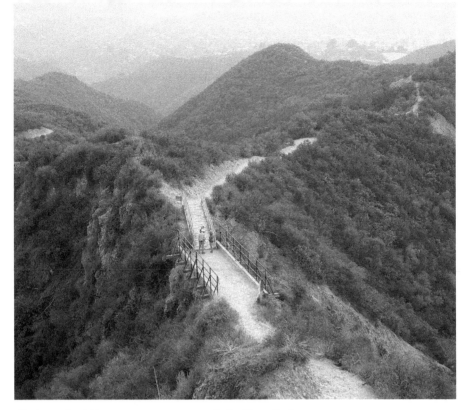

Chicken Ridge Bridge gets your attention on the Backbone Trail.

known variously as Chicken Ridge and Gobbler's Knob. It is also the easternmost small piece of the Backbone Trail, which stretches the length of the Santa Monica Mountains (see Trips 10.2 and 33.4, pages 144 and 449).

At 1.8 miles you cross Chicken Ridge Bridge, spanning a knife-edge saddle between Rivas Canyon on the west and Rustic Canyon on the east. Just ahead at another saddle (2.1 miles), turn right on a trail that wastes no time descending into Rustic Canyon.

On the descent, you make your way through a mini-forest of chaparral, including green-bark ceanothus, mountain mahogany, chamise, manzanita, toyon, sumac, and buckwheat. At 2.7 miles you reach a secluded glade in the bottom of Rustic Canyon, where you might spook a deer if no one else is around to have done it already. A large barn stood here but is in the process of being demolished by the city at the time of this writing.

Upstream, to the left, lies the Boy Scouts' Camp Josepho, named after Will Rogers's friend Anatol Josepho, inventor of the automated photo booth. The trail up the canyon has vanished in places. Our route turns south (downcanyon) past the site of one of Rogers's cabins and an assortment of other structures, burned or abandoned and severely abused with graffiti. Plenty of ornamental trees and shrubs mix with the native live oak and syca-mores along the trickling stream.

On the left a way down stands the concrete shell of a power-generator building. This, along with a diesel-fuel bunker and sheet-metal buildings, was part of the pre–World War II Murphy Ranch, which was protected by a high fence and patrolled by armed guards. Shortwave broadcasts beamed to Germany from the site finally convinced authorities of its true nature and led to the arrest of a German spy. The spy, it seems, had duped a wealthy couple and convinced them to finance construction of this stronghold, which was to serve as a haven for true believers in the Third Reich. After the war, this section of the canyon was sold to the Hartford Artists' Colony, until ravaged by fire and flood. Today it is owned by the City of Los Angeles.

After you pass the Murphy Ranch Road on the left climbing up to Sullivan Fire Road, the canyon narrows and the unmaintained trail becomes merely a muddy track through a tight constriction in the canyon. Walls of conglomerate rock soar eerily on both sides. Watch out for poison oak and slippery rocks; during high water, you may have to wade the creek in places. Some rough use trails climb the east and west walls of the canyon, but are not recommended. At 4.9 miles the canyon abruptly widens. On the right a signed trail curves uphill toward the polo field across from the Will Rogers home, your starting point. Beware of a false trail leading back up to the Backbone; stay in the creek bed as long as possible.

VARIATION

The easiest and most popular (but less scenic) route to Murphy Ranch is from the Capri Trailhead. Park near the junction of Capri and Amalfi Drives. Walk up Capri; then turn left on Casale Road, which soon turns to dirt and becomes Sullivan Fire Road. Pass the Camp Josepho gate and then the narrow unsigned Beehive Trail; then reach a gap in the fence on the left with a staircase. Descend the 531 steps into the canyon bottom. Turn left on the Murphy Ranch Road and descend to the floor of Rustic Canyon. Turn right and hike past the powerhouse and up to the signed trail junction by the old stables. Shortly beyond, veer right onto another part of Murphy Ranch Road and follow it up to Sullivan Fire Road. Stay right and follow it back to the trailhead. This trip is 3.7 miles with 700 feet of elevation gain.

trip 10.9   Sullivan Canyon

see map on p. 142

Distance	10.5 miles (loop)
Hiking Time	4.5 hours
Elevation Gain	1,600'
Difficulty	Moderately strenuous
Trail Use	Suitable for mountain biking, dogs allowed
Best Times	October–May
Agency	Santa Monica Mountains Conservancy
Optional Map	Tom Harrison *Topanga State Park* or Trails Illustrated *Santa Monica Mountains National Recreation Area (253)*

DIRECTIONS Drive 2.3 miles west on Sunset Boulevard from the 40 Freeway, and turn right (north) onto Mandeville Canyon Road in Brentwood. Make a left on the first intersecting street, Westridge Road, and go 1.2 miles to Bayliss Road. Turn left on Bayliss and continue 0.3 mile to Queensferry Road, a dead-end street on the left. Find a place to park on Bayliss near the intersection, taking care to observe the strict parking restrictions.

In serene Sullivan Canyon you can hike for at least an hour without catching sight of any man-made improvements, save for a gravelly service road and some markers indicating a buried pipeline. For a long time it appeared as though Sullivan and neighboring upper Rustic Canyon would become a huge dump site for solid waste. But that threat seems to have passed now, and the land here is now part of Westridge–Canyonback Wilderness Park.

This comprehensive tour goes up along Sullivan Canyon's sycamore-lined bottom and touches upon Mulholland Drive, where on clear days a hiker can view the ocean and the San Fernando Valley from a single stance. It concludes with an easy descent on the long, sinuous ridge just east of the canyon. The route, and variations of it, is ideally suited for runners and mountain bikers as well as walkers.

The route lies almost entirely on a geologic formation called Santa Monica Slate, a gray, bluish-gray, or black rock. These 150-million-year-old rocks of marine origin, the oldest found in the Santa Monica Mountains, are exposed in a broad area stretching almost continuously from Coldwater Canyon and Franklin Canyon behind Beverly Hills into the east half of Topanga State Park.

Since the road in Sullivan Canyon is at best only semishaded, you may want to choose a time that takes advantage of early-morning or late-afternoon shadows. You could, for example, walk up the canyon late in the day, catch the setting sun from Mulholland, and watch the city lights twinkle on as you walk down the east ridge.

Start off by stepping around a gate at the end of Queensferry Road and walk down to the service road going up along the bottom of Sullivan Canyon. Oaks, willows, and sycamores cluster along the usually dry creek bed. At 0.7 mile a narrow path comes down steeply from the left, giving access to Sullivan Canyon's west-ridge fire road, an alternate route used by some people.

The almost imperceptible climb on the canyon-bottom road takes you past thinning sycamores to a fork in the canyon (3.3 miles), where the main canyon branch heads northeast. You follow the road up a smaller, steeper ravine going northwest. Climbing in earnest, you swing around some sharp turns and then hook up with the west-ridge fire road (4.3 miles). Continue north to unpaved Mulholland Drive; then follow Mulholland east along the Santa Monica Mountains divide toward San Vicente Mountain (5.6 miles). When you reach that high point, you'll discover the interpretive site known as San Vicente Mountain Park, which

Dogs and humans alike enjoy hiking in Sullivan Canyon.

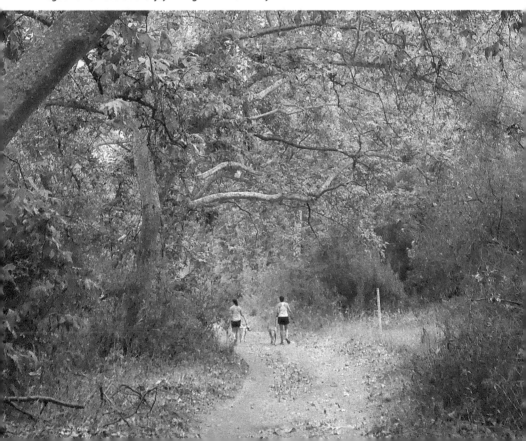

centers on a Cold War–era Nike missile base. The view from here, when not compromised by smog or haze, is undeniably spectacular. Look north to glimpse the Tehachapi Mountains, 70 miles distant, through the gap between the Santa Susana and San Gabriel Mountains.

From San Vicente Mountain Park, head south along the West Mandeville Fire Road. It curves around several rounded bumps on the ridge between Mandeville and Sullivan Canyons, climbing on occasion, but mostly descending. You'll have outstanding views of the L.A. Basin to the east and south, marred only by some foreground power lines. Take care to stay on the main path, not any of the many spurs you pass.

At 9.3 miles you hook up with Westridge Road in a suburban housing development. Walk 0.5 mile down Westridge, turn right on Bayliss, and continue another 0.5 mile down to Queensferry.

trip 10.10   Viewridge Trail

Distance	2.6 miles (semiloop)
Hiking Time	1.5 hours
Elevation Gain	400'
Difficulty	Easy
Trail Use	Dogs allowed, good for kids
Best Times	November–June
Agencies	Mountains Recreation & Conservation Authority, Santa Monica Mountains Conservancy
Optional Map	Tom Harrison *Topanga State Park* or Trails Illustrated *Santa Monica Mountains National Recreation Area (253)*

see map on p. 142

DIRECTIONS From the 101 Freeway in Woodland Hills, take Exit 27B for southbound Topanga Canyon Road (Highway 27). In 3.5 miles turn left onto Viewridge Road. Proceed 0.5 mile and park on the street at the signed trailhead on the right, opposite the gated Summit Point Estates.

The Viewridge Trail passes interesting sandstone formations.

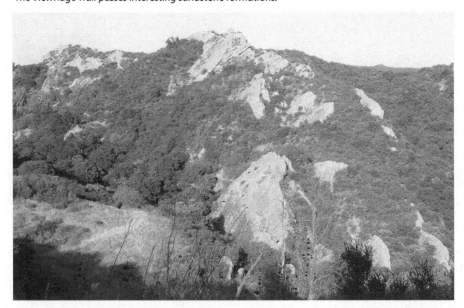

Summit Valley was slated to become a golf course and luxury home development before it was acquired by the Santa Monica Mountains Conservancy in 1994. The 652-acre Summit Valley Edmund D. Edelman Park is named for an L.A. County supervisor who brokered the deal after a long campaign by activists. The rolling hills are an important east–west wildlife corridor and are laced with a disconnected system of short trails. Trip 10.11 (below) explores the grassy western section, while this trip visits the more diverse and less-used eastern section. This trailhead has an advantage of free parking.

Follow the gradually descending trail south through a mixed community of chaparral, oak woodland, and grasslands. Cross the handsome Viewridge bridge over the headwaters of Topanga Creek, pass a bench at a good viewpoint, and admire the sandstone cliffs of Santa Maria Canyon.

In 0.9 mile reach narrow, paved Santa Maria Road. Turn right and go 0.1 mile; then look for the trail resuming on the opposite side. Now you can make a 0.5-mile lollipop loop on the south side of Santa Maria. You'll pass two spurs on the south leading to housing developments and viewpoints. When the trail brings you back to Santa Maria Road, turn left, walk 0.2 mile, and then turn right to retrace your steps uphill to the Viewridge Trailhead.

trip 10.11 Summit Valley

Distance	1.6 miles (out-and-back)
Hiking Time	1 hour
Elevation Gain	450'
Difficulty	Moderate
Trail Use	Dogs allowed, good for kids
Best Times	November–June
Agencies	Mountains Recreation & Conservation Authority, Santa Monica Mountains Conservancy
Optional Map	Tom Harrison *Topanga State Park* or Trails Illustrated *Santa Monica Mountains*
Fees/Permits	$5 parking fee

see map on p. 142

DIRECTIONS From the 101 Freeway in Woodland Hills, take Exit 27B for southbound Topanga Canyon Road (Highway 27). Proceed 4.3 miles south to a sweeping, 180° curve. On the inside of this curve (west side of Topanga Canyon Boulevard) is a dirt parking area for Summit Valley. Pay the day-use fee at the iron ranger.

Named in honor of a county supervisor, Summit Valley Edmund D. Edelman Park spreads across both sides of Topanga Canyon Boulevard south of Woodland Hills and features one easily accessible trail on the west side. Come and see Summit Valley at its best, when it's spring-green and burgeoning with wildflowers (most likely in April); in other seasons, the trail is primarily of interest to locals.

From the parking area, head west down a ravine for 0.2 mile to a south-flowing drainage

*Sugar bush (*Rhus ovata*) is a common plant of the Southern California chaparral.*

(an upper tributary of Topanga Canyon) adorned with coast live oaks and stream-hugging willows. Eucalyptus and California walnut trees dot the slopes higher up in this bowl-like valley. You cross a little stream at the bottom. You may see an unsigned trail forking south to a residential area, immediately followed by a trail forking north up a ravine and then another trail forking north up the ridge alongside the ravine; this hike, however, stays on the better-maintained main path.

Our path turns northwest and climbs a couple of switchbacks so as to gain the top of a linear ridge beside a small park above a residential neighborhood. For a longer walk, turn left or right and join the wide fire road known as the Summit Motorway. Otherwise, enjoy the commanding view from this spot, and then return the way you came.

trip 10.12 Woodland Ridge

see map on p. 142

Distance	2.3 miles (out-and-back)
Hiking Time	1 hour
Elevation Gain	600'
Difficulty	Moderate
Trail Use	Dogs allowed
Best Times	Year-round
Agency	Los Angeles Department of Recreation and Parks
Optional Map	Tom Harrison *Topanga State Park*

DIRECTIONS From the 101 Freeway in Woodland Hills, take Exit 26A for southbound De Soto Avenue, which becomes Serrania Avenue south of the freeway. In 0.8 mile turn right into the Serrania Park lot.

At sunset the weird chorus of sharp-pitched shrieks and howls started up, with echoes that reverberated off the walls of the houses below. The coyotes were defiantly laying claim—or so it seemed when I (Jerry) was there—to one of the dwindling number of open spaces remaining on the San Fernando Valley's south rim. That little patch of public land,

Woodland Ridge is an important wildlife corridor amid the suburban development of Woodland Hills.

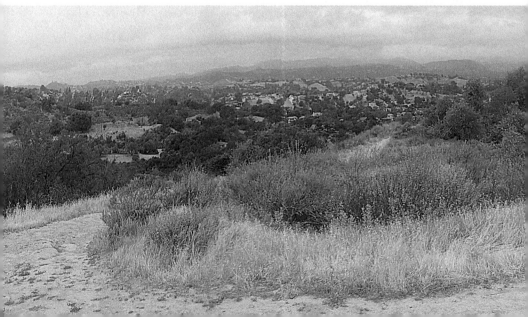

known variously as Woodland Ridge and Serrania Ridge, boasts a ridge-running trail that connects Serrania Park with Mulholland Highway.

The unsigned trail climbs along the park's east fence line, tops a couple of rises offering nice views across the valley, and finally arrives at Mulholland Drive a little below the Santa Monica Mountains crest. To the right as you climb are views of the Woodland Hills Country Club golf course and hillside housing developments characteristic of the 1950s and '60s. On the left is a more recent version of suburbia—a small canyon jam-packed with hulking pseudo-mansions, ridiculously out of proportion to the postage stamp–size lots on which they sit. The contrast between the older and the newer illustrates how valuable even marginally buildable land has become in this well-to-do corner of the valley.

trip 10.13 **Caballero Canyon**

see map on p. 142

Distance	4.5 miles (out-and-back)
Hiking Time	2 hours
Elevation Gain	1,000'
Difficulty	Moderate
Trail Use	Suitable for mountain biking
Best Times	October–June
Agency	Topanga State Park
Optional Map	Tom Harrison *Topanga State Park* or Trails Illustrated *Santa Monica Mountains National Recreation Area (253)*

DIRECTIONS From the 101 Freeway in Tarzana, take Exit 23 for southbound Reseda Boulevard. Proceed 2.3 miles to the trailhead on the left, opposite the Braemar Country Club clubhouse.

Hikers reach the knoll above Caballero Canyon.

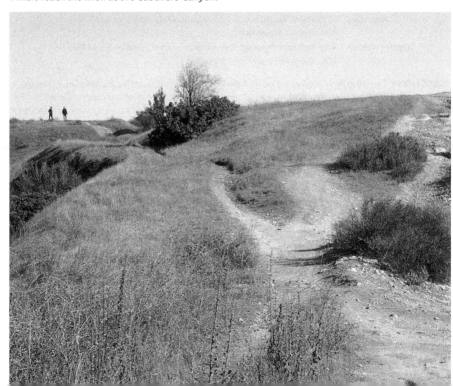

Caballero Canyon's convenient trailhead gives San Fernando Valley hikers easy access to the trails of Topanga State Park without having to drive either the curvy Topanga Canyon Boulevard or the notoriously rutty dirt section of Mulholland Drive. Mountain bikers may travel the Caballero Canyon route as well, but they are restricted to fire roads within the state park and hence are not allowed on the Bent Arrow Trail at the top.

From the trailhead, walk up sycamore-dotted Caballero Canyon on an old fire road. After 1.5 miles and 600 feet of elevation gain, you arrive at a saddle traversed by unpaved Mulholland Drive. The view is good there—but it's much better if you climb a little farther. To the east you'll notice a very steep firebreak going up a ridge. Walk to the base of the firebreak, where you'll notice an unsigned but well-used trail on the right. This narrow path, a segment of the Bent Arrow Trail, takes you on a winding route up a south-facing slope, jogs left as it crosses a firebreak, and finally tops out on a rounded, nearly flat ridge. There's a 1,927-foot knoll immediately to the east, and a slightly higher point overlooking Mulholland Drive 0.4 mile east. Look for Van Nuys Airport in the valley below. Late in the day you can watch evening shadows elongate across the San Fernando Valley, and clouds form along the coast as the chill of evening descends upon the land.

Return the way you came. Or, for a slightly longer trip back, take dirt Mulholland west, and then descend to Reseda Boulevard and loop back to your vehicle.

---

trip 10.14   San Vicente Mountain

see map on p. 142

Distance	1.6 miles (out-and-back)
Hiking Time	1 hour
Elevation Gain	300'
Difficulty	Easy
Trail Use	Suitable for mountain biking, dogs allowed, good for kids
Best Times	October–June
Agencies	Mountains Recreation & Conservation Authority, Santa Monica Mountains Conservancy
Optional Map	Tom Harrison *Topanga State Park* or Trails Illustrated *Santa Monica Mountains National Recreation Area (253)*

DIRECTIONS From the 405 Freeway in Encino, take Exit 61 for westbound Mulholland Drive. The black-top ends after 2.1 miles at an intersection where Encino Hills Drive descends north toward the San Fernando Valley. Continue 0.2 mile up the dirt portion of Mulholland to a parking area beside a gate.

Perched above the San Fernando Valley on one of the more prominent bumps of the Santa Monica Mountains, the Cold War–era Nike missile site at San Vicente Mountain (1,961') has become a popular destination for hikers, dog walkers, and mountain bikers maneuvering over the unpaved section of famed Mulholland Drive. The route is closed 9 p.m.–6 a.m.

Walk or bike past the sturdy gate (open or closed) on dirt Mulholland, heading steeply up the wide dirt roadway. The steady ascent takes you to the old Nike missile installation, which is now a popular interpretive site within Santa Monica Mountains National Recreation Area. Between 1956 and 1968 soldiers from the LA96C battalion manned the site, which was part of a continental system of defensive missile-launch sites to intercept Soviet bombers. The missiles were upgraded to nuclear warheads but were soon rendered obsolete by the development of intercontinental ballistic missiles, which flew too fast to intercept.

At best, the view from San Vicente Mountain Park includes the Tehachapi Mountains to the north, a distant Pacific Ocean horizon to the southwest, and the urban sprawl of the

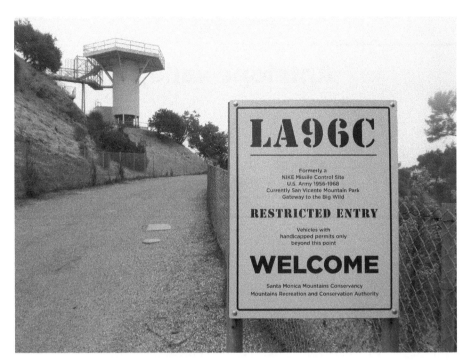

San Vicente Mountain recalls the Cold War days, when Americans feared Soviet nuclear bombers.

Los Angeles Basin and San Fernando Valley lapping at the Santa Monica foothills. The park also serves as a primary trailhead into spacious parcels of undeveloped land to the south: Mulholland Gateway Park and a spread of canyons and ridges becoming known as the Big Wild—20,000 acres of wilderness and wildlife habitat practically on the edge of the West L.A. metropolis.

chapter 11

Antelope Valley

The part of Los Angeles County north of the San Gabriel Mountains and east of the Tehachapi Mountains forms the western tip of the Mojave Desert. It was named Antelope Valley because of pronghorns, antelope-like animals that roamed the area until they were starved and hunted nearly out of existence in the 1880s.

The cities of Lancaster and Palmdale are the major population centers in the valley, but homes and ranches are scattered throughout. Nevertheless, the valley retains a wild charm, especially on account of the plentiful Joshua tree woodlands and wildflowers, as well as the rocky buttes. Protected spaces are increasingly important as the population expands. This chapter covers a sampling of the notable parks in the valley.

trip 11.1 Arthur B. Ripley Desert Woodland State Park

Distance	1.2 miles (loop)
Hiking Time	45 minutes
Elevation Gain	50'
Difficulty	Easy
Trail Use	Good for kids
Best Times	October–April
Agency	California State Parks
Maps	None

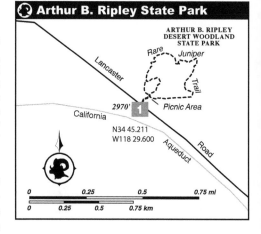

DIRECTIONS From Highway 138 (13 miles east of the 5 Freeway), turn south on 245th Street West, which becomes Lancaster Road. Follow this road south and east through many turns for 4.7 miles; then park on the shoulder, taking care not to block the gate into the signed state park. If you're coming from Antelope Valley California Poppy Reserve, follow Lancaster Road generally west for 7 miles through many turns.

Arthur B. Ripley Desert Woodland State Park is a little-known gem in the Antelope Valley. The small park protects a dense grove of Joshua trees and California junipers in the midst of otherwise stark desert. The land was donated to the state in 1988 by Mr. Ripley, a farmer, to conserve one of the last remaining examples of this woodland community that had once been plentiful in the valley. A short trail is well suited to families, and also makes a great add-on for plant lovers after visiting the nearby Antelope Valley California Poppy Reserve (see next trip).

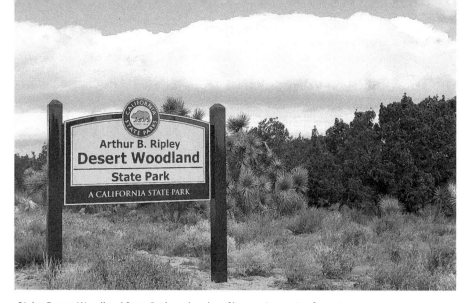

Ripley Desert Woodland State Park packs a lot of beauty into a tiny footprint.

Park on the shoulder of the road and walk in through a gate past the sign for the state park. In 0.1 mile reach a picnic area with interpretive signs. Pick up a brochure for the Rare Juniper Trail if one is available. The Ripley Nature Trail loop departs from the north side of the picnic area. You'll see two paths that rejoin in about 0.1 mile, with the left path being slightly shorter. Take either path and continue north after they rejoin.

The Rare Juniper Trail continues to make a clockwise loop. In the springtime, you might see the Joshua trees in bloom, or striking blue sage alongside many other familiar wildflowers. The interpretive brochure tells a fascinating story of the California juniper. Most grow from a root burl that sends up 2–12 trunks over the 75- to 130-year lifespan of the plant, but several unusual junipers in this area have no root burl and produce only a single trunk, including the beautiful specimen at interpretive marker #1. Female junipers produce berries that stay on the tree for 1.5 years from March or April until August or September of the following year. Hence, in the summer, you will see two crops of berries simultaneously, with the new berries being green and the mature ones being bluish-purple. The berries germinate after being eaten, carried away, and defecated by native animals; juniper seedlings do not normally grow under their mother plant. Male junipers produce tiny brown pollen cones. Curiously, about 3% of junipers change sex each year; watch for unusual trees with both berries and pollen cones that are in the process of a sex change.

Near marker 8, you'll see a field of rabbit-brush in a spot where the land had been cleared for farming until 1972. Watch for brilliant scarlet bugler flowers nearby. Finally, you loop back to the picnic area, where you'll see marker 10 beside "Big Mama," one of the largest and most fertile junipers in the area, with 15 trunks and thousands of berries.

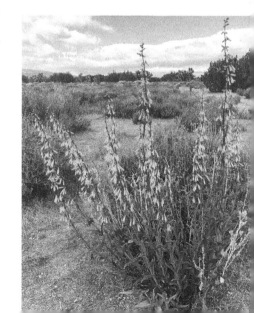

*Scarlet bugler (*Penstemon centranthifolius*) is a striking member of the penstemon family.*

trip 11.2   Antelope Valley California Poppy Reserve

Distance	1–4 miles (many loops possible)
Hiking Time	30 minutes–3 hours
Elevation Gain	200'–500'
Difficulty	Easy
Trail Use	Good for kids
Best Times	March–April
Agency	California State Parks
Optional Map	Free *Antelope Valley California Poppy Reserve* map
Fees/Permits	$10 day-use fee

DIRECTIONS From Highway 138 (13 miles east of the 5 Freeway), turn south on 245th Street West, which becomes Lancaster Road. Follow this road south and east through many turns for 11.6 miles; then turn left into the signed entrance for Antelope Valley California Poppy Reserve, and follow the entry road to the parking area. If the lot is overcrowded in peak season or you don't want to pay the hefty parking fee, you can also park on Lancaster Road and walk in on the park road.

After a good wet winter, the Antelope Valley California Poppy Reserve can be one of the best places in Southern California to enjoy spring wildflowers, especially the iconic state flower, the California poppy. Other common flowers include lupines (purple-blue), goldfields (masses of hundreds of small yellow flowers per square foot), owl's clover (maroon flowers resembling paintbrush), phacelia (tiny blue or lavender flowers with many stamens), blue dicks (tiny six-petaled blue flowers with a yellow center), and fiddleneck (tiny yellow flowers on a curled hairy stalk). The 1,781-acre reserve was established in 1976 on the site of the Munz Ranch. Stop in the Pinheiro Interpretive Center for more information about the wildflowers.

An extensive trail network lets you make a loop of up to 2 miles to the west via Tehachapi Vista Point, or 4 miles to the east via the Antelope Butte Vista Point. The allure of the park, however, is the flowers much more so than the trails, so bring a camera and enjoy the blooms. Please stay on the trail; don't be lured into the meadows to take a selfie that kills the flowers you've come to see. For information on current conditions, visit the park website (parks.ca.gov/?page_id=627), call the Poppy Reserve Wildflower Hotline at 661-724-1180, or check out the California Wildflower Report (desertusa.com/wildflo/ca.html).

Antelope Valley California Poppy Reserve delights hikers of all ages. Photo: Janet Winters

trip 11.3   Saddleback Butte

Distance	3.8 miles (out-and-back)
Hiking Time	2 hours
Elevation Gain	1,100'
Difficulty	Moderate
Best Times	October–April
Agency	California State Parks
Optional Map	Free *Saddleback Butte State Park* map
Permit:	$6 day-use fee

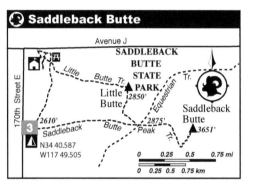

DIRECTIONS From Highway 138, turn north on 165th Street East at a sign for Saddleback Butte State Park. In 2.7 miles the road veers right and becomes 170th Street. In 9.1 more miles, turn right into the campground entrance and park near the signed trailhead.

Saddleback Butte (3,651') is a granite mountain rising from the alluvial plain of the Antelope Valley. The mountain and surrounding Joshua tree–creosote plains were set aside in 1960 as a state park to protect habitat for the native plants and animals. The park will give you a sense of what the valley was like before large-scale development began. A trail from the campground to the summit threads past the Joshua trees and low sand dunes before making a vigorous climb to the rocky summit. Watch for wildlife including the elusive desert tortoise, as well as foxes and rabbits. Beware that rattlesnakes also make their home here, including the especially venomous Mojave green rattler. Between February and April, you might catch a good wildflower display or see the Joshua trees in bloom.

From the signed Saddleback Butte Peak Trailhead, hike east toward the mountain. Walking may be surprisingly difficult because of the deep soft sand. In 1.0 mile cross the Equestrian Trail at a junction with the Little Butte Trail. The trail soon steepens and climbs to a saddle south of the summit before following the ridge to the top. Enjoy the excellent views and then return the way you came.

VARIATION

You can also begin this trip behind the visitor center at the picnic area at the north entrance to the park. Start down the Dic Dowen Nature Trail, but turn left onto the unsigned Little Butte Trail before reaching the concrete portion of the pathway. This route is half a mile longer each way and the views are no better.

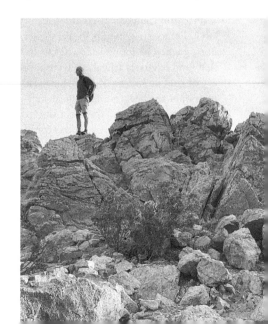

A hiker stands atop the windswept summit rocks of Saddleback Butte.

chapter 12

Desert Gateway

Millions of years of geologic tumult can be read in the frozen stone exposed to casual view as you drive the Antelope Valley Freeway (Highway 14) between the 5 Freeway (I-5) and the Mojave Desert city of Palmdale. The area is chock-full of fault-sliced sedimentary rock formations, twisted and turned into a variety of forms. On a geologic time scale, of course, the rocks are anything but solid and unmoving. The collapse of a freeway ramp over the 5 Freeway near the Antelope Valley Freeway during the 1971 Sylmar earthquake and again during the 1994 Northridge quake were pointed reminders of that.

Some of the most magnificent rock formations in this desert-gateway area of northern Los Angeles County can be found in Vasquez Rocks Natural Area. The Pacific Crest Trail passes through this smallish park as it wends its way from the Mexican border to the Canadian border. In June 1993 a "golden spike" ceremony was held not far away in Soledad Canyon to commemorate the completion of the final link of trail tread in that 2,640-mile-long pathway.

The desert gateway area is also notable as a significant "wind gap" between the coastal valleys of Ventura and Los Angeles Counties and the interior desert. Often on spring and summer afternoons the canyon serves as a conduit for cool, hazy marine air flowing east toward the southwestern Mojave Desert. Less common are the hot, dry Santa Ana winds of fall and early winter that scream through the area in the opposite direction.

Also included in this chapter is Placerita Canyon Natural Area, which nestles comfortably at the foot of one of the more verdant slopes of the San Gabriel Mountains. The park's wild backcountry sector is complemented by a very civilized nature center—the envy of many a national park—housing exhibits on local history, prehistory, geology, plants, and wildlife.

Placerita Canyon's fascinating history is highlighted by the discovery of gold there in 1842. Francisco Lopez, a local rancher, was digging for wild onions after tracking stray horses, when he found yellow flecks in the soil. That event, which touched off California's first (and relatively trivial) gold rush, predated by six years John Marshall's famous discovery of gold at Sutter's Mill in Northern California. When you first arrive at Placerita, you may want to check out the wheelchair-accessible Heritage Trail, which leads to the "Oak of the Golden Dream," the exact site (according to legend) where gold was discovered by a herdsman pulling up wild onions for his after-siesta meal.

In the bucolic early 1900s, Placerita settlers grew vegetables and fruit, raised animals, and tapped some small reserves of a very high-grade "white" oil. Right out of the ground, the fuel was suitable for home heating and lighting purposes—and even for powering a Model T Ford. By the 1950s, Placerita Canyon had become one of the more popular generic Western site locations used by Hollywood's movie makers and early television producers. The canyon was eventually acquired as parkland.

The July 2016 Sand Fire started near Sand Canyon Road and Highway 14 and burned 41,432 acres. Subsequent landslides and mudslides wiped out the backcountry trail system in Placerita Canyon, and the trails are still recovering at the time of writing.

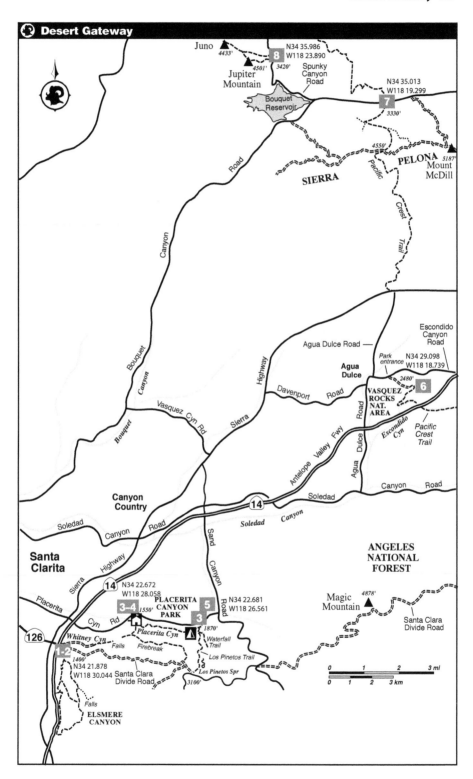

Juno
4433'
4501'
3420'
8
N34 35.986
W118 23.890
Spunky
Canyon
Road
Jupiter
Mountain
Bouquet
Reservoir
N34 35.013
W118 19.299
7
3330'
4550'
Road
Pacific
SIERRA
PELONA 5187'
Mount
McDill
Canyon
Crest
Trail
Bouquet
Canyon
Escondido
Canyon
Road
Agua Dulce Road
Park
entrance
N34 29.098
W118 18.739
Agua
Dulce
2480'
Bouquet
Vasquez Cyn Rd
Highway
Davenport
Road
VASQUEZ
ROCKS
NAT.
AREA
6
Sierra
Escondido
Cyn
Pacific
Crest
Trail
Road
Antelope Valley Fwy
Agua
Dulce
Canyon Country
14
Soledad
Canyon
Road
Soledad
Canyon
Canyon Road
Soledad
Canyon
Road
Soledad Canyon
Road
ANGELES
NATIONAL
FOREST
Santa
Clarita
Highway
Sand Canyon Road
Magic
Mountain
4878'
Santa Clara
Divide Road
Sierra
14
N34 22.672
W118 28.058
PLACERITA
CANYON
PARK
5
N34 22.681
W118 26.561
Placerita
3-4 1550'
3
1870'
Cyn Rd
Placerita Cyn
Waterfall
Trail
126
Whitney Cyn
Falls
Firebreak
Los Pinetos Trail
1-2
1400'
N34 21.878
W118 30.044
Santa Clara
Divide Road
Los Pinetos Spr
3100'
0   1   2   3 mi
0 1 2 3 km
Falls
ELSMERE
CANYON

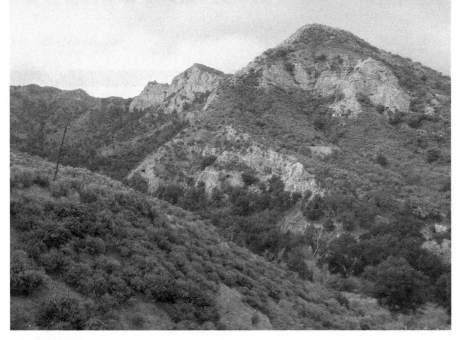

Stunning Elsmere Canyon narrowly escaped becoming a giant landfill.

trip 12.1 Elsmere Canyon Falls

see map on previous page

Distance	2.6 miles (out-and-back)
Hiking Time	1.5 hours
Elevation Gain	300'
Difficulty	Easy
Trail Use	Dogs allowed, good for kids
Best Times	Year-round
Agencies	City of Santa Clarita Open Space Preservation District, Mountains Recreation & Conservation Authority, Santa Monica Mountains Conservancy
Optional Map	Free *Elsmere Canyon Trails* map (available at hikesantaclarita.com/maps)

DIRECTIONS From the 14 Freeway in Santa Clarita, take Exit 2 for eastbound Newhall Avenue. Immediately enter a large Park and Ride lot. Hiker parking can be found at the lower Whitney Canyon Park lot through a gate to the north.

Elsmere Canyon was developed for oil drilling by the Pacific Coast Oil Company in 1889. In 1987, the Los Angeles City Council voted to study converting the canyon into a 1,500-acre landfill, which would be the worlds largest when filled to the brim. Conservationists waged a 20-year battle before land was finally donated to the Mountains & Recreation Conservation Authority to become an open-space preserve. The Elsmere Canyon preserve now contains more than 1,200 acres. Many trails and dirt roads lace the canyon and hills. This trip follows the shortest one through the scenic canyon to a small waterfall. If you have more time, consult the map and pick a different and longer route back.

The canyon's name came into use by the California State Mining Bureau in 1896, which mentioned an early oil field. According to one unconfirmed story, it was named by Ed Lingwood, who settled there in 1889, to commemorate Baron Ellesmere, who founded Lingwood's childhood town in England.

From the entrance to the Whitney Canyon Park lot, find a path signed Elsmere Canyon Open Space and follow it south along a fence around the perimeter of the Park and Ride and southwest up onto a low ridge where you meet the unsigned Santa Clara Divide Road on the left at 0.1 mile. Descend south for 0.1 mile to meet the signed Creek Trail, a broad dirt road on the floor of Elsmere Canyon.

Take the Creek Trail 0.7 mile up the oak-shaded canyon. The high sedimentary cliffs are part of the Towsley Formation that formed about 5 million years ago beneath a shallow sea. This formation is rich in fossils and oil seeps. Shortly after passing a dirt road on the left, the main dirt road you have been following makes a hairpin turn to the right and the Creek Trail becomes a narrow unmaintained path following the creek up the canyon. Take the Creek Trail another 0.4 mile, fording the creek, weaving around fallen trees, and dodging poison oak. When the canyon forks, go 30 yards up the right (south) fork to a seasonal two-tier waterfall with a small pool between the tiers. Return the way you came.

VARIATION

If you have more time, consult the map and pick a different and longer route back. The big loop in Elsmere is 6 miles and is mostly interesting but also has a tedious segment along an old road directly above the 14 Freeway.

---

trip 12.2 Whitney Canyon

see map on p. 167

Distance	3.4 miles (out-and-back)
Hiking Time	1.5 hours
Elevation Gain	300'
Difficulty	Easy
Trail Use	Suitable for mountain biking, dogs allowed, good for kids
Best Times	Year-round
Agencies	Mountains Recreation & Conservation Authority, Santa Monica Mountains Conservancy
Optional Map	Tom Harrison *Angeles Front Country*

DIRECTIONS From the 14 Freeway in Santa Clarita, take Exit 2 for eastbound Newhall Avenue. Immediately enter a large Park and Ride lot. Hiker parking can be found at the lower Whitney Canyon Park lot through a gate to the north.

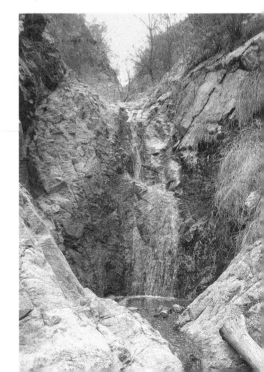

The dry and desolate landscape you behold at the trailhead hides a pleasant thing or two not far up Whitney Canyon.

From the north end of the Whitney Canyon Lot just before a bridge, go east on an unsigned dirt road leading into Whitney Canyon, which remains broad and uninteresting for the first half mile. Stay left as you pass two power-line service roads. You'll pass under some massive high-voltage power lines, and then the scenery improves. The canyon bottom narrows, and massive live

Whitney Canyon Falls is a pleasant surprise.

oaks and sycamores arch overhead, creating inviting pools of shade, even on hot summer days. The excessively gnarled appearance of the trees suggests that they are the survivors of multiple wildfires over decades and centuries.

Past a second set of large power lines. Just beyond an old wall of light-colored masonry on the right, a small tributary canyon opens on the right (south) side, just shy of where the old road peters out, 1.0 mile from the start. Poke 30 yards into this little ravine, and you will soon come upon a cattail-choked freshwater marsh. A covey of quail might explode from this oasis as you approach it. In back of the marsh look for an artesian sulfur spring—a clear pool of water, possibly with sulfurous bubbles coming up.

In the winter and spring, continue 0.7 mile up the canyon on a narrower trail. Even if the lower canyon is dry, you'll likely start to see water flowing. Pass a series of cascades and eventually reach a lovely waterfall blocking farther progress up the canyon.

trip 12.3   Placerita Canyon

see map on p. 167

Distance	3.6 miles (out-and-back)
Hiking Time	2 hours
Elevation Gain	400'
Difficulty	Moderate
Trail Use	Dogs allowed, good for kids
Best Times	Year-round
Agency	Los Angeles County Parks & Recreation
Optional Map	Tom Harrison *Angeles Front Country*

Placerita Canyon boasts bountiful hiking trails.

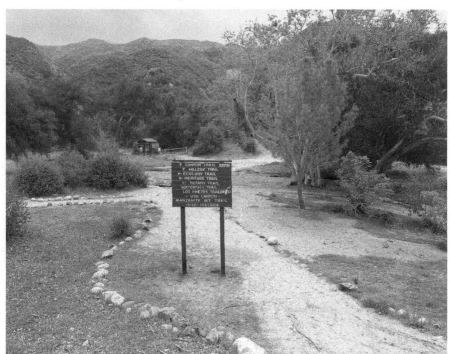

NOTES Placerita Canyon Natural Area burned in the 2016 Sand Fire. A number of its trails remain closed at the time of this writing, with an anticipated 2020 reopening. Call the park office at 661-259-7721 or check "News" at placerita.org for updates.

DIRECTIONS From the 14 Freeway in Santa Clarita, take Exit 3 for eastbound Placerita Canyon Road. In 1.5 miles turn right into Placerita Canyon Natural Area. Continue 0.2 mile to the trailhead parking area by the visitor center.

Placerita Canyon's melodious creek flows decently about half the year (winter and spring), caressing the ears with white noise that echoes from the canyon walls. During the fall, when the creek is bone-dry, you make your own noise instead by crunching through the crispy leaf litter of the sycamores.

Starting at the Placerita Canyon Nature Center, cross a bridge and pick up the Canyon Trail heading east up the canyon's live oak–shaded flood plain. Down by the grassy banks you'll see wild blackberry vines, lots of willows, and occasionally sycamore, cottonwood, and alder trees.

After a while, the canyon narrows and becomes a rocky gorge. Soaring walls tell the story of thousands of years of natural erosion, as well as the destructive effects of hydraulic mining, which involved aiming high-pressure water hoses at hillsides to loosen and wash away ores. Used extensively in Northern California during the later Gold Rush, "hydraulicking" was finally banned in 1884 after catastrophic damages to waterways and farms downstream. At Placerita Canyon, several hundred thousand dollars' worth of gold was ultimately recovered, but at considerable cost and effort.

At about 1 mile you reach a split. The right fork climbs a little onto the chaparral-clad slopes to the south, while the left branch connects with a trail going up to a parking area on Placerita Canyon Road and then goes upstream along the willow-choked canyon bottom. Follow either branch, but try taking the other on the return leg of the hike.

Using either route, you eventually reach the scant remains of some early-20th-century cottages hand-built by settlers Frank and Hortense Walker and some of their 12 children. The area is now the site of a large campground catering to organized groups (drinking water is available here). Amid a parklike setting of live oaks and gentle slopes, you'll discover a sturdy chimney and a cement foundation. Back by the nature center stands another cabin built by Walker but later modified for use in the TV series *Hopalong Cassidy*.

VARIATION

From near the end of the split, take the Waterfall Trail south 0.5 mile to visit Los Pinetos Waterfall (see Trip 12.5, page 173). This variation adds 1.0 mile and 200 feet of elevation gain round-trip.

---

trip 12.4 **Manzanita Mountain to Los Pinetos Canyon**

Distance	7 miles (loop)
Hiking Time	4 hours
Elevation Gain	1,800'
Difficulty	Moderately strenuous
Trail Use	Suitable for backpacking, dogs allowed
Best Times	October–June
Agencies	Angeles National Forest, Los Angeles County Parks & Recreation
Recommended Map	Tom Harrison *Angeles Front Country*

see map on p. 167

DIRECTIONS From the 14 Freeway in Santa Clarita, take Exit 3 for eastbound Placerita Canyon Road. In 1.5 miles turn right into Placerita Canyon Natural Area. Continue 0.2 mile to the trailhead parking area by the visitor center.

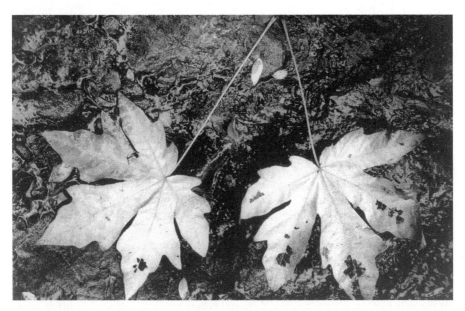

Big-leaf maple (Acer macrophyllum) grows best in moist canyons. Photo: Jerry Schad

NOTES Placerita Canyon Natural Area burned in the 2016 Sand Fire. The Manzanita Mountain Trail is open, but the Los Pinetos Trail, along with several others, remains closed at the time of this writing, with an anticipated 2020 reopening. Call the park office at 661-259-7721 or check "News" at placerita.org for updates.

The grand tour of Placerita Canyon country takes you swiftly up a steep trail and fire-break to the top of a ridge spur of the San Gabriels, and then easily back downward via the Los Pinetos and Canyon Trails. Start the hike early (the park gate opens at 9 a.m.) so you avoid broiling in the midday sun while ascending. If you want to make this an over-night trip, you have the option of making camp on Angeles National Forest lands, subject to fire regulations. Contact the Santa Clara/Mojave Rivers Ranger District (see Appendix D, page 469) for more information about that.

Start by picking up the Hillside Trail just behind the restroom building near the west end of the picnic area in Placerita Canyon Natural Area. Climb past oaks and chaparral to a point just short of the camouflage-painted water tank. There you'll find an unmarked but well-worn trail heading straight up the ridge. After 0.5 mile on this you come to a side trail on the right leading 100 yards to the top of a rounded knoll dubbed Manzanita Mountain. Not much manzanita grows hereabouts, due to repeated wildfires. From this point on, you're on Angeles National Forest lands until you reach the lower part of the Los Pinetos Trail.

Just past the side trail you come to a wide, sandy firebreak. Turn left and tackle the first of several extremely steep pitches you'll encounter on the undulating firebreak during the next 1.8 miles. At 2.6 miles you join Whitney Canyon Road, at the high point in elevation along the route. From there, it's downhill the rest of the way.

Turn left (east) and head for Wilson Canyon Saddle, a popular destination for equestrians and mountain bikers who come up from the San Fernando Valley via Wilson Canyon Road from Olive View Drive in Sylmar. Scramble up either of the two bumps on the ridgeline just east of here for a stupendous view (weather permitting) of the metropolis below. It's quiet here whenever the marine layer gets thick enough to smother the ridgeline in fog. At other times, when sound refracts upward through the inversion layer, the muffled roar of tens of thousands of cars on the network of freeways below comes through loud and clear.

Picking up the Los Pinetos Trail on the north side of the saddle, you begin a pleasant descent through splendid live-oak woodlands, and you lose all sights and sounds of the city. Here and there you'll find nice specimens of the California walnut (black walnut) tree, a small deciduous tree with colorful foliage in the fall. The range of this trademark Southern California tree is limited to the margins of the L.A. Basin and the mountainous interiors of Ventura and Santa Barbara Counties. Much of its habitat in Los Angeles County has been usurped by urbanization.

Down past a couple of switchbacks you come to Los Pinetos Spring, on the right, where non-potable water is stored for firefighting. Continue your descent on the trail ahead, winding amid thick growths of chaparral—ceanothus, scrub oak, chamise, sugar bush, mountain mahogany, manzanita, and sage—along the slope west of Los Pinetos Canyon. At 5.2 miles you reach Walker Ranch Campground (water available here). From there, head west down the well-trodden trail through Placerita Canyon back to the starting point.

trip 12.5   **Los Pinetos Waterfall**

Distance	1.6 miles (out-and-back)
Hiking Time	1 hour
Elevation Gain	350'
Difficulty	Moderate
Trail Use	Dogs allowed, good for kids
Best Times	Year-round
Agency	Los Angeles County Parks & Recreation
Optional Map	Tom Harrison *Angeles Front Country*

see map on p. 167

DIRECTIONS From the 14 Freeway in Santa Clarita, take Exit 3 for eastbound Placerita Canyon Road. In 3.2 miles, by mile marker 5.4, park at a turnout by the gated road leading into the Walker Ranch section of Placerita Canyon Natural Area.

A little hiker explores the canyon near Los Pinetos Falls.

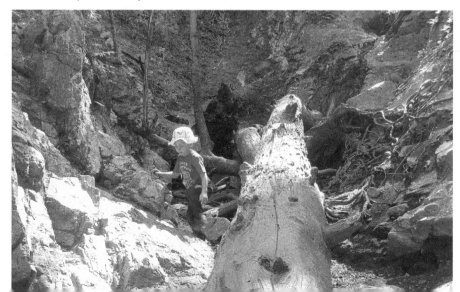

NOTES Placerita Canyon Natural Area burned in the 2016 Sand Fire. A number of its trails remain closed at the time of this writing, with an anticipated 2020 reopening. Call the park office at 661-259-7721 or check "News" at placerita.org for updates.

Nourished by springs, Los Pinetos Canyon harbors at least a tiny trickle of water virtually year-round. About midway up this short tributary of Placerita Canyon is a sublime little grotto, cool and dark except when the sun passes almost straight overhead. If you come here after gully-washing rains, you'll find a true waterfall; otherwise you can just listen to water dribbling down the chute and enjoy the serenity of this private place just 3 miles—and a world away—from the edge of the L.A. metropolis.

Walk down to the Walker Ranch group campground and turn south on the Waterfall Trail into Los Pinetos Canyon. Don't confuse this trail with the signed Los Pinetos Trail going up the slope west of the canyon bottom. The Waterfall Trail momentarily climbs the canyon's steep west wall, then drops onto the canyon's sunny flood plain. Presently you bear right into a narrow ravine (Los Pinetos Canyon), avoiding a wider tributary bending left (east).

Continue, now on an ill-defined path, past and sometimes over water-polished, metamorphic rock. Live oaks and big-cone Douglas-firs cling to the slopes above, and a few big-leaf maples grace the canyon bottom. The big-cone Douglas-fir, a Southern California variant of the Douglas-fir of the Pacific Northwest, is abundant in the San Gabriel Mountains from elevations of about 2,000 feet (as here) up to about 6,000 feet. The big-leaf maple, also common in the Pacific Northwest, has gained a foothold in the San Gabriels as well, especially in moist canyons and ravines.

About 0.2 mile after the first fork in the canyon, there's a second fork. Go right and continue 50 yards to the base of the waterfall—the end of the line in this branch of the canyon. Beware of poison oak that abounds along the trail and near the waterfall, especially in the winter when its bare twigs are difficult to recognize.

trip 12.6   Vasquez Rocks Natural Area

see map on p. 167

Distance	3.5 miles (out-and-back)
Hiking Time	2 hours
Elevation Gain	300'
Difficulty	Easy
Trail Use	Dogs allowed, good for kids
Best Times	Year-round
Agency	Los Angeles County Parks & Recreation
Optional Map	Tom Harrison *Angeles Front Country* or Trails Illustrated *Angeles National Forest (811)*

DIRECTIONS From the 14 Freeway, take Exit 15 for northbound Agua Dulce Road. Go 19 miles to where the road turns east and becomes Escondido Canyon Road. Proceed 0.6 mile east to the Vasquez Rocks Natural Area entrance on the right. Drive in on a dirt road, past the ranger office, to the furthest parking area, 0.56 mile southeast.

A perennial location for filming Old West movies and sci-fi extravaganzas, the distinctive Vasquez Rocks may be familiar to you from episodes of *Bonanza, Star Trek, The Lone Ranger, 24,* and movies such as *Blazing Saddles* and *Austin Powers: International Man of Mystery.* Somehow these tilted slabs look impossibly high and steep when you first see them. But that illusion is dispelled when you try to climb them—none rise more than about 150 feet into the air, and there's almost always an easy way up. The best of the rocks

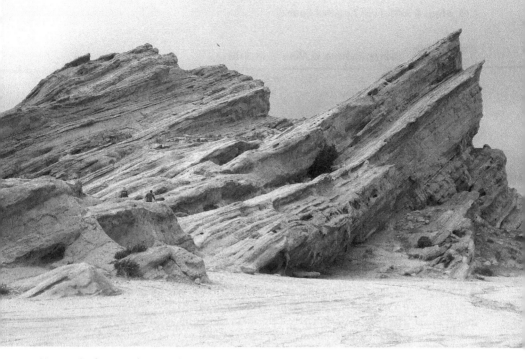

Vasquez Rocks Natural Area's otherworldly atmosphere makes it an ideal movie location.

are included in the 932-acre Vasquez Rocks Natural Area, named after Tiburcio Vasquez, a notorious 19th-century bandito who reputedly used the park's cliffs and caves to hide from vigilantes and sheriffs' posses.

Geologically speaking, the rocks are west-dipping outcrops of sandstone and fanglomerate layers belonging to the Vasquez Formation. Here and in the surrounding area, the Vasquez Formation and the overlying Mint Canyon Formation constitute a 20,000-foot-thick sequence of sediments laid down 8–15 million years ago. The sandstone developed from fine-grained deposits laid down along gentle streams and shallow ponds. The fanglomerate (which resembles conglomerate rock) developed from layers of coarse, broken rock deposited on what were probably alluvial fans at the base of steep mountains.

More recently, faulting uplifted these layers, inclining them roughly 45° horizontally. Erosion put on the final touches, producing the sheer east-facing exposures that you will see throughout the park.

The park includes a large picnic area, a couple of well-trampled nature trails, and a segment of the Pacific Crest Trail. That scenic stretch of the PCT is described here.

Walk through a gate at the end of the parking area. Look for the signed southbound Pacific Crest Trail, which leads southeast and then southwest along a ridge. After 0.7 mile the PCT dives downward off the ridge, reaches the bottom of Escondido Creek, and turns sharply left to follow the canyon uphill (east). A 2007 fire singed the sycamores and incinerated everything else here, but the chaparral regenerated quickly.

Make your way upstream into a lush riparian zone filled with willows and cottonwoods, right underneath the stony gaze of some spectacular overhanging cliffs of sandstone and conglomerate rock. High above on one jutting edge above, you might spot a lone, battered juniper.

Go as far as the point where the PCT drops right in the creekbed, bound for a nearby tunnel that takes the trail under the freeway. This a good spot to turn around and retrace your steps, enjoying a new perspective of the same great scenery.

see
map on
p. 167

trip 12.7 Sierra Pelona & Mount McDill

Distance	12 miles (out-and-back)
Hiking Time	6 hours
Elevation Gain	2,500'
Difficulty	Easy
Trail Use	Dogs allowed, equestrians
Best Times	Year-round
Agency	Angeles National Forest
Maps	None

DIRECTIONS From the 14 Freeway, take Exit 9 for northbound Sand Canyon Road. In 2.0 miles turn right onto Sierra Highway; then, in 0.3 mile, turn left onto Vasquez Canyon Road. In 3.6 miles turn right onto Bouquet Canyon Road. In 13.7 miles park at a turnout on the right (near mile 4.3 according to the mile markers along the road).

Mount McDill (5,187') is the highest point of the Sierra Pelona, a piece of the Transverse Ranges northwest of the San Gabriels. This trip tours the range via the Pacific Crest Trail (PCT) and a fire road along the crest. Sierra Pelona means Bald Mountains, an apt name for the range. The crest is blown clear of trees and shrubs by the 100-mile-per-hour winds that sometimes scour the ridgeline as great masses of air flow from the desert down Soledad Canyon to the Los Angeles Basin. Go on a calm day when you can enjoy the sweeping views.

From the parking area, take a short trail that climbs to meet the PCT. Turn right and step over a gate intended to deter the dirt bikers who illegally use the trail. At 1.0 mile reach a switchback on a ridge above a second gate where the PCT turns east and two lightly used trails wander into the chaparral. The old PCT once went this way toward Big Oak Spring, and bikers still follow the Five Deer Trail, but these trails are now partially overgrown with many unsigned junctions, so our trip stays on the new PCT up the ridge. At 1.6 miles the

A huge canyon live oak (Quercus chrysolepis) *on the Sierra Pelona*

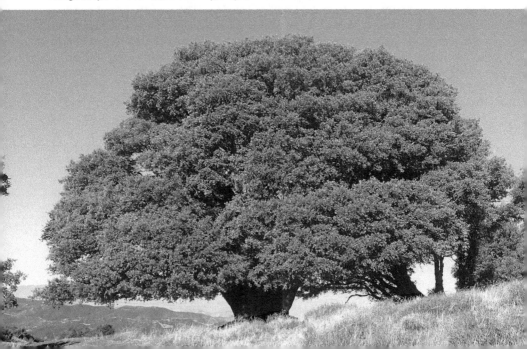

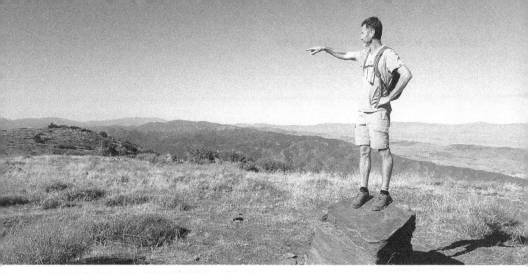

Windswept Mount McDill affords far-reaching views.

PCT leaves the ridge near a third gate, but a steep firebreak continues up (you could follow this firebreak to a saddle on the ridge, shaving off 1.3 miles from the ascent). At 2.3 miles watch for seasonal piped Bear Spring above the trail. The chaparral gives way to canyon live oaks as you climb. At 3.0 miles reach the Sierra Pelona crest.

To reach Mount McDill, turn left and follow the fire road along the crest, veering right or left at times to bypass small hills. Reach a substantial hill; then descend to a saddle where you'll see the obscure firebreak trail coming up from the PCT. The next hill has a magnificent old many-trunked live oak on the summit. Pass a fire road on the left descending to Bouquet Canyon Road and make the final climb to the double-humped summit of McDill. The first hump has a benchmark called Mint, while the second is the true McDill. Historians speculate that the mountain is named for an early homesteader. The rock outcrops are made of Pelona Schist, a 200-million-year-old metamorphic basement rock that makes up the entire Sierra Pelona ridge and underlies much of the San Gabriel Mountains. Return the way you came, or shortcut down the road or firebreak.

VARIATION

For a shorter trip, simply turn around at the Sierra Pelona crest. This trip on the Pacific Crest Trail is 3 miles each way with 1,300 feet of elevation gain.

---

trip 12.8 **Jupiter Mountain**

Distance	3.8 miles (out-and-back)
Hiking Time	2.5 hours
Elevation Gain	1,600'
Difficulty	Moderate
Trail Use	Dogs allowed
Best Times	October–June
Agency	Angeles National Forest
Maps	None

see map on p. 167

DIRECTIONS From the 14 Freeway, take Exit 9 for northbound Sand Canyon Road. In 2.0 miles turn right onto Sierra Highway; then, in 0.3 mile, turn left onto Vasquez Canyon Road. In 3.6 miles turn right onto Bouquet Canyon Road. In 11.5 miles turn left onto Spunky Canyon Road. Go 2.7 miles and park on the left near mile 2.70.

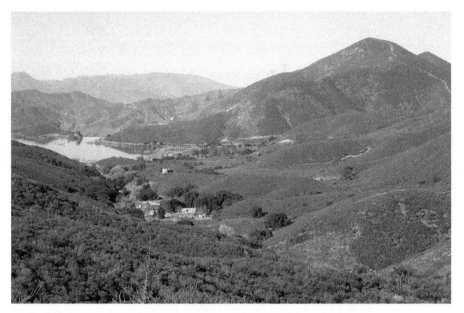

Jupiter Mountain, on the right, presides over Bouquet Reservoir. The view here is from the Pacific Crest Trail below Sierra Pelona.

Clad in chaparral, Jupiter Mountain's swayback summit ridge presides regally over a landscape of fault-churned ridges and linear canyons. A little-known trail cuts along the mountain's cool north slope, giving access to its viewful crest, high above Bouquet Reservoir and the valley and little hamlet that share the name Green Valley.

The trail starts on a saddle by a plantation of pine, cedar, and cypress trees established in 1964. Walk up a service road for 100 yards to a split where you stay left onto a rutted firebreak. Follow this firebreak, steep in places, 1.0 mile to the 4,498-foot summit. From here, you have great views. Looking north and turning counterclockwise brings you views of the Tehachapi mountain wind farms, Sawmill Ridge, the Sespe Wilderness, the Santa Clarita area with the Boney Mountains peeking over the Simi Hills, and the western San Gabriel Mountains beyond Bouquet Canyon reservoir. The Los Angeles Aqueduct runs through a white pipe below, storing water in the reservoir en route from the eastern Sierra Nevada to LA. In the southwest foreground are ridges and canyons overlain by offshoots of the San Andreas Fault. One of these, the San Francisquito Fault (running southwest down Bee Canyon and San Francisquito Canyon), was implicated in one of California's worst disasters: the collapse of the St. Francis Dam in 1928. The culprit in this case was not an actual earthquake, but rather weakness in the rocks of the fault zone that were supporting the huge concrete dam.

This trip runs the ridge northwest to Juno Mountain, a secondary summit at the far end of the ridge, at 2.0 miles. About a third of a way along the ridge, note a trail on the right returning to the trailhead. Take in the view from Juno; then return to this junction and descend the narrow but adequately maintained trail across the brush-smothered north-facing slopes. With barely enough room to get by, you'll get to know intimately several of the most common chaparral plants seen around Southern California: chamise, manzanita, mountain mahogany, scrub oak, and ceanothus.

VARIATION

Doing the loop on Jupiter Mountain alone is 2.4 miles with 1,100 feet of elevation gain.

chapter 13

Glendale & Verdugo Mountains

Like a ship caught fast on a sandbar, the Verdugo Mountains protrude above what would otherwise be an unbroken sheet of alluvial deposits slanting down from the foot of the San Gabriel Mountains toward the San Fernando Valley. The narrow, sloping La Crescenta valley divides the Verdugos from the San Gabriels to the east, while the pancake-flat San Fernando Valley stretches nearly 20 miles to the west.

The Verdugos are, in fact, geologic cousins of the San Gabriels; they're only about half as high, but similar in origin and form. Both are youthful, fault-block ranges of unconsolidated crystalline (granitic and metamorphic) rocks, pushed skyward by vertical movements along faults at their bases.

The Verdugo Mountains stand as a remarkable island of undeveloped land—a haven for wildlife such as deer and coyotes—completely encircled by an urbanized domain. A number of trailheads in and around the city of Glendale provide public access by foot or mountain bike to the mountain slopes. The network of pathways includes wide, smooth fire roads built many decades ago to accommodate fire trucks and to service hilltop antenna installations, plus a number of narrow hiking trails constructed since the 1980s. These routes are your ticket to hours of healthy exercise and enjoyable views whenever the air turns clean and transparent. This chapter lists many hikes in the Verdugos, but the map shows that regular visitors could cobble together other options linking the trails and roads.

The northern end of the mountain range burned to bare earth in the September 2017 La Tuna Fire. The 7,194-acre fire was the largest ever within the city of Los Angeles. The cause was not determined but is not believed to be arson.

In addition to hikes in the Verdugo Mountains, this chapter also includes two destinations at the foot of the San Gabriel Mountains: Deukmejian Wilderness Park, on the northern edge of the city of Glendale, and Haines Canyon, just above the L.A. community of Tujunga.

The Verdugo Hills are laced with trails and fire roads. This photo was taken from Mount Lukens.

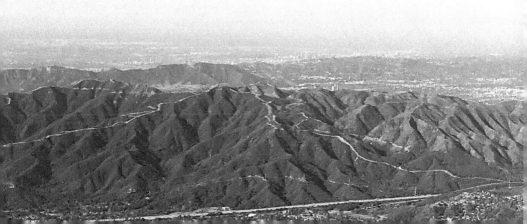

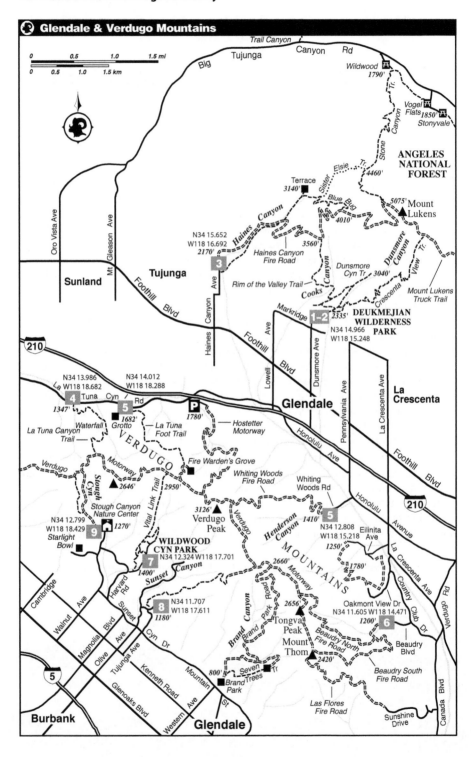

Glendale & Verdugo Mountains

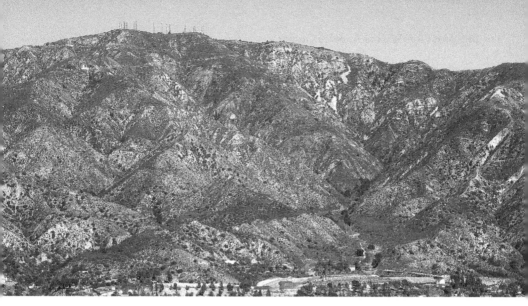

Deukmejian Wilderness Park (canyon at lower right) lies beneath antenna-clad Mount Lukens.

trip 13.1 — Deukmejian Wilderness Park

Distance	2.5 miles (loop)
Hiking Time	1.5 hours
Elevation Gain	800'
Difficulty	Moderate
Trail Use	Suitable for mountain biking, dogs allowed, good for kids
Best Times	Year-round
Agency	Glendale Community Services & Parks
Optional Map	Tom Harrison *Angeles Front Country*

see map opposite

DIRECTIONS From the 210 Freeway in Glendale, take Exit 17A for northbound Pennsylvania Avenue. In 1.4 miles turn left on Henrietta. In 0.3 mile turn left on New York. In 0.2 mile make a forced left onto Markridge. In 0.1 mile turn right into Deukmejian Wilderness Park, and proceed 0.2 mile to the parking area near the old stone barn.

Not many small cities can boast of three mountain ranges within their borders, but Glendale does. Stretching east and north from the San Fernando Valley, the city takes in substantial parts of the San Rafael Hills and the Verdugo Mountains, plus a small slice of the San Gabriel Mountains at the city's northern extremity. At this northernmost spot in Glendale, overlooking the foothill communities of La Crescenta and Tujunga, lies Deukmejian Wilderness Park, named after former California governor George Deukmejian. The park's 700 acres are drained by two steep ravines: Cooks Canyon and Dunsmore Canyon. During the mid-20th century, the area alongside Dunsmore Canyon stream was used by the Le Mesnager family as a vineyard. An old stone barn at the trailhead is reminiscent of that time. The park is open from 7 a.m. until 1 hour after sunset.

From the parking area, take either the gated service road or a trail at a kiosk to its right, both of which soon merge to become the Dunsmore Creek Trail, an old fire road. Pass the signed start of the Mummy Rock Nature Trail, then the McFall Oak, a heritage coast live oak that survived the 2009 Station Fire, which burned many of the other trees in the canyon. After 1.0 mile and 700 feet of relentless and shadeless ascent, the road ends. Duck under the cover of the streamside alders and enjoy the sound of the happy little stream tumbling over and around boulders of various sizes. Major floods occasionally rearrange the streambed rocks, creating mini-cascades that are probably temporary. The crystalline purity of the water at this spot is remarkable. Also, the 3,000-foot elevation here ensures that on many days you can be well above the smog level.

Retrace your steps 0.4 mile to where the Le Mesnager Loop Trail veers right. Take this longer but view-rich route back toward the start, taking advantage of two short spur trails along the way. The spurs lead to points overlooking Dunsmore and Cooks Canyons. Both afford a more distant view of the suburbs below and the rising swell of the Verdugo Mountains beyond. On the Le Mesnager Loop Trail you'll also pass the Rim of the Valley Trail, a winding footpath that crosses the stream in Cooks Canyon and ascends toward Mount Lukens (see next trip).

trip 13.2 Mount Lukens Southern Approach

see map on p. 180

Distance	10 miles (loop)
Hiking Time	5 hours
Elevation Gain	2,800'
Difficulty	Strenuous
Trail Use	Suitable for mountain biking, dogs allowed
Best Times	October–April
Agency	Glendale Community Services & Parks
Optional Map	Tom Harrison *Angeles Front Country*

DIRECTIONS From the 210 Freeway in Glendale, take Exit 17A for northbound Pennsylvania Avenue. In 1.4 miles turn left on Henrietta. In 0.3 mile turn left on New York. In 0.2 mile make a forced left onto Markridge. In 0.1 mile turn right into Deukmejian Wilderness Park, and proceed 0.2 mile to the parking area near the old stone barn.

View of Mount Lukens from the southeast; Big Tujunga Canyon and Condor Peak are behind Lukens.

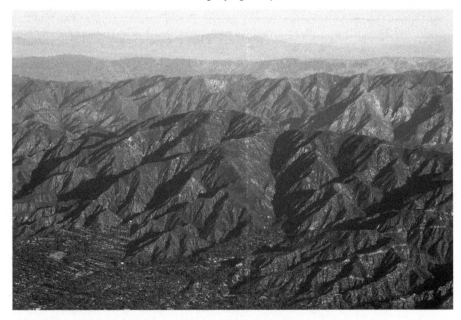

Mount Lukens (5,075') is the westernmost summit of the San Gabriel Mountains and the highest point within the Los Angeles city limits. The mountain was called Sister Elsie Peak in the 1875 Wheeler Survey but was renamed in 1922 for Theodore Lukens, who served as Acting Supervisor of the San Gabriel Timberland Reserve (now Angeles National Forest) in 1906. According to legend, Sister Elsie was a Catholic nun who died while nursing smallpox victims; historians, however, have been unable to confirm that she actually existed. The peak is now blemished by an array of antennas but remains an excellent hike with outstanding city views. The southern approach by way of the Crescenta View and Rim of the Valley Trails offers a terrific workout just minutes from the freeway, and is best done on a clear, cool day. After a winter storm, you might be able to build a snowman on the summit.

From the parking area, take either the gated service road or a trail at a kiosk to its right, both of which soon merge to become the Dunsmore Creek Trail, an old fire road. Pass junctions for the Mummy Rock Nature Trail and Vineyard Trail. In 0.4 mile pass the Le Mesnager Loop/Rim of the Valley Trail on the left, by which you will return. Just beyond, veer right onto the Crescenta View/Vineyard Trail and cross a crib dam. The Vineyard Trail soon loops back toward the trailhead, but you stay on the Crescenta View trail, which climbs unrelentingly through the shadeless sage scrub up a narrow ridge and across a steep face. Mount Lukens, topped by antennas, looms high above to your left. At mile 2.0, pass a circular stone windbreak with great views over the valley. The trail eventually joins the abandoned Pickens Spur road cut (Forest Service Road 2N76C), and tops out at the Mount Lukens Truck Trail (FS 2N76) at 3.4 miles.

Turn left and continue to the summit, at 4.5 miles. Walk around to enjoy the expansive views. To the south and west are the Verdugo Hills, Griffith Park, downtown Los Angeles, Palos Verdes Peninsula, Channel Islands, and Santa Monica Mountains. The San Gabriel range runs to the east, culminating in the towering summit of Mount Baldy.

Continue west on the Mount Lukens Truck Trail, possibly obscure at first. At mile 4.9, turn left onto the abandoned Haines Canyon Motorway, now the upper part of the Rim of the Valley Trail. Pass an unsigned junction with the Old Mount Lukens Trail on the right; then reach an easily overlooked junction at a switchback where a carsonite post marks the lower part of Rim of the Valley Trail on the left (7.5 miles). Switchback south down this trail, passing an unmarked junction with a rougher parallel path that soon rejoins your route. At 9.5 miles turn right onto the Le Mesnager Trail in Cooks Canyon, and follow it down to the Dunsmore Creek Trail and back to where you began.

---

trip 13.3   ## Haines Canyon

Distance	3.4 miles (out-and-back)
Hiking Time	2 hours
Elevation Gain	1,000'
Difficulty	Moderate
Trail Use	Suitable for mountain biking, dogs allowed, good for kids
Best Times	October–June
Agency	Angeles National Forest
Optional Map	Tom Harrison *Angeles Front Country* or Trails Illustrated *Angeles National Forest (811)*

see map on p. 180

DIRECTIONS From the 210 Freeway in Tujunga, take Exit 16 for northbound Lowell Avenue. In 0.6 mile turn left on Foothill Boulevard. In 0.9 mile turn right on Haines Canyon Avenue. Proceed 0.9 mile to the end, briefly jogging right along the way. Backtrack to find a place to park on the shoulder of the street, observing parking restrictions in the area.

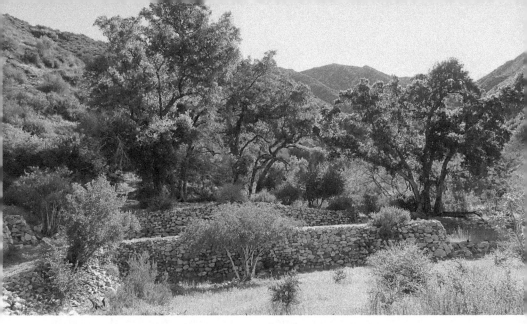

Oak-shaded abandoned terraces in Haines Canyon make great picnic spots.

Coyotes howl, water splashes down a willow-lined creek, hummingbirds flit about in search of nectar. All of this takes place barely a mile from the grid of suburban streets on L.A.'s fringe. It's Haines Canyon we're referring to here, but it sounds a lot like dozens of other small canyon streams that give up their water to the concrete storm channels of the city below. At the mouth of almost every one yawns a debris basin, often 50–100 feet wide, designed to catch the slurry of silt, sand, rocks, and boulders that roar down the mountain slopes during infrequent cloudbursts.

An abandoned fire road ascends Haines Canyon and continues all the way to 5,074-foot Mount Lukens. Our modest goal on this hike is merely to quickly reach a secluded middle section of Haines Canyon, removed from both the improvements of the L.A. County Flood Control District and the sights and sounds of the city.

Walk up the dirt Haines Canyon Motorway continuing from the end of Haines Canyon Avenue. Pass a paved private road on the left; then walk around the vehicle gate and bypass a typical, ugly debris basin and dam. Continue upstream on the dirt road, which soon deteriorates to a singletrack. The sight of civilization quickly fades, except for a dozen check dams (aka crib dams) down along the creek, all constructed of the same kind of precast concrete "logs." Decades of regrowth of native trees such as willows, live oaks, and sycamores have done a lot to soften their visual impact.

After 1.2 miles the abandoned Haines Canyon Motorway curves abruptly right and climbs out of the canyon toward Mount Lukens. You take the old road (now a singletrack maintained by mountain bikers) to the left, up the main branch of the canyon. At 1.6 miles watch for an unsigned trail on the left, which descends toward the seasonal creekbed; here you'll come to an obscure T-junction with an abandoned road, where you'll see patches of asphalt underfoot here and there, hidden beneath the encroaching vegetation. Turn right and thread your way through the brush to a terraced site shaded by large coast live oaks, a great site for a picnic.

On your return, the trail splits just south of the Haines Canyon Motorway junction. A singletrack parallels the Haines Canyon Motorway on the east side of the streambed. Numerous jumps and terrain features attest to its popularity among mountain bikers. The trail ends on Haines Canyon Road near where you parked.

VARIATION ───────────────────────────────────────

Mount Lukens is a 5.4-mile hike one-way with 2,900 feet of elevation gain by way of the Haines Canyon Motorway. Return the way you came, or explore the web of other trails coming off the mountain.

VARIATION ───────────────────────────────────────

If you stay on the singletrack rather than detouring to the oaks on the terraced site, you'll soon reach a spring feeding the creek—beware of poison oak here. The old Sister Elsie Trail crosses the creek and climbs to join the Stone Canyon Trail on the shoulder of Mount Lukens. The path deteriorates quickly to the point of invisibility if not constantly maintained, so only adventurous hikers should attempt to follow it. The well-maintained singletrack, beloved by mountain bikers, continues east and climbs to meet the Haines Canyon Motorway; it's sometimes called the Old Mount Lukens Trail or the Blue Bug Trail (in honor of a striking Volkswagen car wreck near the top). Optionally, you can continue up to Mount Lukens or loop back down onto the motorway.

───

trip 13.4   La Tuna Loop

Distance	9 miles (loop)	
Hiking Time	4.5 hours	
Elevation Gain	1,900'	
Difficulty	Moderately strenuous	
Trail Use	Dogs allowed	
Best Times	October–May	
Agencies	Mountains Recreation & Conservation Authority, Santa Monica Mountains Conservancy	
Optional Map	Tom Harrison *Verdugo Mountains* or *Angeles Front Country*	

see map on p. 180

NOTES The La Tuna Canyon Trail has reopened in the wake of the 2017 La Tuna Fire; at the time of this writing, however, it is overgrown and washed out in spots along the canyon floor due to flash flooding in 2018, potentially making navigation difficult. Call 323-221-9944 for updates on trail conditions.

DIRECTIONS From the 210 Freeway in Glendale, take Exit 14 for westbound La Tuna Canyon Road. Pass the large parking lot at Hostetter Fire Road and a smaller trailhead for the La Tuna Foot Trail before reaching the unsigned trailhead in 1.4 miles. From the west, the trailhead is 3.3 miles east of Sunland Boulevard in Sun Valley.

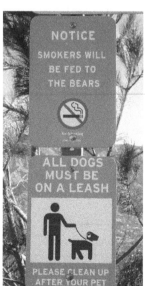

The 1,100-acre La Tuna Canyon Park—basically an open-space area with a roadside picnic table—drapes over the north-facing slopes of the Verdugo Mountains. (In Spanish, *la tuna* refers not to fish but the fruit of the prickly pear cactus.)

Most of the trails in the Verdugos are fire roads, but an ingenious trail was cut through this park in 1989. The slopes once held luxuriant stands of chaparral and the canyons were shaded by oak and sycamore, but the

Verdugo rangers have a good sense of humor.

hillsides were incinerated in the 2017 La Tuna Fire. As of early 2019, the trail is open again, and the regeneration process will be interesting to watch. On clear days, the best part is the walk along the Verdugo ridgecrest.

From the trailhead follow the La Tuna Canyon Trail up along a small canyon about 100 yards to a viewpoint overlooking a natural declivity, where water cascades after a good rain. From there you double back and undertake an easy switchback ascent of the canyon's east wall. At the top of the climb, step left onto a knoll with a good view.

After about 1 mile the trail starts to contour across a slope immediately above La Tuna Canyon Road and then drops quickly to the bottom of Grotto Canyon, parallel to the first. The trail briefly climbs onto the east wall of the canyon to bypass a 20-foot waterfall. The tunnel of arching live oaks that shade the canyon have been badly burned, but some may survive.

At 1.6 miles the narrow trail tread joins traces of an old road that leaves the canyon and quickly gains the ridge between the two canyons and then connects with Verdugo Fire Road. A heart-pounding climb (600 vertical feet in 0.6 mile) puts you on the wide fire road. Turn left and head east toward Verdugo Peak.

The next stop—worth the short side trip if the air is clear—is a 2,646-foot knoll on the right at 2.9 miles. Scramble up the firebreak on the knoll's east side and enjoy what is likely the most complete view of the San Fernando Valley available from any land-based vantage point. The pseudo-aerial perspective reveals flat grids of linear streets slashed by curving freeways, huge complexes of industrial buildings that look like giant computer circuit boards, endless rows of stuccoed single-family homes half hidden in a green haze of street trees, and spiky clusters of high rises. The valley's geographic connection to the main Los Angeles Basin is plainly revealed. In the gap where the connection is made (between the Verdugo and Santa Monica Mountains), sunlight gleams on the concrete banks of the Los Angeles River flood channel.

Farther east you pass several antenna sites and at 4.1 miles skirt the Fire Warden's Grove—scattered pine, cedar, and cypress trees planted for experimental purposes after a major fire in 1927. Clearly out of their natural element on these high and dry slopes, the trees are nonetheless a welcome addition to the scenery, though most perished in the La Tuna Fire.

Turn left at the next road junction onto the Hostetter Motorway, at 4.5 miles. Another 3.4 miles of easy descent takes you down to a large parking area alongside La Tuna Canyon Road. Follow the wide shoulder of that road 1.2 miles to return to your car—an easy half-hour walk or 15-minute jog, or an even shorter trip if you left a car or bicycle.

The Verdugos offer an unsurpassed view of the San Fernando Valley and its connection to the L.A. Basin.

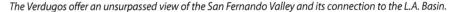

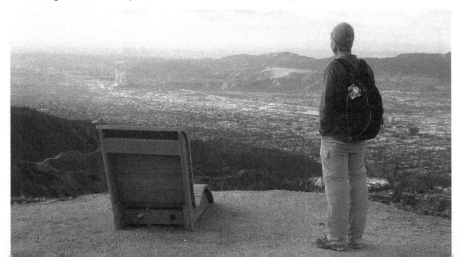

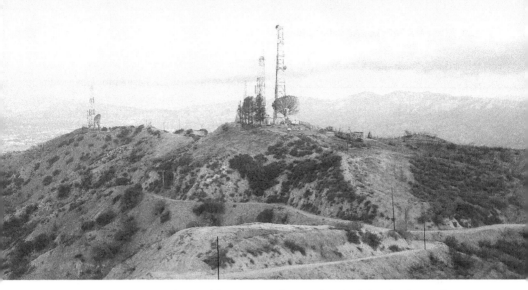

The 2017 La Tuna Fire stripped most of the vegetation from Verdugo Peak, but the chaparral has evolved to regenerate quickly.

trip 13.5   Verdugo Peak Traverse

Distance	6 miles (one-way)
Hiking Time	3 hours
Elevation Gain	1,800'
Difficulty	Moderately strenuous
Trail Use	Dogs allowed
Best Times	November–April
Agency	Santa Monica Mountains Conservancy
Optional Map	Tom Harrison *Verdugo Mountains* or *Angeles Front Country*

see map on p. 180

DIRECTIONS This trip requires a 4.5-mile shuttle between trailheads by car, bicycle, or ride-sharing service. If you plan to leave a getaway vehicle at the Whiting Woods Trailhead, take Exit 17A for Pennsylvania Avenue from the 210 Freeway in Glendale, and drive south 0.6 mile; then turn right on Whiting Woods Road and go 0.3 mile to park at the end by the gated Whiting Woods Motorway.

To reach the Grotto Trailhead, return to the freeway (or Honolulu Avenue, which parallels it), and proceed north. Take Exit 14 west on La Tuna Canyon Road and go 0.9 mile to the (possibly unsigned) Grotto Trailhead, where the La Tuna Foot Trail begins.

With a drop-off-and-pick-up transportation arrangement, you can enjoy a lively traverse across the north end of the Verdugo Mountains, ascending though La Tuna Canyon Park on a rough foot trail and descending toward the finish at Henderson Canyon on a wide, graded fire road. Assuming the skies are crystal clear when you go, you'll have consistently spectacular views the entire way.

From the trailhead, walk 50 yards up the west side of the deeply shaded ravine to visit the base of the small cliff (a waterfall in the wet season) called The Grotto. Return to the trailhead and find the La Tuna Foot Trail on the east side of the ravine. The trail quickly settles into a steady and almost uninterrupted uphill grade, zigzagging when necessary to keep on or near the top of a well-defined ridge trending southeast. The mature chaparral burned to bare earth in the 2017 La Tuna Fire but will likely regenerate quickly.

After 2.1 miles and nearly 1,200 feet of elevation gain, the trail arrives at a wide, graded fire road. To the left and below lies the main part of the Fire Warden's Grove, an experimental forest dating from the 1920s. You turn right, however, and climb 0.3 mile farther to the Verdugo Motorway, where you get your first wide vistas of the vast San Fernando Valley to the west and south.

Turn left on the Verdugo Motorway and follow it east, passing various antenna installations on the crest of the ridge. The highest point (3,126'), at 3.1 miles, is unofficially known as Verdugo Peak. The antenna facility at the top blocks a complete 360° view, but you can walk around to take it all in. The San Gabriel Mountains and La Crescenta Valley to the east are especially striking. On the far side of the valley, subdivisions completely cover most of the classically formed alluvial fans that spill from the foot of the San Gabriels. Debris dams at the apex of nearly every fan do their best (but sometimes fail) to catch the muddy slurry that sweeps down the canyons whenever storms unleash torrents of water on the slopes above.

Look for the Whiting Woods Motorway intersecting at 3.5 miles into the hike. Turn left and follow its twisting course down an east-plunging ridgeline all the way into the shady depths of Henderson Canyon. The traverse ends where the fire road terminates, at the western end of Whiting Woods Road, a residential street.

---

trip 13.6   **Beaudry Loop**

Distance	5.5 miles (loop)
Hiking Time	3 hours
Elevation Gain	1,600'
Difficulty	Moderately strenuous
Trail Use	Suitable for mountain biking, dogs allowed
Best Times	November–May
Agency	Glendale Community Services & Parks
Optional Map	Tom Harrison *Verdugo Mountains* or *Angeles Front Country*

see map on p. 180

DIRECTIONS From the westbound 210 Freeway in Glendale, take Exit 17B south on La Crescenta Avenue. In 1 mile turn right onto Oakmont View Drive. In 0.2 mile turn left (south) onto Country Club Drive. In 0.7 mile turn right onto Beaudry Boulevard, and proceed 0.4 mile to the trailhead where the road veers right. Park on the street.

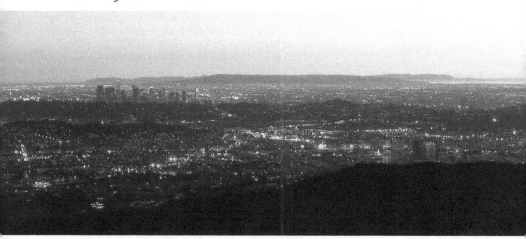

The Beaudry Loop is a great place to take in sunsets and city lights.

From the south end of the Verdugos' summit ridge, your gaze takes in the San Gabriel Mountains, much of the L.A. megalopolis, and even the ocean on occasion. Do this trip late in the day if you want to enjoy both a spectacular sunset and a blaze of lights after twilight fades. At best, try this on any cloud-free, smog-free day that falls within two weeks on either side of the winter solstice (December 21). During that period, the sun sets on the flat ocean horizon behind Santa Monica Bay. At other times of year, the sun's sinking path is likely to intersect the coastal mountains. The seemingly strange fact of the sun setting over land most of the year is a consequence of the east–west orientation of California's coastline in the area upcoast from Los Angeles. The trail is named for the nearby street, which in turn is named for Prudent Beaudry, a businessman who served as mayor of Los Angeles from 1874 to 1876.

From the residential neighborhood at the end of Beaudry Boulevard, walk up a paved segment of fire road, bypass a vehicle gate, and continue on dirt past a debris basin to where the fire road splits (0.3 mile). Choose for your way the shadier but less viewful right branch, Beaudry North Motorway. You'll return to this junction by way of the left branch, the Beaudry South Motorway. About halfway up the north road you come to a trickling spring at Dead Man's Tank nestled in a shady ravine, a good place for a breather. The water tank got its name because a body was found in it.

When you reach the summit ridge (2.3 miles), turn sharply left on Verdugo Motorway and continue climbing another 0.4 mile toward a cluster of brightly painted radio towers atop a 2,656-foot bump called Tongva Peak, the highest point along this hike. For the best view, follow a use trail south along the fence line to a vista point. Continue south along the ridge 0.6 mile to a road junction. The right branch descends to Sunshine Drive in Glendale; you take the left branch and return along an east ridge to the split just above the debris basin.

trip 13.7   Vital Link Trail

see map on p. 180

Distance	3.2 miles (out-and-back)
Hiking Time	2.5 hours
Elevation Gain	1,500'
Difficulty	Moderately strenuous
Trail Use	Dogs allowed
Best Times	November–April
Agency	City of Burbank Parks and Recreation
Optional Map	Tom Harrison *Verdugo Mountains* or *Angeles Front Country*

DIRECTIONS From the 5 Freeway in Burbank, take Exit 146B for Burbank Boulevard. Go north on Burbank for 0.2 mile; then turn right on Third Street. In one block, turn left on Harvard Road. In 1.6 miles turn right into the entrance of Wildwood Canyon Park. Pass a first trailhead parking lot just inside the entrance and continue 0.4 mile to a second trailhead parking area.

The nearly straight-up Vital Link Trail connects popular Wildwood Canyon Park in the Verdugo foothills with the Verdugo Mountains crestline. Almost every step on the trail yields a higher vantage for the panoramic view of the platelike San Fernando Valley floor and the pillowy Santa Monica Mountains beyond. The reverse, downhill leg of the trek is a possibly knee-banging exercise, but the view then lies directly in front of you. The entirely south-facing aspect of this hike mandates that you hike only during the coolest time of year, and preferably not in the midday sunshine. This area was partially burned in the 2017 La Tuna Fire but has reopened.

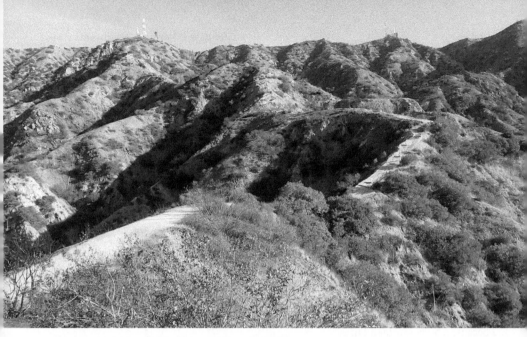

The Vital Link Trail climbs steeply to the ridge near the antenna tower.

From the arched trailhead 0.4 mile into Wildwood Canyon Park (actually the second of a total of four gateways to the park's trail system), head sharply up the canyon wall to the north. The trail initially resembles a maze, but head uphill and all the branches will eventually converge. After a quarter mile, make a right and settle into a moderate grade that will take you up onto the ridgeline. Upon reaching the ridgeline trail, stay right to climb the ridge; then, shortly thereafter, pass a trail on the right leading back down to the park.

Pick up the signed Vital Link Trail on the left, 0.6 mile from the start (not quite as far as a picnic table perched on knoll). The real climb begins now as the trail doggedly sticks to a narrow ridge trending north and goes acutely uphill all the way to the crest. The vegetation along the ridge was incinerated by the 2017 La Tuna Fire. You'll top out at an excellent viewpoint on a service road near an antenna tower. The Burbank airport, Griffith Park, and downtown Los Angeles lie far below. Return the same way for a 3.2-mile round-trip distance.

The service road continues north 0.1 mile to join the Verdugo Motorway, a service road running along the backbone of the hills. Possible extensions include a visit to the nearby Fire Warden's Grove (partially burned), a traverse west and then south into Stough Canyon, or a traverse east ending at any of several trailheads on the north or west sides of the Verdugos. The Vital Link trail truly provides a vital link for all kinds of travel possibilities.

trip 13.8   West Side Loop

Distance	9 miles (loop)
Hiking Time	4 hours
Elevation Gain	2,000'
Difficulty	Strenuous
Trail Use	Dogs allowed
Best Times	November–April
Agency	City of Burbank Parks and Recreation
Optional Map	Tom Harrison *Verdugo Mountains*

see map on p. 180

DIRECTIONS From the 5 Freeway in Burbank, take Exit 146A for Olive Avenue. Follow Olive northeast 1.2 miles to Sunset Canyon Drive. Proceed straight across on what becomes Country Club Drive. After 0.3 mile turn right on Via Montana. Go uphill one long block to the corner of Via Montana and Camino de Villas, where you can find curbside parking.

The West Side loop climbs the abandoned Skyline Mountain Motorway, now trail, to the spine of the Verdugo Mountains, then descends via the Brand Park Motorway. You'll enjoy outstanding views and a vigorous workout along the route. Part of the Skyline route has slid away, leaving a short walk across a steep hillside that might not be enjoyable for some hikers.

From the corner of Via Montana and Camino de Villas, walk north across a grassy lot below a mansion to an old dirt road cut going north, now faded to a singletrack trail. Stay on this well-defined path as it climbs steadily. In 1.5 miles enter the 2017 La Tuna Fire burn zone, and then pick your way across a steep slide before joining a maintained road. At 2.7 miles reach the crest and continue a few yards to a junction with the Verdugo Motorway, as well as a broad firebreak bulldozed along the ridgeline.

Go straight to pick up the southbound Verdugo Motorway (the path on the right is a firebreak that soon ends). Continue 0.3 mile to a junction with Brand Park Motorway, where a wooden bench on the shadeless ridgeline invites you to sit a spell (if it's not too hot) and enjoy the view. Brand Park Motorway, a fairly new addition to the fire-road network and the route of the annual Verdugo Mountains 10K race, is somewhat less scenic than what you've traveled so far. Follow its turns and twists 3.3 miles south to the green lawns of Brand Park in the valley below.

In a corner of Brand Park stands Glendale's architecturally noteworthy Brand Library, a Moorish-style structure built by early-1900s civic booster Leslie Brand. Near the library and for some distance up the canyon behind it are the remnants of the tropical gardens that once graced Brand's estate.

To complete this loop hike, continue out of the south end of the park, turn right, and walk along pleasantly shaded Mountain Street (which becomes Sunset Canyon Drive as you pass into the city of Burbank) for 1.2 miles to Tujunga Avenue. Turn right on Tujunga (which later becomes Camino de Villas) and walk 0.6 mile uphill through a posh neighborhood to Villa Montana and your waiting car.

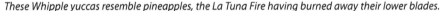

These Whipple yuccas resemble pineapples, the La Tuna Fire having burned away their lower blades.

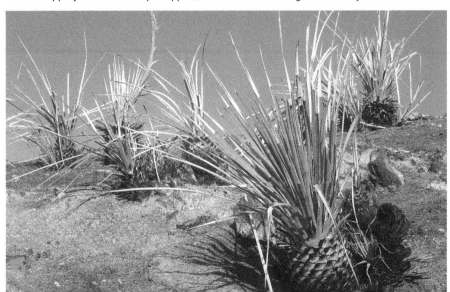

trip 13.9 Stough Canyon Loop

Distance	3.0 miles (loop)
Hiking Time	1.5 hours
Elevation Gain	800'
Difficulty	Strenuous
Trail Use	Dogs allowed
Best Times	November–April
Agency	City of Burbank Parks and Recreation
Optional Map	Tom Harrison *Verdugo Mountains*

see map on p. 180

DIRECTIONS From the 5 Freeway in Burbank, take Exit 146B for Burbank Boulevard. Go east on Burbank for 0.2 mile; then turn left on Third Street. In another 0.2 mile, turn right on Delaware; then make an immediate right onto Glenoaks Boulevard and a left on Walnut Avenue. Follow Walnut 1.9 miles to its end at the Stough Canyon Nature Center.

This trip explores the northern end of the Verdugo Mountains from the Stough Canyon Nature Center. It makes a short but vigorous climb to a pair of viewpoints where you can watch the jets departing Burbank Airport beneath you. If you have time after your trip, stop in the nature center to learn more about the area's plants and wildlife. The area is named for Oliver Stough, who deeded part of his extensive Burbank ranch to the city as a public parkland.

Take the gated dirt Stough Canyon Mountain Way from the nature center. In 0.4 mile, after two hairpin turns, you'll reach a signed trail on the left for The View and Old Youth Campground. Take this trail, and when it splits at 0.6 mile, stay left to the top of the nearby hill where you can enjoy great views. Then return to the split and take the other path, which soon deteriorates to a singletrack. At 1.0 mile watch for a chimney and foundation, the remains of a cabin from the abandoned Old Youth Camp.

At 1.3 miles reach the Verdugo Motorway near the crest. For another great view, turn left (west) and climb to One Tree Hill (1.5 miles), where you can rest at a picnic table beside a lonely tree reminiscent of the Wisdom Tree on Cahuenga Peak.

To finish the trip, go back east until you reach a saddle (2.0 miles); then turn right and follow Stough Canyon Mountain Way back to the nature center.

VARIATION

From the saddle, you can follow the Verdugo Motorway east to the radio towers and then descend the Missing Link Trail to Wildwood Park and walk back along the street. This enjoyable loop is 7 miles with 2,200 feet of elevation gain.

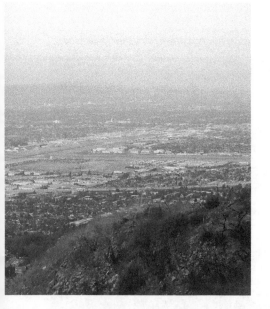

From The View you can watch the planes come and go at Hollywood Burbank Airport.

chapter 14

Griffith Park

Why shouldn't one of the world's most expansive cities boast one of the world's biggest city parks? It does, in fact. Griffith Park's 4,511 acres—about five times the size of New York City's Central Park—rate as the nation's largest municipal park completely surrounded by urban areas. The park was established in 1896 when Welsh developer Griffith J. Griffith donated his Ranch Los Feliz property to the city.

Griffith Park is L.A.'s "park for the people," where Angelenos (and some tourists) come to spread a picnic blanket, visit the homegrown zoo or the observatory and planetarium, and explore the chaparral-covered hills and scenic vistas. More than half of the park's area consists of terrain too steep to be developed as parkland in the conventional manner, so it remains as a kind of in-city wilderness, albeit of a mostly dry and scrubby kind.

More than 50 miles of fire roads and foot trails lure those on foot and horseback; while bicyclists can explore more than 20 miles of twisting pavement, or take to the dirt wherever such use is permitted. The trails are busy on sunny weekends, yet it can be amazingly quiet here as long as you get an early start (the park's several gates swing open at 6 a.m. for access by automobile). By starting early you can also take advantage of the day's coolest temperatures and generally the cleanest air.

The sketch map of Griffith Park in this chapter, though adequate for the purposes of navigating the routes described here, omits some lesser paths and geographic details. At the ranger station and visitor center on the east side of the park, however, you can pick up a

The Wisdom Tree is a popular destination on the west shoulder of Cahuenga Peak (Trip 14.1, page 195).

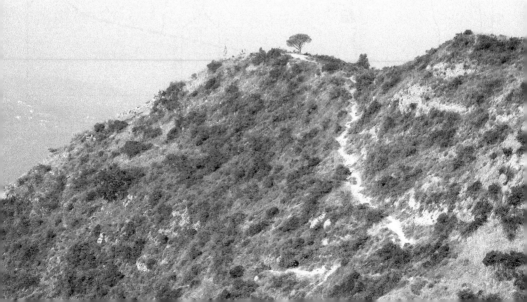

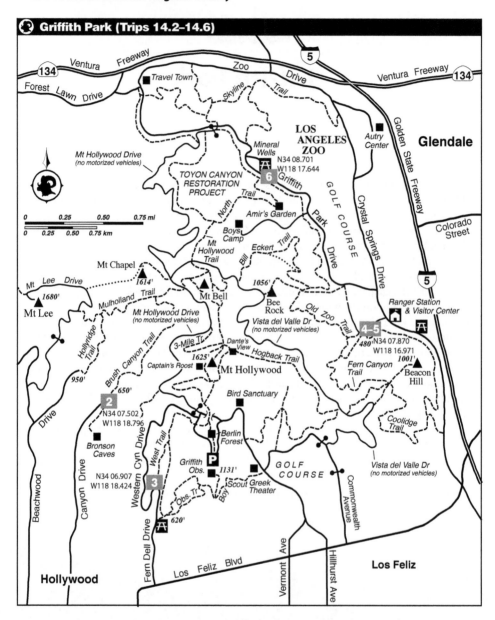

Griffith Park (Trips 14.2–14.6)

copy of an excellent, large-scale color map/brochure showing a wealth of detail. The map is also available online: see tinyurl.com/griffithparkmap1 and tinyurl.com/griffithparkmap2.

The park's interior paved roads—Mount Hollywood Drive and Vista del Valle Drive—are closed to motorized traffic. Cyclists, who are not allowed to ride on the park's trails, can enjoy biking on miles of car-free pavement.

Griffith Park occupies the eastern tip of the Santa Monica Mountains, a fact difficult to discern until you climb one of the park's high points and look west along the crest of the range. The higher and wilder parts of the Santa Monicas, west of Sepulveda Pass, are covered in the Santa Monica Mountains section of this book.

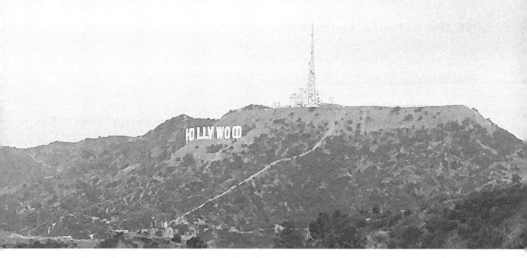

The iconic HOLLYWOOD *sign on Mount Lee is most easily reached from the west.*

trip 14.1   Hollywood Sign via Cahuenga Peak

Distance	2.8 miles (out-and-back)
Hiking Time	2 hours
Elevation Gain	1,000'
Difficulty	Moderate
Trail Use	Dogs allowed, good for kids
Best Times	October–April
Agency	Los Angeles Department of Recreation and Parks
Optional Map	Free *Griffith Park Map*

DIRECTIONS From the 101 Freeway, take Exit 11A for Barham Boulevard. Follow the Cahuenga Boulevard frontage road north for 0.5 mile; then turn right on Barham Boulevard. In 0.3 mile turn right again onto Lake Hollywood Drive, and proceed 0.5 mile to its junction with Wonder View Drive. Park on Lake Hollywood Drive south of the intersection.

Tourists from around the world flock to see the HOLLYWOOD sign, one of the world's most recognized landmarks. Excellent views of the sign abound from Griffith Observatory (see Trip 14.3, page 197) and the neighborhoods below, but this is the most direct route to actually reach the sign itself. The Hollyridge Trail from Beachwood Drive was even more direct, but it was closed in 2017 after a lawsuit from the Sunset Ranch Hollywood Stables, which disliked the heavy hiker traffic on Beachwood.

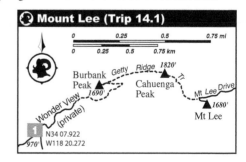

This short but rugged hike follows the ridge over Burbank and Cahuenga Peaks to the HOLLYWOOD sign overlook on Mount Lee. The mountain is named for Don Lee, a TV pioneer who built the early W6AXO broadcast tower here in the 1930s. The ridge was part of a 138-acre parcel purchased in 1940 by Howard Hughes and rezoned in 2008 for luxury estate development. The Trust for Public Land acquired the parcel in 2010 and it is now protected as part of Griffith Park. Tens of thousands of people rallied and donated to purchase the land, with major gifts from Steven Spielberg,

George Lucas, Hugh Hefner, Aileen Getty, and the Tiffany & Co. Foundation. Cahuenga Peak takes its name from a nearby Tongva village called Kawengna, or "place of the mountain."

The trail is open sunrise–sunset. Griffith Park's famous resident mountain lion, P-22, favors these hills and has been spotted here after dark. As a young male, P-22 apparently left the Santa Monica Mountains, crossed two major freeways, and made his way through Beverly Hills to reach Griffith Park, where he was photographed beneath the HOLLYWOOD sign in 2013. As he is cut off from potential mates in his current habitat, the National Wildlife Federation is campaigning to establish a wildlife crossing over the 101 Freeway.

Begin your hike by walking east up Wonder View Drive. Pass through a gate onto a dirt road, and soon join the narrow Burbank Peak Trail at a high-voltage transmission-line tower. Climb steeply to the 1,690-foot summit, where you'll find the solitary Wisdom Tree. According to legend, the pine was originally a Christmas tree and was replanted on the mountaintop by a man who wanted to honor his mother. Look for a box that contains an interesting geocaching register.

The path, now signed as the Aileen Getty Ridge Trail, continues east to the 1,820-foot summit of Cahuenga Peak, the highest summit in Griffith Park, from which you can enjoy splendid views over the Los Angeles Basin. Turning clockwise on a clear day, your views encompass Griffith Park, Mounts Baldy and Wilson, Burbank, the Hollywood Hills, Santa Monica Bay, Hollywood, and downtown Los Angeles.

Continue east to the end of paved Mount Lee Drive, a service road reaching the antennas above the HOLLYWOOD sign. A formidable fence divides the topmost part of Mount Lee from the sheer slope below, which precariously supports the spindly looking whitewashed letters of the famous sign.

trip 14.2 Mulholland Ridge

Distance	3.6 miles (out-and-back)
Hiking Time	2 hours
Elevation Gain	1,000'
Difficulty	Moderate
Trail Use	Dogs allowed
Best Times	Year-round
Agency	Los Angeles Department of Recreation and Parks
Optional Map	Free *Griffith Park Map*

see map on p. 194

DIRECTIONS From the northbound 101 Freeway in Hollywood, take Exit 8C for Gower Street. Immediately turn right onto Beachwood Drive, then right again onto Franklin Avenue. In 0.2 mile turn left (north) onto Canyon Drive. Follow Canyon Drive 1.4 miles to its far end. There's room for parking in a small lot here or back a little way alongside Canyon Drive itself.

If Mulholland Drive/Mulholland Highway, the scenic road that follows the crest of the Santa Monica Mountains, were ever extended eastward, it would probably snake along the sharply defined ridge between Mount Lee and Mount Chapel. But for now—and probably forever—the phenomenal views both north and south from this ridge remain the privilege of self-propelled travelers only.

From the end of Canyon Drive, proceed on foot past a gate and up the dirt-road extension of Canyon Drive, which climbs steadily up the east slope of a ravine known as Brush Canyon. After 1.1 miles you come to an intersection of a fire road known as the Mulholland Trail. Turn right and continue climbing a bit until you reach the paved but closed-to-auto-traffic

Mount Hollywood Drive. Make a sharp left there, walk on pavement for another 0.2 mile, and then cut left on the wide path going up along the southeast slope of Mount Chapel. The path leads to a water tank just north of the peak itself, and you can follow a steep climbers' trail to the 1,614-foot summit.

On Mount Chapel you almost feel as if you're flying as you gaze a thousand feet down on the Hollywood foothills to the south and the serene green spaces of Forest Lawn Memorial Park to the north. When you're finished taking in the complete view, return to Mount Hollywood Drive and head back the same way you came.

Griffith Park supports a resident coyote population.

VARIATION ───────────

A narrow ridgeline trail connects Mount Chapel to Mount Lee. From the water tank, take the rough trail west to the paved Mount Lee service road. From here you can turn right and make a short excursion to the top of the HOLLYWOOD sign. Then you descend to Mulholland Trail and follow it back to Brush Canyon. If you enjoy rough trails, this 6-mile, 1,300-foot-gain loop is much more interesting than just retracing your steps.

VARIATION ──────────────────────────────────

From the same trailhead, you can also walk south 0.4 mile to the Bronson Caves. These caves are actually tunnels quarried by the Union Rock Company between 1903 and 1920 to obtain rock for building city streets. They were named for nearby Bronson Avenue (from which actor Charles Bronson also took his stage name). The conveniently located and wild-looking tunnels have been used in more than 100 films and television shows; most notably, one of them served as the entrance to the Batcave in the 1960s *Batman* series.

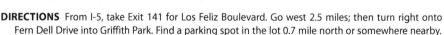

---

trip 14.3 Mount Hollywood

Distance	4.7 miles (loop)
Hiking Time	2 hours
Elevation Gain	1,000'
Difficulty	Moderate
Trail Use	Dogs allowed, good for kids
Best Times	October–May
Agency	Los Angeles Department of Recreation and Parks
Optional Map	Free *Griffith Park Map*

see map on p. 194

DIRECTIONS From I-5, take Exit 141 for Los Feliz Boulevard. Go west 2.5 miles; then turn right onto Fern Dell Drive into Griffith Park. Find a parking spot in the lot 0.7 mile north or somewhere nearby.

The bald, flattish 1,625-foot summit of Mount Hollywood would scarcely be something to write home about except for its strategic location overlooking just about everything. Hikers approach from all directions, but the most popular starting point is the overcrowded

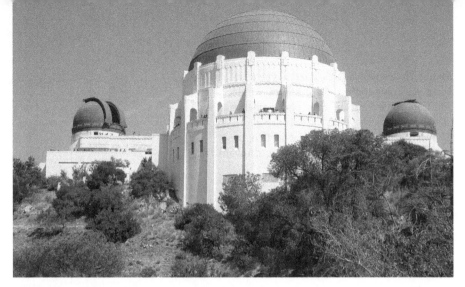

Griffith Observatory is a prominent Los Angeles landmark.

observatory parking lot. On the somewhat longer trek described here, you'll start out below the observatory so you can enjoy the exotically landscaped Fern Dell area, too. The dell features picnic tables, a year-round brook (a part of the observatory's cooling system, but appealing nonetheless), plenty of succulent plants, and shade trees.

From Fern Dell's main parking lot, walk across the lowermost horseshoe curve on Western Canyon Road and continue on the wide dirt fire road heading uphill (north) into sunny chaparral country. Dry and a bit trampled at first, the landscape improves as you climb. Along the trail are larger shrubs, such as toyon, elderberry, laurel sumac, sugar bush, and ceanothus, and smaller ones such as black sage, buckwheat, and fuchsia-flowered gooseberry—all are very typical of the drier south- and west-facing slopes in the park. Here, too, are common noxious invasive plants such as fennel, tree tobacco, and castor bean. Planted eucalyptus and pine trees stand high on the nearby slopes, while a handful of native live oaks tucked into the bigger creases on the sun-seared slopes draw just enough moisture from the soil to survive.

After passing under a couple of shade-giving oaks, the trail curves left and crosses the west observatory road. Soon you're on the ridgeline south of Mount Hollywood, passing high over a road tunnel. Listen for horns blaring as cars barrel through below.

A couple of long, lazy switchback legs up the Charlie Turner Trail take you to a trail junction not far below Mount Hollywood's summit. Make a sharp left, pass the Captain's Roost picnic area (drinking water here), and continue to a wide trail junction just north of the summit. Make a hard right here and walk over to the picnic tables on the top. Your gaze takes in (among many other things) the downtown L.A. skyline and the antenna-topped Mount Lee with its famous HOLLYWOOD sign facing south over Tinseltown. Just beyond Mount Lee is the top of Cahuenga Peak (1,820'), the highest summit in this corner of the Santa Monica Mountains (see Trip 14.1, page 195).

On your return, backtrack to the wide junction and go right, circling Mount Hollywood's east side. Retrace your steps on the two switchback segments or follow a steeper trail straight south; then keep south along the ridgeline after you reach the top of the tunnel. Walk across the observatory parking lot toward the monumental, three-domed building that houses a state-of-the-art planetarium and museum, a massive, antique Zeiss refractor telescope, and various solar instruments. Swing around the back side of the building to discover observation decks offering commanding views of the L.A. Basin.

For the final leg of the trip, follow the trail that descends the slope just east of the observatory. It starts from the left side of the building as you face its grand entrance. After 0.2 mile of descent, swing sharply right on the Observatory Trail. Go either way at the next junction where the trail divides into West Observatory Trail and East Observatory Trail. The two branches meet down below at Fern Dell. After winding past golden-blossomed silk oak trees, you arrive at Fern Dell's bubbling brook. Your starting point is just up the road to the right.

VARIATION

For a grand tour of Griffith Park's most famous attractions, continue to the top of the HOLLYWOOD sign from the summit of Mount Hollywood via the Three Mile Trail, Mount Hollywood Drive, the Mulholland Trail, and Mount Lee Drive. Return on Mount Hollywood Drive to Griffith Observatory rather than climbing over Mount Hollywood a second time. This trip is 10 miles with 2,000 feet of elevation gain.

---

trip 14.4 Beacon Hill

Distance	4.1 miles (loop)
Hiking Time	2 hours
Elevation Gain	800'
Difficulty	Moderate
Trail Use	Dogs allowed, good for kids
Best Times	Year-round
Agency	Los Angeles Department of Recreation and Parks
Optional Map	Free *Griffith Park Map*

DIRECTIONS From I-5, take Exit 141 for Los Feliz Boulevard. Go west a short distance and then turn right (north) on Crystal Springs Drive. After 1.3 miles (next to the visitor center/ranger station) turn left on Griffith Park Drive. Go 0.2 mile to the large parking lot on the right, near the merry-go-round.

Sharply terminated by the Los Angeles River flood channel and the 5 Freeway, Beacon Hill stands as the last eastward gasp of a 50-mile-long mountain range: the Santa Monicas. Back in the early 20th century it served a utilitarian purpose as the site of an illuminated beacon for Grand Central Airport in Glendale. Today it presides over flatlands overrun by

Beacon Hill has a great view of the downtown L.A. skyline.

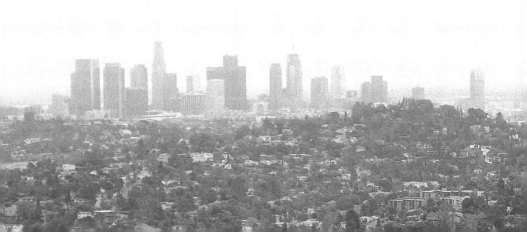

industrial buildings. Commercial air operations have long since shifted to LAX and four other big airports around the L.A. Basin. On this looping trip up to Beacon Hill's summit, you'll have a unique view of Glendale's industrial tracts, its medium-rise downtown skyline, and the looming Verdugo Mountains beyond.

In 2007, this area was burned in an 800-acre fire that was likely caused by arson. The fast-growing chaparral is adapted to fire and has mostly recovered.

From the merry-go-round parking lot, continue up Griffith Park Drive 0.1 mile to the fire road known as Fern Canyon Trail. (Note that this is not the narrower Fern Canyon Nature Trail on the floor of the canyon, which is still under repair at the time of this writing.) From here on, the rule is to stay left at every intersection. The canyon is lush with live oak, laurel sumac, toyon, and other native chaparral.

After 1.0 mile of gentle ascent, you'll come to the Five Points junction. Turn left on the Upper Beacon Trail, which follows a slightly rounded ridgeline for a quarter mile and takes you to Beacon Hill's 1,001-foot summit offering views east over Glendale and south over downtown Los Angeles.

When it's time to go, return to Five Points and turn left again to descend the Coolidge Trail, which loops back to your vehicle. Or if you are in a hurry, just retrace your steps to save a mile.

trip 14.5   East Side Loop

see map on p. 194

Distance	6 miles (loop)
Hiking Time	3.5 hours
Elevation Gain	1,300'
Difficulty	Moderately strenuous
Trail Use	Dogs allowed
Best Times	October–June
Agency	Los Angeles Department of Recreation and Parks
Optional Map	Free *Griffith Park Map*

DIRECTIONS Exit the 5 Freeway at Los Feliz Boulevard. Go west a short distance and then turn right (north) on Crystal Springs Drive. After 1.3 miles (next to the visitor center/ranger station) turn left on Griffith Park Drive. Go 0.2 mile to the large parking lot on the right, near the merry-go-round.

Botanically and geologically, this is perhaps Griffith Park's most interesting hike. It's no slouch when it comes to good views either. The route tops out on the very crest of the park at Mount Hollywood. The large 2007 Griffith Park wildfire burned large sections of the park's east side, but the fast-growing chaparral has recovered quickly.

From the merry-go-round parking lot, cross Griffith Park Drive and start heading southwest up Fern Canyon Trail. Just 0.1 mile ahead turn right on Upper Old Zoo Trail. In the next 0.7 mile you pass the site of the old L.A. Zoo, and a side trail leading left (west) toward Bee Rock, an impressive outcrop of cavernous sandstone poking out of the ridge above. Bee Rock is a good example of the types of marine sedimentary rock that are widely exposed throughout the middle and eastern Santa Monica Mountains. Up around Mount Hollywood, the bedrock consists of volcanic rocks more characteristic of the west end of the Santa Monicas.

Just past the Bee Rock Trail, turn sharply left on the Bill Eckert Trail (aka the East Trail). Bill Eckert, Griffith Park Ranger #1, served from 1965 to 1981 and was famed for his interpretive hikes. You zigzag around a chaparral-covered ridge overlooking the Griffith Park

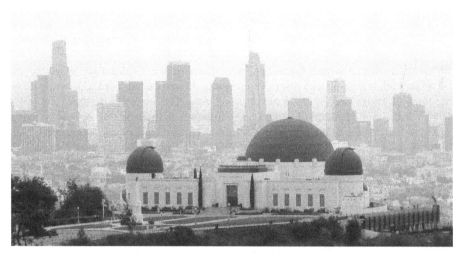

Downtown's skyscrapers loom large over Griffith Observatory.

Boy's Camp and arrive, after 1.2 miles, at Vista del Valle Drive. Swing right, walk about 0.1 mile down the pavement; then veer left on the wide trail that ascends sharply up the slope to the south. Turn sharply left at the next junction, and continue south along the ridge between Mount Bell and Mount Hollywood.

From the wide intersection just below Mount Hollywood's summit, you will eventually go east along the sunny ridgeline. But first pay a visit to the summit itself, where you can enjoy the panoramic view west to the HOLLYWOOD sign, then counterclockwise to the Santa Monica Mountains and Bay, Griffith Observatory, downtown L.A., the San Gabriel Mountains, and the Verdugo Mountains. Later, cool off and refill your water bottle at the irrigated spot east of the summit known as Dante's View. Dante Orgolini, a Brazilian journalist and longtime Griffith Park hiker, built a garden here with hand tools. Charlie Turner became the next garden keeper, and volunteers continue to care for it today. Eucalyptus trees and succulent plants frame a view to the south at this little hideaway.

The view-rich-but-sometimes-steep trail along the ridgeline to the east, Hogback Trail (aka East Ridge Trail), meanders down to meet Vista del Valle Drive. Cross the pavement there, walk down along the shoulder for about 100 feet, and pick up the trail going left past a water tank and down into the upper reaches of Fern Canyon. When you reach the Five Points junction near Beacon Hill, make a hard left and descend Fern Canyon Trail to your starting point below.

trip 14.6 Mount Bell

Distance	5 miles (loop)
Hiking Time	3 hours
Elevation Gain	1,100'
Difficulty	Moderately strenuous
Trail Use	Dogs allowed
Best Times	October–June
Agency	Los Angeles Department of Recreation and Parks
Optional Map	Free *Griffith Park Map*

see map on p. 194

DIRECTIONS This trip starts at the Mineral Wells Picnic Area. From the 134 Freeway, take Exit 4 for southbound Forest Lawn Drive. In 0.2 mile turn left onto Zoo Drive. In another 0.2 mile, turn right onto Griffith Park Drive. In 1.2 miles turn right into the Mineral Wells lot, and park near the entrance.

The Mount Bell Loop tours the lesser-used northern trails in Griffith Park. When the rest of the park is teeming with hikers, you might find some solitude here. The loop features the tranquil Amir's Garden and a mountaintop vista. The mountain is named for Major Horace Bell, a contemporary of Griffith and a historian of Southern California.

From the entrance to the parking lot, walk southwest on a wide and unassuming trail. Within a few yards, you'll cross the Mineral Wells Trail that parallels the road. Continue on the North Trail as it climbs up past a water tank. In 0.4 mile, at a hairpin turn, reach Amir's Garden. The oasis, established in 1971 by Amir Dialameh after a wildfire burned the slopes, is now tended by volunteers.

Our trip stays on the main trail. At 0.9 mile pass the signed Bridal Trail, on the right. At 1.3 miles cross the paved Vista Del Valle Drive (closed to vehicles). At 1.5 miles turn hard right at a junction on the northeast side of Mount Bell. At 1.7 miles turn left at another junction. Follow the trail around the west and south sides of Mount Bell, or take a steep use trail over the summit. At 2.0 miles reach a bench and viewpoint at Taco Peak, the next bump on the ridge southeast of Mount Bell.

After taking in the view, descend a narrow trail south from Taco Peak to rejoin the North Trail. Turn hard left and go north; then, at 2.3 miles, turn right and descend to Vista Del Valle Road at 2.6 miles. Veer right on the road for 0.1 mile to a faucet where you turn left onto the Bill Eckert Trail. At 3.9 miles turn left onto the Mineral Wells Trail, and follow it back to your starting point.

Bee Rock has a fenced viewpoint on top. Beware of the steep, loose social trails beneath the outcrop.

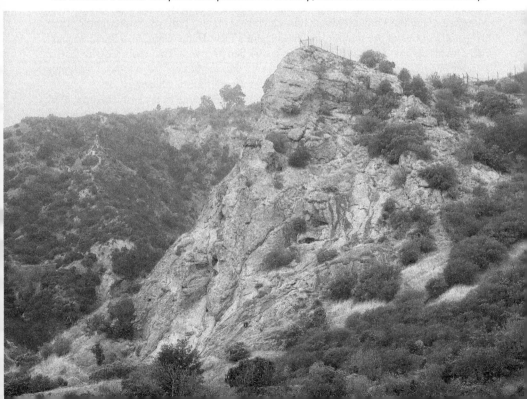

chapter 15

Hollywood Hills

The scraggly ridges and precipitous canyons separating San Fernando Valley from Hollywood and Beverly Hills harbor more than just a tangled net of serpentine streets and the homes of the rich and famous. Here and there, a few pockets of open space remain where one can roam over sage-scented trails and partake, however briefly, of some of the perks—like great vistas on a clear day—afforded to Hollywood's most privileged residents.

The patchwork of parks and open spaces covered here are included within the sinuous boundaries of the Santa Monica Mountains National Recreation Area, a mosaic of federal, state, and local parkland, and private lands stretching from Cahuenga Pass above Hollywood to Point Mugu in Ventura County. The remainder of the national recreation lands will be treated separately in the Santa Monica Mountains section of this book. Here on the east end of the Santa Monicas, even diminutive parcels of land mean a lot for an area whose last unprotected ridges and canyons have for decades been cut and filled in by massive development. Literally minutes away from L.A.'s most congested districts, the hikes described in this chapter offer remarkable opportunities to escape noise, traffic, and low-lying smog.

trip 15.1 Franklin Canyon

see map on next page

Distance	1.8 miles (loop)
Hiking Time	1 hour
Elevation Gain	400'
Difficulty	Easy
Trail Use	Dogs allowed, good for kids
Best Times	Year-round
Agencies	Mountains Recreation & Conservation Authority, National Park Service, Santa Monica Mountains Conservancy
Optional Map	Trails Illustrated *Santa Monica Mountains National Recreation Area* (253)

DIRECTIONS From the intersection of Sunset Boulevard and Beverly Drive in Beverly Hills, go north on Beverly Drive. After 0.7 mile be careful to fork left on the less-traveled north end of Beverly Drive at the intersection where the main road, Coldwater Cañon Drive, goes straight. After another 0.8 mile, bear right on narrow Franklin Canyon Drive. Go 1.2 miles farther to Lake Drive. Turn right and backtrack 0.3 mile south to a small parking area with a kiosk and gated dirt road. If you reach a larger parking area with restrooms by a field and ranch house, you've gone 0.3 mile too far.

From the north via the 101 Freeway, it's easier to take Exit 15 for Coldwater Canyon Avenue heading south. In 2.5 miles cross Mulholland Drive, and veer right onto narrow Franklin Canyon Drive. Continue 1.3 miles through the park, passing the lake and nature center; then veer left onto Lake Drive. Go 0.3 mile to the small parking area.

The Franklin Canyon Ranch park site, a part of the Santa Monica Mountains National Recreation Area, belongs to a complex of open-space units straddling the Santa Monica

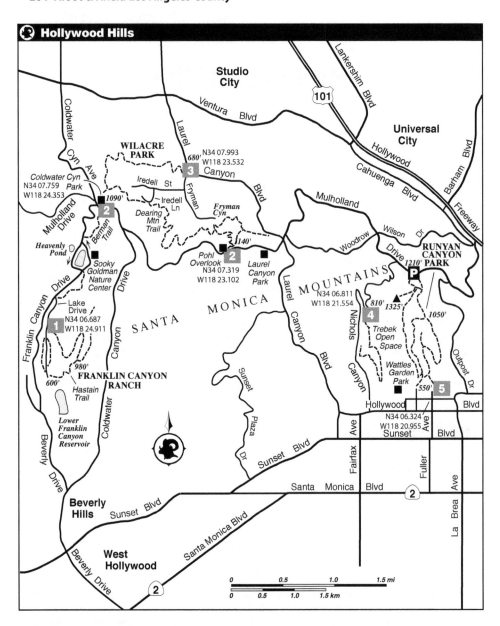

Hollywood Hills

Mountains crest. The other units include Upper Franklin Canyon Reservoir, Coldwater Canyon Park, Wilacre Park, and Fryman Canyon Natural Area. The Franklin Ranch itself was owned by the family of pioneering Angeleno Edward Doheny, who discovered oil in Los Angeles in 1892. The 400-acre ranch property was acquired as parkland in 1981.

From the kiosk at the parking area, walk up the gated fire road, which is unsigned but known as the Hastian Trail. Go 0.9 mile along chaparral-covered slopes to a hairpin turn (980 feet elevation) with a panoramic view of the city. Looking over green-mantled Beverly Hills estates and the office towers and condominiums of the Wilshire Corridor, you can sometimes see a blue horizon beyond.

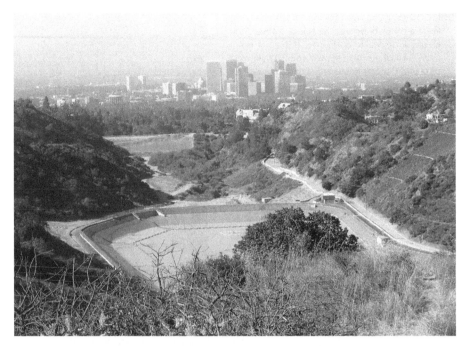

Upper Franklin Canyon Reservoir has been intermittently dry during droughts in the 2000s.

From the hairpin turn, the fire road continues climbing toward Coldwater Canyon Drive. You veer right on the narrow switchback trail, descending a steep half mile to the green lawn and Doheny ranch house below. Somehow the old Doheny spread has managed to retain its rustic, rural charm.

From the ranch house, you can walk back to your car along the pavement or on either of two poorly marked trails that parallel Lake Drive. The trail on the right passes under a shady canopy of live oaks, while the trail on the left meanders among scattered oaks and sycamores down along Franklin Canyon's usually dry streambed.

The park is laced with a ghostly web of other, nearly abandoned trails; poorly signed, many of them dead-end at private property at the park's boundary. Adventurous locals can spend some time exploring them. Families will prefer walking around placid Upper Franklin Canyon Reservoir; visiting Heavenly Pond, a tiny duck pond adjoining the reservoir to the west; and/or checking out the exhibits at the nearby Sooky Goldman Nature Center.

trip 15.2 Coldwater to Fryman Canyon

see
map
opposite

Distance	2.9 miles (one-way)
Hiking Time	1.5 hours
Elevation Gain/Loss	500'/450'
Difficulty	Moderate
Trail Use	Dogs allowed, good for kids
Best Times	Year-round
Agency	Los Angeles Department of Recreation and Parks
Optional Map	Trails Illustrated *Santa Monica Mountains National Recreation Area (253)*

DIRECTIONS If you aren't hailing a ride share back, leave a car or bicycle at the Nancy Hoover Pohl Overlook on Mulholland Drive. This point is 4.9 miles west of the 101 Freeway and 0.8 mile west of Laurel Canyon Boulevard. Continue west on Mulholland Drive for 2 miles; then turn right into Coldwater Canyon Park.

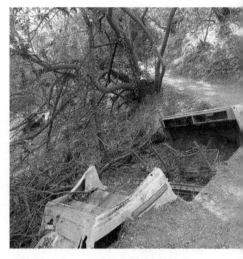

The Betty B. Dearing Mountain Trail commemorates a conservationist (1917–1977) who foresaw a trail stretching from Los Angeles along the mountain crests to the sea. Today's Santa Monica Mountains Backbone Trail is the realization of her dream.

The Dearing Mountain Trail runs roughly parallel to the automotive equivalent of the Backbone Trail: Mulholland Drive. Together with Mulholland Highway to its immediate west, Mulholland Drive winds for 50 miles through Santa Monica Mountains National Recreation Area.

Car wreck along the Betty B. Dearing Mountain Trail

If you don't want to arrange a shuttle, you can do this trip as a rugged out-and-back, or as a loop by walking or jogging back along Mulholland Drive—a good option if you can do the road-walking part very early on a Sunday morning to avoid traffic.

Walk east through the TreePeople complex in Coldwater Canyon Park, descend a staircase, and hook up with the broad Dearing Mountain Trail below. Go right (downhill) 0.5 mile to meet Iredell Lane. Walk 100 yards down the sidewalk, and then veer off on the fire road that slants up to the right. After 0.1 mile turn left onto a signed foot trail. You soon bend right and begin climbing straight up a slope over wooden water bars. The next stretch through Fryman Canyon Park, known as the Rainforest, is particularly lush. Pass a signed spur on the left leading to a formidable gate on Valleycrest Road, watch for a brightly painted car wreck and, in 2 miles, switchback sharply up to a junction. The trail continues to the left (east) for 0.7 mile to a dead end—turn right to immediately reach Pohl Overlook.

trip 15.3	**Wilacre & Coldwater Loop**

Distance	2.7 miles (loop)
Hiking Time	1.5 hours
Elevation Gain	500'
Difficulty	Moderate
Trail Use	Dogs allowed, good for kids
Best Times	Year-round
Agencies	Mountains Recreation & Conservation Authority, Santa Monica Mountains Conservancy
Optional Map	Trails Illustrated *Santa Monica Mountains National Recreation Area (253)*

see map on p. 204

DIRECTIONS From the 101 Freeway in Studio Canyon, take Exit 14 for southbound Laurel Canyon Boulevard. Drive south 1.4 miles; then turn right onto Fryman Road and immediately right again into the Wilacre Park lot. Note that this extremely popular trailhead fills up early. Nonresidential parking is prohibited on Fryman Road and adjacent streets, so you'll have to backtrack if you're looking for street parking.

A heavily used 129-acre island of open space in the midst of Studio City's more lavish residential areas, Wilacre Park—the former estate of silent movie star Will Acres—offers a wide-ranging view of San Fernando Valley. This loop route goes up through Wilacre Park and visits Coldwater Canyon Park, which is the headquarters of TreePeople, a grassroots organization that is spearheading efforts to plant millions of trees in the urban Los Angeles area.

From the trailhead parking lot, walk west up the gated Betty B. Dearing Mountain Trail, named in memory of an advocate of Santa Monica Mountains trails. At first you're on a curving, hardtopped driveway flanked by pine and cypress trees. The road becomes dirt at 0.5 mile. You ascend, more easily now, along north-facing slopes dotted with live oak and native walnut trees. At 1.2 miles reach a high point, where you see the signed Loop Trail on the left. Turn south to stay on the Dearing Mountain Trail, descend slightly, and arrive at a wide junction (1.4 miles) on the edge of Coldwater Canyon Park. Take the Magic Forest Trail on the right, or use some steps a little way to the left to reach the old fire station above that serves as headquarters for TreePeople. Pick up a brochure at the parking lot and make your own self-guided tour of TreePeople's exhibits and nursery.

Return to the wide junction and continue east (downhill) on the Dearing Mountain Trail. At 2.0 miles you hit pavement at Iredell Lane, a cozy residential cul-de-sac. The home stretch is along lightly traveled streets—down Iredell Lane to Iredell Street, down Iredell Street to Fryman Road, and finally down Fryman Road to your starting point.

VARIATION

To avoid the road walk and escape the crowds, return to the Loop Trail (aka U-Vanu Trail) and follow this narrow singletrack path up to the crest of the ridge and then down the ridge's spine. Stay on the main ridge path as you pass various spurs, and eventually rejoin the paved road just above the trailhead. This hike is about the same length.

Young hikers enjoy exploring the Dearing Mountain Trail.

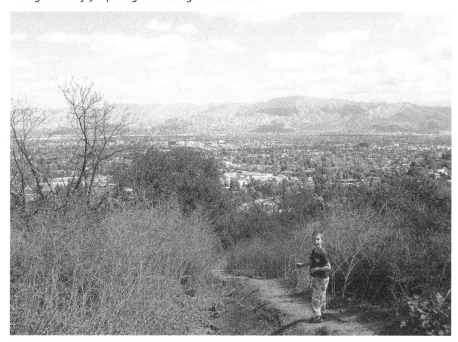

trip 15.4   Trebek Open Space

see map on p. 204

Distance	2.5 miles (out-and-back)
Hiking Time	1.5 hour
Elevation Gain	400'
Difficulty	Moderate
Trail Use	Dogs allowed, good for kids
Best Times	October–April
Agencies	Mountains Recreation & Conservation Authority, Santa Monica Mountains Conservancy
Optional Map	Trails Illustrated *Santa Monica Mountains National Recreation Area (253)*

DIRECTIONS From the 101 Freeway in Hollywood, take Exit 8B for westbound Hollywood Boulevard. In 2.4 miles turn north on Nichols Canyon Road. Go 1.4 miles to a dirt pullout on the right, by a hairpin turn.

Trebek Open Space, just over the ridge from Runyon Canyon, is a good place to find the same million-dollar views but avoid the crowds. The 62-acre park was donated to the Santa Monica Mountains Conservancy in 1998 by Alex Trebek, host of the game show *Jeopardy!* The trails are open sunrise–sunset. This trip describes the aptly nicknamed "Daily Double," an out-and-back hike on the Bantam and Castair Trails.

Pass through the gate and begin by climbing the Bantam Trail, an old fire road. In 0.5 mile reach a junction with another dirt road leading back to Astral Drive. In another 100 yards, reach the end of the road by a coast live oak and enjoy panoramic views over Hollywood to downtown L.A.

A steep trail with more good views continues down the knife-edge ridge for 0.3 mile, reaching the Castair Trail fire road near the end of gated Wattles Drive. Turn right and follow the fire road another 0.5 mile to a locked gate on Castair Drive. Return the way you came.

VARIATION

You could follow the other dirt road from Bantam Trail to Astral Drive, then up Astral and Solar Drives to reach the West Ridge Trail in Runyon Canyon Park in 0.6 mile.

trip 15.5   Runyon Canyon

see map on p. 204

Distance	2.0 miles (loop)
Hiking Time	1 hour
Elevation Gain	500'
Difficulty	Moderate
Trail Use	Dogs allowed, good for kids
Best Times	Year-round
Agency	Los Angeles Department of Recreation and Parks
Optional Map	Trails Illustrated *Santa Monica Mountains National Recreation Area (253)*

DIRECTIONS From the 101 Freeway in Hollywood, take Exit 8B for westbound Hollywood Boulevard. In 1.9 miles turn north on Fuller Avenue. Go 0.3 mile to the north end of Fuller, where you will find the Fuller entrance to Runyon Canyon Park. Parking is a serious problem and you can expect to have to search for parking some distance from the trailhead. You might be better off taking public transit, such as the Metro train to the Hollywood/Highland Station, 0.8 mile east of the trailhead.

Runyon Canyon Park, a narrow strip of open space in the hills just a couple of miles from the heart of Hollywood, counts among its former residents actors John McCormick and Errol Flynn. The canyon is named for Carman Runyon, a businessman who acquired the land in 1919. The now-quiet canyon site was long threatened by proposals to transform it into either a massive resort or a luxury housing development. In 1983, the property was purchased as parkland by the City of Los Angeles. Its popularity has grown among those seeking a little peace from the pressure-cooker pace of life in the metropolis below. Runyon Canyon is open from sunrise to sunset. The park is extremely popular for dog walking, and you can expect crowds.

In the 1930s, McCormick built a mansion here and began to landscape the area around it. Despite the later razing of the mansion and the effects of fire, flood, and general neglect, plenty of palms, pines, eucalyptus, and other exotic vegetation still grow on the site. Native chaparral vegetation thrives as well—dry and unappealing during summer's drought, but verdant and aromatic in the springtime.

The park has three connecting trails, which are unsigned and have acquired a variety of informal names: Runyon Canyon Road, which is graded dirt and easiest; the East Ridge (aka Steps, Star, or Inspiration Point) Trail; and the strenuous West Ridge (aka Spine, Hero, or Western Highway) Trail. This trip introduces you to the park with a loop up Runyon Canyon Road and down the East Ridge.

From the Fuller entrance at the north end of Fuller Avenue, walk north for 0.1 mile to an unsigned junction. Turn left onto Runyon Canyon Road, which later changes from dirt to pavement. Pass the Vista entrance gate at a sharp right turn, and in another 0.1 mile pass the West Ridge Trail on the left (see variation below). Continue up Runyon Canyon Road to the head of the canyon, where you reach a junction on the east ridge.

Runyon Canyon Road veers left and climbs toward Mulholland Drive, but you make a right on the East Ridge Trail and pass over a viewpoint called Cloud's Rest, where the view of the L.A. Basin is spectacular and panoramic. Continue descending about 300 feet of

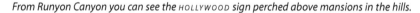

From Runyon Canyon you can see the HOLLYWOOD *sign perched above mansions in the hills.*

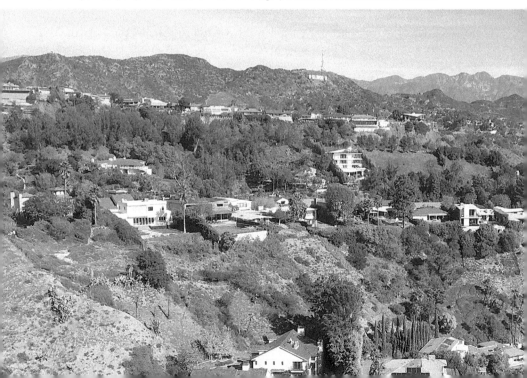

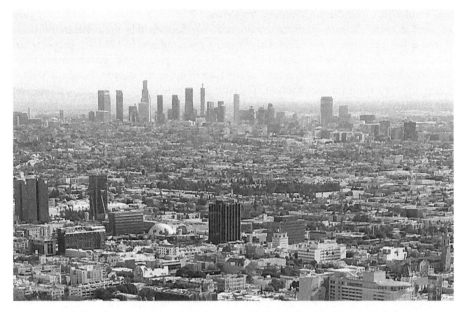

Looking south from Runyon Canyon, you can see past Hollywood to the downtown skyline.

elevation to a second, lower viewpoint called Inspiration Point. On a clear day, your view east will encompass the HOLLYWOOD sign in Griffith Park; the four county high points, San Antonio, San Gorgonio, San Jacinto, and Santiago; and downtown Los Angeles. Work your way down a series of steps built from railroad ties until the grade eases. Pass the remains of a tennis court, and continue down to the Fuller entrance.

VARIATIONS

For a longer, more rugged loop of 3.7 miles with 800 feet of elevation gain, take the West Ridge Trail and continue all the way up to Mulholland Drive. A shorter but still-strenuous loop up the West Ridge Trail to Mulholland Drive and then down the East Ridge Trail is 3.3 miles with 700 feet of elevation gain.

VARIATION

You can also enter Runyon Canyon Park from its uppermost end. On Mulholland Drive you'll find a crowded parking area 1.6 miles west of the 101 Freeway at Cahuenga Pass. From here you can descend toward the Cloud's Rest viewpoint or take a short spur from the West Ridge Trail that leads to the park's 1,325-foot high point, atop a small summit.

chapter 16

Urban Parks

The greater Los Angeles urban area is dotted with a variety of hills, many of which are covered with parks and trails. This chapter covers some of these trails. The San Rafael Hills between Pasadena and Glendale are part of the Transverse Ranges, like their larger neighbors, the Verdugo Hills and the San Gabriel Mountains. Debs Park and Elysian Park flank the Arroyo Seco just north of downtown Los Angeles. These historic but underappreciated parks have a wild feel within the bustling city. The Baldwin Hills, southwest of downtown, offer great views and a place to stretch your legs in the city.

trip 16.1 San Rafael Hills

Distance	5 miles (semiloop)
Hiking Time	2.5 hours
Elevation Gain	900'
Difficulty	Moderate
Trail Use	Suitable for mountain biking, equestrians, dogs allowed
Best Times	November–April
Agency	Glendale Community Services & Parks
Maps	None

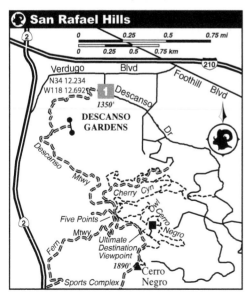

DIRECTIONS From the northbound 2 Freeway, take the connector toward the eastbound 210; then exit onto Verdugo Boulevard. In 0.3 mile turn right onto Descanso Drive. In 0.1 mile, where the road bends left, park on the shoulder near the signed trailhead for the Descanso Trail.

The San Rafael Hills are a low range paralleling the more prominent Verdugo Hills. A popular network of fire roads and trails draws local hikers to enjoy great views while getting a good workout. This trip describes a moderate hike from Descanso Gardens along the crest to two viewpoints. Regular visitors will discover many possible variations. If you have time, consider stopping for a stroll at lovely Descanso Gardens afterward. The hills are named for Rancho San Rafael, a 1784 Spanish land grant to the west.

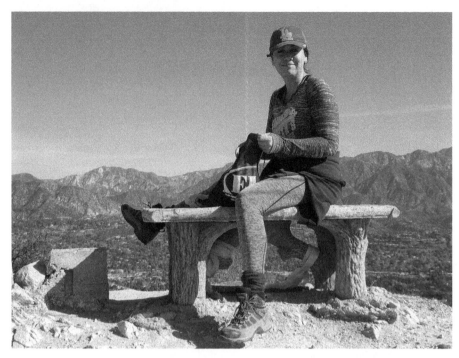

A bench on Cerro Negro provides a place to rest and take in the views.

Find the signed Descanso Trail leading between the fenced gardens and some private homes. The trail soon switchbacks steeply through an oak grove to gain the ridge of the San Rafael Hills, then turns south. In 0.7 mile pass a spur road on the left down to a gate for Descanso Gardens. At 1.6 miles pass Edison Road on the left, following power lines down to Forest Hills Drive. Just beyond, at 1.7 miles, come to a major junction called Five Points. You've come from the north on Descanso Motorway and will continue south on Ridge Motorway. The Cherry Canyon Motorway forks to the northeast, descending to a small trailhead on Hamstead Road. Two paved branches of Pasa Glen Drive lead west to a police shooting range and south to the Glendale Sports Complex. You will return to this point via the southernmost of two unsigned trails between Cherry Canyon and Ridge Motorways.

Continue south on Ridge Motorway. At 1.9 miles pass a signed trail on the left to the modestly named Ultimate Destination Vista Point. At 2.1 miles reach another viewpoint on a clearing just north of the Cerro Negro ("black hill") antenna cluster.

After enjoying the view, pick up the signed Ultimate Destination/Cerro Negro Trail, departing the clearing to the northeast. Pass a spur on the right leading to Sugarloaf Drive; then turn right at a second junction, and promptly reach the Ultimate Destination Vista Point, with a picnic table, water fountain, and namesake views. These hills were slated for development in the 1980s and the clearing here was bulldozed for a house pad. Decades of efforts by activists led to the city of La Cañada Flintridge acquiring the land and protecting it for public enjoyment.

Find an attractive trail continuing down near the picnic table. Take it to a junction with the Cerro Negro Trail, where you turn left. Pass the Owl Trail on the right, and eventually arrive back at Five Points at 3.3 miles. Return the way you came, or descend one of the side trails and follow city streets back to the Descanso Trailhead.

trip 16.2	**Debs Park**

Distance	5 miles (loop)
Hiking Time	2.5 hours
Elevation Gain	1,000'
Difficulty	Moderate
Trail Use	Dogs
Best Times	Any
Agency	Los Angeles Department of Recreation and Parks
Maps	None

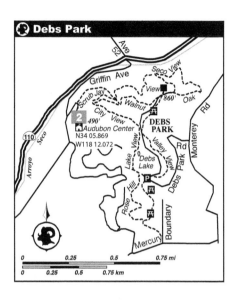

DIRECTIONS From the 110 Freeway north of downtown, take Exit 28A for eastbound Avenue 52, following signs for the Audubon Center; the street name changes from Avenue 52 to Griffin Avenue. In 0.6 mile turn left onto a gated road leading up to the Audubon Center parking area. If the gate is closed or the lot is full, park outside on Griffin and walk in.

rnest E. Debs Park is a little-known 300-acre wilderness area overlooking the Arroyo Seco close to downtown Los Angeles. The city acquired portions of the park as early as 1949, but the facilities remained undeveloped until 1968, and most of the parkland still has a semiwild feel.

Originally named Rose Hill Park, it was renamed in 1994 in honor of Debs, who served as an L.A. city councilman and a county supervisor from 1947 to 1974. Debs was also noted as a fierce foe of the 1960s counterculture movement. (In 1966, the city imposed a 10 p.m. curfew in Hollywood to discourage the emerging rock 'n' roll clubs, provoking the Sunset Strip Curfew Riot.)

The park lacks any trail signs, so either take care to follow these directions carefully, or just roam as you see fit and eventually you'll make your way back to the starting point.

Families may wish to start by exploring the Audubon Center. When you are ready to begin hiking, walk north to a gated dirt road at the hairpin turn in the Audubon Center road. Follow this road (the Scrub Jay Trail), or an adjacent singletrack, through an unusual plant community of black walnut, coast live oak, elderberry, toyon, lemonade berry, and coastal sage scrub. Birds and squirrels are plentiful in this wooded sanctuary. In 0.4 mile reach a four-way junction by a green staircase. You could shortcut up the stairs, but our route turns hard left and climbs to a viewpoint with benches. Turn left again onto the Walnut Forest fire road, which dips before climbing up to meet the paved Summit Ridge Road on the crest, at 1.0 mile. Turn left here and make a short excursion to the north end of the road, where you'll find shaded benches and views up the Arroyo Seco.

Return to the Summit Ridge Road a second time and continue east on the dirt road. You'll

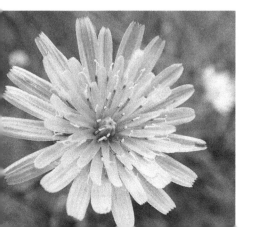

Cliff aster

soon pass the easily overlooked Oak Grove Trail on your right. Descend to a T-junction and turn right on the Seco View Trail. Soon, turn right onto the easily overlooked Oak Grove Trail, an intimate singletrack that threads past poison oak and live oaks. Pass a spur on the left down to a neighborhood, but stay on the Oak Grove Trail as it climbs back up to the aforementioned junction before you return to Summit Ridge Road for the third time (2.0 miles).

Turn south on the paved Summit Road. You'll soon come to a large gazebo. Just beyond, veer left onto the faint Valley View Trail, which parallels the road. At 2.7 miles reach a parking lot at the top of Debs Park Road beside a sprawling picnic area. Walk south through the picnic area until you find an asphalt path continuing south through a gap to a second, smaller picnic area (3.1 miles). At the south end of this second picnic area, you'll see a white gate on an abandoned road. This road leads to the Native American Terrace Garden beside a trailhead at the corner of Boundary and Mercury, but the garden has received little attention and is not particularly worth a detour.

Instead, take an unlikely looking dirt path, the Rose Hills Loop Trail, just to the right of the gated road. The path leads up a hill. Stay right at a T-junction and follow the singletrack under a row of houses and past a bird-watching bench. When you reach a concrete walkway coming up from the main picnic area parking, jog right on it, then immediately turn left up the stairs to reach a field. Continue up a steep hill beyond, which eventually tops out at a pond, where you might catch your breath on a bench and admire the tranquil setting. Our trail continues beyond the pond, stays left, and then soon joins the paved Summit Road. Follow the road north until you can veer left onto the aptly named City View Trail. This trail eventually reaches the three-way junction with the Scrub Jay and Walnut Forest Trails near your starting point. Stay left and retrace Scrub Jay back to your starting point.

Reflections in tranquil Debs Lake

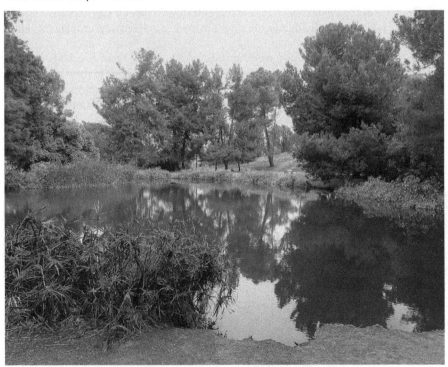

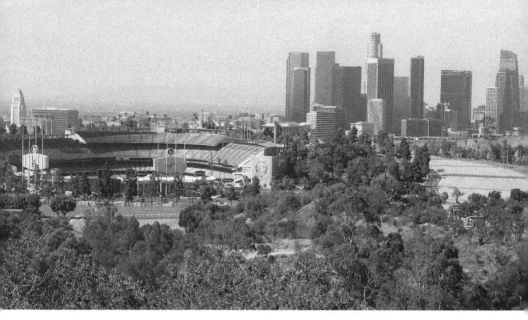

From Elysian Park you get great views of downtown Los Angeles beyond Dodger Stadium.

trip 16.3   Elysian Park

Distance	2.5 miles (loop)
Hiking Time	1.5 hours
Elevation Gain	300'
Difficulty	Easy
Trail Use	Dogs allowed, good for kids
Best Times	October–June
Agency	Los Angeles Department of Recreation and Parks
Maps	None

DIRECTIONS If you're coming from the south, take the 101 Freeway to Exit 4A for Echo Park Avenue. Proceed 0.8 mile; then turn right on Morton Avenue. In 0.2 mile turn right on Academy Road. In 0.3 mile turn left on Stadium Way; then, in 0.5 mile, turn left on Elysian Park Drive, and proceed 0.2 mile to a parking area opposite the Grace Simons Lodge. If you're coming from the north, take the 5 Freeway to Exit 138 for Stadium Way. Go south 0.7 mile; then turn right onto Elysian Park Drive and continue 0.2 mile to the aforementioned parking.

Elysian Park is L.A.'s first and oldest city park. Although it suffers from graffiti, a lack of signage, and insufficient maintenance and is unsafe after dark, the park nevertheless attracts many hikers and dog walkers who enjoy the tree-lined paths and incredible city views. The lot opposite Grace Simons Lodge is a convenient starting point for this hike. Grace Simons (1901–1985), the lodge's namesake, was a newspaper reporter and activist noted for founding the Citizens Committee to Save Elysian Park. The lodge is now a popular venue for weddings and other special events.

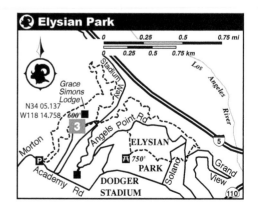

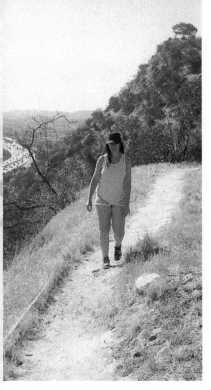

The best-defined trail in the park is a loop on the northwest side of Stadium Way. From the parking area just south of Grace Simons Lodge, walk west through a white gate on a paved but worn road. Follow the road south through a eucalyptus grove for 0.5 mile to reach another trailhead on Academy Road. Make a hard right turn, pass through another gate, and join a dirt path leading back north above the road you just followed. Enjoy views of the downtown L.A. skyline to the south and the San Gabriel Mountains and Verdugo Hills to the north over the 5 Freeway. You'll pass several spurs shortcutting back down, but follow the trail all the way to the north end of the park until it loops back and emerges at a gate near the corner of Stadium Way and Elysian Park Drive. Turn right and follow Elysian Park Drive a short way back to your vehicle.

VARIATION

If you have a good sense of direction, you can make a 3-mile loop on the southeast side of Stadium Way that offers unsurpassed views of the Los Angeles Skyline over Dodger Stadium. From the corner of Stadium Way and Elysian Park Drive, find a narrow gated dirt path leading northeast above Stadium Way. The path turns southeast on a steep hillside overlooking the 5 Freeway. In 1.1 miles, just before you reach paved Grand View Drive, turn hard left and follow the Chavez Ridge Disc

Angelenos love the expansive city views from the loop trail on the southeast side of Stadium Way in Elysian Park.

Golf trail up to a knoll and back down to a complex junction of Grand View Drive and two branches of Park Row Drive—it's almost impossible to give clear directions from here because of the tangle of unsigned roads and trails, but look west and identify the prominent hilltop across a valley. Pick a path on roads or steep trails to gain the hilltop, where benches offer a wonderful view over Dodger Stadium. Follow a trail west along the ridge to a picnic area with a second great vista point; then turn north on paved Park Road. When it ends at Angels Point Road by a huge water tank, turn left. Pass above the Los Angeles Police Academy; then briefly detour left to Angels Point, where a fascinating but tragically defaced sculpture by Peter Shire stands at another viewpoint. Return to the road, now called Elysian Park Drive, and continue back to your starting point at Stadium Way.

---

trip 16.4   **Hahn Park**

Distance	2.6 miles (loop)
Hiking Time	1.5 hours
Elevation Gain	350'
Difficulty	Easy
Trail Use	Suitable for mountain biking, dogs allowed, good for kids
Best Times	Year-round
Agency	California State Parks
Maps	None
Fees/Permits	$6 entrance fee weekends and holidays

see map opposite

DIRECTIONS From the 10 Freeway, take Exit 7B south for Washington Boulevard, and then veer left onto Fairfax Avenue. In 0.3 mile turn left onto La Cienega Boulevard. In 1.1 miles take the exit for Kenneth Hahn State Recreation Area. Continue 1 mile through the park to the Eastern Ridgeline Gateway hilltop lot at the end of paved road. Alternatively, on weekends and holidays, take the Link shuttle from the La Cienega Expo Line Station to Hahn Park for 25¢ each way.

The 401-acre Kenneth Hahn State Recreation Area opened in 1983 on the site of the former Baldwin Hills Reservoir and old oil fields. Part of the California State Park system, the family-friendly park has a small lake, a Japanese garden with a koi pond, extensive playgrounds and picnic areas, and a network of trails with great city views. The park is named for Kenneth Hahn, who served on the Los Angeles County Board of Supervisors for 40 years from 1952 to 1992. Go on a clear winter or spring day to enjoy views of downtown backed by the snow-clad San Gabriel Mountains.

The park is laced with trails, many of which braid and rejoin and are poorly signed, so following a precise route could be frustrating for a first-time visitor. Instead, take your pick of paths to make a loop along the eastern perimeter of the park and back near the picnic grounds. The primary trail network is part of the Park to Playa Trail, a 13-mile trail system under construction from the Baldwin Hills to the mouth of Ballona Creek in Playa del Rey. The portion in Hahn Park is known as the Community Loop Trail.

From the hilltop parking area, walk northwest to Janice's Green Valley and take the Bowl Loop Trail to the right (counterclockwise). This valley is named for Janice Hahn, a former congresswoman, current member of the L.A. County Board of Supervisors, and daughter

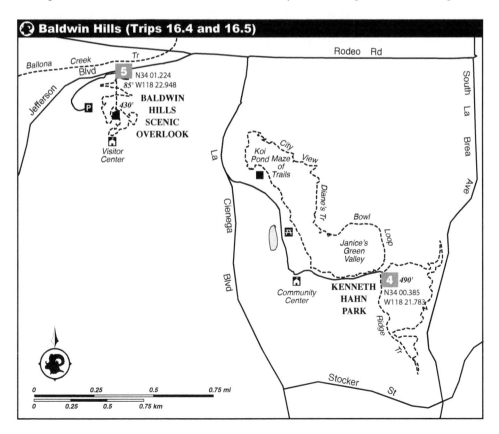

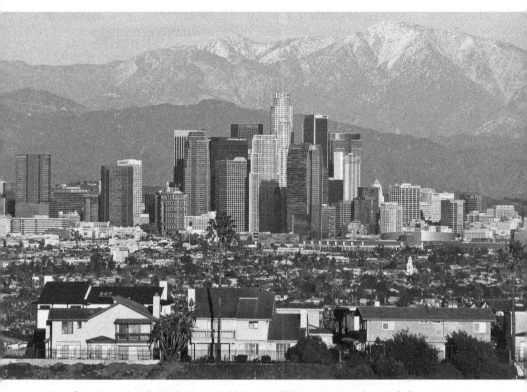

Seen from Kenneth Hahn Park, Mount Baldy's snowy slopes tower over the L.A. skyline.
Photo: BDS2006/CC BY-SA 3.0 US (https://creativecommons.org/licenses/by-sa/3.0/us)

of Kenneth Hahn. The bowl-like depression was formerly the Baldwin Hills Reservoir. Built in 1947 on a spur of the Newport–Inglewood Fault, the dam collapsed in 1963 and released a quarter billion gallons of water, killing five people, washing away 277 homes, and becoming a classic case study in civil engineering. KTLA covered the event live from the air by helicopter, perhaps the first live aerial news coverage of a disaster.

At a signed but confusing junction halfway around the now-tranquil valley, join Park to Playa/Diane's Trail to continue northwest along the ridge. Look west across the park toward the Inglewood Oil Field on the next ridge. Active since 1924, it has produced approximately 400 million barrels of oil and is the largest urban oil field in the United States. Subsidence of the earth due to oil extraction was a factor in the dam collapse.

The path widens into a hilltop dirt service road, and you soon veer right onto the signed City View Trail, which runs east of the dirt road and offers great views of downtown Los Angeles. Perhaps the best view is where City View rejoins the road by the Autumn's Peak picnic shelter. Continue on City View and the Forest Trail to the northwest end; then loop back by way of Randi's Waterfall and the koi pond at Doris's Japanese Gardens. Rejoin the Park to Playa Trail as it leads past playgrounds and picnic areas to the Community Center, then narrows to a concrete sidewalk along the road, climbing back to Eastern Ridgeline Gateway.

VARIATION

If you're looking to add another mile to your walk, head south from the upper parking lot along the Park to Playa/Eastern Ridgeline Trail; then, at any of the several unsigned junctions, loop back on Ron's Trail and then up the Boy Scout Trail.

trip 16.5   Baldwin Hills Scenic Overlook

Distance	1.2 miles (loop)
Hiking Time	1 hour
Elevation Gain	350'
Difficulty	Easy
Trail Use	Suitable for children
Best Times	Year-round
Agency	California State Parks
Maps	None
Fees/Permits	$6 parking fee

see map on p. 217

DIRECTIONS The main park entrance is at 6300 Hetzler Road in Culver City. From the 10 Freeway, take Exit 7B for southbound Washington Boulevard, and then veer left onto Fairfax Avenue. In 0.3 mile turn left onto La Cienega Boulevard. In 0.2 mile turn right on Jefferson Boulevard, and follow it 0.9 mile to the park entrance at the intersection with Hetzler Road. Park along Jefferson; some free spots are available, and you can also find metered parking and a pay lot.

Open space in urban Los Angeles is at such a premium that a 50-acre hillside parcel reclaimed from oil drilling was designated a California State Park and opened to the public in 2009. The short but vigorous hike brings you to the hilltop viewpoint with excellent views over the city, and it has become a popular site for locals to exercise. California Parks has built an elaborate visitor center on the top; this center is presently open on weekends and on Monday, Thursday, and Friday mornings. The Baldwin Hills are named for Elias "Lucky" Baldwin, who made his initial fortune off a silver mine in the Comstock Lode in Nevada and then became a wildly successful land speculator in Southern California. His holdings on Rancho Santa Anita and La Cienega Rancho became the towns of Arcadia, Monrovia, Sierra Madre, and Baldwin Hills, as well as sites for the Santa Anita Park Racetrack and the Montebello Oil Fields.

From the park entrance at the corner of Hetzler Road and Jefferson Boulevard, a concrete sidewalk leads up the hill alongside Hetzler. This trip, however, takes the Hillside Trail, a dirt path to the left. After two switchbacks, reach a steep staircase heading straight up the hill. For the sake of variety, head up the 282 steps, enjoy the view, and then descend on the switchbacking Hillside Trail.

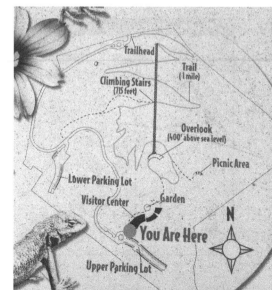

Baldwin Hills Overlook visitor map

chapter 17

Puente Hills

The rambling Puente Hills, overlooking the San Gabriel Valley to the north and Orange County to the south, interrupt what would otherwise be a continuous spread of flat, nondescript suburbs. Rising no higher than 1,500 feet in elevation, they host a collection of hillside homes; the sprawling, mostly undeveloped Rose Hills Memorial Park; the huge Puente Hills Landfill; and several large open-space areas for habitat preservation and public recreation. L.A. County's Skyline Trail skips over the west end of the Puente Hills from one rounded summit to the next, joining a number of spur trails that connect to suburbs below.

Whenever the L.A. Basin is swept clear of smog and moisture by offshore winds, the upper elevations of the Puente Hills offer truly mind-blowing views of almost everything from the mountains to the sea. Don't miss the spectacular sunrises over the San Bernardino and San Jacinto Mountains, and sunsets over the Pacific Ocean.

The Puente Hills Preserve is managed by the Puente Hills Habitat Preservation Authority with representatives from Whittier, Hacienda Heights, and the L.A. County Sanitation District. It is primarily funded by the Puente Hills Landfill as mitigation for the landfill.

Puente Hills Preserve has been drawing increasing throngs of visitors. Lacking adequate trailhead parking, many users must park on city streets, inconveniencing nearby residents. Thoughtless users have left trash and dog poop on the trails and cycled in ways that scare hikers; remember your trail manners. The preserve managers and cities have responded with regulations that discourage visitors from out of the neighborhood.

The Sycamore Canyon, Hacienda Hills, Turnbull Canyon, and Hellman Park Trailheads are open 9 a.m.–5 p.m. October–May (until 6 p.m. June–September). Parking in neighborhoods is heavily restricted. All trails close for 48 hours following rain.

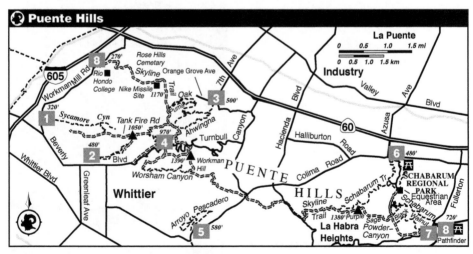

trip 17.1   ## Sycamore Canyon

Distance	2.6 miles (out-and-back)
Hiking Time	1 hour
Elevation Gain	200'
Difficulty	Easy
Trail Use	Good for kids
Best Times	Year-round
Agency	Puente Hills Habitat Preservation Authority
Optional Map	Free *Sycamore Canyon Trailhead and Hellman Park* map (available at habitatauthority.org/trails)

see map on previous page

DIRECTIONS From the 605 Freeway in Whittier, take Exit 16 for eastbound Beverly Boulevard. Go east on Beverly for 0.6 mile and turn left (north) on Workman Mill Road. Go 0.4 mile north to the entrance to Sycamore Canyon on the right. Park at the designated lot. The trailhead is open 9 a.m.–5 p.m. October–May (until 6 p.m. June–September).

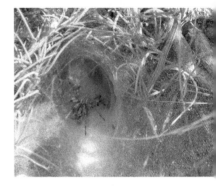

A narrow crease that's incised into the westernmost Puente Hills, Sycamore Canyon harbors some fine riparian habitat overlooked by rather dramatic, eroded cliffs. There are several large and twisted specimens of California sycamore trees to admire, as well as willows, cottonwoods, and toyons—the latter bearing clusters of bright-red berries in late fall and winter. The canyon is filled with the song of birds drawn to the food sources

Funnel-web spiders lurk in the grasslands of Sycamore Canyon.

along the creek. Particularly in the warmer months, watch for funnel-web spiders, which weave their distinctive webs in the grass. Look closely and you may see a spider lying in wait at the mouth of its funnel, awaiting prey.

From the signed trailhead, walk up a short shaded trail to a Y-junction of service roads. Stay left at the Y. You pass a groaning oil well and bend left to join a wider path, which is an old roadbed that currently functions as the Sycamore Canyon Trail. Pass through a

Early-morning sun over the Puente Hills   Photo: Jerry Schad

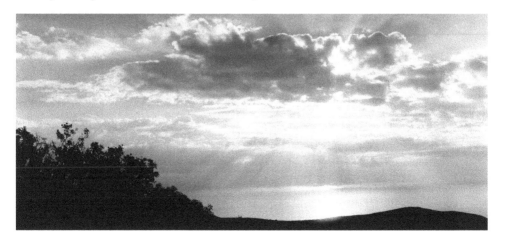

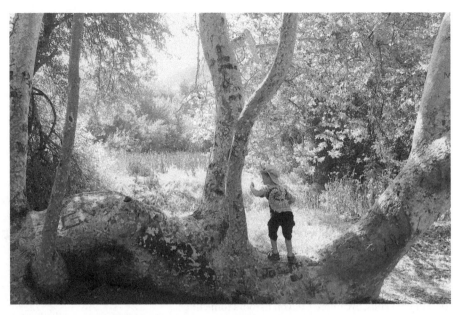

A huge sycamore at the mouth of Dark Canyon attracts a curious visitor.

gate. Note the contrast between the sheer and barren south-facing canyon wall on the left, which bears the full force of sunlight, and the more gently sloping, north-facing, grassy slopes on the right.

After 1.3 miles of travel, the main trail turns sharply right and wastes no time in ascending those grassy slopes. Straight ahead (east) lies a narrow trail that continues up Sycamore Canyon toward a tributary ravine called Dark Canyon, ending in 0.4 mile at the park boundary. This juncture is a good place to turn around and return if your hike is going to be a casual one. If you decide to hike farther into Sycamore Canyon, then watch out for poison oak.

trip 17.2 Hellman Park

see map on p. 220

Distance	2.5 miles (loop)
Hiking Time	1 hour
Elevation Gain	700'
Difficulty	Moderate
Trail Use	Dogs allowed, good for kids
Best Times	Year-round
Agency	Puente Hills Habitat Preservation Authority
Optional Map	Free *Sycamore Canyon Trailhead and Hellman Park* map (available at habitatauthority.org/trails)

DIRECTIONS From the 605 Freeway in Whittier, take Exit 16 for eastbound Beverly Boulevard. Go east on Beverly for 2 miles and turn left (north) on Greenleaf Avenue. Go 0.2 mile north to the Hellman Park Trailhead, on the right. The park is very popular and you are unlikely to find space in the small lot. The surrounding neighborhood has strictly enforced residential parking permits, so you will likely need to drive several blocks south or east to find legal street parking. This popular park is open 9 a.m.–5 p.m. October–May (until 6 p.m. June–September).

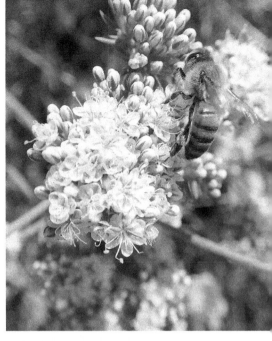

Hellman Park is a patch of open space perched on steep hillsides overlooking the city of Whittier. Whenever crystal-clear skies prevail, a vast sweep of L.A. Basin landscape stretching from skyscrapers of downtown L.A. to Palos Verdes comes into vivid view, along with nearly all of Orange County. At times a distinct Pacific Ocean horizon can be seen, interrupted by the rambling profile of Santa Catalina Island.

It doesn't take much of a lengthy hike to achieve such vistas, but the route is so steep in places that it has been nicknamed "Cardiac Hill." From the Hellman Park Trailhead on Greenleaf Avenue, you start up the fire road (known as the Peppergrass Trail), which leads straight up the ridge to the east.

*California buckwheat (*Eriogonum fascicalatum*), a common sage-scrub species, is popular with bees.*

After 0.4 mile the trail dips slightly, and you have two alternatives: a gradual ascent on the curvy Mariposa Trail to the left, or a continuing steep climb along the spine of the ridge. Pick the left fork—you'll return on the steep path to the right—and thread alongside slopes overlooking a yawning chasm to the north.

At 1.0 mile you rejoin the Peppergrass Trail. Turn left and continue up to the skyline at the junction of the Rattlesnake Ridge fire road and Peppergrass Trail. Turn right and descend Peppergrass.

trip 17.3 West Skyline Loop

see map on p. 220

Distance	4.7 miles (loop)
Hiking Time	2.5 hours
Elevation Gain	1,100'
Difficulty	Moderate
Trail Use	Suitable for mountain biking, equestrians, dogs allowed
Best Times	October–May
Agency	Puente Hills Habitat Preservation Authority
Optional Map	Free *Hacienda Hills Trailhead* map (available at habitatauthority.org/trails)

DIRECTIONS From the 60 Freeway in Hacienda Heights, take Exit 14 for Seventh Avenue. Drive 0.7 mile south to the intersection of Orange Grove Avenue. The small Hacienda Hills Trailhead parking lot is just beyond the intersection, and you can find overflow parking on Seventh Avenue. The trailhead is open 9 a.m.–5 p.m. October–May (until 6 p.m. June–September).

On this looping hike, you'll explore hardy little pockets of oak woodland, and also get a close look at the marine-sedimentary bedrock of the Puente Hills, which dates back 15–30 million years. Mostly this consists of silty, layered deposits, but you'll also find some conglomerate rock in the ravines.

From the informational kiosk at the intersection of Seventh Avenue and Orange Grove Avenue, start hiking south on the unpaved roadway, now called the Ahwingna Trail in honor of a nearby Tongva village site.

In 0.25 mile pass the signed Coyote Trail on the left. This trail—open only to hikers and a recommended alternative if you're on foot—meets the Skyline Trail close to the top of the Ahwingna Trail. If you stay on the Ahwingna Trail, soon veer right up an asphalt strip that leads to an abandoned hillside reservoir. From there, you ascend on switchbacks going up the ridge. At 0.8 mile you reach a junction at a small flat. Keep going straight up the ridge (you'll later return to this spot by way of the Native Oak Trail coming up from the right). At 1.3 miles you arrive at the Skyline Trail, which at this point follows the wide Puente Hills crest.

Turn right and follow the Skyline Trail's right-of-way, fenced on both sides, roughly paralleling some power lines. Long views west (clear air permitting) toward downtown L.A.'s skyline and the Pacific make up for the rather harsh and barren-looking foreground.

At 1.8 miles turn right on the Native Oak Trail. It goes briefly up a little hill and then steadily down along oak-dotted slopes overlooking a deep ravine. Pass a signed junction for the Puma Trail (hikers only), which parallels Native Oak but misses some of the best woodland. After several switchbacks you arrive at the mouth of that ravine (2.7 miles) and traverse to the right around a hillside just above the edge of a subdivision. The trail steers you into another shade-dappled ravine, similar to the first. You ascend moderately along the bottom, veer left (south) up a tributary, and climb switchbacks to the hitching post on the ridge above (3.8 miles). From there retrace your earlier steps past the hillside reservoir to your starting point at Seventh Avenue.

trip 17.4	**Worsham Canyon Loop**

Distance	4.2 miles (loop)
Hiking Time	2 hours
Elevation Gain	1,000'
Difficulty	Moderate
Trail Use	Suitable for mountain biking, equestrians, dogs allowed
Best Times	October–May
Agency	Puente Hills Habitat Preservation Authority
Optional Map	Free *Turnbull Canyon* map (available at habitatauthority.org/trails)

see map on p. 220

Worsham Canyon looks south into Whittier.

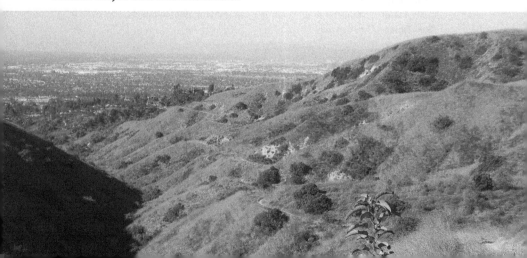

DIRECTIONS From the 605 Freeway in Whittier, take Exit 16 for eastbound Beverly Boulevard, which eventually becomes Turnbull Canyon Road. Park at an easily overlooked turnout on the right by mile marker 4.21, 3.9 miles from the freeway. The trail is open 9 a.m.–5 p.m. October–May (until 6 p.m. June–September).

W hile nearby trails are overcrowded, this loop offers seclusion, a vigorous workout, and some panoramic views. The coastal sage-scrub vegetation has been heavily impacted by invasive plants, including mustard, thistle, and tumbleweeds from the ranching days.

Walk past the gate up the Elderberry Trail and, in 0.4 mile, reach a T-junction with the Workman Ridge Trail. William Workman was the mayor of Los Angeles from 1886 to 1888. He was also a businessman, banker, and real-estate developer, and he subdivided his ranch to create the community of Boyle Heights. To make a counterclockwise loop, turn right and descend Workman Ridge. At 1.0 mile, near a spur coming up from a neighborhood, the main trail turns left and becomes the Worsham Canyon Trail. Curve along the canyon wall as you climb to meet the Skyline Trail at 2.7 miles. Turn left and follow Skyline 0.5 mile to a prominent hill; then turn left again and descend the Workman Ridge Trail back to Elderberry.

trip 17.5   Arroyo Pescadero Loop

Distance	2.8 miles (loop)
Hiking Time	1.5 hours
Elevation Gain	300'
Difficulty	Easy
Trail Use	Equestrians, dogs allowed, good for kids
Best Times	October–May
Agency	Puente Hills Habitat Preservation Authority
Optional Map	Free *Arroyo Pescadero Trailhead* map (available at habitatauthority.org/trails)

see map on p. 220

DIRECTIONS From the 60 Freeway in Hacienda Heights, take Exit 16 for southbound Hacienda Boulevard. Proceed 1.9 miles; then turn right onto Colima Road. In 2 miles turn right into the Arroyo Pescadero Trailhead parking area.

A rroyo Pescadero ("Fishmonger's Ravine" in Spanish) is a gentle canyon on the south side of the Puente Hills. Once torn up by oil wells and grazing, it is now part of a wildlife corridor and nature preserve with an easygoing trail favored by families.

From the trailhead, walk up a short staircase to a T-junction, and turn right on the trail. In 100 yards, reach a second junction—the San Miguel Trail continues straight, while our hike turns left into the arroyo.

The route snakes up the canyon and back on the opposite side on a mix of dirt and crumbling pavement. The vegetation is a mix of native coastal sage scrub and invasives. Look for all four species of native sumacs (laurel sumac, lemonade berry, sugar bush, and poison oak), plus oaks and California pepper trees. Some eucalyptus trees were planted here a century ago by oil companies, although 3,000 others were removed in 2008 to reduce fire danger. Unfortunately, mustard and thistle have overrun the canyon, crowding out many of the natives.

The path eventually zigzags to a junction with the Deer Trail on the right. This 0.8-mile optional loop, included in the mileage of this trip, circles through the southern end of the canyon and returns to the same spot. The Arroyo Pescadero Trail soon weaves back to the starting point.

trip 17.6 Schabarum Loop

see map on p. 220

Distance	6 miles (loop)
Hiking Time	3 hours
Elevation Gain	1,000'
Difficulty	Moderate
Trail Use	Suitable for mountain biking, equestrians, dogs allowed
Best Times	October–May
Agencies	Los Angeles County Parks & Recreation, Puente Hills Habitat Preservation Authority
Optional Map	Free *Powder Canyon Trailhead* map (available at habitatauthority.org/trails; covers only part of the trail)

DIRECTIONS From the 60 Freeway, take Exit 18 for Azusa Avenue. Drive 0.4 mile south to Colima Road, and turn left (east). Just ahead, turn right into Schabarum Regional Park.

Schabarum Regional Park features a green-grass strip extending nearly a mile into the Puente Hills, and lots of steep, brushy hillsides affording some great panoramas of the San Gabriel Valley and the San Gabriel Mountains. You'll share these views with hawks and ravens who ride the hillside thermals. The park and trail are named for Peter Schabarum, who served on the L.A. County Board of Supervisors from 1972 to 1991 after terms in the California State Assembly and on the San Francisco 49ers. He was subsequently charged with embezzlement and convicted of tax evasion.

After parking in any of Schabarum's spacious lots (open during daylight hours), start your hike at a kiosk by the park entrance. Follow the paved path along the greenbelt for 0.1 mile; then turn right onto the signed dirt Schabarum Trail. Pass through a wooded area and across a grassy field to a second trail sign, where you turn left and the trail becomes well-defined. The trail twists and turns along dry, prickly pear–covered slopes west of the park's long strip of green turf; stay on the main trail as you see occasional social trails. Pass above a second trailhead parking area on the left. Just beyond, at 1.0 mile from the park entrance you come

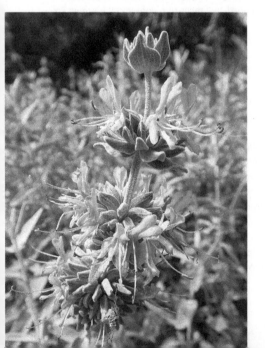

to a split; the left branch goes over to an equestrian ring at the south end of the turf strip, while the right branch, your route, takes you up through dense chaparral toward the Puente Hills crest. The panorama below includes nearby subdivisions in Hacienda Heights, the linear city of Industry (which, unsurprisingly, specializes in industry), and other assorted suburban sprawl stretching to the foot of the San Gabriel Mountains. The winter white-capped summit of Mount San Antonio (aka Old Baldy) floats serenely above it all.

As you approach the ridgeline, you contour below an antenna-topped, 1,416-foot peak. A shortcut to the ridge-running Skyline Trail is possible up and around this. After 2.7 miles from the park entrance, bear left as you

*Purple sage (*Salvia leucophylla) *displays its showy flowers along the Schabarum Loop.*

approach a water tower and antenna site served by a paved service road coming up from below. Follow the dirt road going east, which is the Skyline Trail. You climb some more, passing the 1,416-foot peak, and then descend. To the south you look over the wooded community of La Habra Heights, and across the coastal plains of Orange County. Stay on the main path as you pass some spurs.

After winding down a steep hillside, you reach a north–south dirt road in a saddle (4.3 miles). Ignore the spur turning hard left, and instead go left on the main road and continue down a draw, passing an unsigned trail on the right to Trail View Park, to the equestrian ring (5 miles). Walking through the ring, watch for the signed Schabarum Trail on the right. Follow this trail up onto the hillside and parallel the greenbelt back to the entrance.

VARIATION

The Bobcat Trail is a 2.3-mile subset of the Schabarum Loop that avoids most of the elevation gain. From the junction at 1.0 mile, turn left and shortcut to the equestrian area; then continue on Schabarum as described above.

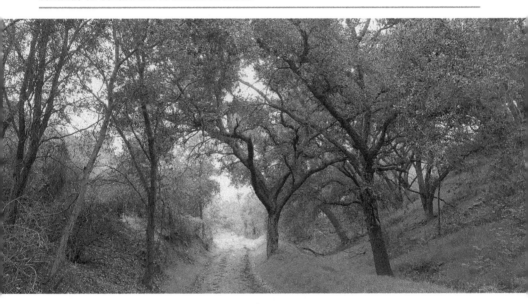

Coast live oaks arch over the Powder Canyon Trail.

trip 17.7 Powder Canyon Loop

see map on p. 220

Distance	4.2 miles (loop)
Hiking Time	2 hours
Elevation Gain	700'
Difficulty	Moderate
Trail Use	Suitable for mountain biking, equestrians, dogs allowed
Best Times	October–May
Agency	Puente Hills Habitat Preservation Authority
Optional Map	Free *Powder Canyon Trailhead* map (available at habitatauthority.org/trails)

DIRECTIONS From the 60 Freeway, take Exit 19 for southbound Fullerton Road. Proceed 2.0 miles; then, immediately past Pathfinder Road, turn right to stay on Fullerton. In 0.1 mile park on the shoulder of the road at a trailhead kiosk.

This loop explores woodsy canyons and viewful ridges at the eastern end of the Puente Hills via the Powder Canyon and Schabarum Extension Trails. Go on a cool spring day to enjoy the green hills, snowcapped mountains, and wildflowers, or anytime for a compact, vigorous workout. Powder Canyon is named for the Union Powder Company, which established a factory nearby around 1913 to manufacture a new explosive called Satanite safely away from town. Satanite was purported to be more stable and powerful than dynamite, but the company went out of business before it could gain a share of the market.

From the trailhead, walk west up the Black Walnut Trail (the main dirt road); don't get distracted by a spur on the right headed toward the Rowland Water District facility. In 0.1 mile turn left onto the Nogales Trail cutting across the hillside; then, in another 0.1 mile, turn right onto the Powder Canyon fire road coming up from a larger trailhead on Fullerton.

At 0.3 mile pass an equestrian staging area. At 0.7 mile pass the signed Gray Squirrel Trail coming down from a third trailhead on Fullerton, and continue up wooded Powder Canyon. At 0.9 mile pass the Black Walnut Trail on the right (which would have also led you here from the trailhead, with a bit more elevation gain and distance). Pass a power-line road on the right and reach a major junction on a saddle at 1.2 miles.

The Purple Sage Trail and another power-line service road depart to the west. A steep unofficial shortcut trail climbs the ridge to the northeast. Our hike continues north on the main fire road descending toward Schabarum Regional Park. At 1.6 mile turn right onto the Schabarum Extension Trail, which makes tight switchbacks out of the canyon. At 2.7 mile pass a spur to a hilltop, where the shortcut rejoins the main trail. Continue east, passing a water tank, as the fire road descends to meet Fullerton Road near its junction with Pathfinder.

trip 17.8   Schabarum–Skyline Trail

see map on p. 220

Distance	16 miles (one-way)
Hiking Time	8 hours
Elevation Gain	2,800'
Difficulty	Moderate
Trail Use	Suitable for mountain biking, equestrians, dogs allowed
Best Times	October–May
Agency	Los Angeles County Parks & Recreation
Optional Map	Free *Puente Hills Habitat Preservation Authority* locator map (available at habitatauthority.org/trails)

DIRECTIONS This trip requires a 16-mile shuttle by car or ride share. From the 605 Freeway, take Exit 18 for Peck Road. Go south 0.6 mile; then turn left onto Workman Mill Road. In 0.1 mile turn left into the parking area—leave a shuttle vehicle here.

To reach the starting point at Pathfinder Park, return to the northbound 605 Freeway and take it to the eastbound 60 Freeway. Take Exit 19 for southbound Fullerton Road. Proceed 2.0 miles; then turn left onto Pathfinder Road. In 0.1 mile turn right into Pathfinder Community Regional Park. Make an immediate left, and follow the road up to parking by the playground.

The Schabarum–Skyline Trail hugs the crest of the Puente Hills all the way from Pathfinder Community Regional Park at the west end to Workman Mill Road Staging Area at the east. Well suited to trail runners, cyclists, and mountain bikers, it provides a grand tour of the hills, with a good chance of seeing wildlife such as deer, coyotes, squirrels, and hawks. The trail mostly follows the right-of-way of huge transmission line towers. It is under the approach path to Los Angeles International Airport, so you can watch a continuous stream of jets descending overhead. The eastern and western trailheads are open sunrise–sunset.

This trail is codesignated as the Juan Bautista de Anza National Historic Trail, which commemorates the 1775–76 overland journey of exploration and settlement traversing 1,800 harsh desert miles between New Spain (now Mexico, south of Tuscon, Arizona) to San Francisco. Anza and the 240 colonists in his expedition established the Presidio and Mission San Francisco de Asís. His actual route traversed the San Gabriel Valley north of the Puente Hills.

From the Pathfinder Park lot, walk back out to the park entrance, turn left, and follow the fenced path east along Pathfinder. At Fullerton Road, you can follow the path as it turns left, dips through a large tunnel under the road, and curves right again, though it is more direct to simply go north and east across the intersection on the crosswalk. Continue north on the fenced trail along Fullerton Road.

At 0.5 mile from the parking area, the Schabarum Extension Trail pulls away from the road and climbs onto the hills, crossing a paved service road to a water tank. In another 1.3 miles, look for an unsigned singletrack leading to the top of the highest hill in the area.

The official Schabarum Trail switchbacks down into a canyon in Schabarum Regional Park, turns north and descends to the equestrian staging area, and then curves west and south to regain the ridge by the KOCE radio antennas in 3.5 miles.

After the paths converge, take a signed dirt path that crosses a paved service road beneath a water tank and then rejoins a fire road. This fire road continues west for 1.4 miles along the ridge before dropping down to Hacienda Boulevard by Leucadia Road. Very little parking is available in this area.

Follow a fenced path north along Hacienda Boulevard for 0.6 mile until you can cross under the road by means of an equestrian tunnel (no parking nearby) that is opposite the Hsi Lai Temple, the second-largest Buddhist temple in the western hemisphere. Courteous visitors are welcome and can take a self-guided audio tour.

The trail climbs back up onto the crest and follows the power-line corridor above some neighborhoods. Beware of many unmarked spurs leading to power-line towers. In 1.1 miles cross a third tunnel under Colima Road (no parking nearby). In 0.4 mile cross Holmes Road, and jog left to where the trail resumes opposite Hermitage Drive. In 0.2 mile cross Frame Road. Neighborhood parking is available near both of these roads.

Leaving the neighborhoods, the trail curves through scenic hills for 1.1 miles to a signed junction with the Worsham Canyon Trail. In another 0.4 mile, it reaches a junction with the Workman Ridge fire road near the 1,391-foot summit of Workman Hill. The area is named

The Schabarum–Skyline Trail is codesignated as the Juan Bautista de Anza National Historic Trail.

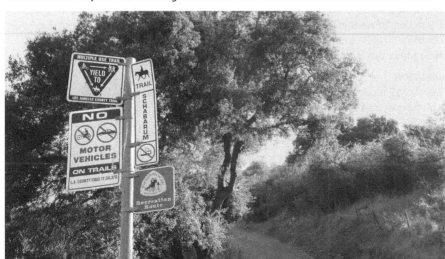

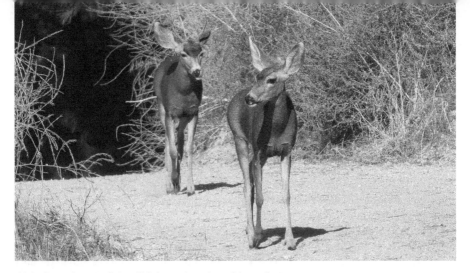

Mule deer take a stroll on a lightly used portion of the trail.

for the Workman family. William "Don Julian" Workman was among the first party of Americans to immigrate overland to Los Angeles, arriving in 1841, and he subsequently became a rancher, banker, and major landowner. His nephew William H. Workman served as mayor of Los Angeles from 1886 to 1888.

Stay right and descend 0.2 mile toward Turnbull Canyon Road. An unsigned singletrack on the left shortcuts down to the road crossing at mile marker 3.24, where parking is available at a turnout. Take the singletrack 0.4 mile down to the floor of the canyon, where you rejoin a fire road at a bend. The Turnbull Canyon trail goes straight, but we turn right and switchback 0.7 mile to regain the crest at a gate.

Turn left (north) and follow the ridge. In 0.2 mile cross a fence on the right through a gate at the top of the Ahwingna Trail, but stay on the crest. In 0.5 mile pass the Native Oak Trail, on the right. You are now squeezing along a narrow strip of trail between the Puente Hills Landfill and the Rose Hills Memorial Park. Follow this strip north 0.6 mile; then briefly join a paved landfill road. The trail veers west and zigzags up a steep fenced route and then along a paved road 0.3 mile to a picnic area near the antennas on Nike Hill. This hill was one of 16 missile bases ringing the L.A. basin to protect Southern California from Soviet bombers with a so-called ring of supersonic steel. Few residents were aware that hundreds of nuclear-tipped warheads were positioned just above their neighborhoods, secured by a chain-link fence and a single soldier with a pistol. The silos on this hill were demolished in 2000.

Follow the paved service road down the far side of the hill. In 0.8 mile veer left at a T-junction. In another 0.4 mile, turn left onto a dirt trail near a sanitation-district warehouse. Continue 0.7 mile to finish your trip at the Workman Mill Road Staging Area. The simplest option to return is to call a ride-sharing service.

VARIATION

Another 15 miles of the trail follow city streets between Schabarum Regional Park and the Antonovich Trail in Corona. Trails also continue westward from Workman Mill to the San Gabriel River and beyond.

chapter 18

San Gabriel Valley

The 1-million-plus residents of the greater San Gabriel Valley area are fortunate to have easy access to dozens of high-country trails in the San Gabriel Mountains. This chapter, however, focuses on hikes on the rim of the valley itself—some right along the base of the San Gabriel Mountains, and others in the San Jose Hills not far from Cal Poly Pomona. Other lowland hikes, in the Puente Hills and the hills near Claremont, are described in the previous and following chapters. All of these hikes make fine winter and spring additions to your repertoire of favorite hiking spots—especially if you're a local resident.

trip 18.1 Monrovia Canyon Falls

Distance	2.6 miles (out-and-back)
Hiking Time	2+ hours
Elevation Gain	600'
Difficulty	Easy
Trail Use	Dogs allowed, good for kids
Best Times	Year-round
Agency	Monrovia Canyon Park
Optional Map	Tom Harrison *Angeles High Country*
Fees/Permits	$5 parking fee ($6 weekends)

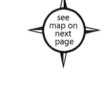 see map on next page

Oak-shaded Monrovia Canyon

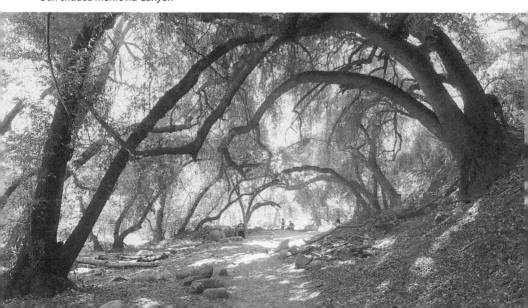

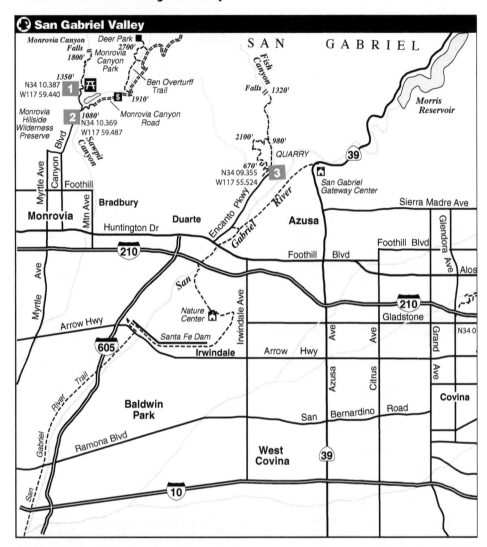

DIRECTIONS From the 210 Freeway in Monrovia, take Exit 34 for Myrtle Avenue. Drive north for 1.9 miles to where Myrtle Avenue ends at Scenic Drive. Turn right and follow Scenic Drive on a meandering eastward course for three blocks; then keep straight as Canyon Boulevard joins from the right. Proceed uphill on Canyon Boulevard, which crookedly ascends alongside the Sawpit Canyon wash to the park entrance. On most pleasant weekends, the small parking lots are overflowing by midmorning, and you'll have to park on Canyon Boulevard well short of the park entrance. Otherwise, pay an entrance fee and park in the small lot near the fee kiosk and ranger station.

Tucked away obscurely in two shady canyons behind the foothill community of Monrovia is one of the most beautiful parks in the Los Angeles area: Monrovia Canyon Park. Adding spice to the rich profusion of riparian vegetation is 40-foot-high Monrovia Canyon Falls, which runs with frothy exuberance for weeks or months after the rainy season ends.

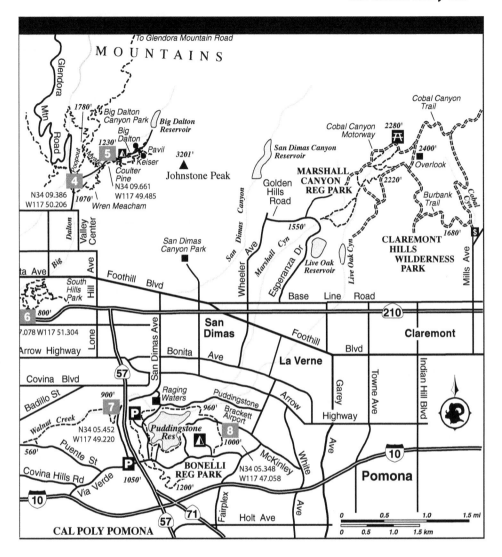

The park is extremely popular, especially on pleasant weekends, so unless you arrive very early or on a weekday, you can expect to park on Canyon Boulevard and walk 0.6 mile up the pavement to the trailhead. The park is closed to vehicles on Tuesdays, but hikers are still permitted. The parking lot is also closed 5 p.m.–8 a.m. weekdays (until 7 a.m. weekends), so don't let your vehicle get locked inside.

Monrovia Canyon was homesteaded in 1874 by the Rankins family, who emigrated from Wisconsin. They made their living by selling wood they cut at Sawpit Canyon, as well as by farming and beekeeping. The four children walked all the way to and from school in Duarte each day, until the eldest son died of typhoid fever at age 19; his two teenage sisters contracted it, too, and died a month later.

The signed Bill Cull Trail begins just above the fee kiosk. A fork on the right parallels and soon joins the road (optional return), but this trip stays left on the Bill Cull Trail, which

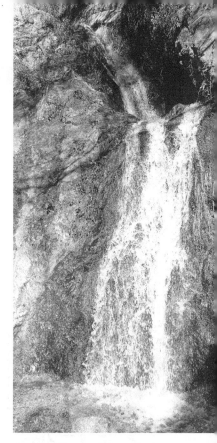

was named for a dedicated volunteer trail-builder. Switchbacks lead 0.2 mile up to a junction in 0.2 mile with the Cunningham Overlook Trail on the left. Stay on the gorgeous main trail, which crosses Monrovia Creek at 0.6 mile to a T-junction. Here, a nature trail leads right to the road, but you stay left. In another 0.1 mile, a second unsigned spur trail on the right leads to the nature center parking lot, but we stay left again.

Your trail mostly sticks close to the canyon's sparkling stream, passing a number of check dams. Alder, oak, and bay trees cluster in the canyon bottom so densely that hardly any sunlight is admitted, even at midday. After 0.6 mile the sound of splashing water heralds your arrival at the falls, where the stream either leaps or dribbles down two distinct declivities on a water-worn cliff face.

Return the way you came, or take one of the spurs back to the park road and walk down the road, which is slightly shorter.

VARIATION

The Cunningham Overlook Trail adds 300 feet of climbing and 0.8 mile round-trip to a bump with good views of the valley below. The trail is named for Ed Cunningham, another volunteer trail-builder who restored the path.

Monrovia Canyon Falls is a big reward after a short hike.

VARIATION

If the parking lots are not full, you can drive all the way to the nature center parking area, shortening your hike to 1.6 miles round-trip but missing out on the scenic lower section.

---

trip 18.2   **Ben Overturff Trail**

Distance	7 miles (loop)
Hiking Time	4 hours
Elevation Gain	1,800'
Difficulty	Moderately strenuous
Trail Use	Suitable for mountain biking, equestrians, dogs allowed
Best Times	October–May
Agency	Monrovia Canyon Park
Optional Map	Tom Harrison *Angeles High Country*
Fees/Permits	$5 parking fee ($6 weekends)

see map on p. 232

DIRECTIONS From the 210 Freeway in Monrovia, take Exit 34 for Myrtle Avenue. Drive north for 1.9 miles to where Myrtle Avenue ends at Scenic Drive. Turn right and follow Scenic Drive on a meandering eastward course for three blocks; then keep straight as Canyon Boulevard joins from the right. Proceed uphill on Canyon Boulevard, which crookedly ascends alongside the Sawpit Canyon wash to the park entrance. On most pleasant weekends, the small parking lots are overflowing by midmorning, and you'll have to park on Canyon Boulevard well short of the park entrance. Otherwise, pay an entrance fee and park in the small lot near the fee kiosk and ranger station.

The more lengthy trek in Monrovia Canyon Park takes you up the Sawpit Canyon drainage to Deer Park, the site of a tourist lodge that was popular during the early 20th century. There you'll see the remains of a stone lodge built by Monrovia contractor Ben Overturff in 1911. Torrential rainfall in 1938 wiped out large sections of Overturff's access trail to the lodge, and by 1948 the lodge and the trail were effectively abandoned. Not until the 1990s would the access trail again come into use; by this time the entire area had become a Monrovia city park.

The park is extremely popular, especially on pleasant weekends, so unless you arrive very early or on a weekday, you can expect to park on Canyon Boulevard and walk 0.6 mile up the pavement to the trailhead. The park is closed to vehicles on Tuesdays, but hikers are still permitted. The parking lot is also closed 5 p.m.–8 a.m. (until 7 a.m. weekends), so don't let your vehicle get locked inside. The trail is occasionally closed on Wednesdays for police target practice at a shooting range.

From the parking lot by the entry kiosk, walk 200 yards up the paved road to the gated Monrovia Canyon fire road, on the right.

Walk uphill on this road (which is paved initially), climbing on zigzags to a point overlooking the small Sawpit dam and reservoir. Continue climbing, more moderately now, past a turnoff for the Trask Boy Scout reservation (1.1 miles) to a gate at a very sharp hairpin turn to the left (1.4 miles), where a sign points to the Ben Overturff Trail.

At the junction, start descending into the ravine on the left using the narrow Ben Overturff Trail. You now experience a terrific 2-mile stretch of narrow footpath densely shaded by live oaks and mature chaparral so thick that it frequently forms a canopy overhead. About halfway through the stretch, the trail passes over the gap in a ridge. Three-fourths of the way through, you traverse a soggy, oak-shaded draw known as Twin Springs Canyon, passing a spur trail on the right leading over to the nearby fire road. Up and over the next ridge, you come to a second trail junction. Go left and hike the final 0.1 mile to the stone cabin ruins and old corral. So serene are the surroundings that it's hard to believe the site was once teeming with tourists.

When it's time to go, retrace your steps 0.1 mile, but turn left to get access to the nearby fire road, where a restroom has been thoughtfully placed. To add some variety, follow the fire road all the way back (3.2 miles of easy walking), passing a Monrovia Police Department shooting range and, later, the aforementioned Overturff Junction.

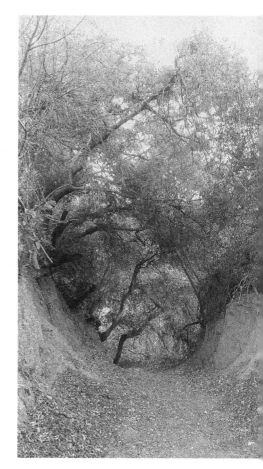

The Gap on the Ben Overturff Trail

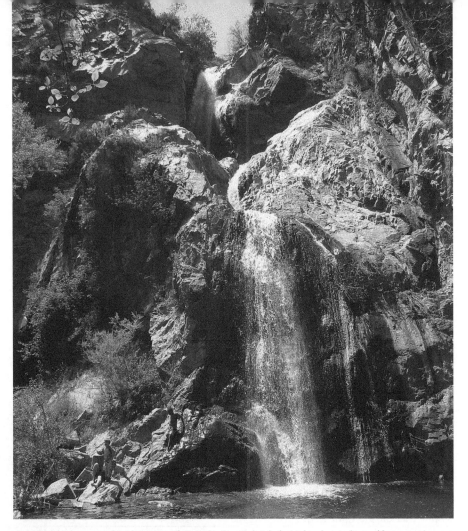

Fish Canyon has one of the best waterfalls in the San Gabriels, but it has been plagued by access issues.

see map on p. 232

trip 18.3   Fish Canyon Falls

Distance	5 miles (out-and-back)
Hiking Time	3 hours
Elevation Gain	800'
Difficulty	Moderate
Trail Use	Dogs allowed, good for kids
Best Times	November–May
Agency	Angeles National Forest
Optional Map	Tom Harrison *Angeles High Country* or Trails Illustrated *Angeles National Forest (811)*

NOTES This trail is closed indefinitely to allow for recovery from the 2016 San Gabriel Complex Fire. Check with Angeles National Forest (626-574-1613, fs.usda.gov/angeles) for updates.

DIRECTIONS From the northernmost end of the 605 Freeway in Duarte, turn east on Huntington Drive. Proceed 0.6 mile east to Encanto Parkway. Turn left and follow Encanto Parkway (and its extension, Fish Canyon Road) northeast for 1.4 miles. Turn left into the dirt parking lot (3901 Fish Canyon Road), which is just short of the Vulcan Materials rock quarry entrance.

Time-traveling visitors from nearly a century ago would have a hard time recognizing Fish Canyon today. Long gone are the dozens of vacation cabins lining the canyon and the dance hall at the canyon's mouth. For the past quarter century, the lower canyon has been chewed apart on an astounding scale by rock quarrying operations. These operations, however, extend only as far into the canyon as the Angeles National Forest boundary. Beyond lies the perennially green Fish Canyon, its sparkling stream, and its magnificent multitiered waterfall.

During the 1980s and most of the 1990s, canyon access was made difficult or impossible by quarry operations. Access was further hampered in 1998, when the City of Duarte opened a trail bypassing the quarry on the canyon's steep west wall. Unfortunately, the devilish climb and descent on this trail—which must be accomplished twice during the round-trip to and from the falls—occupied almost three-fourths of the time and energy expended on the hike.

After years of litigation, the city and Vulcan Materials finally reached an agreement in 2014 and built a fenced trail through the quarry to reach the forest boundary. Shortly thereafter, however, the canyon was swept by the June 2016 San Gabriel Complex Fire. The new quarry trail has been closed ever since, and the old bypass trail was obliterated. That said, Fish Canyon is a breathtakingly beautiful destination, so I (David) have included it here in hopes that the area will be accessible again in the not-too-distant future.

The trail begins at a gate and follows a fenced path across the quarry for 0.7 mile, through a no-man's-land of raw earth and gargantuan machinery, to an upper trailhead at the national-forest boundary. Then, suddenly, you enter a delightful, alder-lined riparian zone with the Fish Canyon stream alongside you and a trail to follow up the canyon. Around the first bend, the trail climbs to a bench on the left, and the ugliness of the quarry is instantly forgotten.

The remainder of the route features a gentle ascent, superb scenery, and many historical reminders. Notice the old cabin foundations, rock-and-mortar walls, and rusty household equipment. Fire and flood wiped out most of the cabins in 1958–59. Check out the botanical evidence: nonnative ivy, vinca, trees-of-heaven, agaves, and ornamental yuccas. Plenty of native vegetation thrives here, too, though—live oaks, big-leaf maples, and bay laurels cling tenaciously to the canyon's precipitous walls. Be alert for poison oak.

After about 1.5 miles of walking on the left bank, you cross the creek to the east bank— a foot- and leg-wetting exercise when the water runs high. A final 0.3-mile stretch leads to a point on the canyonside, offering a fine but not intimately close view of Fish Canyon Falls. The water tumbles nearly 100 feet down a cliff with four separate tiers, slides through riparian vegetation a short way, and makes a final, small leap into a crystalline pool just below the trail. Expect to have plenty of company at the pool.

---

trip 18.4   **Big Dalton Mystic Loop**

see map on p. 232

Distance	3 miles (loop)
Hiking Time	2 hours
Elevation Gain	1,300'
Difficulty	Moderate
Trail Use	Dogs allowed
Best Times	November–April
Agency	City of Glendora Parks and Recreation
Optional Map	Tom Harrison *Angeles High Country*

DIRECTIONS From the 210 Freeway in Glendora, take Exit 44 for northbound Lone Hill Avenue. In 1.0 mile turn left on Foothill Boulevard. In 0.5 mile turn right on Valley Center Avenue. In 0.8 mile turn left on Sierra Madre; then immediately turn right on Glendora Mountain Road. In 0.5 mile park at a turnout on the left immediately beyond Big Dalton Canyon Road.

This loop offers a great workout in a short distance by climbing hills on both sides of the mouth of Big Dalton Canyon. It is an appealing destination for a brisk morning or evening walk, especially in the springtime when the slopes are green, the creek is flowing, and the wildflowers are out. The parking area is outside of Big Dalton Canyon, so the trail is accessible even when the park is closed to vehicles. Some parts of the trail are very steep; shoes with good tread are essential, and a trekking pole might be helpful. The canyon is named for Henry Dalton, an Englishman who came to California in 1843 and established Rancho Azusa de Dalton, which grew to become the region's second-largest landholding.

From the trailhead, walk back south on Glendora Mountain Road for 0.3 mile to the entrance to Linder Equestrian Park. Find the signed Wren Meacham Trail at a bridge over the Big Dalton Wash behind a brick building. Cross both channels on bridges, and then walk upstream along the wash for 0.2 mile to a sign where the trail turns right and begins climbing steeply through the sage scrub and elderberry onto the hillside south of Big Dalton Canyon. Beware of poison oak in places. Weave and climb along the wooded slope; then descend as abruptly as you climbed, and reach the creek at 1.4 miles. The trail leads upstream, crossing the creek three times, to reach the signed north end of Wren Meacham on Big Dalton Canyon Road at 1.6 miles.

Directly across the road, the signed Mystic Trail begins climbing steeply again up the hillside on the north wall of the canyon. At 2.3 miles pass a spur on the left that shortcuts to the Poopout Trail, but continue on Mystic to reach a flagpole at a hairpin turn on the Lower Monroe Fire Road (2N16) at 2.5 miles.

From here, you could take the fire road (now deteriorated to a trail) in either direction to Glendora Mountain Road. Going left leads 2.4 miles down to the mouth of Little Dalton Canyon at mile marker 13.9, while going right climbs 5.0 miles to the ridge at a huge turnout 0.3 mile east of mile marker 5.6. Your route, however, turns hard left and follows the steep Poopout Trail directly down the ridgeline for 0.6 mile to return to your parked vehicle.

Wren Meacham Trail

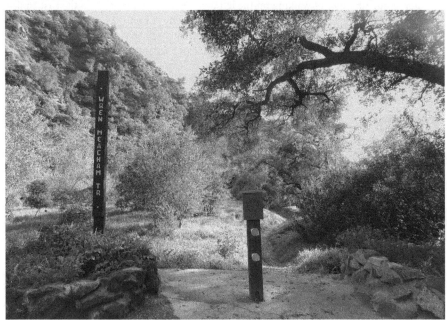

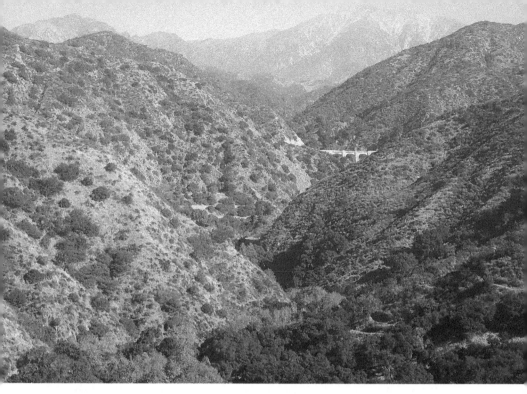

Big Dalton Canyon leads to arched Big Dalton Dam as Mount Baldy rises in the background.

trip 18.5 Big Dalton Canyon

see map on p. 232

Distance	2.1 miles (loop)
Hiking Time	1 hour
Elevation Gain	500'
Difficulty	Easy
Trail Use	Dogs allowed, good for kids
Best Times	November–April
Agency	City of Glendora Parks and Recreation
Optional Map	Tom Harrison *Angeles High Country*

DIRECTIONS From the 210 Freeway in Glendora, take Exit 44 for northbound Lone Hill Avenue. In 1.0 mile turn left on Foothill Boulevard. In 0.5 mile turn right on Valley Center Avenue. In 0.8 mile turn left on Sierra Madre; then immediately turn right on Glendora Mountain Road. In 0.5 mile turn right on Big Dalton Canyon Road. Go 0.7 mile to the signed Coulter Pine Trail on the right near mile marker 0.74.

Big Dalton Canyon, acquired by the City of Glendora from the Glendora Water District in 1964, is maintained as a wilderness park. This trip describes an easy but scenic loop up the wall of the canyon and back along the creek.

The Coulter Pine Trail is named for a small grove of the huge-coned pines at the trailhead. The trail switchbacks up onto the hillside, passing through chaparral, coast live oak, and toyon. Also called California holly, toyon produces striking red berries near Christmastime and is the plant for which Hollywood was named. Look for excellent views of the San Antonio Ridge connecting Mount Baldy to Iron Mountain, as well as glimpses of Big Dalton Dam at the head of the canyon. The mountains north of Big Dalton are maintained as the San Dimas Experimental Forest and are closed to visitors except for researchers studying subjects such as the impact of humans on the lower San Gabriel Mountains.

Stay high, passing two unmarked junctions with trails descending off our path toward Dunn Canyon. Eventually switchback down again on the Keiser Trail to meet the Pavil Canyon Trail on the right at 1.4 miles. In the wet season, you might enjoy following this lightly maintained trail a quarter mile up the canyon to a pair of small cascades. But this trip turns left and drops to a picnic area by the Wilderness Center, then on down to trailhead parking by a gate on Big Dalton Canyon Road.

Cross to the northwest side of the creek on a bridge and turn left on the Big Dalton Canyon Trail. When you reach Big Dalton Canyon Campground, cross back over the creek on another graceful bridge to reach the road; then turn left and walk scant yards back to the Coulter Pine Trailhead.

trip 18.6	**Glendora South Hills Wilderness**

Distance	2.9 miles (loop)
Hiking Time	1.5 hours
Elevation Gain	800'
Difficulty	Moderate
Trail Use	Dogs allowed, good for kids
Best Times	October–May
Agency	City of Glendora Parks and Recreation
Optional Map	Free *South Hills Wilderness Area* map (available at tinyurl.com/glendoratrails)

see map on p. 232

DIRECTIONS From the 210 Freeway in Glendora, take Exit 43 for southbound Sunflower Avenue. In 0.3 mile turn right on Gladstone Street. In 0.5 mile turn right on Bonnie Cove Avenue. In 0.3 mile park at the end of the road at the Bonnie Cove Trailhead.

The 2,200-acre South Hills Wilderness Area is laced with trails and fire roads covering the prominent hill in Glendora. Most of the trails were constructed by Boy Scout troops in the 1990s. The fire roads are open to equestrians and mountain bikers, but most of the narrow trails are exclusively for hikers. The map shows that many short loops are possible; this hike offers a grand tour of most of the park and has many good views.

From the trailhead parking area, look for the signed Bonnie Cove East Trail, to the right. Climb steeply to gain the ridge at 0.3 mile, where you will turn right onto the wide South Hills Backbone Road, which services power lines along the hill. At 0.7 mile turn left onto the attractive Lost Canyon Trail, which switchbacks steeply down to join the Alosta Canyon fire road at 1.1 miles. Turn right and walk down the road; then turn left onto the signed East View Trail at 1.2 miles. The trail promptly splits into a north and south fork—either choice is fine, but this trip assumes that you stay right on the north fork. Watch for posts naming the various native plants growing in the hills.

*The California brush rabbit (*Sylvilagus bachmani*) is the most common cottontail rabbit in chaparral habitat.*

At 1.4 miles come to the end of the North Spur fire road. Jog left and then turn right to join the Toyon Trail. Toyon, or California holly, a shrubby tree with narrow leaves, produces striking red berries in the winter. These berries, bitter before cooking, were made into jelly, porridge, or pancakes by American Indians. Because toyon was long overcollected for Christmas decorations, California state law now forbids collecting the plant on public lands.

At 1.5 miles stay right on Toyon at a signed junction with the Mustard Trail beneath a large oak. Stay on the main path as you bypass some unsigned use trails. At 1.7 miles the Toyon Trail veers right down to South Hills City Park—our loop bears left, onto the Wild Iris Trail. Follow the switchbacks rather than the use trail that goes straight up the hillside. At 1.9 miles veer right onto the Walnut Trail, near a grove of black walnut.

At 2.3 miles rejoin the South Hills Backbone Road, near a large concrete reservoir. Jog right and briefly climb a power-line service road to find an observation bench where you can take in fine views of the San Gabriel Mountains above Glendora, then return and head west on the road. At 2.6 miles turn right onto the signed Bonnie Cove West Trail, and follow it down to the parking area.

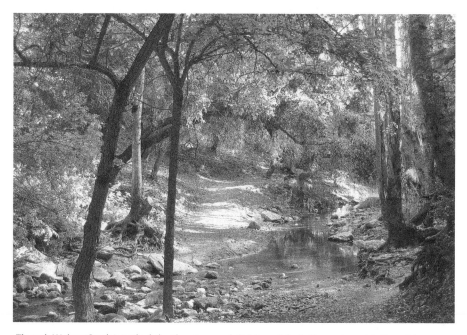

Though Walnut Creek is tucked closely among subdivisions, it feels like you're out in the wilderness.

trip 18.7   Walnut Creek

see map on p. 232

Distance	5 miles (out-and-back)
Hiking Time	2.5 hours
Elevation Gain	350'
Difficulty	Moderate
Trail Use	Suitable for mountain biking, dogs allowed, good for kids
Best Times	Year-round
Agency	Los Angeles County Parks & Recreation
Optional Map	USGS 7.5' *San Dimas*

DIRECTIONS From the 57 Freeway in San Dimas, take Exit 22D for Via Verde. Go a short distance west to San Dimas Avenue, and turn right. Continue 1.0 mile north to a roadside parking area on the left (west) side of San Dimas Avenue.

Walnut Creek County Park is a secluded ribbon of open space stretching through the cities of San Dimas and Covina. A wide and well-traveled bridle trail goes the length of the park, crossing the Walnut Creek stream several times (you'll get your feet wet in winter and spring). Plenty of oaks, sycamores, willows, and assorted nonnative ornamental trees—but relatively few walnut trees—line the banks.

Steep south walls along most of this stretch of Walnut Creek make it a cool haven on all but the hottest days. Often on winter mornings the canyon bottom is a frosty wonderland, since it acts as a sink for cold, dense night air slinking down along the slopes of the nearby San Gabriel Mountains.

From the parking lot, the Walnut Creek Trail zigzags west down the road embankment and arrives at the shady canyon floor. You then go down alongside the creek, where there are several splits in the trail. The first three are merely alternate routes that go along the opposite bank or up onto the steep south slope before returning to the main trail. The fourth splitting trail to the left connects with Puente Street.

Beyond Puente Street there's not much of a trail at all, though the strip of county park land continues about a mile farther to Covina Hills Road. Therefore, Puente Street is a good place to turn around and return the way you came.

trip 18.8   Bonelli Regional Park

see map on p. 232

Distance	8 miles (loop)
Hiking Time	3.5 hours
Elevation Gain	800'
Difficulty	Moderately strenuous
Trail Use	Suitable for mountain biking, equestrians, dogs allowed
Best Times	November–May
Agency	Los Angeles County Parks & Recreation
Optional Map	USGS 7.5' *San Dimas*

DIRECTIONS Park at the Brackett Field Airport terminal at 1615 McKinley Ave. in La Verne. From the 10 Freeway in Pomona, take Exit 43 for northbound Fairplex Drive. In 1.2 miles turn left onto McKinley Avenue, and proceed to the parking area at the end of the road.

Girded by freeways and busy streets, the trails around Puddingstone Reservoir in 2,200-acre Bonelli Regional Park are hardly the place to get away from it all—unless, perhaps, you arrive early on a Saturday or Sunday morning. During those quiet times you can get a sense of how peaceful a spot this was before World War II. In those distant days, the reservoir nestled among serene hills overlooking a patchwork quilt of citrus groves. The park is named for the man who championed its creation: Frank G. Bonelli, a Los Angeles County Supervisor from 1958 to 1972.

Today, the reservoir and the surrounding Los Angeles County–operated regional park are quite popular, with attractions such as Raging Waters aquatic amusement park, a golf course, acres of RV camping and picnic grounds, horse stables, hot tubs, and even motorboat drag races on occasion. For hikers, what remains of the dry, grassy hills above the reservoir can be very attractive in the winter and spring, especially if California poppies brighten the

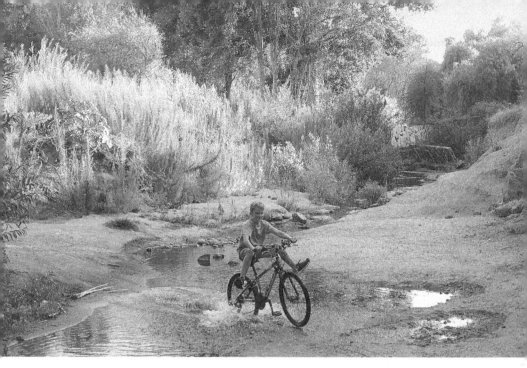

Bonelli Park is popular with cyclists and joggers as well as hikers.

velvety green slopes. The park charges a substantial ($10) vehicle-entry fee, so self-propelled travelers will want to start their hike at the airport, at the Via Verde Park & Ride, or on the north side of Puddingstone Drive.

Although many of the trails at Bonelli Park were designed to serve equestrians, they are popular with hikers, mountain bikers, joggers, and leashed dogs, too. About 14 miles of dirt roads and bridle trails lace the outer perimeter of the park, not even including some pedestrian and bike paths that follow parts of the reservoir's shoreline.

This route starts at Brackett Airport, named for Frank Brackett, a founding professor at Pomona College. In 1911, Calbraith Rodgers landed here on the first trans–United States flight from New York to Long Beach. Consider stopping at the friendly airport café before or after your trip to load up on carbs and watch small planes come and go.

This grand tour of the park circles Puddingstone Reservoir in a roundabout but scenic way, mostly along sometimes-signed Bonelli Trail. You can shorten the trip to about 6 miles by staying closer to the lake, or expand to about 10 miles by following the perimeter of the park. If you have a hard time following the tangle of poorly marked trails, simply make a counterclockwise loop around the lake.

Go west on McKinley through a gate. Pass a trail on the left by which you will return, but continue on the main path. At 0.5 mile stay right on a fence-line trail where the road reaches an RV park. The trail bends right, through a junglelike area nicknamed "Vietnam" by bikers, and passes the departure end of the runway. Ford Live Oak Wash at 0.9 mile, turn right by the picnic grounds, and continue to the northeasternmost corner of the park (1.2 miles), where you cross a paved park road and turn left onto a trail paralleling Puddingstone Drive. The trail crosses three entry roads before reaching a barbed wire fence near the spillway, at 2.1 miles. Turn left here and switchback up to reach paved Ranging Waters Drive at 2.3 miles. Turn left and follow the road over two dams overlooking the water park, passing first a trail that descends near the water park and then a section of the Bonelli Trail that leads into the western reaches of Bonelli Park—take this trail if you want more exercise.

At 3.1 miles turn left into a sailboat launch parking area. Stay right at the kiosk toward the lower parking lot; then, partway down, veer right onto the unsigned Bonelli Trail into the trees. This scenic stretch of trail circles a finger of the lake, passing two trails on the right, before reaching the swim beach at 3.9 miles.

Go up through the parking lot above the swim beach to reach a grassy area with a playground and picnic benches. You'll see a small bridge on the left, which you could cross if you want to make a shorter loop back along the lakeshore—for this hike, though, continue to the end of the grassy area, and turn left onto Via Verde Road.

Look for the Bonelli Trail on the right, which makes a weird gratuitous loop. Instead, stay on Via Verde Road for another hundred yards to catch the Bonelli Trail, a broad fire road, again at 4.5 miles. You now begin the only sustained climb of the loop. At a fork at 5.0 miles, stay right toward the helispot. At a second fork at 5.2 miles, the Bonelli Trail on the right descends toward the freeway—stay left on the Reservoir Trail, toward the crest, for better views of the San Gabriel Mountains and an easier trip. Continue over slopes covered in prickly pear cactus and mustard to a junction. Go left over the hill or right around; the forks soon rejoin.

Continue east on or near the crest toward an orange-and-white tower resembling a bowling pin. This tower is the Pomona Very High Frequency Omnidirectional Radio Beacon, used to guide aircraft navigating this part of the Los Angeles Basin. At 6.3 miles rejoin the Bonelli Trail near Via Verde. Follow the trail up over the hill and through a tunnel under Via Verde to a T-junction by the stables at 6.6 miles. Turn left and circle above the stables to an abandoned restroom at 6.9 miles. Three trails diverge from here, all returning to McKinley Road near the start. The middle one down the valley floor is most direct, reaching the road at 7.5 miles. Turn right and return to the airport where you began.

Puddingstone Reservoir is the centerpiece of Bonelli Park.

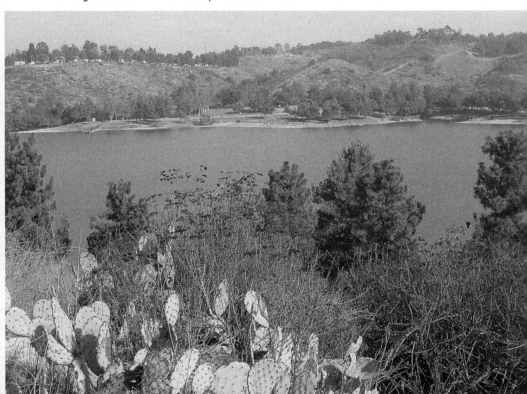

chapter 19

San Dimas–La Verne–Claremont Hills

Residents of communities around San Dimas, La Verne, and Claremont enjoy remarkable hiking, biking, running, bird-watching, and equestrian opportunities at the base of the foothills on the north edge of their towns. In particular, Marshall Canyon Regional Park and Claremont Hills Wilderness Park are extremely popular, and worthy of the occasional visit from hikers who live farther away.

As suburban sprawl has taken over the open space at the base of the foothills, Los Angeles County set aside 678 acres in the oak-filled Marshall and Live Oak Canyons for a regional park. Now, a maze of shady trails tempts hikers, equestrians, and mountain bikers to lose themselves in the canyons. In 1997, the City of Claremont established a wilderness park on the north edge of town with a system of fire roads through the chaparral-clad hills, offering visitors excellent hiking opportunities and panoramic views. These parks form the heart of a 5-mile corridor of protected open space and natural habitat.

This chapter describes several hikes within these parks and on nearby foothills. If you have more time, you can combine several of the hikes into a half-day workout.

trip 19.1 Lower Marshall Canyon

Distance	2.5 miles (semiloop)
Hiking Time	1.5 hours
Elevation Gain	300'
Difficulty	Easy
Trail Use	Suitable for mountain biking, equestrians, dogs allowed, good for kids
Best Times	Year-round but hot in summer
Agency	L.A. County Parks & Recreation
Maps	None

see map on next page

DIRECTIONS From the 210 Freeway in La Verne, take Exit 48 for northbound Fruit Street. Drive 0.1 mile; then turn left on Base Line Road. After 0.3 mile turn right on Esperanza Drive. Follow Esperanza for 1.2 miles; then turn left on Canyon Crest Drive and park near the intersection.

Marshall Creek flows past subdivisions alongside Sierra La Verne Country Club. You might be surprised to discover a trail along the creek, shaded under the oaks, that whisks you away and gives you the feeling of being in the wilderness. Runners, bikers, and hikers all enjoy this short but beautiful loop hike. Beware of poison oak along parts of the trail.

The signed Marshall Canyon Equestrian and Hiking Trail starts on the south side of Canyon Crest Drive. Follow the trail east under the power lines between rows of houses. In 0.3 mile cross Canyon Crest again, and climb a hill for views of the golf course and Sunset

continued on page 248

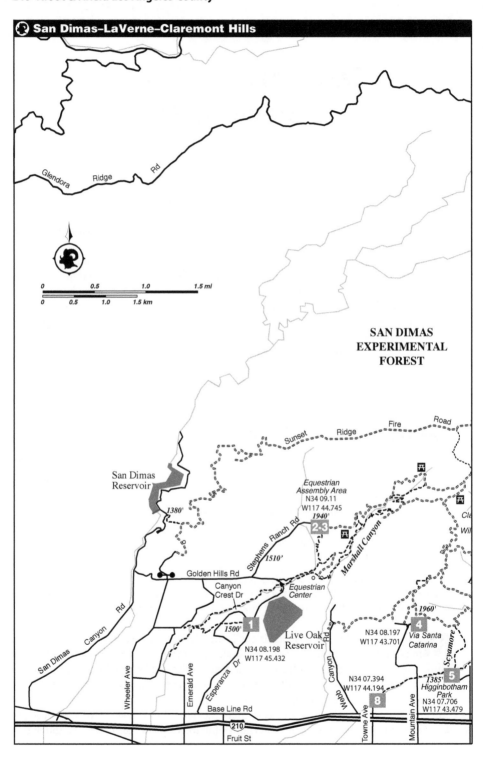

San Dimas–LaVerne–Claremont Hills

SAN DIMAS
EXPERIMENTAL
FOREST

0   0.5   1.0   1.5 mi
0   0.5   1.0   1.5 km

Glendora   Ridge   Rd

Sunset   Ridge   Fire   Road

San Dimas
Reservoir

Equestrian
Assembly Area
N34 09.11
W117 44.745

1380'

1940'

2-3

Stephens Ranch Rd

Marshall Canyon

1510'

Golden Hills Rd

Canyon
Crest Dr

Equestrian
Center

1960'

San Dimas   Canyon   Rd

Wheeler Ave

Emerald Ave

Esperanza Dr

1500'

N34 08.198
W117 45.432

1

Live Oak
Reservoir

N34 08.197
W117 43.701

4

Via Santa
Catarina

Sycamore

Canyon Rd

Webb

N34 07.394
W117 44.194

8

1385'

5

Higginbotham
Park
N34 07.706
W117 43.479

Towne Ave

Mountain Ave

Base Line Rd

210

Fruit St

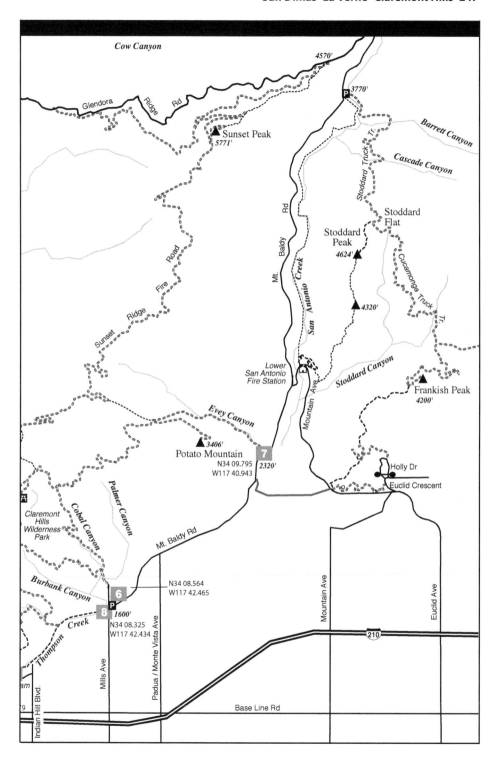

Cow Canyon

4570'

Glendora   Ridge   Rd

P 3770'

Barrett Canyon

▲ Sunset Peak
5771'

Stoddard Truck Tr.

Cascade Canyon

Stoddard
Flat

Mt.   Baldy   Rd

Stoddard
Peak
4624' ▲

Cucamonga Truck

▲ 4320'

Fire   Road

San   Antonio   Creek

Sunset   Ridge

Tr.

Lower
San Antonio
Fire Station

Stoddard Canyon

Frankish Peak
4200' ▲

Evey Canyon

Mountain Ave

▲ 3406'
Potato Mountain
N34 09.795   **7** 2320'
W117 40.943

Holly Dr

Euclid Crescent

Palmer Canyon

Cobal Canyon

A

Claremont
Hills
Wilderness
Park

Mt. Baldy Rd

N34 08.564
W117 42.465

Mountain Ave

Euclid Ave

Burbank Canyon

6
P

8 1600'
N34 08.325
W117 42.434

Creek

Padua / Monte Vista Ave

210

Thompson

Indian Hill Blvd.

Mills Ave

Base Line Rd

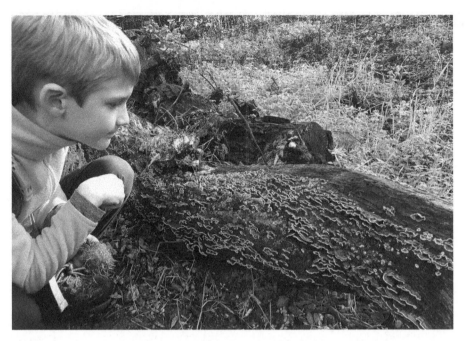

Despite its proximity to suburbia, Lower Marshall Canyon is rife with opportunities to explore nature.

continued from page 245

Ridge beyond the chaparral. In another 0.2 mile reach a junction with another trail coming down from a housing development. Stay right and drop into the oak-lined canyon. When you reach the bottom in 0.2 mile, turn right, and then immediately right again to follow the path upstream for a mile alongside Marshall Creek. The trail crosses the creek at several points and travels alongside the golf course, but for the most part you enjoy the feeling of seclusion. Watch for a rope swing in the canyon. When you reach the tunnel under Esperanza, climb up to the sidewalk. Turn right and walk 0.6 mile southwest alongside Esperanza to return to the starting point.

trip 19.2   **Middle Marshall Canyon**

see map on p. 246

Distance	1.7 miles (loop)
Hiking Time	1 hour
Elevation Gain	300'
Difficulty	Easy
Trail Use	Suitable for mountain biking, equestrians, dogs allowed, good for kids
Best Times	Year-round but hot in summer
Agency	L.A. County Parks & Recreation
Optional Map	Tom Harrison *Angeles High Country*

DIRECTIONS From the 210 Freeway in La Verne, take Exit 48 for northbound Fruit Street. Drive 0.1 mile; then turn left on Base Line Road. After 0.3 mile turn right on Esperanza. Follow Esperanza for 2.1 miles, and then turn right on Stephens Ranch Road. Proceed 1.0 mile past a golf course to the signed Equestrian Assembly Area, a large dirt parking area on the right side of the road.

Marshall Canyon Regional Park, at the top of Live Oak Canyon, is popular with local hikers and riders and features a creek lined with stately oaks. In spring during good rainfall years, wildflowers are in abundant bloom, and on moist days during winter and spring, watch for California newts beneath the oaks. This trip explores a short loop around the middle part of the canyon. There are many possible variations and, if you have time to spare, it is fun to just roam the maze of trails and see where you come out. Poison oak is common in Marshall Canyon, so don't stray off the trail.

From the parking area, head south on a footpath that winds steeply down the hill and passes beneath power lines. The trail crosses a small creek and runs alongside another creek. Although the Marshall Canyon Golf Course is only yards away, the dense trees in the canyon give you the feeling of complete seclusion.

In 0.5 mile reach a T-junction—the right fork leads to the stables at the Marshall Canyon Equestrian Center, but our short loop stays left and begins climbing back up the hill. In 0.2 mile reach a dirt road at the south end of an equestrian training area. Locate a trail that continues east and then north around the perimeter of the training area.

In 0.3 mile descend to the east to join another trail running along Marshall Creek. Turn left again, and hike 0.2 mile north along the creek through the fine oaks. At your first opportunity, stay left,

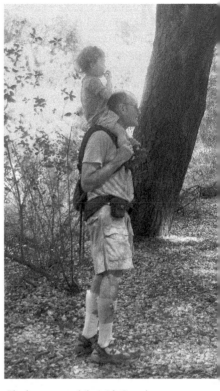

The best way to hike with Grandpa

then left again to work your way out of the canyon to the west through a mazelike area and emerge at the signed Fred Palmer Equestrian Camping and Training facility. From here, a dirt road leads 0.4 mile west back to where you started or, better yet, stay on the pleasant trail paralleling the road.

---

trip 19.3   **Upper Marshall Canyon**

see map on p. 246

Distance	4.5 miles (semiloop)
Hiking Time	2 hours
Elevation Gain	800'
Difficulty	Moderate
Trail Use	Suitable for mountain biking, equestrians, dogs allowed, good for kids
Best Times	Year-round but hot in summer
Agency	L.A. County Parks & Recreation
Optional Map	Tom Harrison *Angeles High Country*

DIRECTIONS From the 210 Freeway in La Verne, take Exit 48 for northbound Fruit Avenue. Drive 0.1 mile; then turn left on Base Line Road. After 0.3 mile turn right on Esperanza. Follow Esperanza for 2.1 miles, and then turn right on Stephens Ranch. Proceed 1.0 mile past a golf course to the signed Equestrian Assembly Area, a large dirt parking area on the right side of the road.

Much like Middle Marshall Canyon, Upper Marshall Canyon is popular with local hikers and riders. It also features a creek lined with stately oaks, locally known as Sherwood Forest. In the spring, wildflowers burst into joyous bloom. This trail through the steep upper part of the canyon is a great way to get exercise while enjoying the outdoors. Poison oak is common in Marshall Canyon, so don't stray off the trail. Los Angeles County Parks and Recreation has "improved" the trails with imposing but hilariously useless trail signs at some junctions.

From the east end of the parking lot, descend to a paved road and follow the trail along the north side of the road. Pass a yellow gate in 0.2 mile, and then come to the signed Fred Palmer Equestrian Camping and Training facility in another 0.2 mile. Turn left at the sign and follow a fire road as it winds generally northeast through shady oaks above the creek. In 0.6 mile come to a three-way junction with two other trails leading to the right. Stay left on the fire road. You will make a loop that returns on the rightmost trail to this point. The middle trail is a shortcut that rejoins the fire road.

As you continue up the fire road, you will soon come to another trail on the right that parallels the fire road for 0.2 mile before rejoining; you may take either path. Soon after, the fire road starts climbing in earnest. Pass a picnic area nestled in the oak trees beside the creek at the head of the canyon. The fire road turns south and comes to another junction where a trail on the right shortcuts back to the three-way junction you passed earlier. But this hike continues east up the fire road 0.4 mile more until it reaches the gate to Claremont Hills Wilderness Park (see Trip 19.6, page 253).

Turn right and follow another broad fire road southwest for 0.4 mile, pass a set of benches, and continue until you can turn right on another fire road that leads back to Marshall Canyon. Descend for 0.5 mile until you reach a trail junction; take the trail right and switchback down the hill and across the creek, returning to the three-way junction. Turn left on the fire road and retrace your steps for a mile back to the parking area.

Marshall Canyon is notable for its enchanting oak tunnels.

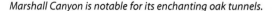

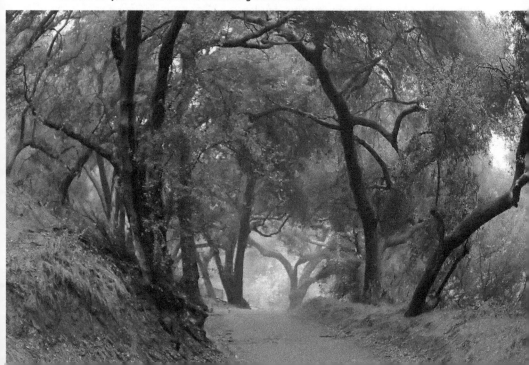

trip 19.4   Johnson's Pasture

Distance	2.2 miles (out-and-back)
Hiking Time	1 hour
Elevation Gain	400'
Difficulty	Easy
Trail Use	Suitable for mountain biking, equestrians, dogs allowed, good for kids
Best Times	Year-round
Agency	City of Claremont Human Services Department, City Parks
Optional Map	Tom Harrison *Angeles High Country*

see map on p. 246

DIRECTIONS From the 210 Freeway in Claremont, take Exit 52 for Base Line Road and drive west. Turn right on Mountain Avenue in Claremont (which is not to be confused with the parallel Mountain Avenue in Upland only a few miles east). Go up the steep hill for a mile to the top, and then make a right on Via Santa Catarina. Park at the end of Via Santa Catarina, taking care not to block private driveways. It's possible that designated trailhead parking will be established by the time you take this trip.

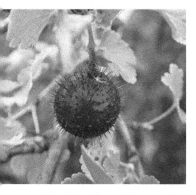

Gooseberry plants (Ribes spp.) bear bright-red fruit with prominent spines.

Johnson's Pasture is a 180-acre plot of land overlooking Claremont, acquired by Claremont pioneer C. C. Johnson and long held in the family. In 2006, city voters passed a bond measure to purchase the land, saving it from development and annexing it to the Claremont Wilderness Park. This short and gentle hike is popular with families and for strolls at sunset.

The trail, actually a dirt road, starts on the north side of the cul-de-sac on Via Santa Catarina. This is a quiet neighborhood—please respect the residents. The trail climbs steeply for the first few yards. In 0.1 mile pass a side road on the right leading to power lines and down to Thompson Creek. In another 0.2 mile, pass a side road on the left leading down to the High Point condominium complex. Straight ahead, you arrive at a pleasant grove of eucalyptus trees, where another power-line road leads left down into Webb Canyon. 0.2 mile later, a short side road on the left climbs up to a hill offering panoramic views of the San Gabriel Mountains, Claremont, and the Inland Empire. But the main road continues, passing yet another side road to an antenna farm on the right, arriving at a switchback junction with the Claremont Hill Wilderness Park loop, 1.1 miles from the start (see next trip). Return the way you came, or wander off to explore some of the side roads (note, though, that none of these side roads return you to the trailhead).

trip 19.5   Sycamore Canyon

Distance	2.3 miles (loop)
Hiking Time	1.5 hours
Elevation Gain	600'
Difficulty	Moderate
Trail Use	Dogs allowed, good for kids
Best Times	Year-round
Agency	City of Claremont Human Services Department, City Parks
Optional Map	Tom Harrison *Angeles High Country*

see map on p. 246

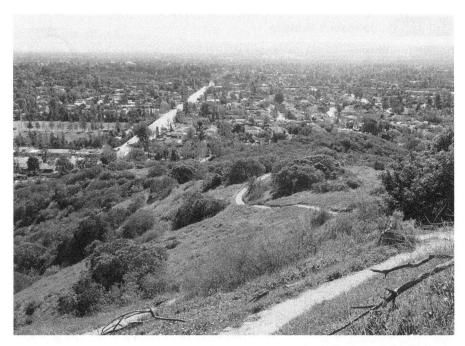

The hillside above Sycamore Canyon is carpeted in green in the spring.

DIRECTIONS From I-10 in Claremont, take Exit 47 for northbound Indian Hill Boulevard. In 3.2 miles turn left on Mount Carmel Drive. In 0.3 mile park on the street along the south side of Higginbotham Park.

Sycamore Canyon Park was established by Claremont in 1972 but remained rather primitive until 2013, when the city built a trail connecting to the Johnson Pasture area. Watch for deer as you ascend the steep but scenic path. This "Claremont Triangle" loop joins the Sycamore Canyon, Pomello, and Thompson Creek Trails.

The Sycamore Canyon Trail branches off the Thompson Creek Trail at the north side of Higginbotham Park, which is popularly known as the Train Park to throngs of local kids. Cross a bridge over the Thompson Creek flood-control channel and immediately come to a fork. The path straight ahead leads 0.1 mile to the ruins of a Boy Scout cabin constructed around 1934. This trip veers right and immediately begins climbing. The slopes are covered with laurel sumac, California sagebrush, and other native sage scrub. Watch for wildflowers in the spring. Be sure to recognize poison oak, which occasionally grows near the path. The vine lacing many of the plants is called wild cucumber or California manroot. The spiky fruits are toxic; they were crushed and thrown into pools by the Kumeyaay people to paralyze fish. After a vigorous 0.8-mile climb, the trail tops out at some benches along the East Pomello Drive fire road. From here, you can enjoy views of three county high points: San Gorgonio, San Jacinto, and Santiago Peaks. You could retrace your steps or make a left to head to Johnson Pasture and eventually on to Claremont Hills Wilderness Park. This trip, however, makes a short loop by turning right and descending on the fire road 0.7 mile to the Thompson Creek Trail. Turn right again and follow the easy path back 0.8 mile to your starting point.

trip 19.6 Claremont Hills Wilderness Park

Distance	5 miles (loop)
Hiking Time	2.5 hours
Elevation Gain	1,000'
Difficulty	Moderate
Trail Use	Suitable for mountain biking, equestrians, dogs allowed, good for kids
Best Times	Year-round
Agency	City of Claremont Human Services Department, City Parks
Optional Map	Tom Harrison *Angeles High Country*
Fees/Permits	Parking fee or annual parking permit required (see tinyurl.com/chwpparking for details)

see map on p. 246

DIRECTIONS From the 210 Freeway in Claremont, take Exit 52 for Base Line Road and drive west. In 0.7 mile turn right on Mills Avenue. Go up the hill 1.2 miles to the large Claremont Hills Wilderness Park trailhead parking area, on the right at the corner of Mount Baldy Road, or an even larger lot beyond at the top of Mills. The lots often fill on busy mornings, and there is no legal street parking nearby. Be aware that the City of Claremont aggressively enforces parking restrictions here. Consider parking on Mills near Base Line and biking to the trailhead.

Claremont Wilderness Park, established in 1997, has become an extremely popular loop for hiking, biking, running, and strollers, receiving an estimated half-million annual users by 2014. On a clear winter day, it offers views of the snowcapped summits of San Jacinto, San Gorgonio, and Ontario Peaks, and out to the skyscrapers of downtown Los Angeles towering beyond countless subdivisions. On a perfect day you can even see Catalina Island. The trail is on a good fire road that is normally well graded, but it can wash out during winter rains. The park can be unpleasantly hot on summer afternoons and is occasionally closed during times of extreme fire danger, including county red-flag warnings.

From the parking lot, walk up Mills Avenue to the start of the trail; then follow the dirt road past the Thompson Creek Dam flood-control basin and across a small creek. The path forks in 0.2 mile—take the right fork up Cobal Canyon, then loop around to return to this junction via Burbank Canyon. Hiking alongside Cobal Creek in the oak-shaded canyon is one of the most pleasant parts of this trip. After 0.8 mile the road leaves the canyon at a switchback and climbs unrelentingly up the ridge. At a water tank in another 0.5 mile, a side road leads east toward Palmer Canyon and Potato Mountain (see next trip)—the Wilderness Park loop veers west and, in 0.5 mile, reaches a saddle at the northernmost point of the park.

The loop continues along an undulating ridge to the southwest. This area burned on Halloween night in 2003, leaving a scorched, barren landscape, but the vegetation has rebounded remarkably well. In 0.1 mile pass a gate on the right at the top of the fire road leading up from Marshall Canyon (see Trip 19.3, page 249). Soon after, hikers will pass shaded benches placed on the hill by the Rotary Club in memory of Claremont mayor Nick Presecan, who helped preserve the park. In 0.4 mile from the last gate, pass a second fire road, again leading to the right down into Marshall Canyon.

In another 0.5 mile, crest the last of the hills and begin the steady descent. In 0.4 mile you reach yet another junction—turn hard left and descend on the switchback. The other path connects to Johnson's Pasture (see Trip 19.4, page 251). Descend the chaparral-covered slopes of Burbank Canyon overlooking Thompson Creek Dam and return to the main fork where you started the loop. Turn right, cross the creek, and reach the parking lot.

trip 19.7 ## Potato Mountain

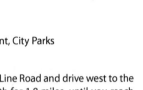

Distance	4.5 miles (out-and-back)
Hiking Time	2.5 hours
Elevation Gain	1,200'
Difficulty	Moderate
Trail Use	Mountain bikes allowed
Best Times	October–May
Agency	City of Claremont Human Services Department, City Parks
Optional Map	Tom Harrison *Angeles High Country*

see map on p. 246

DIRECTIONS From the 210 Freeway in Claremont, take Exit 52 for Base Line Road and drive west to the first intersection, Padua Avenue. Turn right on Padua and travel north for 1.8 miles, until you reach Mount Baldy Road. Turn right and go up Mount Baldy Road for 2.4 miles. Park your vehicle at a gated turnout on the left side of the road, taking care not to block the gate. Parking is very limited and often fills up on weekends. Note that a rash of burglaries has taken place at this trailhead, so exercise caution and don't leave valuables in your car.

Potato Mountain is a seemingly unremarkable bump overlooking the city of Claremont. Though the mountain itself is nothing special, the hike up Evey Canyon is beautiful. The views from the summit on a clear day are far-reaching, and the short but steep trail is popular for exercise. The canyon was formerly part of Pomona College's Herman Garner Biological Preserve, but in 2017 the college donated the land to the City of Claremont to expand Claremont Hills Wilderness Park. Spring is an especially good time to visit because the wildflowers are in bloom. Avoid this hike on summer afternoons, when you are certain to get baked under the unrelenting sun.

The shortest way to reach Potato Mountain is via the fire road up Evey Canyon, which is among the most tranquil canyons in the San Gabriels, with tall oaks branching over the road alongside the stream. The 2002 Williams Fire swept through the foothills and wiped out many trees, but a remarkable number survived and the canyon has returned to its former glory. The dense thickets of streamside white alders mostly burned but have naturally recovered. As the trail climbs above the stream and the canopy opens, watch for wildflowers that the butterflies attract. The coast live oak of the lower reaches, with concave leaves, is replaced by canyon live oak, recognizable by its huge acorns and flat leaves. Watch for California bay, big-leaf maple, big-cone Douglas-fir, and two-petaled ash, all of which attract diverse birdlife, including Lawrence's goldfinches, lazuli buntings, and Western tanagers.

In 1.4 miles the road veers left and reaches a saddle at the top of the canyon. From here, turn left and follow a spur road 0.8 mile to the summit of Potato Mountain. The panoramic view includes the high points of four counties: Mount San Antonio (Baldy) in Los Angeles County, Mount San Gorgonio in San Bernardino County, Mount San Jacinto in Riverside County, and Santiago Peak in Orange County.

VARIATION

At the first bend on Evey Canyon Road, a quarter mile from the trailhead, a steep 0.5-mile use trail on the left ascends the east ridge of Potato Mountain. Beware of the copious poison oak.

ALTERNATIVE FINISH

If you've arranged a car or bicycle shuttle, you can make a fine one-way hike by returning to the saddle, and then following the fire road west for 2.1 miles to Claremont Wilderness Park and another 1.6 mile down to the trailhead at the north end of Mills Avenue (see Trip 19.6, page 253).

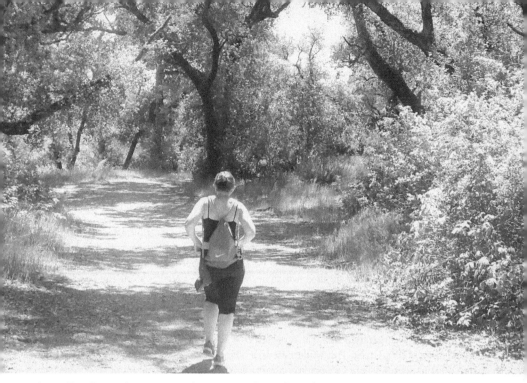

Lower Evey Canyon boasts a marvelous canopy of coast live oak.

trip 19.8   Thompson Creek Trail

see map on p. 246

Distance	4.5 miles (out-and-back)
Hiking Time	2 hours
Elevation Gain	300'
Difficulty	Easy
Trail Use	Suitable for mountain biking, dogs allowed, good for kids
Best Times	Year-round
Agency	City of Claremont Human Services Department, City Parks
Optional Map	Tom Harrison *Angeles High Country*
Fees/Permits	Parking fee or annual permit required (see tinyurl.com/chwpparking)

DIRECTIONS From the 210 Freeway in Claremont, take Exit 52 for Base Line Road and drive west. Proceed 0.7 mile, and then turn right on Mills Avenue. Go up the hill 1.2 miles to the large Claremont Hills Wilderness Park trailhead parking area, on the right at the corner of Mount Baldy Road. The lot often fills on busy mornings, and there is no legal street parking nearby.

Thompson Creek is channeled into a concrete canal to reduce flood risk. The paved Thompson Creek Trail parallels the canal past pleasant landscapes and Higginbotham Park. The popular trail, starts on the west side of Mills Avenue, opposite the parking area. It leads west across the plain beneath Thompson Creek Dam and soon meets the canal. In 0.5 mile, where the trail crosses Pomello Drive, pass the Gail Mountainway Trailhead. In another 0.5 mile, pass a parking area at the north end of Indian Hill Boulevard. Just 0.3 mile farther, reach Higginbotham Park, which has restrooms, a water fountain, and a kids' play area. The Sycamore Canyon Trail departs north here (see Trip 19.5, page 251).

The trail continues west, crossing Mountain Avenue, passing stables, and terminating in 0.9 mile at the north end of Towne Avenue just north of Base Line and the 210 Freeway. Return the way you came.

chapter 20

Piru Creek

Although relatively unknown among hikers, Piru Creek and its tributaries offer a rugged wilderness experience barely an hour's drive from the San Fernando Valley and Santa Clarita Valley suburbs. Los Padres National Forest and Angeles National Forest share administrative responsibilities for the area, which lies west of the 5 Freeway along the Los Angeles–Ventura County line. The area, which has few roads and trails, is managed primarily for its value as watershed and wildlife habitat. The name *Piru* is likely derived from a Native American word of disputed meaning.

In 1992 the gargantuan 220,000-acre Sespe Wilderness was carved out of lands lying mostly west of Piru Creek. This wilderness area includes the Sespe Condor Sanctuary (closed to recreational use), where California condors raised in captive breeding programs have been released into the wild. While you're out exploring the places described below, keep an eye on the skies. Spotting a soaring condor is possible; spotting a golden eagle or a turkey vulture is somewhat probable; spotting common raptors such as red-tailed hawks is virtually certain. In 2009 Congress designated Piru Creek as a Wild and Scenic River, the only so-named waterway in Los Angeles County.

Since the first edition of this book was published in 1991, access to the remote wild section of Piru Creek (aka Piru Gorge) has been made more difficult by the closure of Blue Point Campground at the north end of Lake Piru and the closure (to vehicles) of the paved road around Lake Piru's west shoreline. Trail maintenance has gradually been reduced as well, which makes any journey into the remote section of Piru Creek and its Agua Blanca tributary a true wilderness experience. The Blue Point Campground was closed to protect the endangered arroyo toad.

We begin with a civilized day hike up a slope not far from the 5 Freeway—the Oak Flat Trail. The other two trips are best done as overnight backpacks. Fire regulations apply, and you'll need a fire permit from Los Padres National Forest in order to operate a camp stove.

Aerial view of Piru Lake from the south; Piru Creek continues north from the lake.

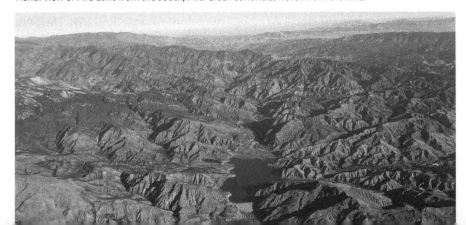

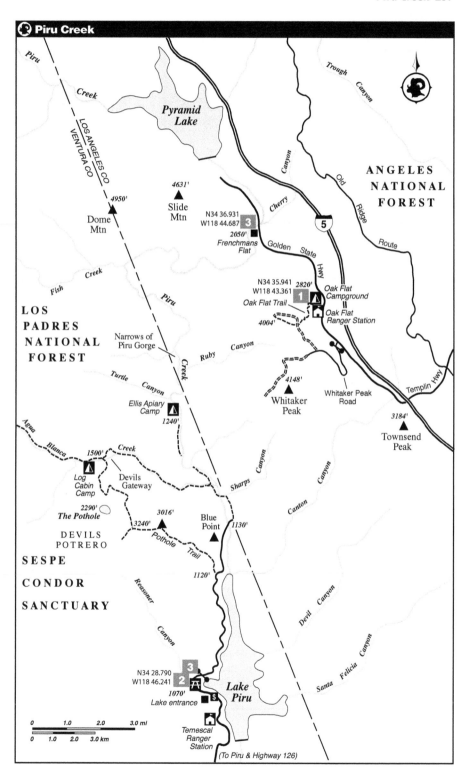

Piru Creek

Piru

Creek

Pyramid Lake

Trough Canyon

LOS ANGELES CO
VENTURA CO

**ANGELES
NATIONAL
FOREST**

4950'

4631'

Dome
Mtn

Slide
Mtn

Cherry

Canyon

Old Ridge Route

N34 36.931
W118 44.687 **3**

2050'
Frenchmans
Flat

Golden State Hwy

5

Fish Creek

Piru

LOS
PADRES
NATIONAL
FOREST

Narrows of
Piru Gorge

N34 35.941
W118 43.361 *2820'*

Oak Flat Trail

Oak Flat
Campground **1**

Oak Flat
Ranger Station

4004'

Creek

Ruby Canyon

Turtle Canyon

Ellis Apiary
Camp
1240'

4148'

Whitaker
Peak

Whitaker Peak
Road

Templin Hwy

3184'

Townsend
Peak

Agua Blanca

1500'

Creek

Log
Cabin
Camp

Devils
Gateway

Sharps Canyon

Canyon

2290'
The Pothole

3016'

3240'

Blue
Point

1130'

Canton Canyon

**DEVILS
POTRERO**

Pothole Trail

SESPE

1120'

CONDOR

Reasoner

SANCTUARY

Canyon

Devil Canyon

N34 28.790
W118 46.241

3
2

1070'
Lake entrance

Lake
Piru

$

Temescal
Ranger
Station

Santa Felicia Canyon

0   1.0   2.0   3.0 mi
0   1.0   2.0   3.0 km

(To Piru & Highway 126)

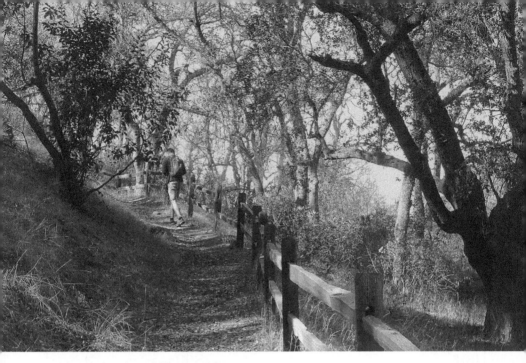

A hiker starts up the trail from Oak Flat.

see map on previous page

trip 20.1   Oak Flat Trail

Distance	2.8 miles (out-and-back)
Hiking Time	1.5 hours
Elevation Gain	1,000'
Difficulty	Moderate
Trail Use	Dogs allowed, good for kids
Best Times	Year-round
Agency	Angeles National Forest
Optional Map	Trails Illustrated *Angeles National Forest (811)*

DIRECTIONS From the 5 Freeway about 45 miles northwest of central Los Angeles, take Exit 183 for Templin Highway. Pick up the frontage road on the west side of the freeway (old Highway 99, formerly the main highway), and drive an additional 3 miles northwest to the Oak Flat Fire Station entrance. Turn left and continue 0.3 mile to a parking area next to the Oak Flat Fire Station, just short of the Verdugo Oaks Boy Scout camp.

The Oak Flat Trail, the only developed trail along the I-5 corridor through the Angeles National Forest, offers ever-widening vistas of fault-tortured canyon country, and a close look on the way up at some interesting outcrops of breccia—a sedimentary rock resembling conglomerate in appearance, except that the embedded stones are sharp, not rounded. The Boy Scouts built the trail and continue to maintain it.

The signed Oak Flat Trail begins on the left side of the big, grassy area just inside Camp Verdugo Oaks. Switchbacks take you under a shady canopy of valley oaks and live oaks. Soon, however, you'll climb to scrub-covered slopes exposed to the morning and midday sun. The area burned in the 2006 Day Fire, which devastated 162,702 acres in the Los Padres

National Forest when an illegal campfire got out of control. The brush has recovered quickly, but you can still see scars.

After surmounting a final set of steeply inclined switchback segments, you reach the Whitaker Spur Road (1.4 miles). From there you can look west into the gorge of Piru Creek and, if it's clear, farther west into the remote Los Padres country where Cobblestone Mountain, White Mountain, and a half-dozen other summits over 5,000 feet raise their shaggy heads. In the foreground is a breccia outcrop with a window in it. Turning north and east, you'll be able to trace the long hogbacks of Liebre and Sawmill Mountains and the gashed face of Redrock Mountain (in the area covered by Chapter 21).

At this point you're standing just east of the San Gabriel Fault, whose trace is not obvious here. The fault continues southeast and east about 70 miles into the San Gabriel Mountains, where it parallels the West and East Forks of the San Gabriel River, roughly dividing the so-called Front Range of the San Gabriels from the High Country.

You'll return down the same trail. In the meantime, you may want to try following the Whitaker Spur Road 0.7 mile west to a 4,004-foot summit offering a nice view of Pyramid Lake to the north. You can also go 0.4 mile south on the same road to see a large outcrop of pockmarked breccia.

trip 20.2   Pothole–Agua Blanca Loop

see map on p. 257

Distance	20 miles round-trip (semiloop, including paved road)
Hiking Time	10 hours
Elevation Gain	3,600'
Difficulty	Strenuous
Trail Use	Suitable for backpacking, dogs allowed
Best Times	November–May
Agencies	Los Padres National Forest, Ojai Ranger District; United Water Conservation District
Recommended Map	Trails Illustrated *Angeles National Forest*
Fees/Permits	Lake Piru Recreation Area use fee (varies; call 805-521-1500 or check camplakepiru.com/pricing for details); campfire permit required for backpackers (see preventwildfireca.org/campfires)

DIRECTIONS From the 5 Freeway, take Highway 126 west for 11 miles. At mile marker 126 VEN 29.34, turn right onto Center Street in Piru, following signs for Lake Piru. In 0.7 mile turn right on Orchard Street. In another 0.2 mile, turn right on Main Street, which becomes Piru Canyon Road. Proceed 6 miles to the entrance gate for Lake Piru Recreation Area, which charges a substantial use fee. Notify the ranger of your hiking plans. Park hours vary by season, and if you arrive before the park opens, you may be able to get in via the leftmost lane. Continue 0.8 mile and park at a day-use lot on the right just before a gate. Even if the gate is open, don't go farther lest you get locked in before your return, unless the ranger tells you that access to the north end of the lake has improved.

Because the area above Lake Piru is seldom visited and is mostly out of range of cell-phone signals, it's imperative to contact Los Padres National Forest (805-646-4348, fs.usda.gov/lpnf, hike lospadres.com) for the latest information on possible flood conditions, wilderness-area rules, trail conditions, and logistics.

The Pothole Trail had been so badly overgrown that it was removed from the last edition of this book; it has recently been cleared, however, and was in good shape in 2018, although it could deteriorate quickly if not regularly maintained. Check with the national forest for the latest conditions.

This trip into the edge of the vast Sespe Wilderness takes you up a ridge for views of the Los Padres National Forest, past an unusual geological formation called The Pothole, and down through a striking sandstone gorge called the Devil's Gateway. You're more likely to see deer tracks and bear scat than other people in this remote country, and you might be lucky enough to glimpse a condor circling above.

Before 2000, this trip was 8.5 miles shorter because you could drive Piru Canyon Road to Blue Point. Piru Creek, however, has been identified as critical habitat for the endangered arroyo toad, and the road is now closed to the public, adding a substantial and dull trip along the paved road to reach the old trailhead. Clever travelers should consider biking those initial miles, although you'll face a stiff hill climb along the way.

From the day-use parking lot, pass through a gate and walk or pedal up the paved road. At 1.3 mile pass a boat launch. (You might be able to drive this far in the spring.) Due to California's prolonged droughts, Lake Piru is presently so low that the boat ramp doesn't reach the lake, and much of the basin formerly occupied by the lake is now covered in bushes and trees. The road then climbs high above the lake, reaching a crest at 2.5 miles. At 4.3 miles arrive at the signed Pothole Trail, at the north end of the lake.

The Pothole Trail makes a demanding 2,000-foot climb directly up the grassy ridge to the northwest. If it has become badly overgrown, you're better off skipping The Pothole Trail and just doing an out-and-back in Agua Blanca Canyon. But if it is still in good shape, you'll enjoy ever-broadening views as you ascend. Look north at the bluish-gray rock of Blue Point and the wildly folded sediments on its adjoining ridge. At 6.2 miles reach Point 3016; then dip slightly and climb back up to the signed Sespe Wilderness boundary at the 3,240-foot-high point of the trip on the shoulder of another hill (6.7 miles).

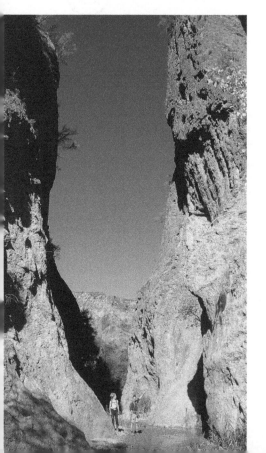

The Pothole Trail now turns north and begins a curving descent to bypass some hidden cliff bands. You'll have interesting views into The Pothole and Devil's Potrero below. The Pothole is an unusual formation created by a landslide that dammed the canyon. The area behind the dam filled with silt to form a flat, round basin, which is now mostly covered with cottonwood trees.

At 8.5 miles traverse a switchback that brings you to the closest point to The Pothole. Unfortunately, reaching The Pothole from here involves a nasty bushwhack through a dense stand of chamise. At 8.7 miles come to a T-junction. Our trail stays right, but you could turn left and wander through a maze of deer trails beneath the oaks in Devil's Potrero (*potrero* is Spanish for "pasture"). At 9.0 miles reach a cabin and campsite near Pothole Spring. William Whitaker established a homestead here in 1891 and hauled farming

Devil's Gateway on Agua Blanca Creek was an easy wade on this day.

tools up here on the back of his mule; some remain. Water generally runs year-round in the nearby creek, which you cross at 9.2 miles.

The trail descends the canyon through a magical grove of coast live oak to reach Agua Blanca Creek at 9.6 miles. *Agua Blanca* is Spanish for "white water," which is only true at times of high flow. Turn left and follow the Agua Blanca Trail upcanyon to Log Cabin Camp at 9.7 miles. The cabin is long gone, but you'll find a great trail camp with a metal stove here on a terrace above the creek. The Agua Blanca Trail was developed here in the 1930s by the Civilian Conservation Corps along the route of an old Chumash footpath. Our hike stops here, but an intrepid backpacker could continue exploring upstream to Hollister Camp, Cove Camp, Big Narrows, and Ant Camp, beyond which the trail is presently unmaintained and overgrown.

Our loop turns back downcanyon. At 9.9 miles pass through Devil's Gateway, a highlight of this trip where the creek fills the 20-foot-wide canyon between the sheer conglomerate walls. During times of high flow in the spring, you might have to wade through waist-deep water. The bypass trail on the north wall was wiped out in the 2007 Ranch Fire and hasn't been rebuilt. The remainder of the trail mostly stays along the steep, shaded south wall of the canyon, but it also fords the creek several times.

At 12.6 miles reach the end of a dirt road. Follow the road out past a cabin to meet dirt Piru Canyon Road at 12.9 miles. Turn right and follow it out, fording Piru Creek twice. Pavement begins at 14.2 miles, you pass the Pothole Trail at 15.6 miles, and you finally get back to your vehicle at 20 miles.

trip 20.3 Piru Creek

see map on p. 257

Distance	21 miles (one-way)
Hiking Time	14 hours/2 days
Elevation Gain/Loss	600'/1,500'
Difficulty	Very strenuous
Trail Use	Suitable for backpacking, dogs allowed
Best Times	October–June
Agencies	Los Padres National Forest, Ojai Ranger District; United Water Conservation District
Recommended Map	Trails Illustrated *Angeles National Forest*
Fees/Permits	Lake Piru Recreation Area use fee (varies; call 805-521-1500 or check camplakepiru.com/pricing for details); campfire permit required for backpackers (see preventwildfireca.org/campfires)

DIRECTIONS This trip requires a 45-minute car shuttle between trailheads. *Note:* Don't count on cell coverage or calling a ride-sharing service in this remote area. From the 5 Freeway, take Highway 126 west for 11 miles. At mile marker 126 VEN 29.34, turn right onto Center Street following signs for Lake Piru. In 0.7 mile turn right on Orchard Street. In another 0.2 mile, turn right on Main Street, which becomes Piru Canyon road. Proceed 6 miles to the entrance gate for Lake Piru Recreation Area, which charges a substantial use fee. If you notify the ranger of your shuttle plans, you might be allowed to bring two vehicles into the park but pay for just one.

Park hours vary by season, and if you arrive before the park opens, you may be able to get in via the leftmost lane. Continue 0.8 mile and park your shuttle vehicle at a day-use lot on the right, just before a gate. Even if the gate is open, don't go farther lest you get locked in before your return, unless the ranger tells you that access to the north end of the lake has improved.

To reach the other end of the trail, return to the 5 Freeway and continue north to Exit 183 for Templin Highway. Go left (west) on Templin; then immediately turn right onto Golden State Highway, the west-side frontage road. Park at Frenchman Flat, where the road ends in 5.2 miles.

Because the area above Lake Piru is seldom visited and is mostly out of range of cell-phone signals, it's imperative to contact Los Padres National Forest (805-646-4348, fs.usda.gov/lpnf, hike lospadres.com) for the latest information on possible flood conditions, wilderness-area rules, trail conditions, and logistics. Efforts are under way to eventually reopen the Blue Point Trailhead, but this may be many years away.

Piru Creek is a federally designated Wild and Scenic River threading through a deep canyon in the Sespe Wilderness. The creek is recognized for its geological significance, as it cuts back in time through a complex series of sedimentary layers that give geologists critical insights into the history of the West Coast. Experienced hikers/backpackers can mount a two-day expedition down Piru Creek, which involves almost no true climbing but rather many miles of riverbank walking and foot-wetting creek crossings. If the water in the creek is flowing too fast, you will want to postpone your trip (Pyramid Reservoir sometimes releases extra water, kayakers run this route during times of high flow, and a flash flood could be lethal). The trip is ideal in April, when the creek is flowing well, the air is warm enough to enjoy getting wet, and the wildflowers are in bloom. No matter what time of year you go, you can expect an epic adventure reminiscent of descending the Zion Narrows.

Wear an old pair of shoes, because you're likely to spend hours in the creekbed. Long pants and sleeves will help protect you from the heavy brush, poison oak, sharp rocks, and ticks; sandals are asking for trouble unless your feet are made of hardened leather. Gaiters may also be helpful. Carry antichafing cream, because your legs may suffer from walking

Of the waterfalls in this book, this enchanting one in the Piru Narrows is the most demanding to reach.

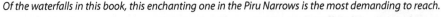

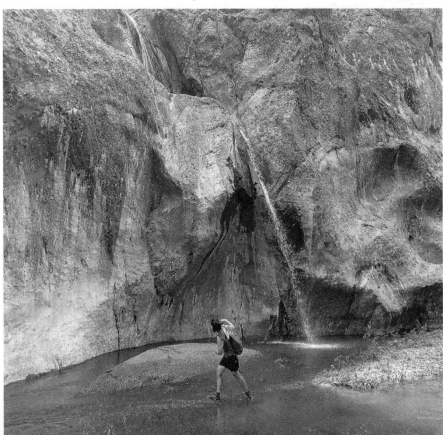

many miles in wet pants. A small pair of pliers might be handy to remove cockleburs that will try to hitchhike on your socks or pants. Line your backpack with a trash bag to hold anything that shouldn't get wet, and tie the bag closed securely. Double- or triple-bag your electronics and car keys with zip-top plastic bags, and also take care to protect your sleeping bag and change of clothes if you're backpacking.

You'll be wading through some pools whose depth can change suddenly, and there is a substantial chance you'll take an unexpected swim. Beware of rattlesnakes, which are plentiful in the canyon and hard to see in the brush.

You'll find flat sandy areas suitable for camping every mile or two along the route. Treat stream water before you drink it. The unmaintained Ellis Apiary trail camp, marked by an old metal camp stove on an oak-shaded bench on the west bank of Piru Creek, is a possible place to spend the night.

From Frenchmans Flat, work your way down the cottonwood- and willow-fringed banks, crossing whenever necessary. (Anglers by the score park at Frenchmans Flat and then hike down along Piru Creek in search of trout fishing holes, so there may be plenty of human company initially. Fishing here is catch-and-release only.) Look for a fisherman's trail on the south bank that leads about 0.7 mile to a campsite before becoming indistinct after the first stream crossing. The stream slips over water-worn boulders, some the size of cars, and collects in silt-bottomed pools. You should resign yourself right away to walking in squishy shoes. Once you get used to it, the interludes of wading will feel refreshing. If you find the stream crossings or obstacles difficult in the first mile or two, go ahead and turn around, because countless tougher challenges lie ahead.

The tilted, seamed, and shattered walls down the length of the gorge ahead, up to 500 feet high, disclose at least five distinct changes in the bedrock as you travel downstream. These rocks reflect a variety of ages, from older than 600 million years (Precambrian metamorphic rocks) to tens of millions of years old (Eocene sedimentary rocks). Several faults cross the route, including the northernmost end of the San Gabriel Fault. If you care to keep apprised of your progress down the canyon, be sure to keep updating your position on a topographic map. The Fish Creek confluence at 5.8 miles into the hike is a major milestone; there you change your general direction of travel from west to south. Travel beyond here may be particularly challenging.

The most interesting part of the canyon is an otherworldly passage of the Piru Narrows starting at mile 9.8. There you make your way between grotesquely sculpted conglomerate-rock walls, wading or swimming most of the time. Watch for a travertine stalactite hanging from an overhang on the right wall as you enter The Narrows. Toward the end, you might be fortunate enough to find a three-tiered waterfall showering down from a tributary into Piru Creek. The Narrows end before you reach the confluence of Ruby Canyon at mile 11.3.

South of that narrow section the canyon widens considerably and you sometimes have the luxury of walking on flat, sandy terraces on either side of the creek. After passing Ellis Apiary at the mouth of Turtle Canyon (12.3 miles), you can follow a remnant of the old Cobblestone Trail on the canyon's west side for some distance before being forced back into the rocky bed of the creek. At 14.5 miles you pick up traces of an old road that will take you past a spur on the right, into Agua Blanca Canyon, and a private ranch near the defunct Blue Point Campground (1,130'), some 16 miles from Frenchmans Flat. The campground was closed in 2000 to protect the endangered arroyo toad, burned in the 2007 Ranch Fire, and was demolished by the U.S. Forest Service in 2018. You're now 6 miles away by paved road, closed to vehicle traffic, from where you can reliably reach a parked automobile: the entrance to Lake Piru. Perhaps you planted a second car there earlier, or someone can meet you at that finish point.

chapter 21

Liebre Mountain & Fish Canyon

I (Jerry) made my first acquaintance with Angeles National Forest as a child, while riding in the family car north of L.A. on Highway 99 (yesteryear's version of the 5 Freeway). The signs said NATIONAL FOREST, but my obvious question—probably voiced by millions before and since—was simply, "Where are the trees?"

There are trees aplenty, if you know where to look for them—high on the ridges, down in the canyons, tucked away on north-facing slopes. If you take literally the poetic name of the chaparral—elfin forest—well, there's plenty of that along I-5 as well. In fact, 78% of the entire Angeles National Forest is covered by either chaparral or sage-scrub vegetation.

The predominance of chaparral is particularly true in the area mapped for this chapter. It is part of a triangular-shaped region bounded by the south edge of Antelope Valley on the north, the 5 Freeway on the southwest, and the 14 Freeway on the southeast. In a geologic sense this triangle is simply an extension of the San Gabriel Mountains, though you don't usually find that name associated with it on maps.

This chapter once included eight trips in this triangular area, but there are now just two. This is because road access over the years has been increasingly restricted and cost-cutting measures have left most trails in the area virtually abandoned, save for the Pacific Crest Trail. Several U.S. Forest Service campgrounds have also been abandoned in recent years.

A few hardy adventurers continue to explore the rugged and forbidding interior spaces around Red Rock Mountain and Cienaga Canyon on the sketchiest of trails. Previous editions of this book may be of help if you wish to do further research on the old, disused trails.

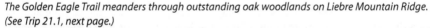

The Golden Eagle Trail meanders through outstanding oak woodlands on Liebre Mountain Ridge. (See Trip 21.1, next page.)

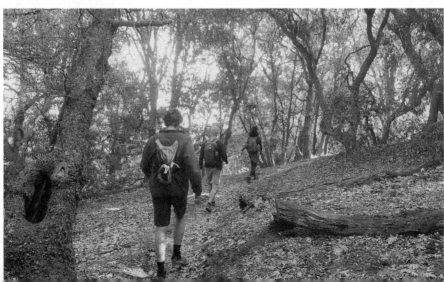

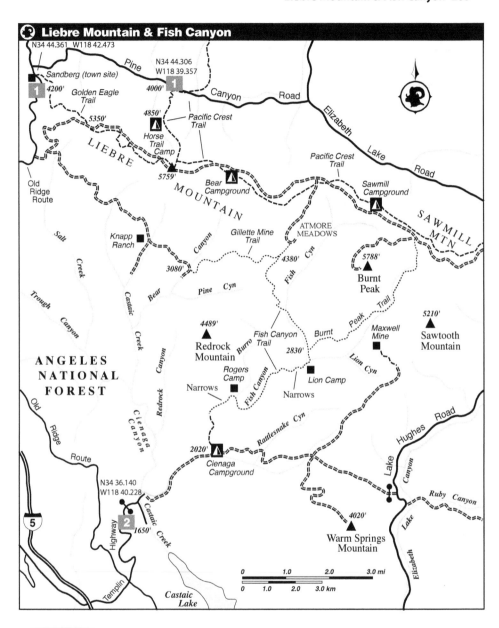

trip 21.1   Liebre Mountain

Distance	10 miles (one-way)
Hiking Time	5 hours
Elevation Gain/Loss	2,000'/1,800'
Difficulty	Moderately strenuous
Trail Use	Suitable for backpacking, dogs allowed
Best Times	October–June
Agency	Angeles National Forest
Recommended Map	Trails Illustrated *Angeles National Forest (811)*

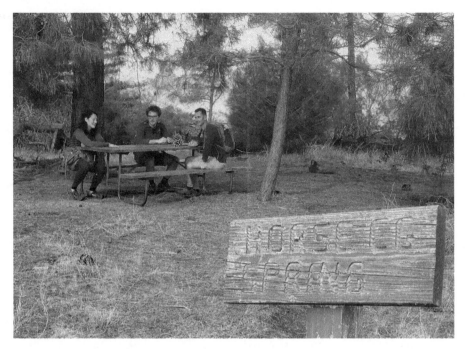

Enjoy a snack break at the Horse Camp picnic bench.

DIRECTIONS This trip requires a 5-mile car or bicycle shuttle. From the 5 Freeway, exit east on Highway 138. Go 4.3 miles; then turn right on the Old Ridge Route (County Road N2). Go 2.2 miles to Pine Canyon Road. Continue 0.5 mile on the Old Ridge Route to a turnout on the right with a plaque marking the site of the historic Sandberg Inn, where you can leave your getaway vehicle.

Return to Pine Canyon Road and turn right (east). In 4.3 miles, at a crest of a hill just beyond mile marker 13.60, turn right (south) on a rutted dirt road. Follow the road 0.1 mile to its end at the Pacific Crest Trail. If the road is washed out and your vehicle has low clearance, consider parking on the shoulder of Pine Canyon instead.

The cool, forested north slopes of Liebre Mountain rear up in stark contrast to the wide, brown Antelope Valley at their feet. The San Andreas Fault, which lies along Liebre Mountain's north base, is responsible for this juxtaposition. Vertical movements have occurred along the fault, as well as the more familiar horizontal movements.

Atop Liebre Mountain's sparsely wooded, mile-high crest you can gaze north to the rolling Tehachapis and the southern Sierra, west toward the Sespe country and the highest (8,000+') summits of Los Padres National Forest, and south and southeast over much of Angeles National Forest. Seemingly at your feet is the flat, arid floor of the Mojave Desert, stretching to a hazy vanishing point on the eastern horizon. The peak is named for the 1846 Mexican land grant Rancho La Liebre (*liebre* is Spanish for "hare").

From the trailhead, take the Pacific Crest Trail (PCT) and begin a leisurely switchback ascent through red-barked manzanitas, wispy gray pines, and deciduous black oaks. Patches of Great Basin sagebrush remind you that the high desert is not far away. The mix of mountain–desert vegetation is soon enhanced by many California buckeye shrubs. Leafless and gray until about April, buckeye becomes one of California's most handsome blooming plants by June, showing off myriad sprays of white blossoms. Buckeye is also known as horse chestnut for its huge seeds, which are mildly poisonous. Botanically, this slope resembles much of Central California's Coast Ranges and the lower Sierra foothills. Here on Liebre Mountain, both buckeye and gray pine are very close to their southern geographical limits. The area bears scars from the 2004 Pine Fire set by an arsonist, but much regrowth has occurred.

At 1.7 miles the trail becomes steeper amidst closely spaced pines. On a little flat to the right, you'll discover Horse Camp, with a picnic table, for hikers on the PCT. The breeze soughing through the long, thin pine needles overhead sets a peaceful mood, and the desert air, whether warm or cool, feels nice on the skin. You might find water seasonally in the canyon to the west, via a short trail from the campsite.

Past the campsite, you continue over the broad top of a 4,923-foot peaklet and descend to a wooded saddle. From there the trail switchbacks up through big-cone Douglas-fir and joins an old road bed. You enter a grassy clearing dotted with black oaks (5,400')—a good place to admire the view of the Antelope Valley while catching your breath. Ahead another half hour (3.5 miles from the start), you arrive at a signed junction where the PCT veers east toward Sawmill Mountain.

The high point of Liebre Mountain (5,760') is just beyond the junction, but the viewless summit is covered in foxtail barley, which has unpleasant barbs that catch in your socks, so you may prefer to skip it. (Dog owners should be especially wary, because the barbs can get into animals' eyes and cause blindness.)

You are almost on the long flat oak-dotted ridge of Liebre, which you will follow west. You have two choices of how to travel. The lightly used Liebre Mountain Truck Trail is easy walking and has good scenery. You can reach it by continuing to the crest and turning right.

Alternatively, an abandoned segment of the PCT called the Golden Eagle Trail parallels the road, first on the north side and later on the south. Originally PCT travelers were to have used this alignment, passing near Quail Lake, to reach the Tehachapis. Later the PCT was rerouted on the path you followed up the hill. The Golden Eagle Trail begins on the right at an easily overlooked junction along a fence line just yards above the sign where the PCT turns left. As of 2018, the delightful trail was in good shape and receives regular use from mountain bikers. However, it could easily become overgrown if it is not maintained. Parts of the trail follow slopes adorned with canyon live oak and mistletoe-studded black

Liebre Mountain is one of the best places in Angeles National Forest to experience oak woodlands.

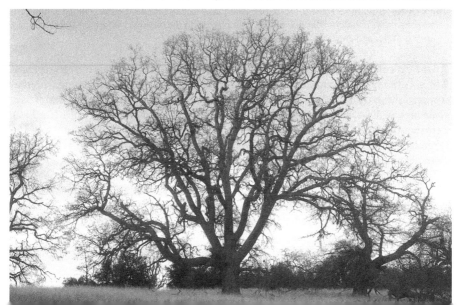

oak, while other parts resemble a tunnel through the tall chaparral. Some old spur roads along the route offer plenty of space for primitive camping.

At mile 6.6 via the road (or a half mile more via the curving Golden Eagle Trail), take the narrow, unmarked but well-maintained Golden Eagle Trail where it crosses to the north side of the road. This point is 0.3 mile east of a 5,345-foot peaklet, labeled Sandberg on the USGS topo map, where the road bends left and starts descending quickly toward Old Ridge Route.

As you descend through the chaparral you'll spot the weathered concrete ribbon of Old Ridge Route winding like a snake down below. This venerable roadway was an important (and dreaded) link in the original Valley Route linking Los Angeles with the Central Valley and points north. Paved with a narrow ribbon of concrete in 1919, the Ridge Route between Castaic and Gorman featured 642 turns in 38 miles, the equivalent of 97 complete circles! Widening and additional asphalt paving in the 1920s eliminated about one-third of the turns. The road was virtually abandoned in 1933 when a new bypass (US 99) opened to the west, and the route finally closed after a 2005 washout. Today a third-generation Ridge Route—the eight-lane 5 Freeway—carries virtually 100% of the through traffic. The trail ends on Old Ridge Route's shoulder, near the defunct townsite of Sandberg, which was a popular stopover on the old highway.

VARIATION

If you lack a car or bike shuttle and don't want to add a 5-mile jog on the road to close the loop, you might prefer to make a 7-mile out-and-back hike on the PCT to Liebre Mountain.

---

trip 21.2   **Fish Canyon Narrows**

see map on p. 265

Distance	10 miles (out-and-back)
Hiking Time	5 hours
Elevation Gain	800'
Difficulty	Moderately strenuous
Trail Use	Suitable for backpacking, dogs allowed
Best Times	October–June
Agency	Angeles National Forest
Recommended Map	Trails Illustrated *Angeles National Forest (811)*

DIRECTIONS From the 5 Freeway north of Castaic, take Exit 183 for eastbound Templin Highway. In 4.3 miles park on the shoulder, in front of a gate that blocks the highway where a private L.A. Department of Water and Power road turns right toward Castaic Lake.

In the trenchlike confines of Fish Canyon, aridity and moisture stand side by side, separated by a matter of a few yards. Mountain mahogany, manzanita, and other drought-resistant chaparral shrubs cling to the walls, while a shallow stream gurgles merrily past a line of oaks, sycamores, willows, and cottonwoods. It's almost as if a little slice of the Pacific Northwest were transplanted to Southern California. Around the time of winter solstice, sunbeams fail to reach the innermost confines of the canyon and frost can linger on the creeping blackberry vines till midmorning.

This trip was once a short excursion from Cienaga Campground, but the campground was abandoned after the access road washed out in 2002. Now it's a longer undertaking starting with a walk up the closed road, but the walk is scenic and the easy miles pass quickly. Although the road is adorned with various NO TRESPASSING signs, the U.S. Forest Service confirms that this trip is open to hikers.

Walk around the gate on Templin Highway and continue up the pavement for 0.6 mile to cross Castaic Creek on a bridge. The road turns south, becomes dirt, and soon forks. Take the left fork toward the mouth of a canyon, and stay left again at a spur just beyond. You'll soon find yourself on an decaying ribbon of concrete threading alongside the creek through the narrow canyon beneath soaring walls of conglomerate rock.

The canyon widens as you pass the remains of the old Cienaga Campground at 2.9 miles. In another 0.1 mile, turn left onto an unsigned trail leading into Fish Canyon. This is a good place to learn to recognize the difference between poison oak and fake poison oak (*Rhus trilobata*), both of which grow side-by-side here. Both have leaves in groups of three, but fake poison oak has smaller leaves with a clublike shape. The oak-shaded trail takes you to a sharp bend to the right at 4.0 miles, where a narrow section of Fish Canyon begins. On the right, you can examine an old mining prospect, called the Pianobox, named for a piano that was once hauled in there by overly enthusiastic miners. You'll find a pleasant campsite beneath a huge coast live oak at Pianobox. Note that campfires are prohibited in Fish Canyon but camp stoves are normally allowed.

The narrow section ahead is flanked by towering walls made of strange, battered-looking, gray- and tan-colored rock. They're part of a 15-mile-wide formation of Precambrian gneiss (or metamorphosed granite) that covers most of Redrock Mountain, Sawmill Mountain, Fish Canyon, and upper Elizabeth Lake Canyon. Keep an eye out for a bolted sport-climbing route on the left soon after you enter the narrows. Only the merest pretense of a trail threads through the narrows, but the going is usually fairly easy along flat benches to either side of the creek. You'll cross the shallow creek two dozen times or more in the next mile, or you may find it expeditious to simply wade parts of it.

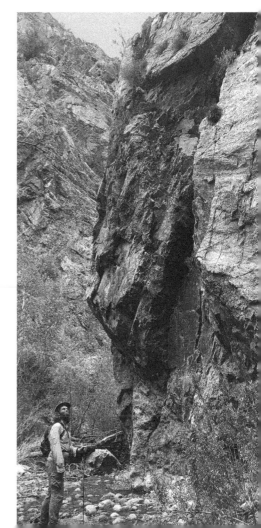

At 5.1 miles you come to a fork where Burro Canyon enters on the left. Look for unmaintained Rogers Camp on a grassy, oak-shaded bench on the left just before the confluence. This is a good turnaround point for a first hike or backpack into Fish Canyon.

Intrepid explorers can press on through an upper narrow section of Fish Canyon and perhaps trace the unmaintained upper Fish Canyon and Burnt Peak Trails, which climb the slopes of mile-high Liebre Mountain and Sawmill Mountain. These trails may have vanished or become badly overgrown in places.

The author enters Fish Canyon Narrows.
Photo: Werner Zorman

chapter 22

Tujunga Canyons

Rising starkly behind the San Fernando and La Crescenta Valley communities of Sylmar, San Fernando, Sunland, and Tujunga, the westernmost ridges of the main San Gabriels have a lean and hungry look—at least from a distance. As seen at closer range—as along Big Tujunga Canyon Road—that impression is certainly reinforced. Canyon walls, some soaring a half mile in height, bear scraggly growths of brush and widely scattered trees. Sharply cut ravines, filled with accumulated rock rubble, appear to sweep down from the rounded ridgelines above. There's an almost palpable sense of violent events past and future. Fires, floods, and landslides keep material on these slopes moving downward even as fault movements heave the whole mountain mass upward.

This dramatic, if unforgiving landscape has a gentler, mostly hidden side, too, discovered off the main roads and especially on the trails. You'll find mile-high peaks (including Mount Lukens, the highest point within L.A.'s city limits), one of the more picturesque waterfalls in the county (in Trail Canyon), riparian glens, and pocket forests of oaks and conifers.

Three large drainage systems penetrate the area. Pacoima Canyon, to the north, stretches east to Mount Gleason and drains the south slopes of the mile-high Santa Clara Divide.

Viewed from Yerba Buena Ridge, Mount Lukens is on the right in the foreground, Strawberry Peak is the highest point on the horizon to the left, and San Gabriel Peak is on the horizon in the center.

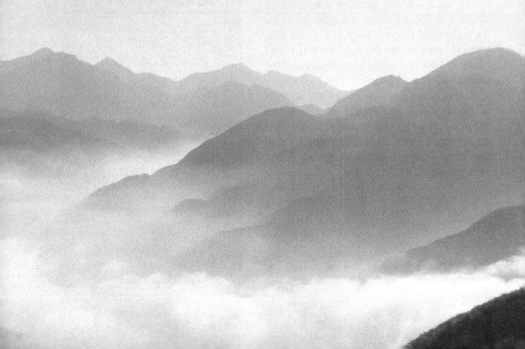

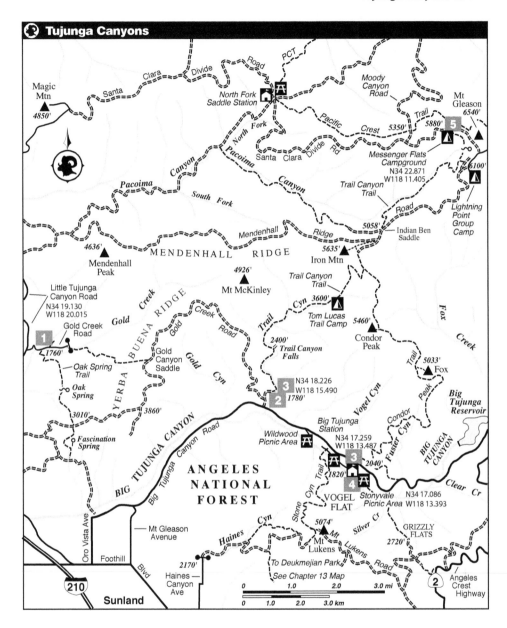

Little Tujunga Canyon, along with its biggest tributary, Gold Creek, drains the rolling foothill country between two prominent ridges: Mendenhall and Yerba Buena. Big Tujunga Canyon, the largest of the three, penetrates deep into the High Country of the San Gabriels. Big Tujunga Canyon Road threads the lower reaches of this canyon, permitting almost instant access to the canyon's lower trails by San Fernando Valley residents.

The Station Fire, which burned about 160,000 acres of the San Gabriel Mountains from August through October 2009, profoundly affected both of the Tujunga canyons. Many homes and trees were lost, but the chaparral and riparian vegetation have adapted well to fire and regrown quickly. The October 2017 Creek Fire scorched parts of the lower canyon.

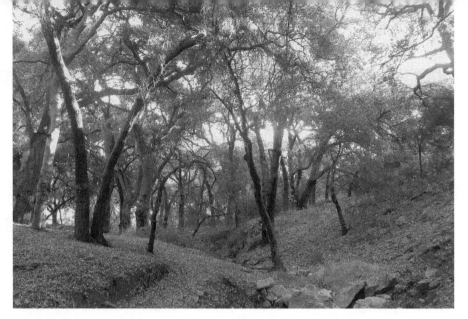

Lovely Oak Spring is tucked away in a crease of chaparral-clad Yerba Buena Ridge.

trip 22.1   Yerba Buena Ridge

see map on previous page

Distance	4.6 miles (out-and-back)
Hiking Time	3 hours
Elevation Gain	1,400'
Difficulty	Moderately strenuous
Trail Use	Suitable for backpacking, mountain biking, equestrians, dogs permitted
Best Times	October–May
Agency	Angeles National Forest
Recommended Map	Tom Harrison *Angeles Front Country* or Trails Illustrated *Angeles National Forest (811)*

DIRECTIONS From the 210 Freeway in Lake View Terrace, take Exit 8 for Osborne Street. The off-ramp will deposit you on Foothill Blvd, which you take one block north until you can turn left onto Osborne Street. After a mile Osborne Street becomes Little Tujunga Canyon Road. At 3.8 miles from I-210, turn right on Gold Creek Road. Continue 0.7 mile to signed Oak Spring Trail on the right, and park on the shoulder of the road or at the Oak Springs Picnic Area, just before the trail.

The Oak Spring Trail, right on the western border of Angeles National Forest, provides a quick escape from the teeming, aging suburban foothill and San Fernando Valley communities down below. This area burned in the 2017 Creek Fire, but the lovely oak grove was unscathed.

From the trailhead on Gold Creek Road, the Oak Spring Trail strikes steadily uphill. It switches back seven times into the burn zone, crosses a hillside, and climbs to a saddle. Here, a spur on the left leads to a hilltop view, but the main trail veers right over a second saddle, and then drops into a bowl containing a live oak grove surrounding Oak Spring (1.4 miles). The spring is one of the sources of the Los Angeles River. From there, the trail contours south for a while and then resumes climbing up ceanothus-smothered slopes that can become waves of white blossoms during the late winter or early spring.

After 2.4 miles of general ascent, you reach the wide, graded fire road following the crest of Yerba Buena Ridge. A rim-of-the-world view of the La Crescenta and San Fernando Valleys unfolds there.

VARIATIONS

You can make a wonderful loop with outstanding views of the Big Tujunga country by turning left and ascending the Yerba Buena Ridge Road (Forest Service Road 3N30). At the 3,892-foot-high point on the ridge, stay left to remain on the main road, and continue down to the wildly eroded Gold Canyon Saddle. Turn left again and descend the Boulder Canyon Road to the unsigned Boulder Canyon Trail. When it ends at gold Creek Road, continue downhill past Repticular Ranch to your vehicle. This loop is 9 miles with 2,400 feet of elevation gain.

You could also turn right, walk 100 yards down the road, and pick up the Fascination Spring trail on the left. Descend, staying left at a fork, 1 mile and 900 feet down to an underwhelming spring. A maze of dirt roads continues south and west, but the exit to Big Tujunga is blocked by private property.

---

trip 22.2　Trail Canyon Falls

see map on p. 271

Distance	4.5 miles (out-and-back)
Hiking Time	2 hours
Elevation Gain	1,000'
Difficulty	Moderate
Trail Use	Dogs allowed
Best Times	December–May
Agency	Angeles National Forest
Optional Map	Tom Harrison *Angeles Front Country* or Trails Illustrated *Angeles National Forest (811)*

DIRECTIONS From the 210 Freeway in Sunland, take Exit 11 for Sunland Boulevard. Go east for 0.7 mile, as the road name changes to Foothill Boulevard; then turn left onto Oro Vista Avenue. Proceed 5.3 miles as the road name changes to Big Tujunga Canyon Road. The trailhead is at mile marker 2.0. Park in the dirt turnout on the left, observing the sign that warns you not to block the gate on Forest Service Road 3N29. If the gate is open, you can drive 0.2 mile uphill to a fork, go right, and continue 0.2 mile down to a parking area, saving 0.8 mile round-trip.

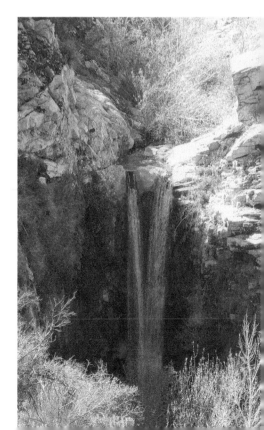

When soaking rains come, the normally indolent flow of Trail Canyon becomes a lively torrent. After it tumbles through miles of rock-bound constrictions and slides across many gently inclined declivities, the water comes to the lip of a real precipice. There the bubbly mixture momentarily attains weightlessness during a free-fall of about 30 feet. If you can manage to ignore the vastly smaller

Trail Canyon Falls can have an impressive flow. This is your best view from the trail—getting to the base can be messy.

scale of this spectacle, you might easily imagine yourself in Yosemite Valley during the spring runoff.

The falls in Trail Canyon are fairly easy to approach, except during the most intense flooding, when the several fords you must cross on the way may be dangerously deep. Sturdy footwear may be helpful at some of the deeper crossings in high water.

If the gate on Forest Service Road 3N29 at Big Tujunga Canyon Road is closed, walk past it and up the hill 0.2 mile to a fork. The Gold Canyon Road climbs to the left, but this trip goes right and descends to a trailhead sign in another 0.2 mile. If the gate is open, you may be able to drive to this point.

Continue up remnants of the same road on foot, passing a few cabins and fording the creek for the first time. The now-very-deteriorated road goes on to follow an east tributary for a while, doubles back, contours around a ridge, and drops into Trail Canyon again (0.6 mile). The old road ends there, and you continue upcanyon on a footpath. The path clings to the banks for 0.5 mile, crossing the stream several times, and then climbs the west wall to avoid a narrow, alder-choked section of the canyon. The falls come into view beneath Mount McKinley as you round a sharp bend about 1.5 miles from the parking area.

Shortly before the falls, you'll notice a use trail descending to the base. This route is potentially dangerous—assess the conditions for yourself before you try to navigate it. Alternatively, you can continue up the main trail to where it reaches the creek above the falls. The granite slabs and shallow pools make a good spot to enjoy a snack. From there, you can walk downstream and carefully peer over the lip of the falls. The Trail Canyon Trail continues on toward Condor Peak (see next trip), but you've already seen the most interesting part of the canyon.

trip 22.3 Condor Peak & Trail Canyon

see map on p. 271

Distance	16 miles (one-way)
Hiking Time	9 hours
Elevation Gain	4,300'
Difficulty	Strenuous
Trail Use	Suitable for backpacking, dogs allowed
Best Times	October–May
Agency	Angeles National Forest
Required Map	Tom Harrison *Angeles Front Country* or Trails Illustrated *Angeles National Forest (811)*

NOTES The segment of trail between Condor Peak and Trail Canyon Falls has been unmaintained since the 2009 Station Fire and is badly overgrown with buckthorn and riparian vegetation at the time of this writing. Before taking this trip, check with Angeles National Forest (626-574-1613, fs.usda.gov /angeles) for updates. If trail conditions haven't improved, you can still enjoy a good 15-mile out-and-back to Condor Peak on the Condor Peak Trail.

DIRECTIONS This trip requires a 2.5-mile car or bicycle shuttle or an unpleasant road walk. Leave a getaway vehicle at the Trail Canyon Trailhead on Big Tujunga Road. From the 210 Freeway in Sunland, take Exit 11 for Sunland Boulevard. Go east for 0.7 mile, as the road name changes to Foothill Boulevard; then turn left onto Oro Vista Avenue. Proceed 5.3 miles as the road name changes to Big Tujunga Canyon Road. The trailhead is at mile marker 2.0. Park in the dirt turnout on the left, observing the sign that warns you not to block the gate on Forest Service Road 3N29. Continue up Big Tujunga Canyon Road with your second vehicle for 2.5 miles to mile marker 4.5 (0.1 mile beyond Vogel Flat), and park in a dirt turnout on the right, taking care not to block another gated fire road.

This all-day trip has a bit of everything: long, winding passages across fragrant chaparral-clothed slopes; outstanding views from the open summit of Condor Peak; and a soothing, foot-wetting descent along Trail Canyon's delightful stream. The elevation gains and losses, however, are punishing to all but well-conditioned hikers and backpackers. Lug soles and long pants or gaiters are recommended. An early start, ideally before sunrise, is advised too. That way you can be off the lower, south-facing slopes before midday's heat. Beware of ticks, especially in the springtime, and watch for poison oak.

Condor Peak is named for the endangered California condor, which once nested on this mountain. At the start of the 20th century, as many as a dozen of the huge birds were reported to circle the peak at once. The condor's population collapsed due to poaching, lead poisoning, and habitat loss, and none have been observed here since World War II.

The unsigned and unlikely looking trail begins on the north side of the road immediately opposite your parking turnout. It climbs steeply, then traverses 0.3 mile to join the main Condor Peak Trail coming in from the east. This 1-mile-long trail was constructed in 1980 after rock slides had closed a section of Big Tujunga Canyon Road. Stay left at the trail junction and continue winding steadily uphill along the ridge between Vogel and Fusier Canyons. In March, thousands of white-flowering ceanothus shrubs burst into bloom on these slopes, suffusing the air with a sublime perfume. Nearly all of the conifers on the south slope have been wiped out by a series of fires.

After 2.2 miles the trail crosses a narrow saddle and begins curving around gullies above Fusier Canyon. The biggest gully you cross (3.2 miles) is a cool, ferny oasis with surface water present until at least April or May. At 5.9 miles (4,600'), the Condor Peak Trail joins an old firebreak coming down from Fox Peak—one of several bumps on the ridge running

The Condor Peak Trail climbs through rugged and lonely country.

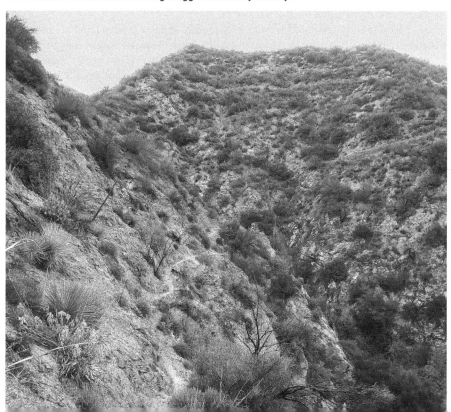

northwest toward Condor Peak. Follow the firebreak up and over the undulating ridge 1.3 miles more to a point just below the east brow of Condor Peak. Leave the trail and scramble 300 feet up the slope on sandy soil and over fractured granite. The westernmost, 5,460-foot peaklet on the windswept summit plateau is the highest and holds the climbers register. A pleasant, but dry camp could be made here on the summit plateau or on any neighboring ridge, if the weather is calm.

From Condor Peak, the Pacific Ocean sprawls more than a quarter of the way around the compass. To the south, barely clearing the broad profile of Mount Lukens, Santa Catalina Island floats in serene splendor on the hazy blue horizon. To the west, over the San Fernando Valley and through the low gap of Santa Susana Pass, rises Santa Cruz Island, the biggest and tallest of the Channel Islands, about 90 miles away.

VARIATION

If time allows, consider scrambling 0.8 mile down the ridge west of Condor Peak to a 5,250-foot knob. From there you can peer almost straight down on upper Trail Canyon, threaded by a dark-green line of riparian vegetation.

After soaking in the view, retrace your way back to the Condor Peak Trail and continue going north on the old firebreak through a sea of buckthorn. At 9.3 miles you come to a 4,840-foot saddle at the head of Trail Canyon and the intersection of the Trail Canyon Trail. Make a sharp left and zigzag steeply down the ceanothus-clad slopes to a dry, sloping bench. At 10.7 miles you reach the line of willow and bay trees making up Big Cienega, the source of Trail Canyon's almost-perennial stream.

This stretch is presently a nasty bushwhack. Tom Lucas Trail Camp was once situated below Big Cienega but was wiped out by the fire. Tom Lucas was an early ranger in the area after the San Gabriel Timberland Reserve was established in 1892. He later had a ranch in Big Tujunga Canyon and hunted grizzly bears.

By 12.5 miles you've escaped the worst of the brush, and you reach a small campsite with a metal fire grate. The trail repeatedly crosses the creek in the trenchlike canyon. At 13.3 miles cross again on a granite slab near a shallow pool above Trail Canyon Falls. Shortly beyond, look back for views of the falls. Stay on the main path as it eventually joins an old road, passes cabins, and drops to the trailhead at Big Tujunga Canyon.

VARIATION

Fox Peak (5,033') is an easy climb from the saddle to the northwest, with 350 feet of elevation gain over 0.2 mile on a use trail. Iron Mountain, the highest point in the vicinity (5,635'), is somewhat more work, with 800 feet of elevation gain over 0.7 mile via a steep climbers' trail branching off the firebreak.

---

trip 22.4 Mount Lukens & Grizzly Flats Loop

see map on p. 271

Distance	13 miles (loop)
Hiking Time	8 hours
Elevation Gain	3,400'
Difficulty	Strenuous
Trail Use	Suitable for backpacking, dogs allowed
Best Times	October–May
Agency	Angeles National Forest
Recommended Map	Tom Harrison *Angeles Front Country* or Trails Illustrated *Angeles National Forest (811)*

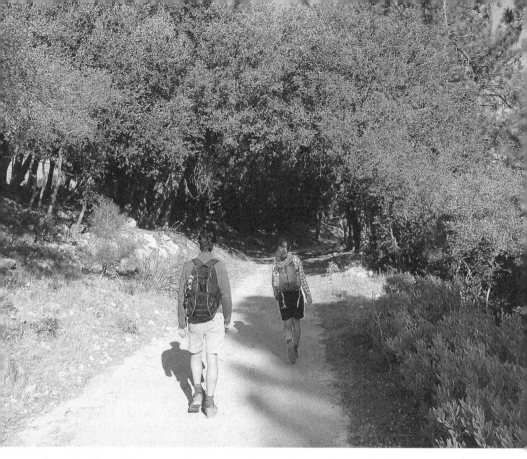

The trail to Mount Lukens passes through a small grove of canyon live oaks just below the summit.

DIRECTIONS From the 210 Freeway in Sunland, take Exit 11 for Sunland Boulevard. Go east for 0.7 mile, as the road name changes to Foothill Boulevard; then turn left onto Oro Vista Avenue. Proceed 7.7 miles as the road name changes to Big Tujunga Canyon Road. Turn right onto Vogel Flat Road; then veer left at the bottom of the hill onto Stonyvale Road, and go 0.2 mile to its end at the Stonyvale Picnic Area.

This all-day adventure lets you walk on the wild side of the Tujunga canyon-and-peak country. After a grueling climb up the north slope from Big Tujunga Canyon, circle back by way of a long, gradually descending route that passes through secluded Grizzly Flats. The hike feels best on a cool day, but beware of periods following heavy rain: the trip begins and ends with crossings of Big Tujunga Creek, which can be hazardous in high water. If you're in doubt, contact Angeles National Forest to check on flood conditions. The trail and homes around Vogel Flat burned in the 2009 Station Fire. The route has reopened and chaparral has regrown, but most of the big old trees are gone. This is a wild hike, with steep narrow sections of lightly maintained trail, but is highly rewarding for those who wish to escape the crowds.

Grizzly Flats is named for the grizzly bear, which is California's state mammal and is featured on the flag. Some 10,000 grizzlies roamed the state at their peak in the early 19th century. Many were shot for sport, but many others were killed when they threatened humans and livestock. In 1916, Cornelius Johnson, a Big Tujunga fruit rancher, killed the last known grizzly bear in Southern California, after the bear spent three nights ransacking his orchard. By 1924, the grizzly was extinct in California.

On foot, head west on Stonyvale Road 0.3 mile to the Vogel Flat Picnic Area, and continue down the narrow, paved road (private, but with public easement) through the cabin community of Stonyvale. When the pavement ends after 0.7 mile, continue on dirt for another quarter mile or so. Choose a safe place to ford Big Tujunga Creek, wade across, and find the Stone Canyon Trail on the far bank. From afar you can spot this trail going straight up the sloping terrace just left (east) of Stone Canyon's wide, boulder-filled mouth. Settle into a pace that will allow you to persevere over the next 3 miles and 3,200 feet of vertical ascent.

From the vantage point of the first switchback, you can look down on the thousands of storm-tossed granitic boulders filling Stone Canyon from wall to wall. Although the boulders are frozen in place, you can almost sense their movement over geologic time. Indeed, floods continue to reshape this canyon and many others in the San Gabriels during every major deluge.

Ahead, you turn along precipitous, chaparral-covered slopes. At or near ground level, a profusion of ferns, mosses, and herbaceous plants forms its own pygmy understory. The dizzying view encompasses a long, obviously linear stretch of Big Tujunga Canyon. This segment of the canyon is underlain by the San Gabriel Fault and its offshoot, the Sierra Madre Fault. The latter fault splits from the former near Vogel Flat and continues southeast past Grizzly Flat, following a course roughly coincident with the final leg of this loop hike.

According to current understanding, the San Gabriel Fault is presently inactive and not likely to be the cause of major movement or earthquakes in the near future. The depth of Big Tujunga Canyon and the steepness of its walls are due primarily to stream cutting following uplift of the whole mountain range.

Between 2.4 and 3.3 miles (from the start), the trail hovers above an unnamed canyon to the east, nearly equal in drainage to Stone Canyon, but very steep and narrow. Down below you can often hear, and barely glimpse, an inaccessible waterfall. Long and short switchback segments take you rapidly higher to a steep, bulldozed track leading to the bald summit ridge of Mount Lukens. Go 0.5 mile farther, connecting with Mount Lukens Road along the way, to reach the 5,075-foot highest point on the ridge (5.1 miles), which is occupied by several antenna structures.

Lukens's summit technically lies within the city limits of Los Angeles and is the highest point in any incorporated city in the county; Glendale almost claims this honor, as its corporate limit reaches within 300 yards of the summit. Both cities encompass parts of the Angeles National Forest, of course. The view can be fabulous on a clear day.

The remaining two-thirds of the hike is almost entirely downhill—a little monotonous, but mostly easy on the knees. Follow Mount Lukens Road southeast down the main ridge. At 6.1 miles stay left at a junction with an abandoned road that descends to Deukmejian Wilderness Park (see Trip 13.1, page 181). At 8.1 miles stay left again at a junction with a service road leading 4 miles down to the Angeles Crest Fire Station. At 10.1 miles reach a four-way junction at a saddle—the Upper Dark Canyon Trail, on the right, descends to Highway 2, and the abandoned fire road ahead also continues to the Grizzly Flat Trailhead on Highway 2. Our trip turns left and descends on a zigzag course to Grizzly Flats (11.3 miles) near a ravine called Vasquez Creek.

The trees that once graced this area are mostly gone after the Station Fire, and a maze of roads and trails also vanished, including the old Dark Canyon Trail from Angeles Crest Highway to Big Tujunga Canyon—roughly the escape route used by the outlaw Tiburcio Vasquez and his unsuccessful pursuers during a hot chase more than a century ago.

Follow the trail down to a creek, eventually descend sharply down a ridge overlooking the pitlike gorge of Silver Creek, and finally reach a wildflower-dotted bench along Big Tujunga Creek. Watch for signs of former homesteads. Head downstream, crossing the creek three times in the next mile, to reach your car at Stonyvale Picnic Area.

VARIATIONS

The shortest way up Mount Lukens is from the Wildwood Picnic Area on the Stone Canyon Trail. This route is 8 miles out-and-back with 3,300 feet of elevation gain.

Mount Lukens can also be approached from the Angeles Crest Highway to the east. Park at the Grizzly Flats Trailhead (mile marker 2 LA 30.60), Dark Canyon Trailhead (2 LA 30.00), or Angeles Crest Fire Station (2 LA 27.65). The map shows many potential loops.

---

trip 22.5 Messenger Flats

see
map on
p. 271

Distance	3.3 miles (loop)
Hiking Time	2 hours
Elevation Gain	800'
Difficulty	Moderate
Trail Use	Dogs allowed, good for kids
Best Times	March–November
Agency	Angeles National Forest
Optional Map	Tom Harrison *Angeles Front Country* or Trails Illustrated *Angeles National Forest (811)*

NOTES Santa Clara Divide Road (Forest Service Road 3N17) has been closed since the 2009 Station Fire and remains so at the time of this writing. Check with Angeles National Forest (818-899-1900, fs.usda .gov/angeles) for updates; if it hasn't reopened, you face a very long walk or bike ride to the trailhead.

DIRECTIONS Exit the Antelope Valley Freeway (Highway 14) at Angeles Forest Highway, 5 miles south of Palmdale. Follow Angeles Forest Highway south into the San Gabriel Mountains. After about 10 miles of uphill driving, you reach the Mill Creek summit. Turn right (west) there on Mount Gleason Road (aka Santa Clara Divide Road/FS 3N17). After another 10 miles on this mostly paved but narrow national-forest roadway, you'll arrive at the trailhead, at Messenger Flats Campground.

Tucked amid a lovely grove of pines on the remote north ridge of the San Gabriel Mountains is pint-size Messenger Flats Campground, an Angeles National Forest facility available on a first-come, first-served basis. The Pacific Crest Trail (PCT), the 2,650-mile "gorilla" of all hiking trails in the West, passes right through, and you can use a section of it to piece together a scenic 3.3-mile hike overlooking the vast Mojave Desert, which lies to the north.

Note that Messenger Flats Campground is seasonally closed due to snow at some point during the winter season. Also, if you're interested in mountain biking in this area, be aware that you must stay on any of the numerous forest roadways in the area. The PCT is off-limits to all mechanized transport, including bicycles.

The PCT parallels Santa Clara Divide Road at a point 20 yards north of the campground entrance. Go left (west) and follow the trail as it veers away from the road and starts to descend along steep, north-facing slopes. This is a narrow, rough-cut, seldom traveled section of the PCT. Conifers and oaks provide welcome shade at frequent intervals. Far below is Soledad Canyon, the broad east–west gash separating the main block of the San Gabriel Mountains from outlying ranges to the northwest. In the hills beyond Soledad Canyon, the tilted sedimentary slabs known as the Vasquez Rocks glow a bright beige amid the otherwise muted gray-green and brown land.

After 1.5 miles the PCT dips into a shady ravine and crosses Moody Canyon Road. Leave the trail and follow the road 0.2 mile uphill to Santa Clara Divide Road. Turn left there and return to Messenger Flats, uphill all the way.

chapter 23

Arroyo Seco & Front Range

Three miles from Barley Flats is the Red Box on the divide between the head of the West Fork Cañon and the cañon of the Arroyo Seco. . . . Here is the parting of the ways for many points—for the Arroyo Seco, for the Upper Tujunga, for Mount Wilson, for Eaton's Cañon, for the camps of the San Gabriel River. Four miles and the man in a hurry may be at Alpine Tavern on Mount Lowe, whence an electric car will whisk him in two hours to Los Angeles.

—Charles Francis Saunders, *The Southern Sierras of California, 1923*

The Front Range has drawn recreational visitors for over a century. In this chapter and the next, we'll cover a host of trail trips featuring fantastic views from high ridges, passages through lush forests, and visits to sparkling waterfalls and mirrorlike pools.

Although hardly qualifying as wilderness by bureaucratic standards (there are too many roads through it), much of the Arroyo Seco area has the look and the feel of wilderness. Most of the fire roads that were carved into the mountainsides decades ago are now blocked to unauthorized vehicle traffic. Once off the pavement, travelers must get around on their own power, much as people did during the so-called Great Hiking Era of the early 1900s. Then, the Front Range and high country beyond were regarded as a local frontier for weekend exploration and recreation. Scenic trails were constructed, and dozens of trailside camps

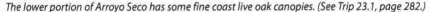

The lower portion of Arroyo Seco has some fine coast live oak canopies. (See Trip 23.1, page 282.)

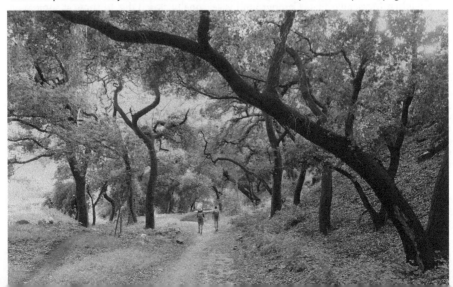

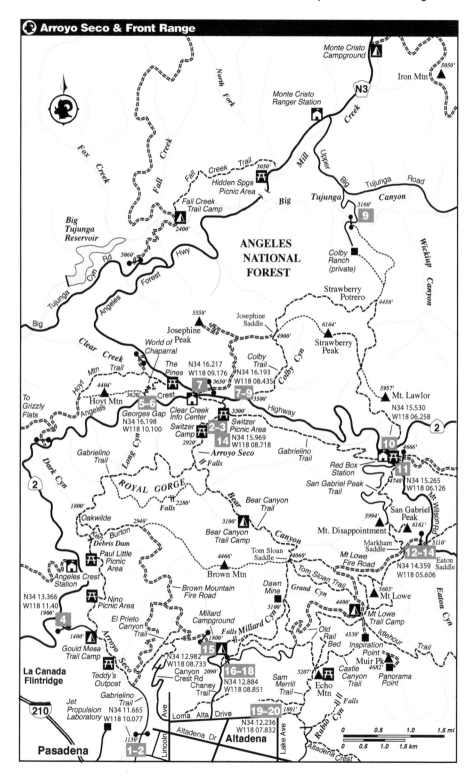

and hostelries sprang up to serve the needs of overnight guests. The road-building era that followed in the late 1930s and '40s ended that idyllic chapter of the mountains' history.

There's a renewed interest in rambling the mountains of the Front Range today, with the focus on day hiking. Volunteers have teamed up with the U.S. Forest Service to refurbish the old trails and construct new ones. Several of the old resorts have been replaced by trail camps that are popular on weekends among youth groups and backpackers.

A clear advantage of the Front Range trails is that many of them can be reached so quickly and easily from the metropolitan basin below. Down in the canyon recesses, a hiker can quickly forget the sights and sounds of L.A., hardly aware that his or her peaceful, uncrowded world lies only a few miles from the edge of one of the world's largest cities.

The Station Fire, which swept through about 160,000 acres of the San Gabriel Mountains from August through October 2009, profoundly affected nearly all of the trips in this chapter. Riparian vegetation in the canyon and ravine bottoms and chaparral zones on the slopes have recovered quickly, but the conifers at the higher elevations may never return. Many of the trails were closed for years, with the Arroyo Seco finally fully reopening in 2018.

trip 23.1   Lower Arroyo Seco

see map on previous page

Distance	5 miles (out-and-back)
Hiking Time	3 hours
Elevation Gain	300'
Difficulty	Moderately strenuous
Trail Use	Suitable for backpacking, suitable for mountain biking, equestrians, dogs allowed, good for kids
Best Times	October–June
Agency	Angeles National Forest
Optional Map	Tom Harrison *Angeles Front Country* or Trails Illustrated *Angeles National Forest (811)*

DIRECTIONS From the 210 Freeway in Pasadena, take Exit 22B for northbound Windsor Avenue. In 0.8 mile park at a busy lot on the left, where Windsor meets Ventura Street.

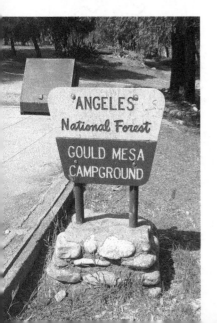

The popular lower portion of the Arroyo Seco Trail draws scores of hikers, mountain bikers, joggers, and even parents pushing strollers. Despite the name Arroyo Seco ("Dry Wash")—which the Spanish gave because the waters sink into the sand in the Los Angeles basin below Devil's Gate—in the winter and spring you can expect a lively, flowing creek lined with lush vegetation. This out-and-back trip takes you to a popular trail camp. You can easily shorten or extend the trip to your liking (also see the next trip to go the whole way).

From the parking area, you walk north onto a gated paved road signed as the Gabrielino Trail. The white buildings of Caltech's famed Jet Propulsion Laboratory (JPL) are prominent on the far side of the Arroyo Seco. In 0.7 mile come to a junction with the Altadena Crest

A man named Will Gould homesteaded in the 1890s on land that is now a campground named in his honor.

Trail on the right and a bridge to the JPL on the left—continue straight through a second gate. Shortly thereafter, cross a bridge over a tributary creek and then a second bridge over the Arroyo Seco as the canyon narrows and the scenery greatly improves. You can easily access the creek here to play in the water, or sit on a bench and take in the view. Beware of poison oak, which is plentiful along the entire route.

Riparian and coastal sage-scrub habitats mingle along the canyon, offering a diverse and beautiful environment. Alder, willow, and mule fat are most common along the creek, while graceful coast live oaks grow on the banks pleasantly shading the trail. Prominent shrubs include ceanothus, elderberry, laurel sumac, and bush poppy, while California sagebrush and sage are common ground cover. Wild cucumber vines entwine all of the plants. Spring wildflowers include wild pea, purple nightshade, bush poppy, bush lupine, and many more. Various invasive plants, especially periwinkle, Scotch broom, and eupatory, have further displaced native species after the fire.

Cross a third bridge, and then, at 1.3 miles, pass Lower Brown Mountain Road on the right—stay left on Forest Service Road 2N70A, the main track up the canyon. Shortly thereafter, pass some private residences and a drinking fountain. At 1.7 miles cross a fourth bridge to reach Teddy's Outpost Picnic Area, with a shady bench and easy access to a pleasant part of the creek. The outpost was once a tourist camp with a store and cabins built by Theodore Sylvertson in 1914, but it was condemned in 1925 by the City of Pasadena Water Department. This is a good turnaround point for a short trip.

The trail narrows as you cross three more bridges and enter Angeles National Forest. At 2.3 miles ford the creek; then reach Gould Mesa Camp at 2.6 miles. The well-situated campsite has many tent sites, an outhouse, and various out-of-place trees and agaves. At the far end of the camp, signed, partially paved Gould Mesa Road (FS 2N69) climbs a mile to meet Angeles Crest Highway at mile marker 2 LA 26.47. This is a good turnaround point, but if you wish to keep going, the Nino and Paul Little Picnic Areas are, respectively, 0.5 and 1.7 miles farther upcanyon, and the artificial waterfall of Brown Mountain Dam is shortly beyond these.

VARIATION

You can extend this trip into an excellent 15-mile loop by continuing up the Arroyo Seco to the former Oakwilde Campground, turning right on the signed Ken Burton Trail (6 miles), and climbing to a saddle at the north end of the Brown Mountain Road (8.2 miles). Follow the road until it splits on a saddle at 11.0 miles; then stay right on FS 2N66 and follow it down to the mouth of El Prieto Canyon (13.6 miles). Turn right and continue 0.2 mile to rejoin the Arroyo Seco Trail, where you turn left and return to the trailhead. This variation has 2,200 feet of elevation gain. Mountain bikers prefer to do it in reverse, climbing the Brown Mountain Road before making a fun descent of Ken Burton and Arroyo Seco.

---

trip 23.2   Down the Arroyo Seco

see map on p. 281

Distance	10 miles (one-way)
Hiking Time	5 hours
Elevation Gain/Loss	300'/2,300'
Difficulty	Moderately strenuous
Trail Use	Suitable for backpacking, suitable for mountain biking, dogs allowed
Best Times	October–June
Agency	Angeles National Forest
Optional Map	Tom Harrison *Angeles Front Country* or Trails Illustrated *Angeles National Forest (811)*

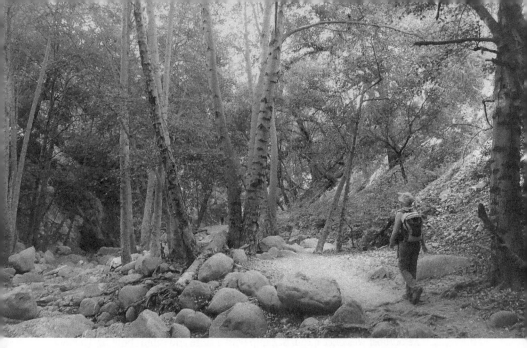

Riparian trees line the banks of the Arroyo Seco between Switzer Picnic Area and the falls.

DIRECTIONS This trip requires a 15-mile car shuttle or ride-sharing trip. Leave your getaway vehicle at the south end of the hike: From the 210 Freeway in Pasadena, take Exit 22B for northbound Windsor Avenue. In 0.8 mile park at a busy lot on the left, where Windsor meets Ventura Street.

   To reach the north end, return to the 210 and go west to Highway 2, then 10 miles north to the turnoff for Switzer Picnic Area, on the right (mile marker 2 LA 34.2). Continue 0.5 mile down the paved access road to the parking lot next to the picnic area. (If the lot is full or the access road happens to be closed and gated, you can park at the top and walk down into the picnic area—250 feet of elevation loss in a half mile.)

The Spanish colonists who christened Arroyo Seco ("dry creek") evidently observed only its lower end—a hot, boulder-strewn wash emptying into the Los Angeles River. Upstream, inside the confines of the San Gabriels, Arroyo Seco is a scenic treasure—all the more astounding when you consider that its exquisite sylvan glens and sparkling brook lie just 12–15 miles from L.A.'s city center. If you haven't yet been freed from the notion that Los Angeles is nothing but a seething megalopolis, walk down the canyon of the Arroyo Seco. You'll be persuaded otherwise.

A botanist's and wildflower seeker's dream, the canyon features generous growths of canyon live oak, Western sycamore, California bay, white alder, big-leaf maple, big-cone Douglas-fir, and arroyo willow. A quick census one spring day—in a dry year, no less—yielded for me (Jerry) the following blooming plants: golden yarrow, prickly phlox, Western wallflower, Indian pink, live-forever, wild pea, deerweed, bush lupine, Spanish broom, baby-blue-eyes, yerba santa, phacelia, chia, black sage, bush poppy, California buckwheat, shooting star, Western clematis, Indian paintbrush, sticky monkey flower, scarlet bugler, and purple nightshade. On other spring days, I've also seen yellow monkey flower, California bells, California poppies, pointed cryptantha, blue dicks, pearly everlasting, larkspur, miners' lettuce, Chinese houses, bluehead gilia, white nightshade, and Humboldt lilies. Watch for seasonal waterfalls along the canyon; in the summer, watch for scarlet monkey flower by the water. This is one of the best trails in the San Gabriels to see woolly mullein, a striking but invasive plant with wide, fuzzy leaves that sends up a tall stalk with small yellow flowers. Beware of poison oak, which is plentiful near the trail.

You'll be traveling the westernmost leg of the Gabrielino Trail, one of four routes in Angeles National Forest designated as National Recreation Trails. The Arroyo Seco stretch of the Gabrielino Trail receives considerable use by (and much-needed maintenance from) mountain bikers. The upper and middle portions, narrow in places with steep drops to one side, are challenging even for expert riders, but they aren't at all hard for hikers. The lower end consists of remnants of an old road built as far up the canyon as Oak Wilde resort in the 1920s.

Bob and Elizabeth Waterman first raised awareness of Arroyo Seco's recreational opportunities when they spent a month-long honeymoon exploring the canyon in 1883. They laboriously chopped a horse trail up the canyon, guarded their packs from hungry bears, built a rock stairway around the waterfall later known as Switzer Falls, and spent several days camped at a lovely spot above the falls. Upon the Watermans' return, "Commodore" Perry Switzer, a Los Angeles carpenter, heard their tale of adventure and built a resort at the aforementioned lovely spot.

Switzer's Camp, established in 1884 and comanaged by the Watermans, was the first of many mountain camps in the San Gabriel Mountains. To escape the summer heat of the valley, throngs of tourists would ride temperamental burros for 8 miles up the Arroyo Seco, crossing the creek 60 times before reaching the camp. Guests would blow a cow horn as they neared the camp, and the cook would listen for the number of blasts to prepare the proper amount of trout for the hungry visitors. Food and lodging cost $1.50 per night.

But in spite of its popularity, the resort was never financially successful, and Switzer retired in 1894. An 1896 wildfire burned most of the Arroyo Seco, including the resort. Lloyd Austin, a former YMCA director, took over and rebuilt the resort in 1912, turning "Switzer-Land" into the leading wilderness retreat in the San Gabriels, drawing church groups, Boy Scouts, and Hollywood stars. He constructed a splendid chapel on a cliff above Switzer Falls, designed by architect Arthur Benson of Mission Inn fame. The camp's glory began to fade, however, when the Angeles Crest Highway to Red Box was finished in 1934, opening the wilderness to cars.

The trip is a testament to the San Gabriel Mountains' awesome powers to wipe itself clean of man's imprint through fire, flood, and avalanche. In the early 1900s, many tourist camps and cabins were erected along the canyon. Virtually all of the structures were either destroyed by flooding in 1938 or removed through condemnation proceedings (based on water and flood-control needs) in the 1920s, '30s, and '40s. Many of these sites were converted to picnic sites and trail camps, but the 2009 Station Fire obliterated some of them.

The trail was badly damaged after the Station Fire but reopened in 2018 following extensive repairs led by mountain bike clubs.

*Woolly mullein (*Verbascum thapsus*) is a striking European plant that has become naturalized in the Arroyo Seco. The tall stalk produces hundreds of small yellow flowers.*

Some kind of car shuttle or drop-off-and-pick-up transportation arrangement is obviously required for this long one-way hike or backpack trip. It's easy to hail a ride-sharing service at the bottom trailhead, and that may be less expensive than bringing a second vehicle. Carry along whatever drinking water you'll need for the duration of the trip; there may be piped water at one or another of the rest stops along the way, but don't count on it. Pleasantly shaded Gould Mesa Campground is the best place to stay if you're backpacking the route.

From the west end of the Switzer Picnic Area, start hiking on the Gabrielino Trail at a sign for Switzer Falls. Make your way across the bridge and along a road past outlying picnic tables, and then down along the alder-shaded stream. Soon nothing but the clear-flowing stream and rustling leaves disturb the silence. Remnants of an old paved road are occasionally underfoot. In a couple of spots you ford the stream by boulder-hopping—no problem except after heavy rain.

One mile down the canyon you come upon the foundation remnants of Switzer's Camp, now a trail campground. The main trail crosses to the west side of the creek at Switzer's Camp. Don't be lured onto one of the use trails continuing down the east side to crumbling cliffs above Switzer Falls, where many fatal accidents have occurred. Watch for the foundations of Christ Chapel on the cliff high above the falls.

Walk down to a fork in the trail at 1.3 miles. You will probably hear, if not clearly see, the 50-foot cascade known as Switzer Falls, to the east. It's worth the short detour if the water is running well. Our trip continues on the right fork (Gabrielino Trail), which now begins a mile-long traverse through chaparral. This less-than-perfectly-scenic stretch avoids a narrow, twisting trench called Royal Gorge, through which the Arroyo Seco stream tumbles and sometimes abruptly drops.

At 2.6 miles the trail joins a shady tributary of Long Canyon and, later, Long Canyon itself, replete with a trickling stream. The trail mostly clings to a narrow ledge cut at great effort into the east wall of the canyon. Alongside the trail you'll discover at least five kinds of ferns, plus mosses, miner's lettuce, poison oak, and Humboldt lilies (in bloom during early summer).

At 3.9 miles the waters of Long Canyon swish down through a sculpted grotto to join Arroyo Seco. At 5.2 miles pass the signed Ken Burton Trail on the left, favored by mountain bikers. The trail descends to Arroyo Seco canyon's narrow floor and stays there, crossing and recrossing many times over the next few miles (count on getting your feet wet in the spring). The trail may disappear in the wash, but just continue downstream through the gorgeous gorge, flanked by soaring walls and dappled with shade cast by the ever-present alders.

Big-leaf maples put on a great show here in November, their bright yellow leaves boldly contrasting with the earthy greens, grays, and browns of the canyon's dimly lit bottom. Camp Oak Wilde, operated by J. R. Phillips, stood here from 1911 until it was destroyed by flooding in 1938. Oakwilde Campground was rebuilt in the same place but was wiped out by the Station Fire.

The canyon widens a bit. At 5.9 miles your way is abruptly blocked by the large Brown Canyon Debris Dam. Built in the 1940s to reduce the flow of detritus into Pasadena, it has completely filled up and no longer serves its purpose, but it remains as a scar on the canyon that will take nature many more years to demolish. Just short of the dam, the trail climbs onto the east wall of the canyon, bypasses the dam, and descends steeply to reach the canyon bottom at a sign for the Paul Little Memorial Picnic Area.

The hardest work is over, and a decent path takes you down the remainder of the gently sloping canyon. Pass the Nino Picnic Area. The trail gradually improves into a road and crosses eight bridges in varying states of repair. At 8.1 miles pass busy Gould Mesa Campground, named for Will Gould, a homesteader who lived here in the 1890s. After Teddy's Outpost Picnic Area and the south end of the burn area, watch for a gauging station on the right and some U.S. Forest Service residences on the left. The last segment of the trail is paved and you are likely to run into cyclists, joggers, parents pushing strollers, and even skateboarders. Pass the imposing complex of Caltech's Jet Propulsion Laboratory on the right and eventually emerge at the Arroyo Boulevard trailhead.

trip 23.3 Switzer Falls

see map on p. 281

Distance	3.8 miles (out-and-back)
Hiking Time	2 hours
Elevation Gain	700'
Difficulty	Moderate
Trail Use	Suitable for backpacking, dogs allowed, good for kids
Best Times	Year-round
Agency	Angeles National Forest
Optional Map	Tom Harrison *Angeles Front Country* or Trails Illustrated *Angeles National Forest (811)*

DIRECTIONS Exit the 210 Freeway at Angeles Crest Highway (Highway 2) in La Cañada Flintridge. Drive 10 miles north to the turnoff for Switzer Picnic Area on the right (mile marker 2 LA 34.2). Drive 0.5 mile down the paved access road to the parking lot next to the picnic area where the road makes a hairpin turn. (If the access road happens to be closed and gated, you can park at the top and walk down into the picnic area—250 feet of elevation loss in a half mile.)

Amid a precarious setting of crumbling rock walls, the waters of the upper Arroyo Seco slide some 50 feet down a steep incline known as Switzer Falls. Normally a modest dribble, but occasionally an exuberant cascade, the falls are tantalizingly secretive—they can be approached at close range only by some foolhardy scrambling over unstable or slippery rock (definitely not recommended, as many people have been killed or seriously hurt this way). This route takes you by trail around the main falls and down to a lesser cascade in the canyon below.

Take the signed Gabrielino Trail toward Switzer Falls, past outlying picnic tables and then down along the alder-shaded stream. Soon nothing but the clear-flowing stream and rustling leaves disturb the silence. Remnants of an old paved road are occasionally underfoot. In a couple of spots, you ford the stream by boulder-hopping—no problem except after heavy rains.

One mile down the canyon, you come upon a picnic area at the foundation remnants of Switzer's Camp. Established in 1884 by "Commodore" Perry Switzer, the camp became the

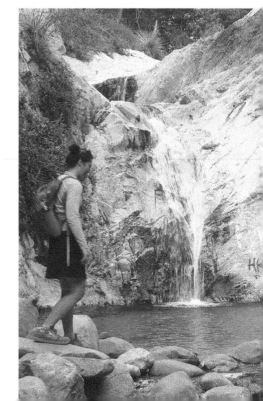

Lower Switzer Falls is a popular destination on a nice spring day.

San Gabriels' premier wilderness resort in the early 1900s, patronized by Hollywood celebrities along with anyone who had the gumption to hike or ride a burro up the tortuous Arroyo Seco trail from Pasadena. After the completion of Angeles Crest Highway as far as Red Box in 1934, and then a severe flood in 1938, the resort lost its appeal. It was finally razed in the late 1950s, but you can still picnic here.

Below Switzer's Camp the stream slides 50 feet over Switzer Falls—but don't go that way. Instead, continue on the Gabrielino Trail as it edges along the canyon's right (west) wall. To the left are glimpses of the falls, a dark pit below them, and the crumbled foundation of a miniature stone chapel (a part of the resort) that perched on a ledge above the falls. Continue 0.3 mile to a trail junction. Take the left fork (the trail to Bear Canyon) and descend to the canyon bottom (1.7 miles). There's a severe, unfenced drop-off on the left on the way down, so watch your step and that of your kids.

Turn left at the canyon bottom and walk along the banks, or rock-hop through the stream itself, 0.2 mile upcanyon. You'll come upon a dark, shallow pool, fed by a 15-foot-high cascade just below the main Switzer Falls. This is a peaceful and secluded spot for a picnic. Climbing farther upcanyon is hazardous.

trip 23.4　Royal Gorge

Distance	13 miles (out-and-back)
Hiking Time	8 hours
Elevation Gain	1,800'
Difficulty	Strenuous
Trail Use	Suitable for backpacking, dogs allowed
Best Times	October–July
Agency	Angeles National Forest
Recommended Map	Tom Harrison *Angeles Front Country* or Trails Illustrated *Angeles National Forest (811)*

see map on p. 281

The Arroyo Seco makes long meanders as it squeezes through rugged Royal Gorge.

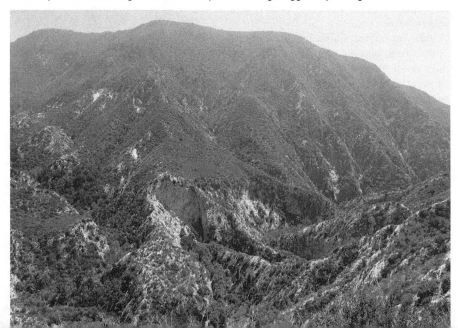

DIRECTIONS Exit the 210 Freeway at Angeles Crest Highway (Highway 2) in La Cañada Flintridge. Drive 2 miles north to a turnout on the right, at mile marker 2 LA 26.47 near paved, gated Forest Service Road 2N69 leading down to Gould Mesa Campground.

Easy trail hiking, then moderate boulder-hopping, and finally some knee-deep wading will take you far into the sublime hideaway of the Royal Gorge, the narrow, rock-walled section of Arroyo Seco that has repelled trail builders for over a century. There you'll come upon a small waterfall and a deep, dark, swimmable pool whose setting suggests the name "Royal Pool" or perhaps "King's Bathtub."

From the parking area, step around the locked gate and descend 1 mile on a paved service road to reach the Gabrielino Trail, just upstream from Gould Mesa Campground. Follow the Gabrielino Trail upstream (north) past Oakwilde Trail Camp (3.7 miles) to the point where the Gabrielino Trail leaves Arroyo Seco and starts going up Long Canyon (5.0 miles). Abandon the trail at this point and start boulder-hopping up the main stream to the right—this is Royal Gorge. (*Note:* Forget about reaching the Royal Pool if the first couple of creek crossings are difficult; that would indicate that the water level is extraordinarily high.)

After following the stream around several horseshoe bends for at least an hour, you enter a section of the gorge where the sheer walls pinch in tight. Clamber over some boulders and wade through a couple of pools to reach the Royal Pool ahead. Fed by water that slides about 8 feet down a 45° incline, then 10 feet more almost vertically, the rock-bound pool measures about 50 feet long and 30 feet wide under optimal conditions, though it can dry up to almost nothing.

Rock climbers can bypass the falls with a Class 4 traverse on the south wall. Note that the rock can be slimy and a slip would lead to a nasty fall.

VARIATION

It's possible to approach the upper lip of the falls from the upstream side (a 1.5-hour boulder-hop and bushwhack through alders from the Bear Canyon Trail). Bring a 25-meter (about 80-foot) rope, some long slings, and rappelling gear if you wish to descend the waterfall. A small rock ledge juts from the base of the falls near the pool's surface. Anyone using the falls as a waterslide would probably experience a very hard (possibly fatal) landing.

---

trip 23.5 World of Chaparral Trail

Distance	2.8 miles (out-and-back)	
Hiking Time	1.5 hours	
Elevation Gain	700'	
Difficulty	Easy	
Trail Use	Dogs allowed	
Best Times	October–June	
Agency	Angeles National Forest	
Optional Map	Tom Harrison *Angeles Front Country*	

see map on p. 281

DIRECTIONS Exit the 210 Freeway at Angeles Crest Highway (Highway 2) in La Cañada Flintridge. Drive 8 miles north the Georges Gap parking area, at mile marker 2 LA 32.82.

The World of Chaparral Trail (11W03) connects the Georges Gap trailhead to the abandoned Pines Picnic Area by way of Clear Creek. This short but strenuous trail has good views of Josephine and Strawberry Peaks and is especially pleasant in the spring when the chaparral is in bloom and the creek is flowing. Avoid it on warm days, when the canyon becomes a furnace.

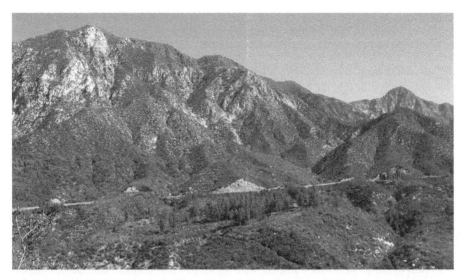

Viewed from the World of Chaparral Trail, Josephine Mountain (left) and Strawberry Peak (right) have imposing granite faces.

From Georges Gap, glance south to view the skyline of Los Angeles, sometimes crystal clear but other times shrouded in smog. Turn north and begin the switchbacks descending to Clear Creek. Watch for clematis, a vine with showy yellow and white flowers that turn into odd hairballs, weaving through the scrub oak, ceanothus, and other chaparral. The top of the trail has the best views of rocky Josephine Peak to the north, with Strawberry Peak to its right.

At 0.8 mile, just before reaching Clear Creek, pass a turnoff for the Hoyt Mountain Trail (11W04) on the left leading up to Grizzly Flat Road—our route continues down to the creek, crossing it just above a small pool and cascade that runs only in the wet season. This is a good turnaround point for families. Otherwise, continue up a narrow ridge and stay on the main path to reach a parking area for the abandoned Pines Picnic Area. Return the way you came.

trip 23.6	**Hoyt Mountain**

see map on p. 281

Distance	3.4 miles (loop)
Hiking Time	2 hours
Elevation Gain	1,300'
Difficulty	Moderate
Trail Use	Dogs allowed
Best Times	October–June
Agency	Angeles National Forest
Optional Map	Tom Harrison *Angeles Front Country*

DIRECTIONS Exit the 210 Freeway at Angeles Crest Highway (Highway 2) in La Cañada Flintridge. Drive 8 miles north the Georges Gap parking area, at mile marker 2 LA 32.82.

Lightly climbed but surprisingly fun, Hoyt Mountain (4,404') has great views and is a short drive along the Angeles Crest Highway. This rugged loop climbs the mountain via a firebreak on the east ridge, then descends the west ridge to Hoyt Saddle and loops back via the poorly maintained Hoyt Mountain Trail. Go on a cool day. If you don't like bushwhacking, check with Angeles National Forest beforehand to inquire if the Hoyt Mountain Trail has been cleared recently. The mountain is named for Silas Hoyt, who homesteaded in Big Tujunga Canyon around 1883.

From the Georges Gap parking area, find the steep firebreak going straight up the east ridge of Hoyt Mountain. Beware of Whipple yucca as you make this short but demanding climb, gaining 800 feet over 0.7 mile. On the summit, you may find a curious tepee made of yucca stalks. Looking west and then turning clockwise, your views encompass antenna-clad Mount Lukens, the deep trench of Big Tujunga Canyon, Condor Peak, burned-out Mount Gleason, rocky Josephine and Strawberry Peaks, Mount Lawlor, Mount Disappoint-

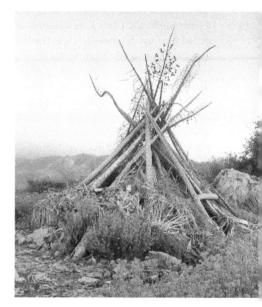

ment, Mount Lowe, the Arroyo Seco, Pasadena, the Los Angeles Skyline, and possibly Catalina Island.

Find a trail descending the west ridge to Hoyt Saddle (1.1 miles), where you meet the overgrown Grizzly Flat Road, which services high-voltage transmission lines. Turn right (north) and follow an abandoned road cut, now known as the Hoyt Mountain Trail (11W04). Parts of this fun trail cling to the rocky mountainside below decomposing cliffs, while others thread through a tunnel of tall ceanothus. This path was first cut as a power-line road by the Southern California Edison Company in 1925–26. If the trail is unmaintained, it could quickly become a nasty bushwhack in places.

At 2.5 miles, just before the old road crosses Clear Creek, turn sharply right onto a narrow, unmarked trail. Climb to a junction with the World of Chaparral Trail (11W03) at 2.6 miles. Stay right and follow the switchbacks up sunbaked slopes back to Georges Trail.

Somebody built a yucca shelter on Hoyt Mountain.

VARIATION

Hoyt Mountain can also be climbed from the Grizzly Flats Trailhead via the Grizzly Flats Road to Hoyt Saddle. This route is 4.8 miles round-trip with 1,500 feet of elevation gain and avoids some of the possible brushy spots, but follows an ugly set of power lines.

---

trip 23.7   **Josephine Peak**

Distance	8 miles (loop)
Hiking Time	4 hours
Elevation Gain	2,100'
Difficulty	Strenuous
Trail Use	Dogs allowed
Best Times	October–June
Agency	Angeles National Forest
Recommended Map	Tom Harrison *Angeles Front Country* or Trails Illustrated *Angeles National Forest (811)*

see map on p. 281

DIRECTIONS Exit the 210 Freeway at Angeles Crest Highway (Highway 2) in La Cañada Flintridge. Drive 9.4 miles north to the junction with the Angeles Forest Highway at mile marker 33.80, where you could leave a car or bicycle shuttle at a large dirt turnout on the north side of the road. Continue 0.8 mile on the Angeles Crest Highway to the Colby Canyon Trailhead, at an unpaved turnout on the left at mile marker 34.55.

Josephine Peak (5,558') offers a vigorous but straightforward climb to great views over the Front Range. Historians debate whether the peak was named for the daughter of Phil Begue, an early ranger in the area, or for the wife of J. B. Lippencott, a USGS surveyor who mapped the San Gabriel Mountains from the summit in 1894. This route makes a loop up the beautiful Colby Canyon Trail to Josephine Saddle and Josephine Peak, then back down a fire road to the Clear Creek Ranger Station. It involves a 0.8-mile walk along the shoulder of the busy highway to close the loop; consider bringing a bicycle or second vehicle to avoid the road walk. Go on a clear cool day to enjoy this shadeless hike through the high chaparral. Mountain bikers may prefer to go up and down the Josephine Fire Road rather than climbing the steep and exposed Colby Canyon Trail.

The lower Colby Canyon Trail is masterfully designed, leading through a gorgeous canyon with year-round water, then along narrow ridges and across a cliff face. This scenic stretch eventually gives way to switchbacks climbing through the chaparral to reach Josephine Saddle at 2.1 miles.

A trail continues north over the saddle to Strawberry Potrero and Strawberry Peak (see Trips 23.8 and 23.9, pages 293 and 295), but our route turns left along a ridgeline trail. At 2.6 miles join Josephine Fire Road (2N64) at a hairpin turn. Turn right and follow this road to the summit (4 miles). The fire lookout that once stood here burned in the 1976 Big Tujunga Fire, but the road is still maintained to service an antenna station.

To make a loop, descend the fire road 4 miles back to the Clear Creek Fire Station, and then turn left and follow the Angeles Crest Highway back to the Colby Canyon Trailhead. You could also pick up the Nature's Canteen Trail at the ranger station parking lot, which runs just below the south side of the highway for half the way before ending at the Switzer Picnic Area road.

Hulking Josephine Mountain, as seen from Hoyt Mountain, towers over the Angeles Forest Highway.

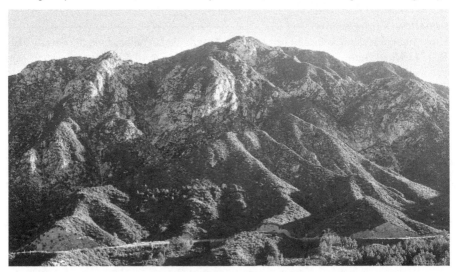

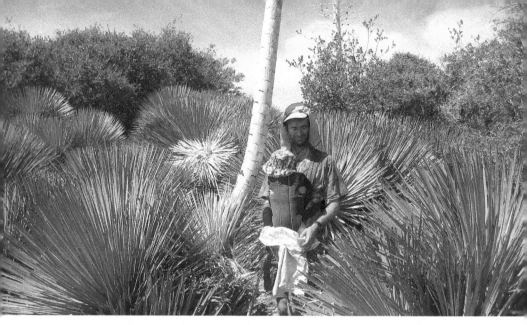

The author navigates a maze of Whipple yucca on the way to Strawberry Peak. Careful—don't poke the sleeping baby. Photo: Evan Harris

trip 23.8 Strawberry Peak

Distance	7 miles (out-and-back)
Hiking Time	6 hours
Elevation Gain	2,700'
Difficulty	Strenuous
Trail Use	Dogs
Best Times	October–June
Agency	Angeles National Forest
Recommended Map	Tom Harrison *Angeles Front Country*

see map on p. 281

DIRECTIONS Exit the 210 Freeway at Angeles Crest Highway (Highway 2) in La Cañada Flintridge. Drive 10.2 miles north to the Colby Canyon Trailhead, at an unpaved turnout on the left at mile marker 34.55.

> *A well-worn trail followed the crest of one of the several ridges that radiate from the peak, and brought me to the base of an apparently perpendicular cliff a couple of hundred feet high and forming the last stage to the summit. A close scanning of the cliff's broken face showed plainly that the only way up was to scale it as best I could; so, holding on by fingers and toes, and carefully testing the stability of the jutting rocks, root-ends, and clinging bushes which served me as pegs to climb by, I got on pretty well.*
>
> —Charles Francis Saunders, The Southern Sierras of California, *1923*

Strawberry Peak's 6,164-foot summit beats by a smidgen 6,161-foot San Gabriel Peak, thus claiming the honor of being the highest peak in the Front Range, as well as the most fun. Although its profile appears rounded as seen from most places, in reality its flanks fall away sharply on three sides, leaving only one relatively easy route to the top. The peak was named by guests at Switzer's Camp, who felt its profile resembled a strawberry. Switzer himself would lead his guests on a favorite hike up Strawberry by way of the airy ridge in the 1880s. He carried a Winchester rifle on his saddle to defend against grizzly bears.

In March 1909, Strawberry Peak garnered national attention when a gas balloon and gondola carrying six passengers over Tournament Park in Pasadena was swept by violent gusts into storm clouds over the San Gabriel Mountains. After being tossed to as high as 14,000 feet, the balloon descended in white-out conditions and crash-landed just below Strawberry's snow-covered summit—its gondola coming to rest just 10 feet from a vertical precipice. Nearly three days later, a telephone call from Switzer's Camp brought news to the world below that the riders had survived.

This hike takes the most fun route to the summit by way of Colby Canyon and the steep west ridge. It is not the easiest route (see the variation below) and is not recommended for hikers who are uncomfortable with heights or scrambling. Long pants are recommended because of the sharp vegetation. You'll be traveling mostly along hot, south-facing slopes and open ridges exposed to the sun, so an early-morning start is best.

The lower Colby Canyon Trail is masterfully designed, leading through a gorgeous canyon with year-round water, then along narrow ridges and across a cliff face. This scenic stretch eventually gives way to switchbacks climbing through the chaparral to reach Josephine Saddle, 2.1 miles.

From the saddle, trails depart west toward Josephine Peak and north toward Strawberry Potrero. Head north about 20 yards; then look for a prominent climbers' trail on the right that follows a ridge directly to Strawberry Peak. Follow this route, which is generally in good condition because of heavy use. In 0.2 mile reach the first obstacle: a steep step of decomposing granite. The trail may be vague here, but it's worth finding because getting off route takes you across dangerous crumbling rock. Beyond this step, dodge prickly Whipple yuccas for 0.7 mile of easy ridge walking. Then pick a path across a talus field to the steep ridge where the climbing gets fun.

Start just right of the crest and look for faded painted arrows or flagging marking the route. The climbing is Class 2–3—fun but nowhere near as difficult as Saunders described— so long as you stay on the easiest route. However, straying from the route quickly leads you to sheer cliffs, and deaths and rescues have occurred here. Pay close attention so you can retrace your route on the descent.

Scattered Coulter pines and big-cone Douglas-firs struggle for existence near the summit, their windblown limbs swept back in gestures that seem defiant. The view from the top is panoramic, but not so exciting as from peaks such as Mount Lowe or Mount Lukens. On the other hand, Strawberry often basks in clean air while the basin-bordering ramparts are wreathed in smog.

VARIATIONS

One could avoid descending the steep rocks and could make a loop around the mountain by descending the trail on the east side to the saddle between Lawlor and Strawberry, then turning north and circling back to Josephine Saddle. This area burned badly in the Station Fire, but the trail has been repaired and stays in good shape thanks to mountain bikers. A flat beneath the north face has great views and camping possibilities beneath a surviving stand of Coulter pines. This loop is 12 miles with 3,500 feet of elevation gain.

Enthusiastic hikers can make a side trip to Josephine Peak from Josephine Saddle (see previous trip). This adds 4 miles out-and-back.

Strawberry Peak can also be climbed from Red Box Gap by way of the saddle between Lawlor and Strawberry. This trail is in good condition all the way and is substantially easier but not nearly as fun. The out-and-back trip is 7 miles with 1,700 feet of elevation gain.

trip 23.9   Colby Canyon to Big Tujunga

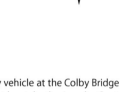

see map on p. 281

Distance	7 miles (one-way)
Hiking Time	5 hours
Elevation Gain/Loss	1,700'/2,000'
Difficulty	Moderately strenuous
Trail Use	Suitable for backpacking, dogs allowed
Best Times	October–May
Agency	Angeles National Forest
Recommended Map	Tom Harrison *Angeles Front Country*

DIRECTIONS This trip requires an 11-mile car shuttle. Leave your getaway vehicle at the Colby Bridge trailhead: To reach Colby Bridge from the 210 Freeway in La Cañada Flintridge, take the Angeles Crest Highway (Highway 2) north for 9.5 miles to the Clear Creek Ranger Station; then turn north on Angeles Forest Highway. Proceed 8.4 miles and turn right on Upper Big Tujunga Road. Continue 1.3 miles and turn right on a dead-end road to Colby Camp. Follow narrow and sharply twisting pavement to a large U.S. Forest Service parking area immediately beyond a bridge over Big Tujunga Creek.

    To reach the starting point, return to Clear Creek Ranger Station and proceed east 0.9 mile on the Angeles Crest Highway to the Colby Canyon trailhead at an unpaved turnout on the left at mile marker 34.55.

A newer bypass of the old Colby Trail through Colby Ranch allows hikers to swing by Strawberry Peak and descend all the way to the bank of Big Tujunga Canyon's creek. (Formerly, the trail ended inside the ranch property—now a private Methodist camp.) For the most part you'll be following a route hewn over the mountains in the 1890s by pioneer Delos Colby. The trail connected Switzer's Camp in the Arroyo Seco with Colby's ranch in Coldwater Canyon, a tributary of Big Tujunga. Around the turn of the 20th century, the ranch catered to hikers, hunters, and fishermen independent and determined enough to travel beyond the fancy resorts of the Arroyo Seco and Mount Lowe areas.

    The highlight of the trip is Strawberry Potrero, a series of gentle depressions tucked under the granite cliffs and talus of Strawberry Peak's sheer north flank. Beyond Strawberry Potrero, the route tends to be less maintained and possibly overgrown and sketchy.

    From the turnout on Angeles Crest Highway, head up the Colby Trail. In the first half mile you'll be charmed by the woodsy atmosphere and (in season at least) the brook trickling down the narrow canyon bottom. All too soon you're struggling up slopes thickly grown with chaparral and punctuated by the giant white plumes of blooming yuccas. The well-graded but at times rock-strewn trail zigzags expeditiously to Josephine Saddle, 2.1 miles. There you meet a trail going west toward Josephine Peak, but our route continues north over the saddle. Almost immediately you'll notice the well-worn climbers' route to Strawberry's summit veering right up the ridge (see previous trip)—stay on the main trail.

    For 2 more miles, the trail stays close to the 5,000-foot contour, bending around precipitous gullies that often serve as chutes for rockfall. Unlike Strawberry Peak's wind-beaten, nearly barren top (unseen more than 1,000' above), oaks, pines, and big-cone Douglas-firs cling tenaciously to this level of the mountain—wherever they survived the Station Fire and the soil is stable enough to retain moisture. Clusters of prickly phlox and Indian paintbrush brighten the muted tones of earth and forest.

    Following a moderate descent, you arrive (4.5 miles) at the westernmost clearing of Strawberry Potrero (the Spanish word *potrero* means "pasture"), a sandy basin ringed by live oaks and Coulter pines. The sheer, granite cliffs and talus of Strawberry Peak's north face preside over this superb camping or picnic spot. In the spring, water might be obtained from runoff or snowmelt on the slopes above.

Continue east along the base of the talus slope, pass through a second clearing, and descend through a shady ravine to a third, open basin—this one a true meadow filled with sedges and grasses.

At a signed trail junction, 5.1 miles from the start, go left (north). When you come to the next fork, 0.2 mile farther, keep right (northeast) on the trail down to Colby Bridge at Big Tujunga rather than the private trail to Colby Camp.

The route ahead was badly damaged by the fire and has not been repaired at the time of this writing. You may find an overgrown path staying east of the ridgeline, but it is easier to remain on the ridge. When the ridge splits, stay left and follow a better-defined path northwest down to meet the paved road to Colby Camp at a gate. Turn right and follow the paved road down to the Colby Bridge trailhead.

trip 23.10 Mount Lawlor

see map on p. 281

Distance	6 miles (out-and-back)
Hiking Time	3 hours
Elevation Gain	1,300'
Difficulty	Moderately strenuous
Trail Use	Dogs allowed
Best Times	October–June
Agency	Angeles National Forest
Recommended Map	Tom Harrison *Angeles Front Country*

DIRECTIONS Exit the 210 Freeway at Angeles Crest Highway (Highway 2) in La Cañada Flintridge. Drive 14 miles north and east to Red Box Station (mile marker 2 LA 38.38, at the intersection of Mount Wilson Road). Park in either the ranger station or picnic-ground lots.

Mount Lawlor (5,957') is one of the underappreciated summits of the San Gabriels, but it offers a fun moderate climb and a panoramic view on a cool clear day. The mountain was named in 1890 by the U.S. Forest Service in honor of Oscar Lawler, a prominent Los Angeles lawyer and conservationist, and the spelling became corrupted. The chaparral-clad slopes burned in the 2009 Station Fire but have largely recovered.

From the Red Box parking area, cross the highway and walk east a few dozen yards to an abandoned service road that has now deteriorated into a trail. Follow this path for 0.8 mile until the road becomes impassable and a good trail veers off to the left. Take this trail, reaching a saddle at 1.1 miles and a second, more prominent saddle, at 2.4 miles.

The main trail continues north, but climbers' trails split off west and east from here to Strawberry Peak and Mount Lawlor. Turn right and follow the path east to the summit of Mount Lawlor. The ridge-hugging route is rocky in places and occasionally brushy, but it receives enough use that it is not overgrown.

Horned lizards (Phrynosoma coronatum) are skilled at camouflage, so it's satisfying to spot one along the trail.

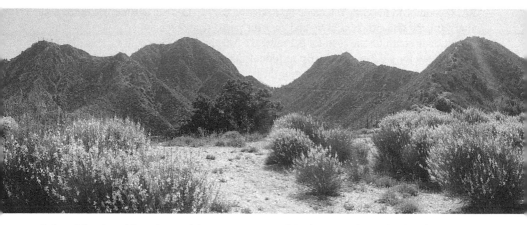

(Left to right, viewed from the west) Disappointment Peak (with towers), San Gabriel Peak, Markham Saddle, Mount Markham, and Mount Lowe

trip 23.11 San Gabriel Peak

Distance	3.7 miles (out-and-back)
Hiking Time	2.5 hours
Elevation Gain	1,400'
Difficulty	Moderate
Trail Use	Dogs allowed
Best Times	Year-round
Agency	Angeles National Forest
Optional Map	Tom Harrison *Angeles Front Country* (trail not shown)

see map on p. 281

DIRECTIONS Exit the 210 Freeway at Angeles Crest Highway (Highway 2) in La Cañada Flintridge. Drive 14 miles north and east to Red Box Station and the intersection of Mount Wilson Road at mile marker 2 LA 38.38. Turn right on Mount Wilson Road and proceed just 0.4 mile to a turnout at the gated Mount Disappointment Forest Service road (FS 2N52) on the right. This is also the trailhead for the San Gabriel Peak Trail.

The San Gabriel Peak/Bill Riley Trail, built by JPL (Jet Propulsion Laboratory) Hiking Club volunteers in 1987–88, bypasses a less-interesting paved service road to Mount Disappointment used by hikers in the past.

Disappointment was the name given to the peak in 1875 by surveyors who were trying to establish a triangulation point on the area's highest promontory. After a laborious struggle through brush, they discovered that they'd reached a false summit: San Gabriel Peak (6,161') lay just beyond and 200 feet higher.

Today's Mount Disappointment is a disappointing shadow of its former self. The U.S. Army blasted off its top in the 1950s, installed a Nike missile base, and built a service road to the top. Currently the flattened summit serves as an antenna site. San Gabriel Peak's summit is not so abused, and makes a fine destination for a high-country hike anytime. The gorgeous canyon live oaks along the trail escaped the 2009 Station Fire, but the top of the peak burned.

From the trailhead, the San Gabriel Peak Trail wastes no time in zigzagging straight up the steep, oak- and conifer-shaded slopes to the west. Starting at about 0.5 mile, the trail comes abreast of and parallels for a while a stretch of the service road. It then resumes switchbacking, offering occasional conifer-framed views of Mount Wilson and the West Fork (San Gabriel

River) country to the east. You come up alongside the service road again at 1.2 miles. Soon afterward, the trail switchbacks up and joins the paved service road.

Continue south on the road for 0.2 mile to a hairpin turn. You could turn north on the service road for a 0.3-mile side trip to Mount Disappointment. Our route to San Gabriel Peak, however, continues southeast over the broad saddle between Mount Disappointment and San Gabriel Peak where the trail resumes near an old heliport. You promptly come to a trail junction: the right branch goes south, dropping to Markham Saddle. Take the left branch, going east up San Gabriel Peak's flank, gaining 400 feet in about 0.4 mile. The view from the top is panoramic, but not quite so impressive as that from Mount Lowe, which is about a mile closer to the great L.A. Basin below.

VARIATION

San Gabriel Peak can also be climbed by way of Eaton Saddle and Markham Saddle—a shorter and slightly easier (3 miles, 1,000' gain) but less scenic approach through the chaparral.

---

trip 23.12   **Mount Lowe**

see map on p. 281

Distance	3.2 miles (out-and-back)
Hiking Time	1.5 hours
Elevation Gain	500'
Difficulty	Moderate
Trail Use	Dogs allowed
Best Times	Year-round
Agency	Angeles National Forest
Optional Map	Tom Harrison *Angeles Front Country*

DIRECTIONS Exit the 210 Freeway at Angeles Crest Highway (Highway 2) in La Cañada Flintridge. Drive 14 miles north and east to Red Box Station and the intersection of Mount Wilson Road at mile marker 2 LA 38.38. Turn right on Mount Wilson Road and proceed 2.4 miles to a roadside parking area at Eaton Saddle.

Mount Markham, here viewed from Eaton Saddle, has one of the more imposing faces in the San Gabriel Mountains.

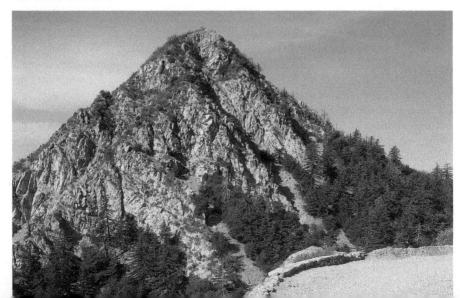

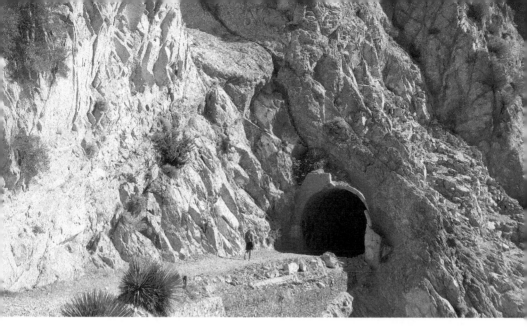

Firefighting in the San Gabriels is so important that the U.S. Forest Service dedicated resources during World War II to build the Muller Tunnel, which connects Mount Lowe Fire Road to Eaton Saddle.

Late in the year, when the smog lightens but temperatures still hover within a moderate register, come up to Mount Lowe to toast the setting sun. You can sit on an old bench, pour the Champagne, and watch Old Sol sink into Santa Monica Bay.

From Eaton Saddle, walk past the gate on the west side and proceed up the dirt road (Mount Lowe Fire Road) that carves its way under the precipitous south face of San Gabriel Peak. Enjoy striking views of Mount Markham's summit pyramid across the canyon. At 0.3 mile pass through the Muller Tunnel, built by the U.S. Forest Service in 1942 to access the fire road. The tunnel is named for A. J. Muller, head of the Angeles National Forest Construction Division, who carved fire roads across the range trying to prevent a repeat of a devastating 1924 wildfire.

At Markham Saddle (0.6 mile) the fire road starts to descend slightly—don't continue on the road. Instead, find the Mount Lowe Trail on the left (south). You contour southwest above the fire road to cross a saddle between Markham and Lowe (1.2 miles), and then start climbing south across the east flank of Mount Lowe without much change of direction. Peak-baggers can climb Markham from here via a climbers' trail up the southwest ridge (0.5 mile, with 400' of climbing to the 5,742' summit). The summit is named for Henry Markham, who served as California's governor from 1891 to 1895.

At 1.4 miles make a sharp right turn at a sign for Mount Lowe. Proceed 0.2 mile uphill; then go left on a short spur trail to Mount Lowe's barren summit (5,603'), where a small grove of canyon live oaks miraculously survived the 2009 Station Fire. Mount Lowe was the proposed upper terminus for Professor Thaddeus Lowe's famed scenic railway (see Trip 23.20, page 310). Funding ran out, however, and tracks were never laid higher than Ye Alpine Tavern (later named Mount Lowe Tavern), 1,200 feet below. During the railway's heyday in the early 1900s, thousands disembarked at the tavern and tramped Mount Lowe's east- and west-side trails for world-class views of the basin and the surrounding mountains. Some reminders of that era remain on the summit of Mount Lowe and along some of the trails: volunteers have repainted, relettered, and returned to their proper places some of the many sighting tubes that helped the early tourists familiarize themselves with the surrounding geography.

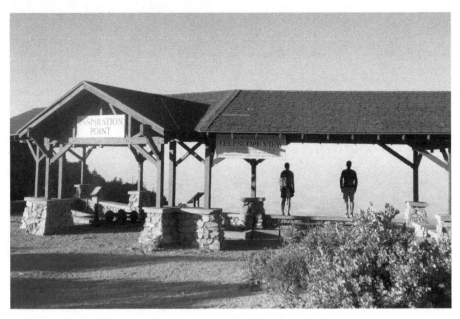

Inspiration Point is aptly named. The ramada was rebuilt on the original 1925 foundations.

trip 23.13 **Inspiration Point**

see map on p. 281

Distance	6 miles (loop)
Hiking Time	3.5 hours
Elevation Gain	1,600'
Difficulty	Moderately strenuous
Trail Use	Suitable for backpacking, dogs allowed
Best Times	October–June
Agency	Angeles National Forest
Optional Map	Tom Harrison *Angeles Front Country*

DIRECTIONS Exit the 210 Freeway at Angeles Crest Highway (Highway 2) in La Cañada Flintridge. Drive 14 miles north and east to Red Box Station and the intersection of Mount Wilson Road at mile marker 2 LA 38.38. Turn right on Mount Wilson Road and proceed 2.4 miles to a roadside parking area at Eaton Saddle.

This trip rambles down to Inspiration Point the back way—via Mount Lowe. It's a down-and-up route, so save most of your energy for the trip back. On the way down and later back, you'll have a chance to use both the east and west trails on the slopes of Mount Lowe. These were among the best-used trails during the era of the railway, and both were brought back into service in the late 1980s.

From Eaton Saddle, walk past the gate on the west side and proceed up the dirt road (Mount Lowe Fire Road) that carves its way under the precipitous south face of San Gabriel Peak. Enjoy striking views of Mount Markham's summit pyramid across the canyon. At 0.3 mile pass through the Muller Tunnel, built by the U.S. Forest Service in 1942 to access the fire road. The tunnel is named for A. J. Muller, head of the Angeles National Forest Construction Division, who carved fire roads across the range trying to prevent a repeat of a devastating 1924 wildfire.

At Markham Saddle (0.6 mile) the fire road starts to descend slightly—don't continue on the road. Instead, find the Mount Lowe Trail on the left (south). You contour southwest above the fire road to cross a saddle between Markham and Lowe (1.2 miles), and then start climbing south across the east flank of Mount Lowe without much change of direction.

At 1.4 miles stay straight at a trail junction to remain on the east trail. You will return to this point via the west trail later. Circle around the south side of Mount Lowe. As you make a switchbacking descent, watch for but don't take a steep firebreak that bypasses some of the switchbacks. Stay left at a junction, following the sign to Inspiration Point. Rejoin the Mount Lowe Fire Road at 2.5 miles.

Turn left and go south on the dirt road, passing a five-way junction, to reach Inspiration Point at 2.9 miles. The shade structure was first built in 1925 and then rebuilt in 1996 on the original foundations. The view is especially inspiring whenever the marine inversion layer lies low across the L.A. Basin, a fairly common occurrence early in the day. On very clear days the ocean horizon can be seen behind the gap at Two Harbors on Santa Catalina Island, and San Clemente Island sprawls indistinctly just left of the leftmost tip of Santa Catalina.

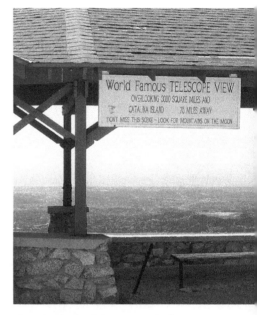

If you're interested in side trips, climb the 4,714-foot peaklet west of Inspiration Point. Better yet, visit Muir Peak (4,682') for even closer views over Eaton Canyon. To get there, continue southeast on the fire road for 0.5 mile; then pick up the signed but easily overlooked Muir Peak Trail climbing 0.1 mile to the summit. Starting around 1915, tourists could travel this stretch aboard a mule-pushed observation car that rolled along narrow-gauge rails. This so-called One Man and a Mule Railroad became a popular side attraction for Mount Lowe Tavern guests and day-trippers.

Alternatively, stay on the fire road to its end at a concrete water tank, an overlook known as Panorama Point. Views of the L.A. Basin from here are unsurpassed by any other land-based vantage point. From this close-in point, less than 2 beeline miles from the edge of the city,

From Inspiration Point, you can look across most of the L.A. Basin and all the way to Catalina Island.

the soft droning of a hundred thousand engines, accented now and again by an accelerating motorcycle or unmuffled car, floats upward on the updrafts.

Return the way you came, except in circling Mount Lowe. From Inspiration Point, walk back north on the Mount Lowe Fire Road for 0.6 mile. Shortly after the point where you joined it, watch for signs to the Mount Lowe East Trail and Mount Lowe Trail Camp; then, a few yards later, pick up the signed Mount Lowe West/Upper Sam Merrill Trail, which curves around the west and north sides of the peak with a worthwhile short detour to the summit. Continue to the junction with the east trail, and return the way you began.

VARIATION

Many hikers reach Inspiration Point via the Sam Merrill and Castle Canyon Trails, a splendid 10-mile loop with 3,000 feet of elevation gain.

trip 23.14 Bear Canyon

Distance	8 miles (one-way)
Hiking Time	4 hours
Elevation Gain/Loss	800'/2,800'
Difficulty	Moderately strenuous
Trail Use	Suitable for backpacking, dogs allowed
Best Times	Year-round
Agency	Angeles National Forest
Recommended Map	Tom Harrison *Angeles Front Country* or Trails Illustrated *Angeles National Forest (811)*

see map on p. 281

DIRECTIONS This trip requires a 6-mile shuttle. Leave one vehicle at the Switzer Picnic Area: To get here from the 210 Freeway in La Cañada Flintridge, take the Angeles Crest Highway (Highway 2) 10 miles north and east to the Switzer Picnic Area (mile marker 2 LA 34.2). Drive 0.5 mile down the paved access road to the parking lot next to the picnic area where the road makes a hairpin turn, and leave a vehicle here.

Take your other vehicle to Eaton Saddle by returning to the Angeles Crest Highway and continuing east 4 miles to Red Box Station. Turn right on Mount Wilson Road and proceed 2.4 miles to a roadside parking area at Eaton Saddle. If you wish to use a bicycle shuttle instead, consider doing the hike in reverse so your ride is downhill.

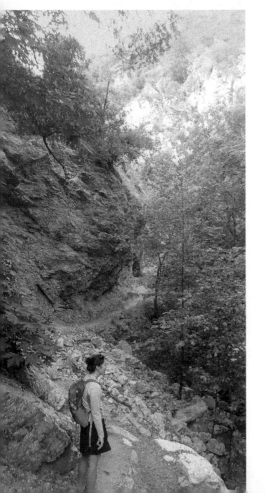

Bear Canyon, as secluded and beautiful as any small canyon in the Front Range country, enjoys the added benefit of trail access from two sides. Graced with a sparkling rivulet of water with numerous small cascades and pools, and shaded by beautiful sycamore, alder, big-cone Douglas-fir, big-leaf maple, and bay trees, the canyon's innermost confines are scarcely disturbed at all by the recently improved historic Tom Sloan Trail, built in 1923 to serve the needs of hikers traveling between Mount Lowe Tavern and Switzer's Camp.

Tom Sloan was a district ranger here around 1918. The stretch through the canyon is a special delight in November, when the leaves of the maples turn crispy yellow, and you scuff through leaf litter so thick it's hard to recognize the path. Wear long pants and long sleeves because poison oak is nearly unavoidable between Bear Canyon Campground and Tom Sloan Saddle. Ticks may be plentiful in March–April. The chaparral-clad slopes west of Tom Sloan saddle burned in the 2009 Station Fire, but the creek itself largely

Bear Canyon is a great place to escape the crowds in the popular Front Range.

escaped damage. The one-way hike suggested here adds some driving logistics, but it makes the hiking/backpacking part a lot easier than hoofing it in both directions. Don't mix up this Bear Canyon with Bear Creek in the San Gabriel River Canyon (see Trip 27.5, page 359).

From the start at Eaton Saddle, take the Mount Lowe Fire Road west to Markham Saddle (0.5 mile). Continue southwest and west without leaving the fire road until you reach a hairpin turn to the left (1.8 miles) atop the long west ridge coming down from Mount Lowe's summit. Leave the road there and continue, on the trail now, westward along the same ridge. Here and there along the way you can look south over Millard Canyon and across the often hazy lowlands to Palos Verdes and Santa Catalina Island. Upper Bear Canyon lies to the north, its fire-scarred, chaparral-clad slopes hardly suggesting the beauty that exists down along the hidden stream. After a few downhill switchbacks, you arrive at Tom Sloan Saddle (3.1 miles), where several trails meet: the east leg of the Tom Sloan Trail from the Mount Lowe Tavern site (with an immediate split down to Dawn Mine), and the west leg of the Tom Sloan Trail (aka the Bear Canyon Trail) coming up from Bear Canyon. The Dawn Mine and Tom Sloan East Trails were rebuilt in 2018 after vanishing in the fire. There is also a ridgetop firebreak, sometimes followed by hikers, leading west to the summit of Brown Mountain.

From Tom Sloan Saddle, you go north, descending switchbacks through chaparral until you reach Bear Canyon's stream (3.9 miles). There you'll discover the remains of a small, stone shed and cabin foundations.

The trail deteriorates as you turn downcanyon, and progress slows. Poison oak hangs close to the trail. From time to time, boulder-hopping may become the way to travel until you reach Bear Canyon Trail Camp at 4.9 miles, on an oak-shaded terrace to the left. Beyond here the pathway becomes easier to follow. A section of trail carved precariously into a sheer wall on the right (mile 6.1) heralds your arrival at Bear Creek's confluence with Arroyo Seco. From here on, the path is wide and obvious, and you'll be climbing almost all the way. You follow Arroyo Seco upstream past some sparkling mini-falls and rock-bound pools. A half mile later you start an ascent up the slope to the left, and soon thereafter join the Gabrielino Trail. You pass Switzer Falls, skirt Switzer's Camp, and finally arrive at Switzer Picnic Area.

VARIATION

For a delightful but strenuous 16-mile loop with 3,500 feet of elevation gain, continue up the Gabrielino and San Gabriel Peak Trails and back to Eaton Saddle, optionally visiting San Gabriel Peak. Consider doing the trip in reverse, starting at Switzer, to do the uphill while you're fresh.

---

trip 23.15 **Millard Canyon Falls**

Distance	1.4 miles (out-and-back)
Hiking Time	1 hour
Elevation Gain	300'
Difficulty	Moderate
Trail Use	Dogs allowed, good for kids
Best Times	Year-round
Agency	Angeles National Forest
Optional Map	Tom Harrison *Angeles Front Country*

see map on p. 281

DIRECTIONS From the 210 Freeway in Pasadena, take Exit 23 for Lincoln Avenue. Go north on Lincoln for 1.8 miles, and turn right on Alta Loma Road. Proceed 0.6 mile east to Chaney Trail (a paved road) on the left. Drive 1.7 miles to the road's end at a large parking lot along Millard Creek, passing a sturdy gate, typically open 6 a.m.–8 p.m., and crossing Sunset Ridge.

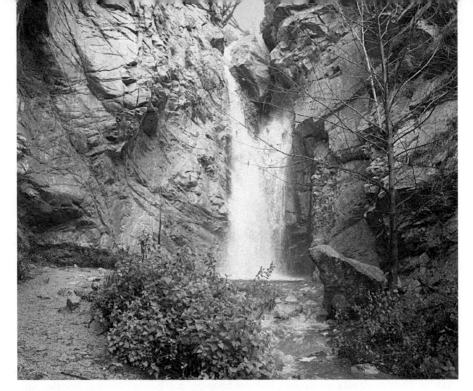

Millard Canyon Falls can be impressive during a rainy winter. Photo: Kyle Kuns

During heavy rains, Millard Canyon's modest watershed gathers enough runoff to stage a real spectacle near its lower end: Millard Canyon Falls. Even in the dry season, when the water dribbles over the rock by way of several serpentine paths, the steep-walled grotto containing the falls is pleasantly cool, and worth a visit. The canyon is named for Henry Millard, who homesteaded here in 1862 with his family, raising bees and hauling wood to Los Angeles.

From the parking lot, hike upstream, past a vehicle gate, and through Millard Campground (a walk-in facility). Continue up the canyon, boulder-hopping from time to time, beneath oaks, bay laurels, and alders, until you reach the falls. It's difficult to take a photograph that does justice to this cool, dark or sun-dappled, pleasant place. You may notice three bolted aid routes on the left where climbers ply their craft.

trip 23.16   Dawn Mine Loop

Distance	6 miles (loop)
Hiking Time	3.5 hours
Elevation Gain	1,600'
Difficulty	Moderately strenuous
Trail Use	Dogs allowed
Best Times	October–June
Agency	Angeles National Forest
Optional Map	Tom Harrison *Angeles Front Country*

see map on p. 281

DIRECTIONS From the 210 Freeway in Pasadena, take Exit 23 for Lincoln Avenue. Go north on Lincoln for 1.8 miles, and turn right on Canyon Crest Road. Proceed 0.6 mile east to Chaney Trail (a paved road) on the left. Drive past a sturdy gate, typically open 6 a.m.–8 p.m., and proceed sharply uphill 1.1 miles to the road crest at Sunset Ridge, where there's parking space by the roadside.

Millard Canyon's happily splashing stream, presided over by oaks, alders, maples, and big-cone Douglas-firs, is the main attraction on this hike. But you can also do a little snooping around the site of the Dawn Mine, one of the more promising gold prospects in the San Gabriels, worked intermittently from 1895 until the early 1950s. The mine was named for Dawn Ehrenfeld, the daughter of a friend of an early prospector, Bradford Peck.

An early start is emphatically recommended. That way you'll take advantage of shade during the climbing phase of the hike, and you'll be assured of finding a place to park your car at the trailhead (which is as popular with mountain bikers as with hikers).

Start by walking east on the gated, paved Sunset Ridge fire road. After 0.1 mile you pass a foot trail on the left leading down to Millard Campground. Continue another 0.3 mile to a second foot trail on the left (Sunset Ridge Trail). Take it. On it you contour north and east along Millard Canyon's south wall, passing above a sometimes-vociferous 50-foot waterfall. You soon reach a trail fork at 0.8 mile. The left branch (your return route) goes down 100 yards past a historic cabin (presently owned by the Altadena Mountain Rescue Team) to the canyon bottom. You go right, uphill. Switchbacks long and short take you farther up along the pleasantly shaded canyon wall. Watch for seasonal Saucer Branch Falls on the opposite side of the canyon. At 2.7 miles reach Sunset Ridge fire road, just below a rocky knob called Cape of Good Hope.

Turn left on the fire road, and walk past Cape of Good Hope. To your right (east), near a large locked gate, is the beginning of the Sam Merrill Trail to Echo Mountain. This trail and the fire road ahead are both part of the original Mount Lowe Railway bed (see Trip 23.20, page 310)—now a self-guided historical trail. Continue your ascent on the fire road/railway bed to Dawn Station on the left (3.0 miles). There you'll find a trail descending to Dawn Mine in Millard Canyon. This is a reworked but primitive version of the path once used by Michael Ryan and his mules, Jack and Jill, to haul ore from the mine to the railway above. On the way down you may encounter a dicey passage where the narrow trail hangs

The old water pump remains at Dawn Mine.

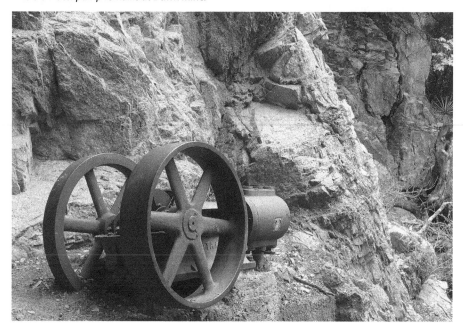

on a steep cliff. The volunteer Restoration Legacy Crew spent countless hours rebuilding this trail and others after the Station Fire.

Reach the gloomy canyon bottom at 3.8 miles. Directly across the canyon is a rusty engine once used to move ore. The entrance to the adjacent shaft was sealed in 2017 by order of the U.S. Forest Service. A second, taller adit can be found on the north wall of the canyon by boulder-hopping up the creek for 0.1 mile. On the southeast side of the canyon, look for the foundation and metal stilts that supported the Ryan House on an airy promontory above the creek.

From the mine, head downcanyon past crystalline mini-pools, the flotsam and jetsam of the mining days, and storm-tossed boulders. Much of the original trail in the canyon has been washed away or damaged by the 2009 Station Fire, but volunteer trail crews have beaten down a pretty good semblance of a path.

After swinging around an abrupt bend to the right, the canyon becomes dark and gloomy once again. At 5.1 miles you'll come to the aforementioned exit trail climbing up to the left. Pass the private cabin and hook up with the Sunset Ridge Trail, which will take you back to the Sunset Ridge fire road and your car.

VARIATION

It's possible to continue down a rough path from the cabin to the top of Millard Canyon Falls. A climbers' path exits to your left and follows a ledge until you can work your way carefully down to the canyon floor below the falls. Part of the path is washed out, so this variation is recommended only for adventurous hikers. Continue down to Millard Campground, and then take the signed trail on the left up to Sunset Ridge near your vehicle.

---

trip 23.17   Upper Millard Canyon

see map on p. 281

Distance	11 miles (loop)
Hiking Time	6 hours
Elevation Gain	2,700'
Difficulty	Strenuous
Trail Use	Suitable for backpacking, dogs allowed
Best Times	October–May
Agency	Angeles National Forest
Recommended Map	Tom Harrison *Angeles Front Country*

DIRECTIONS From the 210 Freeway in Pasadena, take Exit 23 for Lincoln Avenue. Go north on Lincoln for 1.8 miles, and turn right on Canyon Crest Road. Proceed 0.6 mile east to Chaney Trail (a paved road) on the left. Drive past a sturdy gate, typically open 6 a.m.–8 p.m., and proceed sharply uphill 1.1 miles to the road crest at Sunset Ridge, where there's parking space by the roadside.

On this longer version of the Dawn Mine loop described just above, you'll climb all the way to Tom Sloan Saddle at the head of Millard Canyon, and then circle around to Mount Lowe Trail Camp (the site of the historic Mount Lowe Tavern). If this is your first visit to the area, it's better to travel around the loop in a clockwise direction as we describe here, returning via the Mount Lowe Railway bed.

Begin by walking up the Sunset Ridge fire road and veering left onto the Sunset Ridge Trail after 0.4 mile. Bear left at 0.9 mile (where the Sunset Ridge Trail climbs right), descend to Millard Canyon's stream, and work your way up along the banks to Dawn Mine (2.2 miles).

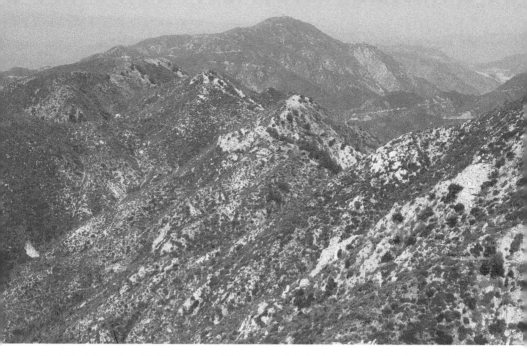

The historic Tom Sloan Trail (foreground right) was rebuilt in 2018, connecting Tom Sloan Saddle (center) to the Mount Lowe Fire Road. Brown Mountain is in the left foreground, accessed by a climbers' trail from Tom Sloan Saddle. Mount Lukens is on the center horizon.

Continue upstream another 0.4 mile to a confluence where a large tributary, Grand Canyon, branches east. The trail turns left and switchbacks up northward to Tom Sloan Saddle (3.7 miles) atop the high ridge shared by Brown Mountain and Mount Lowe.

Five trails converge at the saddle: the one you came from, the Brown Mountain climbers' trail, the Bear Canyon Trail, a firebreak up the east ridge, and the Tom Sloan Trail. Turn right onto the Tom Sloan Trail, which was wiped out by the 2009 Station Fire and rebuilt in 2018. When you reach the Mount Lowe Fire Road, at 5.5 miles, turn right. At 5.8 miles turn right on a signed but easily overlooked trail shortcutting down to Mount Lowe Trail Camp, at 5.9 miles. You may find stream water here seasonally; treat it before using it.

From the trail camp it's downhill virtually all the way back. Follow the fire road/old rail bed west and south, down past a couple of hairpin turns, to Cape of Good Hope, where the pavement begins, at 8.6 miles. Just below the Cape, use the Sunset Ridge Trail to return to the starting point. Alternatively, you can walk down the paved Sunset Ridge fire road, which is slightly shorter but sun-exposed and a lot less scenic.

trip 23.18 Brown Mountain Traverse

Distance	12 miles (loop)
Hiking Time	8 hours
Elevation Gain	3,200'
Difficulty	Strenuous
Trail Use	Dogs allowed
Best Times	October–May
Agency	Angeles National Forest
Recommended Map	Tom Harrison *Angeles Front Country*

see map on p. 281

DIRECTIONS From the 210 Freeway in Pasadena, take Exit 23 for Lincoln Avenue. Go north on Lincoln for 1.8 miles, and turn right on Canyon Crest Road. Proceed 0.6 mile east to Chaney Trail (a paved road) on the left. Drive past a sturdy gate, typically open 6 a.m.–8 p.m., and proceed sharply uphill to the road crest at Sunset Ridge, where there's parking space by the roadside, 1.1 miles.

Brown Mountain (4,472′) is not as tall as many of its neighbors but nevertheless occupies a commanding position above Altadena near the Angeles Crest Highway. This hike traverses the mountain, climbing Millard Canyon to Tom Sloan Saddle, running the Brown Mountain ridge from east to west, and returning via the Brown Mountain Fire Road. The east ridge receives plenty of use from hikers coming from Eaton Saddle and is easy walking. The west ridge is somewhat brushy but generally receives enough use to stay passable.

Brown Mountain was named by Owen and Jason Brown in memory of their father, abolitionist John Brown. The Brown brothers moved to Southern California in 1884 and built a cabin in El Prieto Canyon, where they enjoyed roaming the mountains. Owen died in 1889 and was buried on Little Round Top by El Prieto Canyon.

From the trailhead, follow the Sunset Ridge fire road 0.4 mile; then turn left onto the Sunset Ridge Trail and descend into Millard Canyon. Hike up the canyon past Dawn Mine (2.2 miles) and switchback up to Tom Sloan Saddle (3.7 miles).

Find the climbers' trail leading up the ridge to the west. Watch for a small burn area along the ridge caused by a December 2017 lightning strike. At 4.3 miles pass over a false summit, and at 4.9 miles reach the cairn marking the true summit of Brown Mountain.

If you wish to make the traverse, continue northeast along the ridge through fields of yerba santa and other sage scrub. Near the end of the ridge, briefly stay right to avoid a steep brushy slope before you switchback left and descend to a saddle (6.4 miles) where you meet

David Baumgartner, a leader of the volunteer Restoration Legacy Crew, at the Brown Mountain summit cairn. The RLC has devoted incredible efforts to repairing trails in the wake of the 2009 Station Fire.

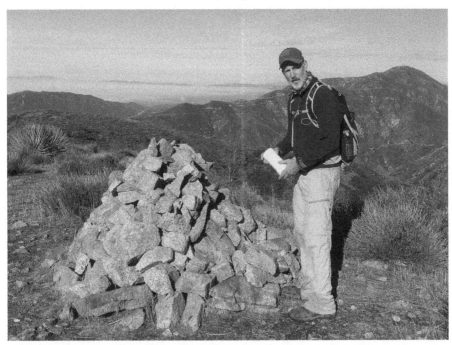

the Ken Burton Trail. (This trail, popular with mountain bikers, descends to Oakwilde Camp in the Arroyo Seco.)

Head south on the fire road, now deteriorated to a singletrack trail. Weave around the mountain, staying left at each fork as you pass various other dirt roads. Finally pass some cabins and the Millard Canyon Campground to find the Sunset Ridge Trail, which climbs the last 300 feet back up to the ridge where you parked.

VARIATION

Brown Mountain is more easily climbed from Eaton Saddle. This out-and-back route is 8.5 miles with 2,400 feet of elevation gain, mostly on the return.

---

trip 23.19 **Echo Mountain**

Distance	5.5 miles (out-and-back)	
Hiking Time	3 hours	
Elevation Gain	1,400'	
Difficulty	Moderate	
Trail Use	Dogs allowed	
Best Times	October–May	
Agency	Angeles National Forest	
Optional Map	Tom Harrison *Angeles Front Country* or Trails Illustrated *Angeles National Forest (811)*	

see map on p. 281

DIRECTIONS From the 210 Freeway in Pasadena, take Exit 26 for Lake Avenue. Drive north on Lake Avenue for 3.6 miles to where the street bends left and becomes Loma Alta Drive. Find any available curbside parking space nearest this intersection.

The Sam Merrill Trail to Echo Mountain is an extremely popular hike, offering a vigorous workout with terrific views from an easily accessible trailhead. The summit draws many hikers to enjoy the sunset, although at least one has taken a fatal fall from the trail during the nighttime descent. The trail has been recognized in many national publications, including the 1996 *USA Today* article "10 Great North American Hikes" and *Sunset* magazine's "Top 44 Hikes in the West." The hike climbs from the historic Cobb Estate to the ruins of White City, a four-story resort hotel built by Professor Thaddeus Lowe in 1894. Painted striking white and illuminated at night with a 3-million-candlepower searchlight, it was a prominent landmark across Los Angeles. Guests reached the hotel by way of a funicular railroad from Rubio Canyon with a grade up to 62%, or from a nearby station on the Mount Lowe Railway. Lowe ran out of money and lost control of the property in 1989. The underinsured hotel burned to the ground in 1900 after a kitchen fire spread out of control. A flash flood wiped out the Rubio station in 1909. The trails lacing the mountains were mostly washed away in the Flood of 1938, but a Sierra Club leader and retired court clerk named Sam Merrill dedicated his retirement to repairing and maintaining the Echo Mountain trail until his death in 1948 at age 80. After his death, the trail was renamed for Merrill.

The Sam Merrill Trailhead lies on the grounds of the long-demolished Cobb Estate, at the north end of Lake Avenue in Altadena. Walk east past the stone pillars at the entrance and continue 150 yards on a narrow, blacktop driveway. The driveway bends left, but you keep walking straight (east). Soon you cross the Altadena Crest Trail at a water fountain on the rim of Las Flores Canyon and a sign indicating the start of the Sam Merrill Trail. Be sure to stay on the Sam Merrill Trail, which goes left over the top of a small debris dam and begins a switchback ascent of Las Flores Canyon's precipitous east wall.

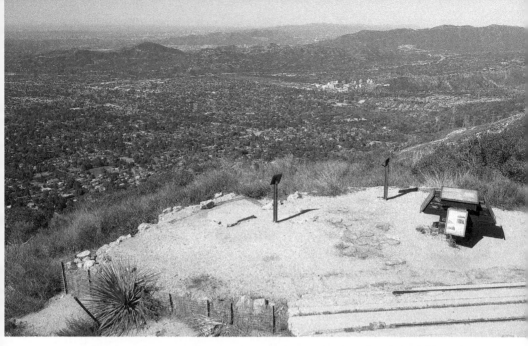

Spectacular views abound over Pasadena, Sierra Madre, and the L.A. Basin from Echo Mountain.

At 2.4 miles, after many switchbacks and excellent views, the trail levels out on the ridge. The Mount Lowe Railway bed turns left, but this trip goes right toward Echo Mountain, a 3,207-foot bump on the southwest ridge of Mount Lowe. Immediately pass more junctions for the Sam Merrill Trail's continuation to Mount Lowe Campground, and for the Castle Canyon Trail to Inspiration Point before reaching the remains of White City.

Return the way you came, or follow the web of nearby trails for a longer adventure (see the next trip for Mount Lowe Railway).

trip 23.20   Mount Lowe Railway

Distance	11 miles (loop)
Hiking Time	6 hours
Elevation Gain	2,700'
Difficulty	Moderately strenuous
Trail Use	Suitable for backpacking, dogs allowed
Best Times	October–May
Agency	Angeles National Forest
Optional Map	Tom Harrison *Angeles Front Country* or Trails Illustrated *Angeles National Forest* (811)

see map on p. 281

DIRECTIONS From the 210 Freeway in Pasadena, take Exit 26 for Lake Avenue. Drive north on Lake Avenue for 3.6 miles to where the street bends left and becomes Loma Alta Drive. Find any available curbside parking space nearest this intersection.

An engineering marvel when built in the 1890s, the Mount Lowe Railway has had a checkered past full of both glory and destruction. Before its final abandonment in the mid-1930s, the line carried over 3 million passengers—virtually all of them tourists. Unheard of by most Southland residents today, the railway was for many years the most popular outdoor attraction in Southern California.

Today hikers are taking a new interest in the old road bed; the Rails-to-Trails Conservancy (which promotes the conversion of abandoned rail corridors into recreation trails) ranked the Mount Lowe Railway as one of the nation's 12 most scenic and historically significant recycled rail lines.

The line consisted of three stages, of which almost nothing remains today. Passengers rode a trolley from Altadena into lower Rubio Canyon, then boarded a steeply inclined cable railway that took them 1,300 feet higher to Echo Mountain, where two hotels, a number of small tourist attractions, and an observatory stood. At Echo Mountain, nonacrophobic passengers hopped onto the third phase: a mountain trolley that climbed another 1,200 vertical feet along airy slopes to the end of the line—Ye Alpine Tavern (later Mount Lowe Tavern), on whose ruins stands today's Mount Lowe Trail Camp.

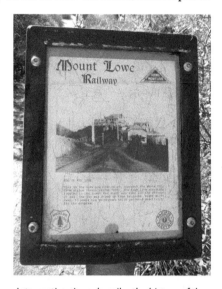

Interpretive signs describe the history of the Mount Lowe Railway.

The U.S. Forest Service (USFS) and volunteers have put together a self-guiding trail, featuring 10 markers fashioned from railroad rails, along the route of the mountain trolley. The middle portion of the old railway bed can be reached by hiking either the paved road or the trail coming up from the Chaney Trail above Millard Canyon. The more direct, easy, and exciting way to reach Station 1 at Echo Mountain, however, is to go by way of the Sam Merrill Trail from Altadena. The first part of this trip coincides with the Echo Mountain hike (see Trip 23.19, page 309).

The Sam Merrill Trailhead lies on the grounds of the long-demolished Cobb Estate, at the north end of Lake Avenue in Altadena. Walk east past the stone pillars at the entrance and continue 150 yards on a narrow, blacktop driveway. The driveway bends left, but you keep walking straight (east). Soon you come to a water fountain on the rim of Las Flores Canyon and a sign indicating the start of the Sam Merrill Trail. This trail goes left over the top of a small debris dam and begins a switchback ascent of Las Flores Canyon's precipitous east wall, while another trail (the Altadena Crest equestrian trail) veers to the right, down the canyon.

Inspired by the fabulous views (assuming you're doing this early on one of L.A.'s clear winter days), the 2.5 miles of steady ascent on the Sam Merrill Trail may seem to go rather quickly. Turn right at the top of the trail and walk south over to Echo Mountain, which is more like the shoulder of a ridge. There you'll find a historical plaque and some picnic tables near a grove of incense cedars and big-leaf maples. Poke around and you'll find many foundation ruins and piles of concrete rubble. An old bull wheel and cables for the incline railway were thoughtfully left behind after the USFS cleared away what remained of the buildings here in the 1950s and '60s. After visiting Echo Mountain, you'll go north on the signed Echo Mountain Trail, where you'll walk over railroad ties still embedded in the ground.

The rail bed is now marked with a series of interpretive signs, highlighting the following. Numbers in parentheses refer to hiking mileage starting from Echo Mountain.

Station 1 (0.0): Echo Mountain This was known as the White City during its brief heyday in the late 1890s, but most of its tourist facilities were destroyed by fire or windstorms in the first decade of the 1900s. The mountain remained a transfer point for passengers until the mid-1930s.

Station 2 (0.5): View of Circular Bridge You can't see it from here, but passengers at this point first noticed the 400-foot-diameter circular bridge (Station 6) jutting from the slope above. As you walk on ahead, you'll notice the many concrete footings that supported trestles bridging the side ravines of Las Flores Canyon.

Station 3 (0.8): Cape of Good Hope You're now at the junction of the Echo Mountain Trail and Sunset Ridge fire road where the route crosses from Las Flores to Millard Canyon. The tracks swung in a 200° arc around the rocky promontory just west—Cape of Good Hope. (Walk around the Cape, if you like, to get a feel for the experience.) North of this dizzying passage, riders were treated to the longest stretch of straight track—only 225 feet long. The entire original line from Echo Mountain to Ye Alpine Tavern had 127 curves and 114 straight sections. The Cape of Good Hope also marks the edge of the vast burn area from the 2009 Station Fire. *Note:* Many mountain bikers use this section of the old railroad grade. They mostly arrive by way of the Sunset Ridge fire road.

Station 4 (1.0): Dawn Station/Devil's Slide Dawn Mine lies below in Millard Canyon. Gold-bearing ore, packed up by mules from the canyon bottom, was loaded onto the train here. Ahead lay a treacherous stretch of crumbling granite, the Devil's Slide, which was eventually bridged by a trestle. (The current fire road has been shored up with much new concrete, and cement-lined spillways seem to do a good job of carrying away flood debris.)

Station 5 (1.2): Horseshoe Curve Just beyond this station, Horseshoe Curve enabled the railway to gain elevation above Millard Canyon. The grade just beyond Horseshoe Curve was 7%—steepest on the mountain segment of the line.

Station 6 (1.6): Circular Bridge An engineering accomplishment of worldwide fame, the Circular Bridge carried startled passengers into midair over the upper walls of Las Flores Canyon. Look for the concrete supports of this bridge down along the chaparral-covered slopes to the right.

Station 7 (2.0): Horseshoe Curve Overview Passengers here looked down on Horseshoe Curve, and could also see all three levels of steep, twisting track climbing the east wall of Millard Canyon.

Station 8 (2.4): Granite Gate A narrow slot carefully blasted out of solid granite on a sheer north-facing slope, Granite Gate took 8 months to cut. Look for the electric wire support dangling from the rock above.

Station 9 (3.4): Ye Alpine Tavern The tavern, which later became a fancy hotel, was located at Crystal Springs, the source that still provides water (which now requires purification) for backpackers staying overnight at today's Mount Lowe Trail Camp. The rails never got farther than here, although it was hoped they would one day reach the summit of Mount Lowe, 1,200 feet higher. The Station Fire thankfully spared this splendid forest of canyon live oak and big-cone Douglas-fir here.

Station 10 (3.9): Inspiration Point From Ye Alpine Tavern, tourists could saunter over to Inspiration Point along part of the never-finished rail extension to Mount Lowe. Sighting tubes (still in place there) helped visitors locate places of interest below.

Inspiration Point is the last station on the self-guided trail. The fastest and easiest way to return is by way of the Castle Canyon Trail, which descends directly below Inspiration Point. After 2 miles you'll arrive back on the old railway grade just north of Echo Mountain. Retrace your steps on the Sam Merrill Trail.

chapter 24

Mount Wilson & Front Range

In the lush and shady recesses of Big Santa Anita Canyon, Eaton Canyon, and other drainages at the foot of Mount Wilson, you can easily lose all sight and sense of the hundreds of square miles of dense metropolis lying just over a single ridge. With very easy access, by city street or mountain road and then by trail, these are perfect spots to discover the San Gabriel Mountains' beguiling charms.

The flattish, rambling summit of Mount Wilson, a sort of centerpiece for the area covered in this section, is hardly notable for its elevation of about 5,700 feet. But its long history of use, dating back to 1864, has made it a major node in the trail network of the San Gabriels. Today the drive to Mount Wilson is an easy one—half an hour at best from the 210 Freeway at La Cañada Flintridge. You can play tourist by visiting Skyline Park (open daily, 10 a.m.–4 p.m., April–November) and Mount Wilson Observatory, or you can get serious and set off on one of the steep trails down its flank.

Chantry Flat, above Arcadia, is the hikers' hub on the lowland side. Chantry Flat is also the jumping-off spot for cabin owners who must walk down to their homes away from home in Big Santa Anita Canyon. At Chantry Flat, you'll find spacious (although often inadequate) parking space, a ranger station, a picnic ground, and a mom-and-pop refreshment stand. There's also a freight business: the Adams Pack Station, established in 1936, is the last such establishment operating year-round in California. Almost daily, horses, mules, and burros carry building materials and other supplies to canyon residents.

A sturdy gate on Santa Anita Avenue just above Arcadia clangs shut every night at 8 p.m. and doesn't open till 6 a.m. the next morning. On weekends it's wise to arrive early at Chantry Flat; otherwise parking is hard to come by. It's also worth noting that—if the recent past is any guide—the road to Chantry Flat could be closed to cars due to any combination of fire, flood, or mudslide.

In August and September 2009, Mount Wilson was the scene of dramatic battles between firefighters and the ever-shifting flames of the Station Fire. Mount Wilson Observatory and a large telecommunications facility nearby were saved during this effort. Santa Anita Canyon and Chantry Flat were untouched by the fire, though most of the area north of the Mount Wilson summit was thoroughly incinerated. Some trails remained closed until 2018.

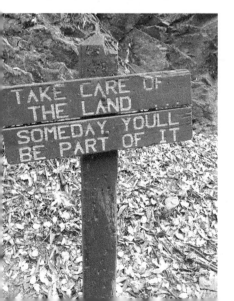

The sentiment expressed on this trail sign in Santa Anita Canyon is all too true.

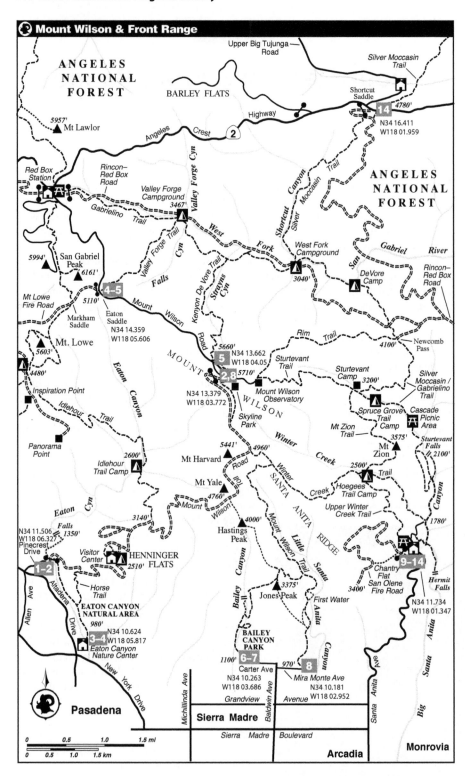

Mount Wilson & Front Range

trip 24.1 Henninger Flats

Distance	5 miles (out-and-back)
Hiking Time	3 hours
Elevation Gain	1,400'
Difficulty	Moderately strenuous
Trail Use	Suitable for backpacking, suitable for mountain biking, dogs allowed, good for kids
Best Times	October–June
Agency	Los Angeles County Fire Department, Forestry Division
Optional Map	Tom Harrison *Angeles Front Country* or Trails Illustrated *Angeles National Forest (811)*

see map opposite

DIRECTIONS From the eastbound 210 Freeway, take Exit 28 for northbound Altadena Drive. (From the westbound 210, take Exit 29A for Sierra Madre and follow the frontage road to Altadena Drive.) Proceed 2.7 miles; then turn right onto Crescent Drive and immediately right again onto Pinecrest Drive, where you will find the gated trailhead (2260 Pinecrest Drive). Parking is heavily restricted in this area, so carefully observe the signs; you may have to return to Altadena Drive to find parking.

Parklike Henninger Flats is a pleasant surprise to come upon after the sunny, often sweaty climb up the lower end of the Mount Wilson Toll Road. The bench is named for "Captain" William Henninger, a gold miner who homesteaded here from 1884 until his death in 1894.

The flats and slopes hereabouts have been the site of an experimental forest since 1903, with seedlings of pine, cypress, cedar, and other trees raised for reforestation projects. Run by the Los Angeles County Fire Department, the area encompasses four delightful camp and picnic areas, a visitor center, a pioneer museum, a short nature trail, and a seedling nursery. The visitor center displays a large relief model of the Mount Wilson/Front Range area, and outside there's a diminutive lookout structure that stood on Castro Peak in the Santa Monica Mountains from 1925 to 1971. Henninger Flats' 0.5-mile-high elevation perched directly over the edge of the city gives it a commanding view—by day and especially by night. Backpackers register with

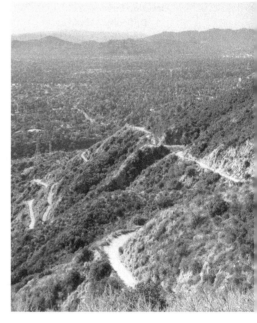

The Mount Wilson Toll Road switchbacks steeply as it climbs to Henninger Flats.

the ranger on duty; campfire permits and wood are usually available. Although this is a wonderful hike on a pleasant spring evening, beware of being trapped when the Pinecrest gate is locked at sunset. Finally, watch out for poison oak along the trail.

The old toll road is now a fire road used by fire department or forestry trucks, and plenty of self-propelled travelers of all sorts. Walk through the gate on Pinecrest Drive (typically open sunrise–sunset) and proceed down across a bridge over Eaton Canyon. Dogged determination, and hopefully the inspiration of fabulous views over the big city below, will get you up the moderately steep and steady grade ahead. This well-engineered road/former trail was built and improved (among other reasons) to haul telescope parts to the summit of Mount Wilson, including those of the 100-inch Hooker Reflector—the world's largest telescope for 31 years. Benches are positioned at scenic locations along the ascent.

You can easily use up a couple of extra hours at Henninger Flats poking around the museum and the visitor center and taking short side trips to check out the groves of trees. For the best view of the surroundings, try climbing a little higher to Henninger Ridge: continue upward on Mount Wilson Toll Road another 0.6 mile, and turn left on the dirt road that loops around to a heliport. This puts you on the shoulder of a ridge perched 400 feet above the groves of Henninger Flats, where the view of the city below stretches 180°. From the north side of the ridge, Mount Wilson rears up starkly, 2.5 miles away. After a winter storm, the spike-shaped antennas on its crest look exactly like upside-down icicles.

trip 24.2 Mount Wilson Toll Road

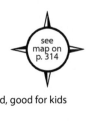

see map on p. 314

Distance	9 miles (one-way)
Hiking Time	4 hours
Elevation Loss	4,200'
Difficulty	Moderate
Trail Use	Suitable for backpacking, mountain biking, dogs allowed, good for kids
Best Times	October–June
Agency	Angeles National Forest
Optional Map	Tom Harrison *Angeles Front Country* or Trails Illustrated *Angeles National Forest (811)*

DIRECTIONS This one-way trip requires a 45-minute shuttle between trailheads; unless you're using a ride-sharing service, leave one car near the Pinecrest Drive trailhead. From the eastbound 210 Freeway, take Exit 28 for northbound Altadena Drive. (From the westbound 210, take Exit 29A for Sierra Madre and follow the frontage road to Altadena Drive.) Proceed 2.7 miles; then turn right onto Crescent Drive and immediately right again onto Pinecrest Drive, where you'll find the gated trailhead (at 2260 Pinecrest Drive). Parking is heavily restricted in this area, so carefully observe the signs; you may have to return to Altadena Drive to find parking.

To reach the upper trailhead, return to the 210 Freeway and continue 8 miles west to the Angeles Crest Highway (Highway 2) in La Cañada Flintridge. Drive 14 miles north and east to Red Box Station and the intersection of Mount Wilson Road (mile marker 2 LA 38.38). Turn right on Mount Wilson Road, and proceed 5 miles to the gate outside Mount Wilson Observatory Skyline Park. The top of the Mount Wilson Toll Road is now a gated dirt Forest Service road, signed 2N45.

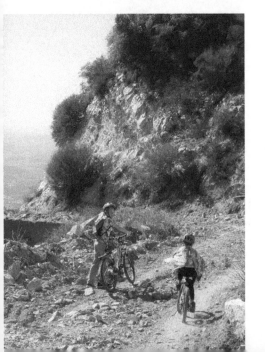

This one-way trip descends from Mount Wilson to Pasadena by way of the historic Mount Wilson Toll Road. Along the way, enjoy

For a great family outing, get dropped off at the top of the Mount Wilson Toll Road with your kids and their bikes.

sweeping views over the L.A. Basin as well as intimate passages through shady groves of canyon live oak and big-cone Douglas-fir. If you're looking for a more strenuous undertaking, hike the trip in reverse or combine it with one of the mountain's many other wonderful trails.

The Mount Wilson Toll Road was first proposed by Judge Benjamin Eaton in 1889. He and other investors formed the Pasadena and Mount Wilson Toll Road Company. A crew hacked a narrow horse trail to the summit in just five months of work, opening in 1891. In 1917, when Carnegie Observatory began building the 100-inch Hooker Telescope, the world's largest at the time, the path was widened to 12 feet to haul parts up the mountain. The white-knuckle drive was legendary in Southern California until it became obsolete when Angeles Crest Highway opened in 1935. Today, it is U.S. Forest Service property and is enjoyed by hikers and mountain bikers.

From the gate at the top of 2N45/Mount Wilson Toll Road, begin your long switchbacking descent. Watch for signs of the 50-acre 2017 Wilson Fire. After 1.0 mile stay left at a fork where you meet a service road to Mount Harvard and a footpath descending from Skyline Park. At 1.5 miles stay right at an intersection with the Mount Wilson Trail that leads down to Sierra Madre (see Trip 24.8, page 324) or Chantry Flat (see Trip 24.13, page 332). At 5.1 miles stay left again as you pass the Idlehour Trail (see Trip 24.4, page 318). Continue down through Henninger Flat (6.2 miles; see Trip 24.1, page 315), where you can find pleasant camping and picnic grounds shaded beneath an experimental forest. Finally, cross the toll road bridge at the mouth of Eaton Canyon and arrive at the Pinecrest Drive trailhead.

trip 24.3   Eaton Canyon Falls

see map on p. 314

Distance	3.8 miles (out-and-back)
Hiking Time	1.5 hours
Elevation Gain	400'
Difficulty	Moderate
Trail Use	Dogs allowed, good for kids
Best Times	Year-round
Agency	Los Angeles County Parks & Recreation
Optional Map	Tom Harrison *Angeles Front Country* or Trails Illustrated *Angeles National Forest (811)*

DIRECTIONS From the eastbound 210 Freeway, take Exit 28 for northbound Altadena Drive. (From the westbound 210, take Exit 29A for Sierra Madre and follow the frontage road to Altadena Drive.) Proceed 1.7 miles to the nature center parking on the right, or the nearby overflow area.

Eaton Canyon Natural Area is a well-known gem at the foot of the San Gabriel Mountains. On a pleasant spring weekend, thousands of people gather at the busy trailhead for a stroll. The canyon burned to ash in the 1993 Altadena Fire but has completely recovered. The rebuilt Nature Center is full of knowledgeable volunteers who share their passion about the outdoors.

Upstream from the 190-acre park, where the waters of Eaton Canyon have carved a raw groove in the San Gabriel Mountains, you'll discover Eaton Canyon Falls. Impressive only during the wetter half of the year, the falls possesses, as John Muir once put it, "a low sweet voice, singing like a bird." The falls are well worth visiting, especially in the aftermath of a larger winter storm, if only to witness the power of large (by meager Southern California standards anyway) volumes of falling water. The canyon is named for Judge Benjamin Eaton, who tapped water here for his Fair Oaks Ranch (now north Pasadena).

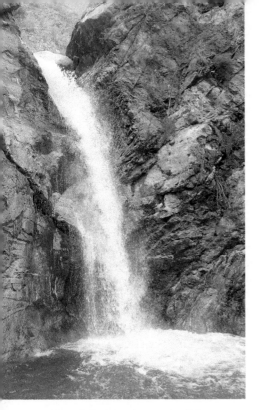

From the parking lot at Eaton Canyon Nature Center, follow the Eaton Canyon Trail upstream. The trail promptly splits—both branches run parallel and then rejoin before crossing to the east side of the canyon. After crossing the canyon's cobbled bottom, the trail sticks to an elevated stream terrace, passing some beautiful live-oak woods.

At 1.2 miles you rise to meet the Mount Wilson Toll Road bridge over Eaton Canyon. Just before the bridge, veer left onto a narrow track at a sign for Eaton Canyon Falls. The rough path leads up the canyon, crossing the creek eight times. Expect plenty of boulder hopping, and you may get your feet wet if the stream is lively. This is not a place to be when the creek is in flood. Except for a line of alders along part of the stream and some live oaks on terraces just above the reach of floods, the canyon bottom and the precipitous walls are desolate and desertlike. After 0.7 mile of canyon-bottom travel, you come to the falls, where the water slides and then free-falls a total of about 35 vertical feet down a narrow chute in the bedrock.

Eaton Falls draws thousands of hikers on nice spring weekends.

VARIATION

The walk can be shortened to 1.4 miles out-and-back by starting from the lower gate of the Mount Wilson Toll Road on Pinecrest Drive in Altadena. Make sure to observe the strict parking restrictions in that neighborhood.

---

trip 24.4   Idlehour Descent

see map on p. 314

Distance	12 miles (one-way)
Hiking Time	5.5 hours
Elevation Gain/Loss	1,300'/5,300'
Difficulty	Strenuous
Trail Use	Suitable for backpacking, dogs allowed
Best Times	October–June
Agency	Angeles National Forest
Optional Map	Tom Harrison *Angeles Front Country* or Trails Illustrated *Angeles National Forest* (811)

DIRECTIONS This one-way trip requires a 45-minute shuttle between trailheads; unless you're using a ride-sharing service, leave one car at Eaton Canyon Natural Area. From the eastbound 210 Freeway, take Exit 28 for northbound Altadena Drive. (From the westbound 210, take Exit 29A for Sierra Madre and follow the frontage road to Altadena Drive.) Proceed 1.7 miles to the nature center parking on the right.

To reach the upper trailhead, return to the 210 Freeway and continue 8 miles west to the Angeles Crest Highway (Highway 2) in La Cañada Flintridge. Drive 14 miles north and east to Red Box Station and the intersection of Mount Wilson Road at mile marker 2 LA 38.38. Turn right on Mount Wilson Road and proceed 2.4 miles to a roadside parking area at Eaton Saddle.

Not an idle descent at all, this one-way hike passes through some of the most varied and interesting terrain in the Front Range. From shady canyon to mountainside view, the landscape is ever changing along the way. The lush and lightly visited middle portion is also a promising area to spot wildlife. Over a distance of almost 11 miles on roads and trails, you journey 4 air miles from the crest of the Front Range at Eaton Saddle all the way down to the edge of the L.A. Basin at Eaton Canyon County Park. The name *Idlehour* comes from Idlehour Trail Camp, formerly a trail resort, passed at the midway point of the hike. Much of the Mount Lowe area burned in the 2009 Station Fire, but the chaparral recovers quickly and the verdant canyons escaped the inferno.

From Eaton Saddle, follow Mount Lowe Fire Road 0.5 mile west to Markham Saddle, where trails intersect left and right. Leave the fire road and bear left on the Mount Lowe Trail. Cross a second saddle at 1.2 miles, where a climbers' trail follows a ridge northeast to Mount Markham. At a trail junction ahead (1.4 miles), the Mount Lowe summit trail comes in acutely from the right. Unless you want to detour to the peak, keep straight to remain on the shorter, better-maintained east-side route down along the flank of the mountain. At 2.4 miles you can either drop to the fire road on your right or stay on the trail another 0.2 mile to meet the same fire road farther south. Briefly continue walking south on the fire road to a five-way junction (2.7 miles).

Turn left onto the Idlehour trail and descend through scattered north-slope groves of live oak and big-cone Douglas-firs to a crossing of a west fork of Eaton Canyon, at 4.6 miles. You then climb a bit to cross a chaparral-covered divide to the east, and begin a switchback descent into Eaton Canyon. Look for the faultlike discontinuity in the igneous rock exposed on Eaton Canyon's sheer east wall.

At the bottom (5.8 miles) the trail goes downcanyon and becomes intermittently lost in a refreshingly chilly wonderland of crystal-clear cascades, overarching oaks and maples, and crispy carpets of orange and brown leaf-litter. Cabin-foundation ruins can be found under the trees, a reminder that even in this inviting hideaway, no construction is spared for long the ravages of fire and flood—or, in this case, removal by the Pasadena Water Department. You soon come to Idlehour Trail Camp (6.4 miles), nestled on an oak-shaded flat lying next to a rock fin with vertical striations, dividing Eaton Canyon from its aforementioned west fork. Naturally, this is the best place for a picnic if you're day-hiking, or for a place to pitch a tent and call it a night if you're backpacking the route.

The narrow, wild section of Eaton Canyon below the camp was eschewed by trail builders in favor of a route up the east canyon wall to Mount Wilson Toll Road. (Some people have followed the lower canyon route, including John Muir, who later described the front face of the San Gabriels as "rigidly inaccessible." Many rescues and fatalities have occurred here, and the desert is suitable only

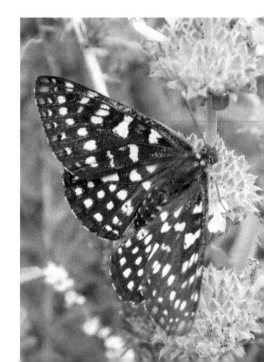

*The variable checkerspot butterfly (*Euphydryas chalcodona*) is commonly found on chaparral during the spring in the San Gabriel Mountains.*

for experienced canyoneers—see ropewiki.com for details.) The safe and easy Idlehour Trail goes east up a tributary (Harvard Branch) momentarily, then climbs up and over a ridge to meet Mount Wilson Toll Road (8.2 miles).

Descend on the old toll road past Henninger Flats (9.4 miles) to a hairpin turn (11.2 miles), where an equestrian trail takes off down the slope to the left into Walnut Canyon. Switchbacks, steep at times, take you down 0.5 mile to the wide Eaton Canyon Trail following Eaton Canyon wash. Turn left and complete the remaining 0.6 mile to the nature center at Eaton Canyon Natural Area.

| trip 24.5 | **Valley Forge & DeVore Trails** |

Distance	7 miles (one-way)
Hiking Time	4 hours
Elevation Gain/Loss	1,700'/2,100'
Difficulty	Moderately strenuous
Trail Use	Suitable for backpacking, dogs allowed
Best Times	October–June
Agency	Angeles National Forest
Optional Map	Tom Harrison *Angeles Front Country* or Trails Illustrated *Angeles National Forest (811)*

DIRECTIONS If you wish to avoid a 2-mile walk or bike ride along between trailheads, leave one vehicle at the west (lower) end at Eaton Saddle. Exit the 210 Freeway at Angeles Crest Highway (Highway 2) in La Cañada Flintridge. Drive 14 miles north and east to Red Box Station and the intersection of Mount Wilson Road at mile marker 2 LA 38.38. Turn right on Mount Wilson Road and proceed 2.4 miles to the large but busy parking area at Eaton Saddle.

To reach the east (upper) trailhead, continue 2.0 miles to where the road splits and becomes a one-way loop around the antenna-spiked Mount Wilson ridgeline. Parking is available in a roadside turnout to the west.

The Falls Canyon Research Natural Area on the north slope of Mount Wilson helps protect a steeply sloping, 1,000-acre block of land covered by magnificent stands of big-cone Douglas-fir and canyon live oak. The point-to-point route described here circumnavigates that area by way of the Kenyon DeVore (formerly Rattlesnake), Gabrielino, and Valley Forge Trails, completing about four-fifths of a circle. (You can make this a full-circle hike by walking some 2 miles along the narrow shoulder of possibly busy Mount Wilson Road, or pre-position a bike at the upper trailhead and do the loop in reverse.) The strenuous hiking and lightly maintained trails make it likely that you can escape the throngs who visit many of the other trails in the vicinity. The 2009 Station Fire swept through the canyon but spared most of this hike. The narrow trail clings to steep slopes in places, so it's not recommended for the acrophobic.

From the turnout on Mount Wilson Road, the Kenyon DeVore Trail descends on long and sometimes poorly maintained switchbacks. Kenyon DeVore (1911–1995) was a long-time mountain man and U.S. Forest Service ranger who grew up at his parents' resorts of Camp West Fork and Valley Forge Lodge in the canyon that this trip visits.

You're following the drainage of Strayns Canyon, crossing the stream of the main canyon or tributaries at least four times. (The canyon's name is apparently a corruption of the name of A. G. Strain, who operated a tourist camp on Mount Wilson's north slope in the 1890s.) Deeply shaded by alders and big-leaf maples down along the stream, this is a thoroughly enjoyable stretch.

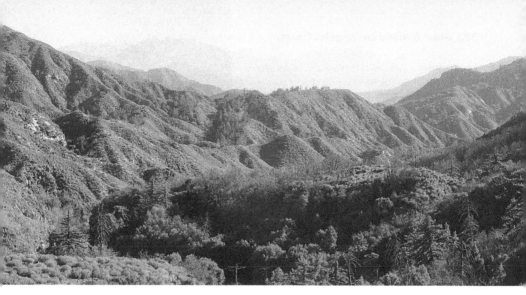

Looking down the West Fork of the San Gabriel River canyon near Valley Forge

At 2.7 miles there's an easy-to-miss junction. The combined DeVore/Gabrielino Trail continues downcanyon, on the right-hand side of the stream, to Rincon–Red Box Road and West Fork Camp—go left, across the stream, westbound on the Gabrielino Trail. On it you contour, more or less, through shady glens or through sunny thickets of chaparral.

At 4.1 miles you come to an intersection with the Valley Forge Trail, which is your route back up to Mount Wilson Road. On the Gabrielino Trail, 0.1 mile beyond this junction, there's a side path to Valley Forge Campground down along the bank of West Fork San Gabriel River. This makes a good overnight campsite for trail travelers, as the road from Red Box is now gated year-round and there's always peace and quiet here. The Valley Forge Lodge was a popular resort here from 1922 until 1938, when a great flood wiped out nearly every canyon resort in the San Gabriels.

On the Valley Forge Trail you go up through the semi-shade of oaks, bay laurels, and tall chaparral—first on switchbacks, then on a straighter course high on the west wall of Falls Canyon. Finally arrive at Eaton Saddle, where you may have left a getaway vehicle.

VARIATION

For a more strenuous and even more attractive loop, descend the DeVore Trail as above; then turn right and hike down to the West Fork Trail. Follow the trail or road up to Newcomb Pass, and then take the Rim Trail back up to Wilson. This route is 11 miles with 2,700 feet of elevation gain.

---

trip 24.6   **Bailey Canyon**

Distance	1.2 miles (out-and-back)
Hiking Time	1 hour
Elevation Gain	300'
Difficulty	Easy
Trail Use	Dogs allowed, good for kids
Best Times	Year-round
Agency	City of Sierra Madre
Optional Map	Tom Harrison *Angeles Front Country* or Trails Illustrated *Angeles National Forest (811)*

see map on p. 314

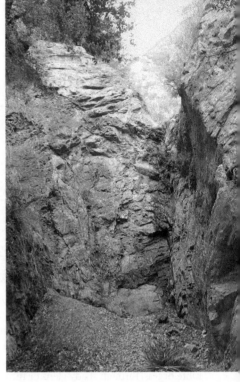

DIRECTIONS From the 210 Freeway in Arcadia, take Exit 31 for Baldwin Avenue. Drive 1.6 miles north; then turn left on Carter Avenue. Proceed 0.5 mile west to reach the small day-use parking lot at Bailey Canyon Park.

Sierra Madre's impeccably maintained Bailey Canyon Park includes a small, shady picnic area, and the lower part of a trail that now goes all the way to the Mount Wilson Trail above Orchard Camp. This little excursion within the park visits the narrow bottom of Bailey Canyon, which hosts an easy-to-reach small, seasonal waterfall. The park is named for R. J. Bailey, who ran a ranch here from 1857 to 1881.

From the west side of the parking lot, walk west under shade-giving trees to a gap in a chain-link fence. Pick up a paved service road just beyond, and follow it uphill and around a debris basin lying at the mouth of Bailey Canyon. Follow the narrow Bailey Canyon Trail onward into the canyon.

At 0.3 mile the undermaintained Live Oak

Bailey Canyon Falls will probably look like this unless you arrive during a rainstorm.

Nature Trail forks right over a bridge, and you stay straight on the Canyon View Nature trail toward the waterfall. In another 0.1 mile, the Bailey Canyon Trail veers right toward Jones Peak (see next trip), but you veer left into the sandy stream bottom. In a quarter mile you'll come to the end of the line for easy hiking. A dike of dark, intrusive igneous rock, squeezed between lighter granite walls, lies ahead. This natural barrier forces any water flowing in the canyon to plunge about 15 feet over a precipice. The waterfall trills like a bird only after significant rain has fallen.

A use trail on the left leads to the top of the falls. Canyoneers with ropes have followed the canyon all the way to the cabin ruins (see the next trip for Jones Peak).

trip 24.7 **Jones Peak**

see map on p. 314

Distance	6 miles (out-and-back)
Hiking Time	4 hours
Elevation Gain	2,300'
Difficulty	Moderately strenuous
Trail Use	Dogs allowed
Best Times	October–May
Agency	City of Sierra Madre
Optional Map	Tom Harrison *Angeles Front Country* or Trails Illustrated *Angeles National Forest (811)*

DIRECTIONS From the 210 Freeway in Arcadia, take Exit 31 for Baldwin Avenue. Drive 1.6 miles north; then turn left on Carter Avenue. Proceed 0.5 mile west to reach the small day-use parking lot at Bailey Canyon Park. Be sure to turn your wheels toward the curb at the trailhead, as the City of Sierra Madre issues tickets.

Jones Peak (3,375') is nowhere near the loftiest of the many named summits you can climb in the sharply rising Front Range of the San Gabriel Mountains. But its elevated position— barely 1 mile as the crow flies from the fringe of the vast Los Angeles Basin metropolitan sprawl—affords a 180°-plus view of a big chunk of Southern California. That view is nothing less than commanding during the best clear-air episodes characteristic of the late fall and winter seasons. The peak is named for C. W. Jones, who served as the first mayor of Sierra Madre from 1907 to 1914.

From the west side of the Bailey Canyon Park lot, walk west under shade-giving trees to a gap in a chain-link fence. Pick up a paved service road just beyond, and follow it uphill and around a debris basin lying at the mouth of Bailey Canyon. Follow the narrow Bailey Canyon Trail onward into the canyon.

At 0.3 mile the undermaintained Live Oak Nature Trail forks right over a bridge, and you stay straight on the Canyon View Nature Trail toward the waterfall. In another 0.1 mile, the nature trail veers left into the creek—go right on the Bailey Canyon Trail and commence a crooked, unforgivingly steep ascent up the east wall of the canyon. As you climb, note the distant downtown Los Angeles skyline positioned over the Mission-style buildings of a Passionist Fathers monastery right down below.

At 0.6 mile pass a bench, and at 0.8 mile pass a second bench signed INDIAN LOOKOUT POINT, offering an outstanding view. You've climbed 500 feet so far, and this is a fine turnaround point if you are looking for a shorter hike. Watch for amusing but historically dubious plaques on this bench and elsewhere along the trail.

At 2.1 miles the trail reaches a level about even with the seasonal stream flowing in the upper reaches of Bailey Canyon. A cabin foundation lies just below the trail on a small flat just above the stream. That's a good place to take a breather, since the remaining 1.3 miles of the hike are again steep. Proceed generally east up a series of tight switchbacks, and arrive at Jones Saddle. Swing right and scamper up a sketchy path to the Jones Peak summit, where you can take in the comprehensive view.

On the clearest days, the tree-dotted urban plain rolls out like a shaggy carpet toward the Pacific Ocean, which takes on a silvery sheen in late fall and winter. Look for as many as three of the Channel Islands punctuating the horizon: Santa Catalina Island (often obvious); San Clemente Island (sometimes glimpsed to the left of the leftmost tip of Santa Catalina); and tiny Santa Barbara Island (well to the right of Santa Catalina).

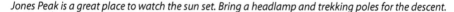

Jones Peak is a great place to watch the sun set. Bring a headlamp and trekking poles for the descent.

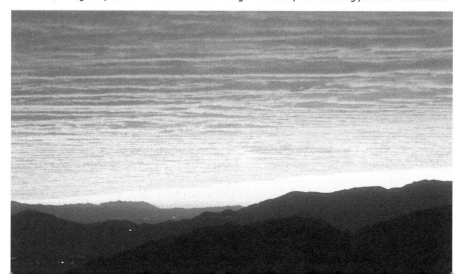

VARIATIONS

It's possible to hike north on a firebreak trail 0.2 mile from Jones Saddle, then descend tight switchbacks on the Jones Peak Connector Trail to meet the Mount Wilson Trail and follow it down. Follow Carter Avenue back to the start.

The good firebreak trail also continues north from Jones Peak over 4,000-foot Hastings Peak (not labeled on all maps) to meet the Mount Wilson Toll Road, enabling a variety of strenuous but enjoyable loops. The peak is named for Charles Hastings, who acquired a 1,100-acre ranch between Pasadena and Sierra Madre in 1882.

Jones Peak can also be climbed from the Mount Wilson Trail via a steep firebreak up the south-southeast ridge, known locally as Bastard Ridge. Start at the fork where the Mount Wilson Trail rounds a bend into the main canyon, and follow Charlie's New Trail on the left, up past a bench and on up the ridge.

---

trip 24.8	**Mount Wilson to Sierra Madre**

see map on p. 314

Distance	7 miles (one-way)
Hiking Time	3.5 hours
Elevation Gain/Loss	100'/4,800'
Difficulty	Moderately strenuous
Trail Use	Suitable for backpacking, dogs allowed
Best Times	November–May
Agency	Angeles National Forest
Optional Map	Tom Harrison *Angeles Front Country* or Trails Illustrated *Angeles National Forest (811)*

DIRECTIONS This trip requires a 1-hour car (or ride-sharing service) shuttle. To reach the lower trailhead from the 210 Freeway in Arcadia, take Exit 31 for Baldwin Avenue. Go north 1.5 miles; then turn right on Mira Monte Avenue. Go two blocks east on Mira Monte to reach the Mount Wilson Trailhead, on the left—leave a shuttle vehicle here. Be sure to turn your wheels toward the curb at the trailhead, as the City of Sierra Madre issues tickets.

To reach the upper trailhead, return to the 210 Freeway and drive west 10 miles to Angeles Crest Highway (Highway 2) in La Cañada Flintridge. Drive 14 miles north and east to Red Box Station and the intersection of Mount Wilson Road at mile marker 2 LA 38.38. Turn right on Mount Wilson Road and proceed 4 miles to the parking lot at the end of the road.

On the Mount Wilson Trail you can almost feel the weight of history. This is the oldest and most direct route connecting Mount Wilson's 5,710-foot summit and the San Gabriel Valley floor, and the first of many trails that were built to something resembling modern standards in the San Gabriel Mountains. In 1864, Benjamin Wilson widened and improved this former Indian path in order to exploit timber resources near the summit. Very little timber was actually cut, but the precipitous trail soon became popular among hikers and horsemen. By 1889, the first instrument placed on the mountaintop that would someday host the world's foremost observatory was hauled up in pieces on the same trail—a process that took a month to accomplish. By 1891, a "new" Mount Wilson trail from the mouth of Eaton Canyon (Mount Wilson Toll Road) was constructed, largely preempting the shorter but steeper older trail. Still in use today, the old trail remains passable only by virtue of volunteers who maintain it.

The lower part of the Mount Wilson Trail, which lies in the city of Sierra Madre, may close during periods of high fire danger, so check first with the U.S. Forest Service or the City of Sierra Madre, whose website (cityofsierramadre.com) lists current information about the city's recreational areas.

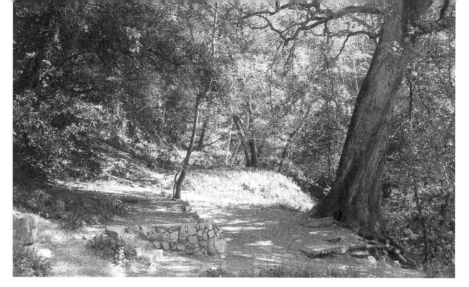

Orchard Camp foundations halfway up the Mount Wilson Trail

From the south edge of the parking lot at the end of Mount Wilson Road, take the signed Mount Wilson Trail, which immediately starts zigzagging down a steep slope through the 50-acre burn zone of the 2017 Wilson Fire. Beware of poodle dog bush, a purple-flowered plant that grows for up to a decade after a fire and can cause severe skin irritation. After 0.7 mile you join Mount Wilson Toll Road. Continue on the old toll road 0.5 mile to the intersection of the Mount Wilson Trail on the left, just as the toll road begins curving west. Follow a firebreak down about 100 yards; then pick up a narrow trail to the right offering a gentler descent. At 1.7 miles the Mount Wilson Trail forks right and starts descending through chaparral into the headwaters of Little Santa Anita Canyon. Live oaks, sycamores, big-leaf maples, alders, and big-cone Douglas-firs cluster about the canyon bottom below. You cross the canyon bottom and descend along a shady, west-side slope for a while. Next, a set of tight switchbacks takes you down to a wooded glen along the canyon stream at 3.5 miles. There you'll find the foundation ruins of Orchard Camp (a resort), earlier known as Halfway House because it was located almost exactly halfway between Mount Wilson and the foot of the trail in Sierra Madre.

After a more-or-less-level stretch under oaks, look for a side path to the left (4.3 miles) leading to an open spot—a sometime heliport—on the shoulder of a ridge overlooking the canyon. Then watch for the signed Jones Peak Connector Trail on the left. Thereafter, you begin an almost constant, steep descent across dry chaparral slopes. In spring, sweet alyssum (a nonnative escapee from foothill gardens) blooms along the path, along with many native wildflowers, including ceanothus, prickly lupine, blue dicks, purple nightshade, phacelia, and wild pea.

At a sharp bend, an unsigned trail descends Lost Canyon to the bottom of Little Santa Anita Canyon, where Quarter Way House and Camp Nomad drew visitors from 1888 through the 1930s. A footpath continues downstream for a quarter mile to a cascade, pool, and picnic bench at First Water before climbing back to rejoin the main trail at a signed junction at 5 miles.

Shortly beyond, come to another unsigned fork at a switchback. Turn left to stay on the official trail; the unmaintained path on the right rejoins the main trail in 0.5 mile, where a rough firebreak climbs Bastard Ridge, the south-southeast ridge of Jones Peak. The trail becomes a dirt road at 7.0 miles. Just beyond this point, take the path to the right, because the road ahead is private. You end up on a paved drive, and after 0.1 mile more reach the trailhead on Mira Monte Avenue in Sierra Madre.

trip 24.9   **Santa Anita Ridge**

Distance	7 miles (out-and-back)
Hiking Time	3.5 hours
Elevation Gain	1,300'
Difficulty	Moderately strenuous
Trail Use	Suitable for mountain biking, dogs allowed
Best Times	November–May
Agency	Angeles National Forest
Optional Map	Tom Harrison *Angeles Front Country* or Trails Illustrated *Angeles National Forest (811)*

see map on p. 314

DIRECTIONS From the 210 Freeway in Arcadia, take Exit 32 for Santa Anita Avenue. Drive north 5 miles to the parking lots at Chantry Flat, passing a vehicle gate that's open 6 a.m.–8 p.m.

Winding its way lazily upward from the crowded parking lots at Chantry Flat, San Olene Fire Road leads to a shoulder of Santa Anita Ridge—the scenic divide between Big and Little Santa Anita Canyons. From the top of the road, the sweeping view takes in the Santa Anita Park race track (only 3 miles to the south), a good chunk of the San Gabriel Valley, and parts of the San Gabriel Mountains' High Country to the north and northeast.

The ridge and road are named for Rancho Santa Anita, a 13,319-acre Mexican land grant carved from a part of Mission San Gabriel's property and given to Hugo Reid in 1845. Two years later, Reid sold the ranch to his neighbor Henry Dalton for $2,700. This was a good price, considering that the land now comprises much of Arcadia, Monrovia, Sierra Madre, Pasadena, and San Marino. In 1875, Elias "Lucky" Baldwin purchased the ranch for $200,000 and established the race track that still bears the same name.

The road climbs 3.5 miles at an almost steady 6% grade—a bit tedious at walking pace, it's probably better for running or mountain biking. On clear days the scenery is uniformly pleasant, especially after winter storms have dusted the surrounding summits. Edging along north-facing slopes much of the way, the road twists and turns through stands of mature chaparral and mini-groves of bay and maple. From the top you could catch a winter sunset, watch the city lights turn on, then return by the light of a three-quarter or full moon (but remember, the gate below Chantry Flat closes at 8 p.m. daily).

Route finding could scarcely be more simple. From the upper end of the parking area, walk up the gated paved service road (signed 2N41/UPPER WINTER CREEK TRAIL). At 0.7 mile you pass the Chantry Flat Heliport, where the pavement ends and a dirt road continues. (Those who would prefer a much shorter, but gut-busting, approach can follow an old but periodically maintained firebreak straight up the ridge west of the heliport. It leads to the uppermost hairpin turn on San

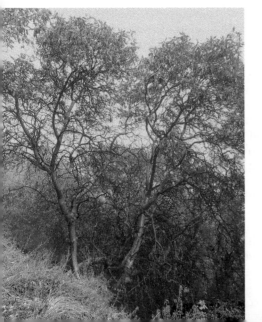

Madrone (Arbutus menziesii), instantly recognizable by its smooth, red bark, resembles manzanita in tree form.

Olene Fire Road. It replaces 2.5 miles of fire road with 0.6 mile of unrelenting ridge.) At 3.5 miles the road levels. There's a microwave reflector structure on the left and a water tank signed SANTA ANITA RIDGE on the right. Proceed 0.15 mile down the ridge to the south to the road's end for the best view of the valley below.

VARIATION

A firebreak known as the Manzanita Ridge or Goat Trail climbs Santa Anita Ridge from the water tank to the Mount Wilson Trail near its confluence with the Winter Creek Trail. Vigorous hikers could envision many various strenuous trips using this path.

---

trip 24.10   **Hoegees Loop**

Distance	5.5 miles (loop)
Hiking Time	2.5 hours
Elevation Gain	1,300'
Difficulty	Moderate
Trail Use	Suitable for backpacking, dogs allowed
Best Times	Year-round
Agency	Angeles National Forest
Optional Map	Tom Harrison *Angeles Front Country* or Trails Illustrated *Angeles National Forest (811)*

see map on p. 314

DIRECTIONS From the 210 Freeway in Arcadia, take Exit 32 for Santa Anita Avenue. Drive north 5 miles to the parking lots at Chantry Flat, passing a vehicle gate that's open 6 a.m.–8 p.m.

The canyons of Big Santa Anita and Winter Creek exist in a time warp. On foot is the only way in for the owners of the 82 cabins on Forest Service land here, dating from the early 1900s. Typical cabin amenities include kerosene lamps, drinking water carried in by the jugful, and one-hole privies. This ramble on rustic trails takes you through both of these secluded canyons, where trickling streams and rustling leaves make you forget you're anywhere near a big city.

On this looping hike to and from Hoegees Trail Camp on Winter Creek, you'll get a good feel for the riparian splendor that attracted early residents and day-trippers, and that still attracts legions of hikers today. (Since there are about a dozen stream crossings on the route without benefit of bridges, you'll want to avoid this trip after a heavy rain.) Native alders, oaks, bays, and willows cluster along the bubbling, cascading streams. Ivy and vinca, planted by the early settlers, have run rampant in some areas, climbing high into the trees in a fashion reminiscent of the kudzu-vine invasion of the American Southeast. Poison oak is plentiful here as well.

Both canyons have been plugged in many places with so-called crib dams—check dams constructed of precast concrete logs—but many decades of steady regrowth have softened their visual impact.

Start at the south edge of the lower parking lot at Chantry Flat, where a gated, paved road (the Gabrielino Trail) starts descending into Big Santa Anita Canyon. After rounding the first sharp bend at 0.2 mile, veer right onto the narrow and precipitous First Water Trail. This was once a lateral branch of the original Sturtevant Trail between the San Gabriel Valley and Sturtevant Camp (see Trip 24.12, page 330). Descend on precipitous switchbacks—watch your step!—to the stream below, where an appropriately named First Water Camp welcomed hot and footsore hikers in the 1920s and '30s. Turn left (upstream) and follow the rudiments of a trail amid streamside cabins and boulders to the confluence

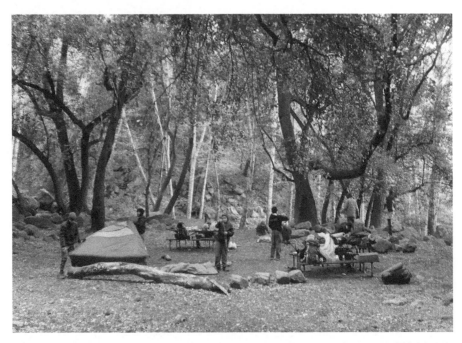

Hoegees Camp is popular with youth groups because of the short approach and wild setting.

of Big Santa Anita Canyon and Winter Creek, where the paved trail comes down from Chantry Flat. A small restroom building occupies a flat area nearby (1,780') where the largest resort of the area, Roberts' Camp, sprawled in the early 1900s. During the peak of its popularity, a branch of the L.A. County Library and a post office were established here to serve guests and passing hikers.

From the confluence, head west into the steep-walled confines of Winter Creek. Winter Creek is named for Sturde's Winter Camp, a work camp that Wilbur Sturtevant built in 1895 while developing his trail up Big Santa Anita Canyon. The well-traveled trail snakes upward, sometimes along the stream, otherwise up on the canyon walls in order to bypass crib dams or to swing by cabins. After 1.5 miles (from the confluence) you come to Hoegees Trail Camp (tables, stoves), tucked into a shady nook on Winter Creek's south bank. Nearby are the scattered foundation ruins of the original Hoegees Trail Camp (later called Camp Ivy), a hikers' resort with a store, dining room, tent cabins, and stable, established in 1908 by Arie Hoegee Jr., and destroyed by wildfire in 1953. Today, Hoegees is one of the more popular trail camps in the San Gabriels: charming, rustic, and easy to reach by either leg of our loop hike.

If you plan to camp here, beware that black bears sometimes raid the camp at night, looking for food. They're highly skilled at getting food hanging from trees, so a bear canister is the only reliable solution. Also note that the Environmental Protection Agency forced the U.S. Forest Service to close the pit toilet at the campground, so you'll need to walk into the woods at least 100 feet from the stream and any cabins or campsites to relieve yourself and then dig a hole 6–8 inches deep to bury solid waste.

Your return is by way of the Upper Winter Creek Trail. From Hoegees, continue upstream on the north bank, passing the Mount Zion Trail on the right. Presently, the trail swings left to cross the stream and climb obliquely up Winter Creek's south canyon wall. In a short

while you reach a signed junction—right toward Mount Wilson and left back to your starting point, a crooked 2.4 miles away. About 0.3 mile from the end, the trail joins a paved
section of San Olene Fire Road; it will take you down past the picnic area to the upper
parking lot at Chantry Flat.

VARIATION

From the bottom of the First Water Trail, you can turn right and walk downstream through
the beautifully forested canyon to Hermit Falls (interesting but vandalized, and less impressive than Sturtevant Falls). They were named for Frank Volvin, "The Hermit of Big Santa
Anita," who built a small cabin near here around 1898. Note that the falls have been the site
of multiple fatal slips and cliff-jumping accidents, so be careful here. This excursion adds
1 mile round-trip with 200 feet of elevation gain.

---

trip 24.11   **Sturtevant Falls**

Distance	3.4 miles (out-and-back)
Hiking Time	1.5 hours
Elevation Gain	700'
Difficulty	Moderate
Trail Use	Dogs allowed, good for kids
Best Times	Year-round
Agency	Angeles National Forest
Optional Map	Tom Harrison *Angeles Front Country* or Trails Illustrated *Angeles National Forest (811)*

see
map on
p. 314

DIRECTIONS From the 210 Freeway in Arcadia, take Exit 32 for Santa Anita Avenue. Drive north 5 miles
to the parking lots at Chantry Flat, passing a vehicle gate that's open 6 a.m.–8 p.m.

At Sturtevant Falls, the waters of Big Santa Anita Canyon leap (or dribble, depending
on the season) over a 50-foot precipice into a shallow pool. Sturtevant Falls ranks,
along with falls of a similar stature in Millard and San Antonio Canyons, as one of the
more impressive and yet easily reached waterfalls in Southern California. A local attraction
since the days of the early resorts, it still draws hundreds of visitors on some fair-weather
weekends. To avoid the crowds and gain some feeling of majesty in this special spot, it's
best to pay a visit on a weekday. Better yet, come on an overcast day, when flat lighting
enhances the subdued colors of the rocks, the trees, and the frothing water. The falls are
named for Wilbur Sturtevant (see the next trip for more about him). Watch out for poison
oak along the trail.

From the south edge of the lower parking lot at Chantry Flat, hike the first paved segment
of the Gabrielino Trail down to the confluence of Winter Creek and Big Santa Anita Canyon
(0.6 mile). Pavement ends at a metal bridge spanning Winter Creek. Pass the restrooms
and continue up alder-lined Big Santa Anita Canyon on a wide road bed following the left
bank. Edging alongside a number of small cabins, the deteriorating road soon assumes the
proportions of a foot trail.

At 1.4 miles, amid a beautiful oak woodland, you come to a four-way junction of trails.
Take the right fork and continue upstream, boulder-hopping over the clear-flowing stream
part of the way (and perhaps getting your feet wet for the first time), to the foot of the
falls. Don't be tempted to climb the side walls; the two trails going left back at the four-way
junction can take you safely past the falls if you want to press on farther up the canyon.

trip 24.12 **Santa Anita Canyon Loop**

see map on p. 314

Distance	8.5 miles (loop)
Hiking Time	5 hours
Elevation Gain	2,200'
Difficulty	Moderately strenuous
Trail Use	Suitable for backpacking, dogs allowed
Best Times	October–June
Agency	Angeles National Forest
Optional Map	Tom Harrison *Angeles Front Country* or Trails Illustrated *Angeles National Forest (811)*

DIRECTIONS From the 210 Freeway in Arcadia, take Exit 32 for Santa Anita Avenue. Drive north 5 miles to the parking lots at Chantry Flat, passing a vehicle gate that's open 6 a.m.–8 p.m.

Sturtevant Camp is both the oldest (1893) and the only remaining resort of the Big Santa Anita drainage. Now renting cabins to the public, the camp remains accessible only by foot trail. Supplies are packed in from Chantry Flat on the backs of pack animals, not unlike a century ago. Today's pack trains ply the Gabrielino Trail up Big Santa Anita Canyon past Sturtevant Falls. Around the turn of the century, however, travelers and supplies came by way of a trail hacked out by Wilbur M. "Sturde" Sturtevant (1841–1910) and some associates. Beginning in Sierra Madre, this original Sturtevant Trail worked its way along the high, west wall of lower Big Santa Anita Canyon; crossed a shady spot later known as Chantry Flat; traversed Winter Creek at a point near today's Hoegees Trail Camp; ascended a hot, dry slope to a notch just below Mount Zion; and finally slanted downward to Sturtevant's camp in Big Santa Anita's headwaters. Be sure that you can recognize poison oak, which grows beside many parts of the trail.

In this scenic loop trip from Chantry Flat, you'll climb by way of the newer Gabrielino Trail to Sturtevant Camp, and return by way of the Mount Zion and Upper Winter Creek Trails—the original Sturtevant route. Do it in a day, or take your time on an overnight backpacking trip, with a stay at Spruce Grove Trail Camp or Sturtevant Camp. The trail camp is a popular one, so plan to get there early to secure a spot on the weekend—or go on a weekday. With advance reservations, you can stay at a historic cabin at nearby Sturtevant Camp (sturtevantcamp.com) and even have the pack train carry in your gear.

From the south edge of the lower parking lot at Chantry Flat, hike the first paved segment of the Gabrielino Trail down to the confluence of Winter Creek and Big Santa Anita Canyon (0.6 mile). Pavement ends at a metal bridge spanning Winter Creek. Pass the restrooms and continue up alder-lined Big Santa Anita Canyon on a wide road bed following the left bank. Edging alongside a number of small cabins, the deteriorating road soon assumes the proportions of a foot trail.

At 1.4 miles, amid a beautiful oak woodland, you come to a four-way junction of trails. The right branch goes upcanyon to Sturtevant Falls; the middle and left branches bypass the falls and join again about a mile upstream. If the creek is flowing well, consider a 0.3-mile side trip to the falls, and then return here. The left, upper trail is recommended for horses. Take the middle, or lower, trail—the more scenic and exciting alternative—unless you dislike heights. The lower trail slices across a sheer wall above the falls and continues through a veritable fairyland of miniature cascades and crystalline pools bedecked with giant chain ferns.

A half mile past the reconvergence of the upper and lower trails, you come upon Cascade Picnic Area (2.8 miles—tables and restrooms here), named for a smooth chute in the stream bottom just below. Press on past a hulking crib dam to Spruce Grove Trail Camp (3.2 miles), named for the big-cone Douglas-fir trees that attain truly inspiring proportions hereabouts.

In another 0.3 mile, the Gabrielino Trail forks right to climb toward Newcomb Pass (see Trip 24.14, page 334). You go left on the signed Sturtevant Trail and enter Sturtevant Camp in 0.1 mile. The camp was established by Wilbur Sturtevant in 1893. Sturtevant, a Civil War veteran from Ohio, abandoned his wife and daughters and came west seeking gold. He reworked an old logging trail and built a store, dining room, and cabins and tents. His resort became one of the most popular in the San Gabriel Mountains. Its fame drew the attention of Sturtevant's family, who moved to Sierra Madre and converted him to Christianity and alcoholism.

The ranger cabin in the camp was constructed in 1903 and is the oldest standing ranger cabin in the Angeles National Forest. On the far side of camp, the trail veers left and crosses the creek to the Upper Mount Zion Junction, where you take the Mount Zion Trail (3.6 miles). This restored version of Sturtevant's original trail (reconstructed in the late 1970s and early '80s) winds delightfully upward across a ravine and then along timber-shaded, north-facing slopes.

When you reach the trail crest, in a notch just northwest of Mount Zion, take the side path up through manzanita and ceanothus to the summit (4.6 miles), where you get a broad if unremarkable view of surrounding ridges and a small slice of the San Gabriel Valley.

Return to the main trail and begin a long switchback descent down the dry north canyon wall of Winter Creek—a sweaty affair if the day is sunny and warm. At the foot of this stretch you reach the cool canyon bottom and a T-intersection with the Winter Creek Trail (6.0 miles), lying just above Hoegees Trail Camp. Backpackers staying at Hoegees should bring bear canisters, because nightly visitors are skilled at procuring your food if it's unguarded or hung from a tree. But we turn right, going upstream momentarily, follow the trail across the creek, and climb to the next trail junction in 0.2 mile. Bear left on the Upper Winter Creek Trail, which briefly climbs and then gradually descends for 2.3 miles through the cool woods overlooking Winter Creek. Upon reaching the paved service road, follow it down 0.3 mile past a water tank and picnic grounds to reach the Winter Creek Trailhead at the upper Chantry Flat parking area.

Chantry Flat has been a popular gateway to Big Santa Anita Canyon since Sturtevant Camp was established in 1893.

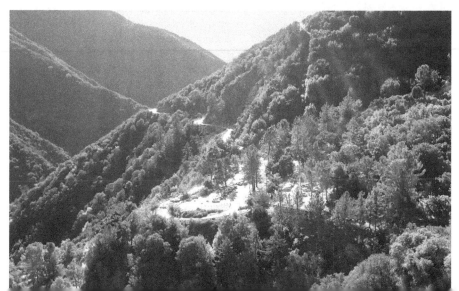

trip 24.13 Mount Wilson Loop

Distance	13.5 miles (loop)
Hiking Time	8 hours
Elevation Gain	4,100'
Difficulty	Strenuous
Trail Use	Suitable for backpacking, dogs allowed
Best Times	October–June
Agency	Angeles National Forest
Optional Map	Tom Harrison *Angeles Front Country* or Trails Illustrated *Angeles National Forest (811)*

see map on p. 314

DIRECTIONS From the 210 Freeway in Arcadia, take Exit 32 for Santa Anita Avenue. Drive north 5 miles to the parking lots at Chantry Flat, passing a vehicle gate that's open 6 a.m.–8 p.m.

Basically an extension of the previous trip, this loop hike from Chantry Flat will take you all the way to Mount Wilson, where a host of roads and trails converge. Completion of the entire loop is a respectable achievement, even for those in excellent physical condition. Of course, those with a penchant for downhill walking only, and the wherewithal to arrange the necessary transportation, can utilize either the uphill or the downhill segments described here as a strictly one-way downhill route. Watch out for poison oak along the trail.

From the south edge of the lower parking lot at Chantry Flat, hike the first, paved segment of the Gabrielino Trail down to the confluence of Winter Creek and Big Santa Anita Canyon (0.6 mile). Pavement ends at a metal bridge spanning Winter Creek. Pass the restrooms and continue up alder-lined Big Santa Anita Canyon on a wide road bed following the left bank. Edging alongside a number of small cabins, the deteriorating road soon assumes the proportions of a foot trail.

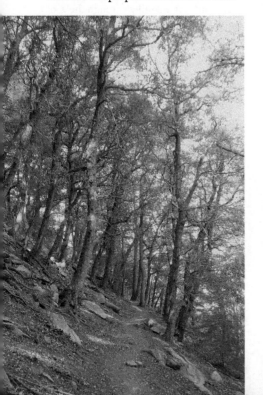

At 1.4 miles, amid a beautiful oak woodland, you come to a four-way junction of trails. The right branch goes upcanyon to Sturtevant Falls; the middle and left branches bypass the falls and join again about a mile upstream. The left, upper trail is recommended for equestrians. Take the middle, or lower, trail—the more scenic and exciting alternative—unless you're afraid of heights. The lower trail slices across a sheer wall above the falls and then continues through a veritable fairyland of miniature cascades and crystalline pools, bedecked with giant chain ferns.

A half mile past the reconvergence of the upper and lower trails, you reach Cascade Picnic Area (2.8 miles; tables and restrooms here), named for a smooth chute in the stream bottom just below. Press on past a hulking crib dam to Spruce Grove Trail Camp (3.3

The upper Sturtevant Trail climbs relentlessly through live oak and big-cone Douglas-fir.

miles), named for the big-cone Douglas-fir trees that attain truly inspiring proportions in this neck of the woods.

A little higher, the Gabrielino Trail forks right to climb toward Newcomb Pass (see Trip 24.14, page 334)—go left on the signed Sturtevant Trail, and reach historic Sturtevant Camp in 0.1 mile; with advanced reservations, you could rent a cabin here (visit sturtevant camp.com for details). At the far end of camp, the trail resumes and crosses the creek to the Upper Mount Zion junction. Here (3.9 miles), the Mount Zion Trail branches left, but you stay right on the Sturtevant Trail, continuing on through upper Big Santa Anita Canyon, in deep shade most of the while.

A series of switchbacks begins at about 4.9 miles as the trail tackles a steep slope consisting of crumbling outcrops and decomposed granite soil. Halfway Rest, at 5.2 miles, features a log bench in a restful, sylvan setting overlooking the uppermost reaches of Big

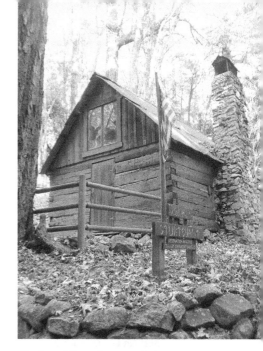

Sturtevant Camp has operated as a hike-in resort since 1893. Rental cabins are available to the public.

Santa Anita Canyon. You're now exactly halfway between Sturtevant Camp, 1.4 miles below, and the top of the trail at Echo Rock on Mount Wilson's east shoulder. Switchbacks continue on the upper 1.4-mile segment, mostly mercifully shaded by canyon live oak and huge big-cone Douglas-fir trees.

At the crest (6.6 miles), step right onto the short fenced path leading to Echo Rock, where you can enjoy a grandstand view of ridges marching east toward Mount San Antonio and south into the usual haze or smog blanket over the San Gabriel Valley. Continue west about 100 yards to a paved service road, turn left, and follow it west past the domes of the historic 60-inch and 100-inch reflector telescopes (each having held the distinction of being the world's largest telescope for a long period), the 150-foot-high solar telescope, and assorted smaller instruments. It was here that astronomer Edwin Hubble, using the great 100-inch Hooker Reflector in the 1920s and '30s, gathered evidence that supported the notion of an expanding universe populated by billions of galaxies—the accepted modern view. Today, operations at the observatory have diminished—light pollution has hampered its effectiveness—but the observatory still maintains a small museum (on your right, open 10 a.m.–4 p.m.) for the convenience of visitors and travelers like yourself.

At 7.0 miles you'll come to the centerpiece of Skyline Park: the Pavilion, a small picnic-and-sightseeing facility, generally open to public access by road April–November. A seasonal snack-bar concession may be found here, and you can get tickets for weekend 1 p.m. observatory tours (closed in winter). To the west lies a string of towering radio and TV antennas. Virtually every major broadcasting station in the L.A. area transmits its signal from here.

Descend to the large, circular parking area and pick up the signed Mount Wilson Trail that switchbacks downward 0.7 mile to join the old toll road on the saddle between Mount Wilson and Mount Harvard. Little remains of Camp Wilson (aka Martin's Camp), a popular resort for hikers and sportsmen based here in the late 1800s and early 1900s. Continue downward on the old Mount Wilson Toll Road 0.5 mile to the intersection of the Mount Wilson Trail on the left, just as the toll road begins curving west. Follow the trail, which crisscrosses a steeper firebreak. It follows the sunny ridgeline between Winter Creek and Little Santa Anita Canyon, known variously as Manzanita Ridge and Santa Anita Ridge. At 8.8 miles stay left atop the ridge as the Mount Wilson Trail forks right and descends into Little Santa Anita Canyon. You're now on the Winter Creek Trail. At 9.6 miles this trail veers left off the ridge and starts a long, crooked descent down Winter Creek's canyon wall. Hearty growths of live oak and big-cone Douglas-fir make this a cool and agreeable stretch, even though there's no relief from the jarring descent. Big-leaf maples near the bottom of the canyon herald your arrival at the junction (11 miles) with the trail to Hoegees on the left. Keep straight at this intersection and finish up the easy way—on the Upper Winter Creek Trail.

trip 24.14 Angeles Crest to Chantry Flat

Distance	12 miles (one-way)
Hiking Time	7 hours
Elevation Gain/Loss	1,800'/4,400'
Difficulty	Strenuous
Trail Use	Suitable for backpacking, dogs allowed
Best Times	October–June
Agency	Angeles National Forest
Recommended Map	Tom Harrison *Angeles Front Country* or Trails Illustrated *Angeles National Forest (811)*

DIRECTIONS This trip requires a 1-hour car shuttle. Leave one vehicle or arrange to be picked up at Chantry Flat: From the 210 Freeway in Arcadia, take Exit 32 for Santa Anita Avenue. Drive north 5 miles to the parking lots at Chantry Flat, passing a vehicle gate that's open 6 a.m.–8 p.m.

   To reach the start of the hike, return to the 210 Freeway and continue west to the Angeles Crest Highway (Highway 2) in La Cañada Flintridge. Drive 19 miles north and east to Shortcut Saddle at mile marker 2 LA 43.3.

This wide-ranging and very scenic traverse takes you from Shortcut Saddle to Chantry Flat, through wooded and fern-draped canyons, and over a major divide. The closure of Rincon–Red Box Road to motor vehicles has made this area effectively more remote from civilization (and any form of help in an emergency) than it has been for decades. The initial portion of this trail burned in the 2009 Station Fire but has been repaired. This route crosses the West Fork of the San Gabriel River 10 times, which means you're likely to get your feet wet if you do the hike in the spring.

   The drive between start and end points takes well over an hour at best, so a good arrangement would be to line up someone to drop you off on Angeles Crest Highway and later pick you up at Chantry Flat. Be sure to watch out for poison oak along the trail.

   Shortcut Saddle is considered to be on the nebulous dividing line between the Front Range of the San Gabriels, south and west, and the High Country, of which Charlton–Chilao Recreation Area (see Chapter 25), just north, is a part.

   You start off on the Silver Moccasin Trail, which dates from 1942, when Boy Scouts mapped out what is now a 52-mile route from Chantry Flat to Vincent Gap near Mount Baden-Powell. Today it combines with parts of the Pacific Crest and Gabrielino Trails. The part of the Silver Moccasin Trail you'll be traveling on was originally Newcomb's Trail, a turn-of-the-century shortcut route for hikers and sportsmen between Big Santa Anita Canyon and the High Country. It was built in 1897 by Lewis Newcomb, a mountain man who homesteaded near Chilao in the 1890s. Newcomb became one of the first forest rangers in 1898 in the new San Gabriel Forest Reserve.

From Shortcut Saddle, follow the southbound Silver Moccasin Trail as it zigzags down 120 vertical feet to a dirt road. Turn right, go 0.1 mile along the road, and then turn left on the continuation of the trail. You now descend hot, south-facing, chaparral-covered slopes, finally settling into the aptly named Shortcut Canyon (1.5 miles). There's only a trickle here from winter through spring, but there's more and more water ahead. Blackberry brambles and willows grow along the stream. At the bottom of Shortcut Canyon cross the West Fork of San Gabriel River to reach West Fork Campground (3.4 miles) and the site of a historic ranger station built in 1900, now removed to Chilao. Either this camp or DeVore Camp ahead is good for an overnight layover if you're backpacking the route.

From West Fork Campground, go east (downstream), fording the river again almost immediately. The sometimes-obscure trail meanders down one of the most beautiful riparian stretches in the county. The stream slides over and around smooth boulders, while sunlight filtering though the tall alders and maples glances off lenslike convexities and concavities on the water surface.

At DeVore Camp (4.6 miles), you turn away from the river and head south—very steeply at first—up along a shady draw to the south. Endless switchbacks take you 1,300 vertical feet up past a crossing of Rincon–Red Box Road to Newcomb Pass (6.1 miles), where a couple of picnic tables have been thoughtfully placed. Ignoring both the Rim Trail to Mount Wilson to the right, and the spur of a fire road to the left, continue south into the watershed of Big Santa Anita Canyon.

The gradual descent across a sun-baked chaparral slope (great views from here on a clear day), then through oak and bay woods, leads to a trail junction (8.3 miles), deep in the shaded bowels of Big Santa Anita. Turning downstream on a now-well-traveled stretch of the Gabrielino Trail, you pass Spruce Grove Trail Camp, Cascade Picnic Area, and Sturtevant Falls. From the Winter Creek confluence, follow the crowds up the paved road to Chantry Flat.

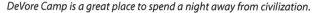

DeVore Camp is a great place to spend a night away from civilization.

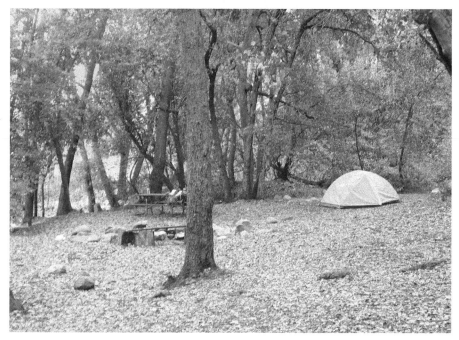

chapter 25

Charlton–Chilao Recreation Area

The gateway to the High Country of the San Gabriel Mountains, Charlton–Chilao Recreation Area draws a good fraction of the travelers headed east on Angeles Crest Highway from Los Angeles. On the way up there are scattered trees aplenty along the highway, but at Charlton Flats the traveler first comes upon what looks like true forest—stately pines, firs, and cedars. It's plain to see that the U.S. Forest Service has gone all-out to accommodate large numbers of visitors. Charlton Flats is named for Angeles National Forest supervisor Rush Charlton, who commissioned a two-year survey of the range in 1918. The surveyor Don McLain held the philosophy that "mountains should be monuments to the men who have treasured and protected them," and coined many of the place-names that persist today.

Three miles beyond Charlton Flats is a turnoff for the Chilao Visitor Center, open Saturday and Sunday, spring–fall, 10 a.m.–4 p.m. Here you'll find exhibits, free printed information, books for sale, scheduled summer activities, and knowledgeable rangers on duty.

The blacktop road to the visitor center continues past spacious camp and picnic grounds, and returns to the highway. Newcomb's Ranch Cafe, the first commercial establishment on Angeles Crest Highway up from La Cañada Flintridge, is around the corner from the visitor center.

Important note: Your car should be gassed up before driving to the High Country—there are no service stations on the 60-mile stretch between La Cañada Flintridge and Wrightwood.

Winter snows may block access (by car) from the highway to Charlton Flats and part of the Chilao complex, but that's no reason not to come. Both areas, with their meandering, gently graded access roads, are perfect for cross-country skiing after the bigger winter storms. Unplowed Santa Clara Divide Road from Three Points is another good bet. (*Hint:* Go on a weekday, or arrive early in the morning on weekends and holidays.)

---

trip 25.1 **Vetter Mountain**

Distance	3.6 miles (loop)
Hiking Time	1.5 hours
Elevation Gain	700'
Difficulty	Moderate
Trail Use	Dogs allowed, good for kids
Best Times	Year-round
Agency	Angeles National Forest
Optional Map	Tom Harrison *Angeles Front Country*

see map opposite

DIRECTIONS Exit the 210 Freeway at Angeles Crest Highway (Highway 2) in La Cañada Flintridge. Drive 23 miles north and east to the turnoff for Charlton Flats Picnic Area on the left at mile marker 2 LA 47.54. After turning into the picnic area, swing right at the first intersection and continue on pavement 0.6 mile to a gate. Park just short of the gate observing signed parking restrictions.

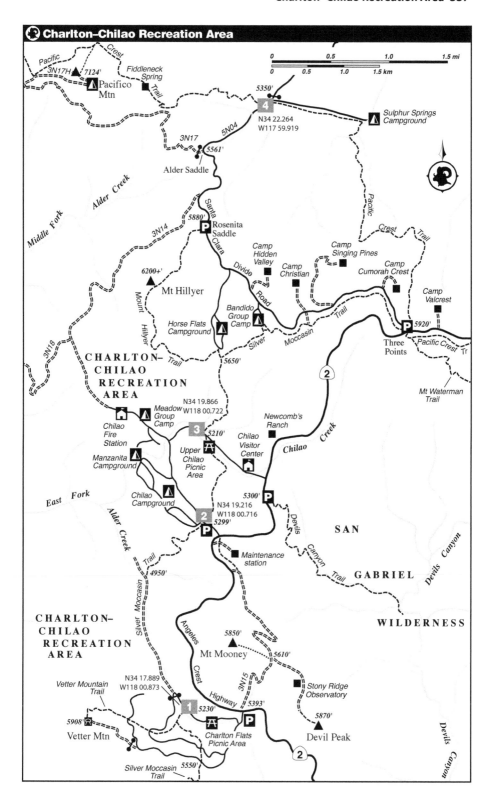

Vetter Mountain's pint-size fire-lookout building—before it was destroyed in the 2009 Station Fire—perched atop Vetter's rounded 5,908-foot summit and offered a 360° view over the midsection of the San Gabriels. The historic lookout building, which was reopened for service in 1998 after an 18-year hiatus, was a popular weekend destination for hikers of all ages. Today, the same panoramic summit is one of the best places to fully appreciate the extent of the Station Fire burn across the western half of the mountain range. There is considerable interest in historic fire lookouts in most of the national forests, and efforts to build this one are underway but moving slowly. The mountain is named for Victor Vetter, a ranger and dispatcher active around 1930.

Aside from visiting Vetter's summit, this loop hike also swings around through Charlton Flats' formerly lush, heterogeneous forest of live oak, Coulter pine, ponderosa pine, incense cedar, and big-cone Douglas-fir. In the years to come it will be interesting to observe the pattern of plant succession, and to learn just how much of the forest has survived, and which kinds of trees will be favored in the post-fire environment.

Look for the signed trail to Vetter Mountain, starting up the south side of a ravine. About 200 yards up the path, the Silver Moccasin Trail swings left—don't take it; this is your return route. Keeping straight, you ascend through mixed forest and then scattered pines, crossing paved service roads twice. A final switchbacking stretch through chaparral leads to the lookout site, 1.3 miles from the start.

Looking north and east from the lookout perch, you'll spot Pacifico Mountain, Mount Williamson, Waterman Mountain, Twin Peaks, Old Baldy, and other High Country summits. The Front Range sprawls west and south, blocking from view most of the city.

When it's time to descend, follow the dirt road downhill instead of the trail. After 0.7 mile you'll meet a paved service road. Continue straight (east) on the pavement for another 0.6 mile and look carefully for the crossing of the Silver Moccasin Trail. Turn left on the trail, cross pavement again, and complete the final, mostly level stretch across a forested slope.

The Vetter Mountain Fire Lookout burned in the 2009 Station Fire. A temporary shelter has been established while the new lookout is being built.

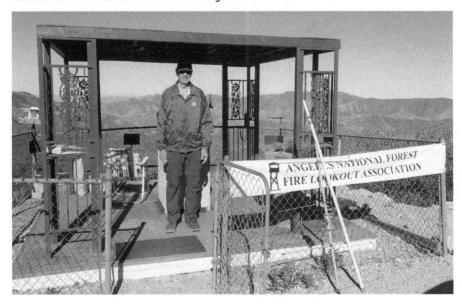

trip 25.2   Chilao & Charlton Loop

Distance	5.5 miles (loop)
Hiking Time	3 hours
Elevation Gain	800'
Difficulty	Moderately strenuous
Trail Use	Suitable for mountain biking, dogs allowed, good for kids
Best Times	October–June
Agency	Angeles National Forest
Optional Map	Tom Harrison *Angeles Front Country*

see map on p. 337

DIRECTIONS Exit the 210 Freeway at Angeles Crest Highway (Highway 2 in La Cañada Flintridge. Drive 25 miles north and east to the turnoff for Chilao Campground on the left at mile marker 2 LA 49.69. Take this road 0.2 mile to a small parking area where the signed Silver Moccasin Trail crosses the road.

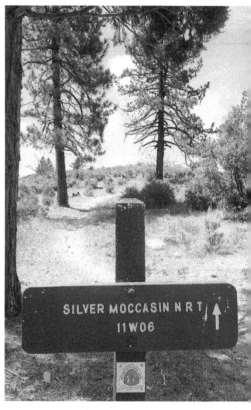

This trip makes use of a variety of dirt roads, paved roads, and trails to accomplish a circumnavigation of Mount Mooney, one of several small summits rising above the flats of Charlton–Chilao. If the air is crystal-clear, an optional side trip to either Mount Mooney or Devil Peak (involving extra mileage) is highly recommended as well. Almost all of this hike burned in the 2009 Station Fire, but the chaparral has largely recovered.

Charlton Flat was named for R. H. Charlton, supervisor of the Angeles National Forest from 1905 to 1925. The name *Chilao* may come from *chillia*, (Spanish for "chili pepper" or, colloquially, "hot stuff"), a nickname purportedly given to a member of the Tiburcio Vasquez gang who killed a bear with some fancy knifework.

On the Silver Moccasin Trail, go south up along a brushy hill overlooking Little Pines Campground and then crookedly down along a brushy ravine. At 0.8 mile you reach a valley, East Fork Alder Creek. Here you turn left

This loop incorporates part of the Silver Moccasin National Recreation Trail (see Trip 33.1, page 439).

to join a dirt road (Forest Service Road 3N86) and continue south up along the East Fork to join a hairpin curve on a paved service road (1.9 miles) just below the edge of Charlton Flats Picnic Area. Bear left on 3N16B and continue on pavement to a gate at the edge of the picnic area, where the Silver Moccasin Trail diverges. Our trip continues on the paved road out of the picnic area. Near the entrance, bear left toward the Angeles Crest Highway. Cross the highway and jog left; then walk up a short paved loop to join dirt Forest Service Road 3N15, which takes you up to a saddle (3.6 miles) located on the ridge between Mount Mooney and Devil Peak.

The optional side trip to Devil is 0.8 mile each way, first on a dirt road past the historic Stony Ridge Observatory, built and operated by amateur astronomers, and then on a steep firebreak. Mooney's ascent from the saddle is just 0.4 mile by way of a steep trail unpleasantly littered with burned trees. The view from Devil is far superior as it includes more of the rugged San Gabriel Wilderness and also (when the smog is lying low) Santa Catalina Island.

From the saddle, your circle route continues north on the fire road down a sparsely wooded slope. After two hairpin turns and a stretch through chaparral, the road swings back to Angeles Crest Highway (5.0 miles). Cross the highway, turn right, and carefully walk up the shoulder for 0.4 mile until you can turn left on the entrance road to Chilao Campground and continue 0.2 mile to the trailhead. Beware that inattentive drivers have killed hikers along this highway.

trip 25.3 Mount Hillyer

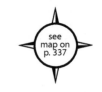

Distance	6 miles (loop)	
Hiking Time	3 hours	
Elevation Gain	1,100'	
Difficulty	Moderately strenuous	
Trail Use	Dogs allowed, good for kids	
Best Times	Year-round	
Agency	Angeles National Forest	
Optional Map	Tom Harrison *Angeles Front Country*	

DIRECTIONS Exit the 210 Freeway at Angeles Crest Highway (Highway 2) in La Cañada Flintridge. Drive 26 miles north and east to the turnoff for the Chilao Visitor Center on the left at mile marker 2 LA 50.60. Take this road 0.6 mile (passing the visitor center) to a small parking area for the Silver Moccasin Trail on the right.

Lovers of the high Sierra Nevada may get some sense of déjà vu atop the rounded ridge known as Mount Hillyer. The summit is named for Mary Hillyer, a clerk in the office of Angeles National Forest supervisor William Mendenhall in the 1920s. The breeze sings in the branches of sugar pines, Jeffrey pines, Coulter pines, and big-cone Douglas-firs. In the spring, expect to see red paintbrush, yellow wallflower, and purple lupine and penstemon. Angular outcrops and large boulder piles lie on the slopes, attracting almost as many rock climbers as hikers. The granite here is not so fractured and pulverized as it is in other parts of the San Gabriels. Mount Hillyer mostly escaped the Station Fire, which burned so much of the surrounding country, and the walk through its fine forests is now the best hike in the area. The view is only fair; the main attractions are the peace and quiet, and the pine-scented air.

Start hiking north on the Silver Moccasin Trail, using switchbacks to gain a slope covered by scattered pines and dense, sweet-smelling chaparral. From just southeast of Horse Flats Campground (1.1 mile), the Silver Moccasin Trail continues over a low ridge to the east, but you veer left (west) toward Mount Hillyer's south ridge on the signed Mount Hillyer Trail, passing a trailhead at the south end of the campground. Well-beaten, sometimes steep switchbacks take you to a rounded summit area, where two high points (6,200+') lie. Continue down the ridge to the northeast, passing a 6,162-foot knoll labeled Mount Hillyer on the topo map.

Due north of the knoll, an old road bed goes sharply downhill. Follow it to the signed Rosenita Saddle Trailhead on the paved Santa Clara Divide Road (3.5 miles), which carries no traffic during the off-season, and light traffic otherwise. Turn right, walk south on

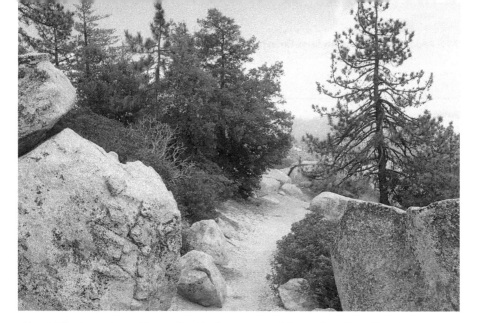

Mount Hillyer's granite boulders and conifer forests are reminiscent of the Sierra Nevada.

the road 0.5 mile to the Horse Flats Campground turnoff; then go 0.7 mile to the south end of the campground. There you can pick up the Silver Moccasin Trail and retrace your steps to Chilao.

VARIATIONS

This route can be challenging in places, especially for families with young kids. Except when the Santa Clara Divide Road is closed in winter, you can shorten the hike by starting closer. The loop from Horse Flats Campground is 3.6 miles with 700 feet of elevation gain. Out-and-back from the Rosenita Saddle is 1.8 miles with only 400 feet of elevation gain, though this route bypasses some of the best scenery.

---

trip 25.4   ## Pacifico Mountain

Distance	10 miles (out-and-back)
Hiking Time	5 hours
Elevation Gain	1,700'
Difficulty	Strenuous
Trail Use	suitable for backpacking, dogs allowed
Best Times	April–June, September–November
Agency	Angeles National Forest
Optional Maps	Tom Harrison *Angeles Front Country* and *Angeles High Country* or Trails Illustrated *Angeles National Forest (811)*

see map on p. 337

DIRECTIONS From the 210 Freeway in La Cañada Flintridge, take the Angeles Crest Highway (Highway 2) north and east 28.2 miles to Sulphur Springs Road at mile marker 2 LA 52.85. Turn left onto Sulphur Springs Road and go 3.9 miles to a fork at Alder Saddle; then turn right on paved one-lane Forest Service Road 5N04. In 1.0 mile park at a clearing on the right, immediately beyond the turnoff for Sulphur Springs Campground.

You can also drive to Pacifico Mountain Campground from the west or east via dirt FS 3N17. This could facilitate a one-way trip or a campout for a youth group. Check with the U.S. Forest Service before relying on the road, because it sometimes washes out.

Pacifico Mountain (7,124') is the westernmost high summit along the Angeles Crest. Its summit offers unsurpassed views of the range. According to historian John Robinson, Tiburcio Vasquez and his gang of horse thieves hid out here in the 1870s, and Vasquez supposedly gave the peak its name because he could see the Pacific Ocean from the top. *Pacifico* is Spanish for "peaceful," and you're likely to enjoy a peaceful time on this lightly visited but attractive summit.

Part of the area burned in the 2009 Station Fire, leaving a crazy quilt of new growth and pristine forest. Backpackers can spend the night at a small campground on the boulder-studded summit, a perfect spot for watching the sunrise (but bring your own water).

From the parking area, walk back along the road for 150 yards to find the signed Pacific Crest Trail (PCT). Follow it west-northwest as it winds above a drainage. The rather unimpressive, partially burned hill on the skyline is Pacifico Mountain. The PCT gradually climbs through scrub oak and mountain mahogany and the occasional Coulter pine. This area is notable for flannel bush, which lights up the trail with vivid yellow flowers in the spring.

Pass through a burn zone, and then round a bend onto the west side of a ridge. At 2.5 miles reach a prominent saddle. At 3.0 miles pass seasonal Fiddleneck Spring, surrounded by ferns and shaded by an incense cedar. At 3.6 miles pass Fountainhead Spring, which is more robust but still not reliable after springtime.

At 4.3 miles reach a flat on the pine-covered north ridge of Pacifico Mountain. Depart the PCT and make a cross-country ascent to the summit, weaving past the granite boulders on the ridge. Your climb ends abruptly at Pacifico Mountain Campground, where you'll find 10 walk-in tent sites shaded beneath the Jeffrey and sugar pines, white firs, and incense cedars. The true high point is a 20-foot boulder. The climb is tricky and a fall would have nasty consequences. Most hikers will be satisfied by taking a snack break at the base.

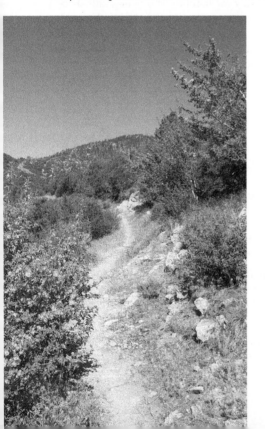

You can return the way you came or make a loop by returning on dirt roads. The road walk adds a mile but is fast and easygoing. Follow the campground-access road, Forest Service Road 3N17H, 1.6 miles down to FS 3N17. Turn left and go 3.2 miles to Alder Saddle. Turn left again on FS 5N04 and follow it 1.0 mile back to your vehicle.

VARIATION

Pacifico can also be climbed by way of the PCT from Mill Creek Summit on the Angeles Forest Highway. This round-trip is 13 miles with 2,300 feet of elevation gain. The lower portion is rather desolate after the Station Fire, but the upper part tours a lovely forest. Follow the PCT up to a saddle where the trail meets FS 3N17H. Turn left and follow the road 1.1 miles to the summit. Return to the junction; then follow FS 3N17H down to FS 3N17. Turn right and follow the road back to Mill Creek Summit.

*Flannel bush (*Fremontodendron californicum), *plentiful near the start of the trail, produces striking spring blooms.*

chapter 26

Crystal Lake Recreation Area

Historian and author John Robinson compares the form of the San Gabriel River's mountain watershed to a "colossal live oak, standing squat on a stout trunk, with an erect center limb and long horizontal branches extending outward in both directions." The West and East Forks form the horizontal branches, while the center branch, the North Fork, drains the top of the tree—Crystal Lake Recreation Area. Highway 39 goes north from the 210 Freeway at Azusa and travels up the "trunk" and the center limb—the main San Gabriel Canyon—and then dead-ends just beyond the Crystal Lake turnoff.

The spacious, oak- and conifer-dotted flats that make up Crystal Lake Recreation Area are quite a rarity in the tectonically active San Gabriels. Here, too, is found bantam-size Crystal Lake, the only permanent natural lake on the south slopes of the San Gabriels. The area was first opened to visitors as a county park in 1932; after World War II, it reverted to U.S. Forest Service administration. Now, as then, it caters mostly to day-trippers and campers seeking a quick escape from the big city.

As you drive up San Gabriel Canyon toward the Crystal Lake Basin, it may be interesting to recall some of the canyon's tortured history. John Robinson's book *The San Gabriels* covers in fascinating detail the efforts to exploit and tame the canyon for mineral riches, water resources, flood control, electrical power, transportation, and recreation. Many of these attempts ended in monumental failures that could easily be blamed entirely on so-called acts of God—fire, flood, and landslide—were it not for human arrogance and stupidity.

During the droughts of the 1860s and 1870s, ranchers Henry Roberts and Cornelius Potter drove their cattle from the parched lowlands to the Crystal Lake area. Grizzly bears, common at the time, poached so many animals that Roberts abandoned the pasture. By 1916, the last grizzly in Southern California was shot in Big Tujunga Canyon.

Perhaps the biggest fiasco was the abortive and costly attempt in the late 1920s to erect below the West and East Forks what would have been (for a time) the world's largest dam. A massive landslide during construction put that project to rest. (Later, the much smaller San Gabriel and Morris Dams were successfully completed downstream.)

The history of California Highway 39, the only road link between Crystal Lake and the

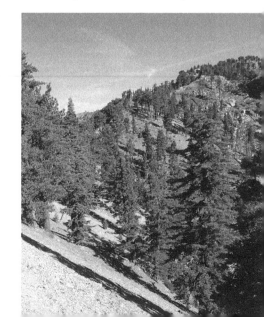

Hawkins Ridge is a beautiful place to escape the crowds. (See Trip 26.5, page 350.)

Crystal Lake Recreation Area

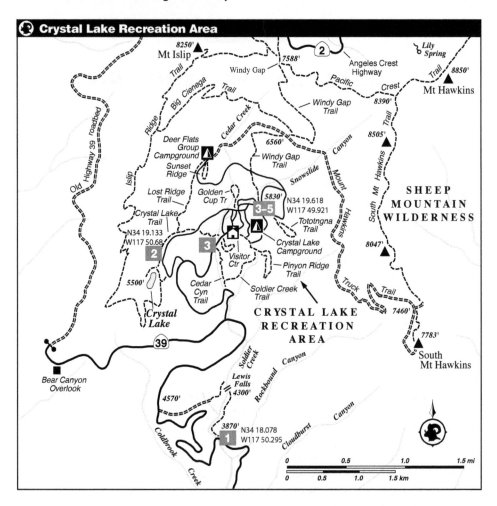

outside world, is a story of dashed hopes as well. The original road washed out nearly every winter, and it took one-and-a-half years to rebuild this highway after torrential flooding in 1938. An ambitious effort to realign a narrow, cliff-hanging section of the highway south of Crystal Lake was aborted when road crews bored through 200 feet of canyon wall without finding solid bedrock suitable for anchoring a bridge. You can see the ugly scars of this experiment below the recreation area near Coldbrook Campground.

A dubious scheme to extend Highway 39 northward to Angeles Crest Highway by way of the sheer, unstable upper slopes of Bear Canyon actually came to fruition in 1961. The road remained in service intermittently until 1978, when a landslide swept away a 500-foot-long section. Since then, hundreds of other slides have occurred in the area. The debate continues today about whether to reopen this part of the road, and the only certainty is that slides will continue.

Meanwhile, the Crystal Lake area—and Highway 39—have suffered from the effects of the 2002 Curve Fire and subsequent flooding and earth movements. Access to Crystal Lake was cut off until 2011. Be prepared for road closures in the future. Nearly the entire Crystal Lake Basin burned in the Curve Fire, and you can still see the scars of the fire on singed trunks, downed trees, and cabin foundations.

trip 26.1 **Lewis Falls**

Distance	0.8 mile (out-and-back)
Hiking Time	30 minutes
Elevation Gain	300'
Difficulty	Easy
Trail Use	Dogs allowed, good for kids
Best Times	Year-round
Agency	Angeles National Forest
Optional Map	Tom Harrison *Angeles High Country* or Trails Illustrated *Angeles National Forest* (trail not shown)

DIRECTIONS From the 210 Freeway in Azusa, take Exit 40 north for Azusa Avenue (Highway 39). Go north on Azusa Avenue, which becomes San Gabriel Canyon Road. Continue a total of 20 miles. Use the roadside mileage markers to identify the starting point: a small, shaded turnout on the right at mile 34.8, where Soldier Creek tumbles through a culvert under the highway.

On the precipice called Lewis Falls, Soldier Creek shoots (or cascades, or merely dribbles) some 50 feet down a two-tiered rock face. The volume of water splattering on rocks and sand below is seldom dramatic; but the cool spray and the sounds of falling water are refreshing. The hike to the base of the falls is short, a manageable adventure (with some assistance) for small children.

From the turnout, make your way up a well-beaten trail on the east side of the creek, under shade-giving oaks, bays, and big-cone Douglas-firs. Many summer cabins once lined the creek, but only a few now remain.

In 0.3 mile the main trail virtually disappears in the flood-scoured bed of Soldier Creek. A final, 200-yard scramble along the stream over rocks and logs takes you to the base of the falls.

Most of the year, Soldier Creek is tame and easily forded by adults. But a major storm, or a rapid thaw in the snowpack above, could produce runoff deep and swift enough to be hazardous, especially for children.

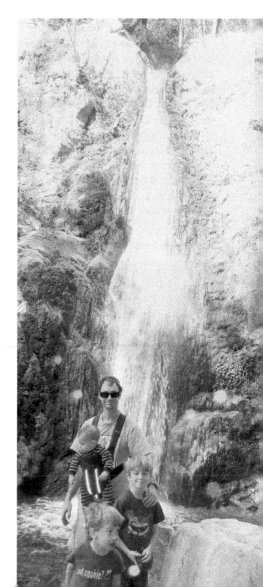

Kids will enjoy the rough trail to Lewis Falls.

trip 26.2	**Mount Islip: South Ridge**

see map on p. 344

Distance	10 miles (loop)
Hiking Time	6 hours
Elevation Gain	2,800'
Difficulty	Moderately strenuous
Trail Use	Suitable for backpacking, dogs allowed
Best Times	May–November
Agency	Angeles National Forest
Optional Map	Tom Harrison *Angeles High Country*

DIRECTIONS From the 210 Freeway in Azusa, take Exit 40 north for Azusa Avenue (Highway 39). Go north on Azusa Avenue, which becomes San Gabriel Canyon Road. Continue a total of 24 miles to the CRYSTAL LAKE RECREATION AREA sign. Turn right into the recreation area and drive 1.1 miles; then turn left onto Forest Service Road 3N09 toward Crystal Lake. In 0.2 mile park at a trailhead lot.

The south ridge of Mount Islip is prominent from many directions and offers great views. The Mount Islip Ridge Trail that ascends this ridge from Crystal Lake had fallen into disrepair after the Curve Fire but is now in good shape again thanks to the volunteer efforts of the San Gabriel Mountain Trailbuilders. It is the longest and most strenuous of the three trails to the summit, but is well worth the effort. With the southern exposure, this trail may be unpleasant on a hot summer day but can be climbed in the edge season when much of the high country is covered in snow.

The unmarked and easily overlooked Islip Ridge Trail starts at the south end of the parking lot. In a minute, pass a prominent wooden sign that would have more logically been located at the start of the trail. The trail climbs to a point immediately south of Crystal Lake, which at the time of this writing has been reduced by drought to a tiny fraction of its historic size.

Switchbacks lead through the Curve Fire burn zone to gain the toe of Islip Ridge in 1.3 mile; follow the ridge upward. To the east, you have fine views of the Mount Hawkins

Gaining the crest of Islip Ridge

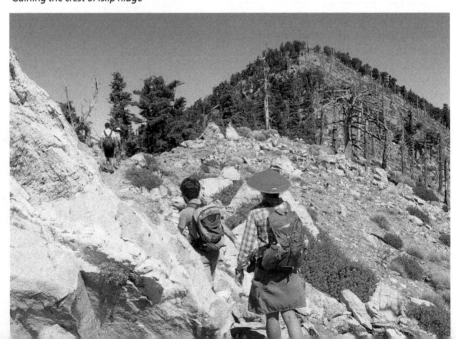

ridge over the Crystal Lake Basin. To the west, Twin Peaks and Mount Waterman are most prominent, with Mount Wilson in the distance. At about 6,700 feet, the canyon live oaks, big-cone Douglas-fir, and ponderosa pines of the lower slopes give way to Jeffrey and sugar pines that favor the cooler, higher mountainside. At this point, you may note ponderosa and Jeffrey pines growing side-by-side. The trees have similar stature, bark, and needles in bundles of three but can be most easily distinguished by the cones: ponderosa cones grow 3–4 inches long, while the much larger Jeffrey cones are 4–8 inches long.

At 4.0 miles reach a signed junction with the Big Cienega Trail. Continue 0.9 mile up the ridge to a junction with the Windy Gap trail, where you turn left and climb the last 0.2 mile to the 8,250-foot summit of Mount Islip.

If the north-facing slopes are icy, you may need to return the way you came or use the Big Cienega Trail. Otherwise, you can make a loop by descending east 0.9 mile to Windy Gap. Just before the gap, you'll notice an unsigned trail on the left shortcutting to Little Jimmy Trail Camp, a great place to spend the night if you are backpacking. From Windy Gap, descend south for 1.4 miles, passing the east end of the Big Cienega Trail just before reaching the Mount Hawkins Fire Road. Take this dirt road 0.6 mile west to the gated entrance of Deer Flats Group Campground; then continue 0.2 mile southwest on the paved campground road. At the southernmost campsites, watch for the signed Lost Ridge Trail. Take this attractive but lightly used trail south for 1.0 mile until it ends at a T-junction with the Lake Trail. Turn right and go 0.4 mile to the upper Crystal Lake parking area; then follow the paved road 0.1 mile down to the lower lot where you began this hike.

trip 26.3   Crystal Lake Nature Trails

Distance	0.5 mile–1.5 miles (per trail)
Hiking Time	Varies
Difficulty	Easy to moderate
Trail Use	Dogs allowed, good for kids
Best Times	Year-round whenever accessible
Agency	Angeles National Forest
Optional Map	Tom Harrison *Angeles High Country*

see map on p. 344

DIRECTIONS From the 210 Freeway in Azusa, take Exit 40 for northbound Azusa Avenue (Highway 39), which becomes San Gabriel Canyon Road. Continue a total of 24 miles to the Crystal Lake Recreation Area on the right. Drive in 1.9 miles and park near the visitor center.

Briefly stated, the several short nature trails of Crystal Lake Recreation Area offer one of the best introductions to the high, forested country of the San Gabriel Mountains. You won't ever get very far away from the sounds of auto traffic or happy campers on these trails, but you can certainly learn quite a bit about the area's natural features. Stop by the visitor center to obtain detailed maps of the trails and campground access roads of the Crystal Lake area. The trails are conveniently located near most of the campsites so campers may be able to take a stroll on the closest path without driving to a trailhead. The Golden Cup Trail is the easiest choice for families with preschool children. The Tototngna Trail has the most diverse scenery. The Soldier Creek–Cedar Canyon Trail is the only steep and strenuous nature trail.

The **Tototngna Trail**, a self-guiding 0.7-mile walk, starts from the main trailhead parking area 0.5 mile beyond (northeast of) the visitor center. Walk east on a paved, gated road for 0.15 mile until you see the signed trail on the right. Tototngna, "place of the stones" in the

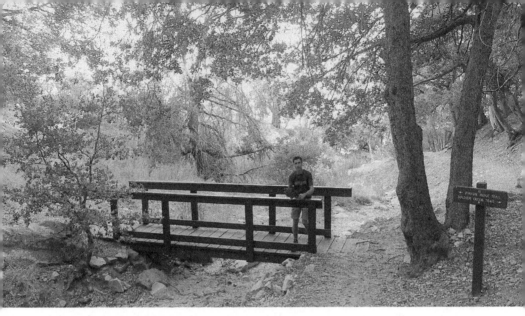

The Soldier Creek and Pinyon Ridge Trails split at this footbridge.

Gabrielino tongue, refers to the boulder-filled gullies sweeping down toward the Crystal Lake Basin from the steep mountain walls surrounding it. On this oak-shaded walk, you'll discover such minutiae as lichens, oak galls, and a small geologic fault.

The **Golden Cup Trail,** starting halfway between the visitor center and the main trailhead parking lot, loops for 0.3 mile through a grove of golden cup oaks, better known as canyon live oaks. The more colorful of the two names comes from the golden color of the shallow pod cup that holds the acorn. Other names for this tree are iron oak and maul oak, allusions to the great density and durability of its wood.

The **Pinyon Ridge Trail** is located southeast of the visitor center. Drive 0.1 mile down the short picnic area road and park before the gate blocking access to campground loop E. Walk another 0.1 mile down the paved road until the Loop E road turns left across a bridge. You'll find the Pinyon Ridge/Soldier Creek Trail sign just left of the outhouse. The trail loops 1.1 mile through habitats ranging from the lush oak-and-conifer forest to barren, sun-baked slopes. Watch for an isolated colony of pinyon pines on the high and dry ridge. These stunted pines seem quite at home in their local microhabitat, but actually they're quite far from their normal range on the desert-facing slopes of the San Gabriel Mountains.

The **Soldier Creek Trail** diverges from the Pinyon Ridge Trail at a small footbridge just below the starting point. You can make a 1.5-mile loop by descending the Soldier Creek Trail to its junction with the **Cedar Canyon Trail,** climbing the Cedar Canyon Trail to meet the main entrance road into the recreation area, and following the entrance road east past the visitor center over to where you started. Both trails are deeply shaded by live oaks, incense cedars, and other trees. *Soldier Creek Trail* is a bit of a misnomer because the trail actually follows a tributary of Soldier Creek. Both this creek and Cedar Creek turn into delightful, tumbling brooks during times of snowmelt—typically winter through early spring.

Just east of the starting point for the Pinyon Ridge Trail, on the lower entrance road to campground loop C, is a 100-yard-long side trail to the Goliath Oak. Set amid a thicket of lesser oaks, this giant canyon live oak measures 20 feet in trunk circumference and 82 feet in height.

The **Half Knob Trail** starts on the south side of the entrance road, just west of the visitor center. It loops halfway around and then back (0.6 mile total) along the side of a wooded knoll, or knob, if you prefer.

The **Lake Trail** allows you to hike from the visitor center to Crystal Lake, 1.0 mile one-way. On the way you'll pass the Lost Ridge Trail, which climbs along a sharply defined ridgeline before joining the paved access road to Deer Flats Group Campground. If you follow the Lost Ridge Trail, you could loop back to the visitor center by way of the access road and the Windy Gap Trail.

The **Sunset Ridge Trail** begins at Deer Flats Campground and makes a 0.5-mile loop to a bench on the end of the ridge, a perfect destination for an evening stroll.

trip 26.4	Mount Islip via Windy Gap

see map on p. 344

Distance	7 miles (out-and-back)
Hiking Time	4 hours
Elevation Gain	2,500'
Difficulty	Moderately strenuous
Trail Use	Suitable for backpacking, dogs allowed
Best Times	May–November
Agency	Angeles National Forest
Optional Map	Tom Harrison *Angeles High Country*

DIRECTIONS From the 210 Freeway in Azusa, take Exit 40 for northbound Azusa Avenue (Highway 39), which becomes San Gabriel Canyon Road. Continue a total of 24 miles to the Crystal Lake Recreation Area on the right. Drive in 2.4 miles to the main hikers' parking lot, 0.5 mile beyond the Crystal Lake Recreation Area visitor center.

The south approach of Mount Islip feels a bit like mountain climbing versus hiking, despite the rather straightforward ascent by way of marked trails. You begin amid spreading oaks and tall conifers in the Crystal Lake Basin, rise through progressively smaller and sparser timber, and finally reach the nearly bald and often windblown summit. There, a comprehensive view both north over the Mojave Desert and south over the metropolis is offered on clear days.

For the slight effort of nearly a mile on the way up or down, you can spend the night at Little Jimmy Campground, one of the finest trail camps in the San Gabriels. Mount Islip is named not for its poor footing, but for George Islip, a Canadian prospector and mountain man who established a homestead in San Gabriel Canyon sometime before 1880.

From the trailhead, follow the Windy Gap Trail north. You cross Mount Hawkins Truck Trail twice, and then tackle the steep upper

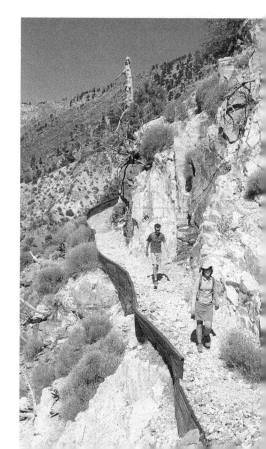

The trail below Windy Gap required extensive engineering to hold it on the mountainside.

slopes of the cirquelike rim overlooking the Crystal Lake Basin. At 2.5 miles you reach Windy Gap, which is the lowest spot on the north side of that rim.

At Windy Gap you meet the Pacific Crest Trail, which joins from the right (east). Continue briefly north on the PCT to the next junction. Going left takes you more directly to the summit of Mount Islip, while going right would lead you to Little Jimmy Campground and a more roundabout ascent of the mountain. In either case, you'll end up on the trail that follows the sunny east ridge of Mount Islip to its summit. (*Note:* Hard snow or ice can linger on the steep, north-facing slopes north of Windy Gap until sometime in May. You might avoid that stretch if need be by going straight up the east shoulder of Mount Islip from Windy Gap; that route becomes snow-free earlier in the season.)

On the 8,250-foot summit (3.5 miles), you'll discover the shell of an old stone cabin and the footings of a fire lookout tower that stood on Islip from 1927 to 1937, when the lookout was moved to a better site to the southeast, South Mount Hawkins. That structure was completely destroyed in the 2002 Curve Fire.

On your return, for the sake of variety, you can follow the Islip Ridge and Big Cienega Trails. Two switchbacks below the summit of Mount Islip, turn right on the Islip Ridge Trail, which goes down Islip's south ridge. A future extension of that trail may go south and east all the way to Crystal Lake. You, however, travel just 1.0 mile down Islip Ridge Trail and then veer east on Big Cienega Trail. After another 2.0 miles of gradual descent along wooded south-facing slopes, you join the Windy Gap Trail just north of the upper crossing of Mount Hawkins Truck Trail. Turn right and return to the hikers' parking lot.

trip 26.5   Mount Hawkins Loop

Distance	11 miles (loop)
Hiking Time	7 hours
Elevation Gain	3,000'
Difficulty	Strenuous
Trail Use	Suitable for backpacking, dogs allowed
Best Times	May–November
Agency	Angeles National Forest
Recommended Map	Tom Harrison *Angeles High Country*

see map on p. 344

DIRECTIONS From the 210 Freeway in Azusa, take Exit 40 for Azusa northbound Avenue (Highway 39), which becomes San Gabriel Canyon Road. Continue a total of 24 miles to the Crystal Lake Recreation Area on the right. Drive in 2.4 miles to the main hikers' parking lot, 0.5 mile beyond the Crystal Lake Recreation Area visitor center.

The Mount Hawkins ridge, forming the high east rim of the Crystal Lake Basin, offers swell views. The Forest Service named the mountain for Nellie Hawkins, who worked as a waitress at the Squirrel Inn near Crystal Lake from 1901 to 1906 and who, according to author and historian John Robinson, "charmed and attracted miners, hunters, campers—just about every mountain man for miles around." The completion of the South Mount Hawkins Trail along the ridge in the late 1980s made the popular traverse between Mount Hawkins and South Mount Hawkins considerably easier than before. On this trip you'll start at the main Windy Gap Trailhead down in the basin, climb to South Mount Hawkins, head north along the Hawkins ridge, and return by looping back on the Pacific Crest and Windy Gap Trails.

Most years, the route becomes snow-free sometime in May. Don't be fooled if the slopes visible from the Crystal Lake Basin appear to be clear of snow in April or early May; icy

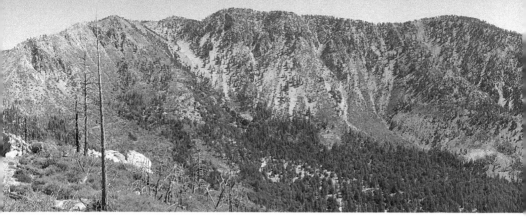

Mount Hawkins Ridge forms the eastern wall of the horseshoe-shaped Crystal Lake Basin.

passages with seemingly bottomless runouts could still await you on the high, north end of the Hawkins ridge. Check first at the visitor center, or with a ranger.

Start by taking the Windy Gap Trail north through a lovely grove of canyon live oak. Cross a paved campground access road at 0.4 mile; then turn right onto the dirt Mount Hawkins Truck Trail at 1.1 miles. This road once serviced a fire lookout tower, but now is rocky and washed out in places, perfect for hiking. At 1.5 miles you'll pass an alder-filled draw where a spring may be running. Scarlet monkey flower grows by the water. This stretch of the road is one of the most accessible places in the San Gabriels to see blazing star, a striking yellow flower. The dirt road climbs steadily and moderately across the steep slopes east of Crystal Lake Basin. If it's summer, it's best if you can cover this road-walking before the morning sun breaks over the high crest to the east.

On a sparsely wooded saddle at 4.4 miles, you'll get your first glimpse east into some of the rugged canyons of Sheep Mountain Wilderness. You could make a dry camp here. From the saddle, you can take the Hawkins Ridge Trail going south along the ridge to the South Hawkins summit (4.6 miles), rather than staying on the road. The whitewashed fire lookout tower once perched here burned in the 2002 Curve Fire.

The South Hawkins summit presides over a wrinkled landscape of dry, sinuous ridges and steeply plunging canyons. One way or another, nearly all of the mountainous terrain in your field of view sheds water into the San Gabriel River.

After your visit to South Hawkins, retrace your steps back to the saddle (5.2 miles). Continue north on the recently reworked Hawkins Ridge Trail, which climbs through parklike scenery of Jeffrey pine mixed with occasional sugar pine and white fir. Early-season lupine gives way to yellow rabbitbrush later in the summer. You could find occasional flat spots suitable for camping. As you pass north of Middle Hawkins, look for a short use trail to the summit.

At 7.5 miles you reach a junction with the Pacific Crest Trail (PCT). Just to the east, you'll see Mount Hawkins, one of several rounded summits defining the crest of what's known as the middle High Country—Mount Islip to Mount Baden-Powell.

Return to Crystal Lake by way of the shortest route—west on the Pacific Crest Trail to the trail junction at Windy Gap (9.0 miles), then left down the Windy Gap Trail. Backpackers could camp at a secluded site at the edge of the burn area 0.4 mile east of Windy Gap, or at the superb but busy Little Jimmy Trail Camp 0.4 mile west of Windy Gap. Little Jimmy has water available from a nearby spring.

VARIATIONS

From the junction with the PCT, Mount Hawkins is a 0.76-mile side trip with 500 feet of elevation gain. Middle Hawkins is a 0.1-mile side trip with 200 feet of elevation gain.

chapter 27

San Gabriel Wilderness

San Gabriel Wilderness was first set aside as the Devils Canyon–Bear Canyon Primitive Area in 1931—well before the advent of the National Wilderness Preservation System in 1964. Its 36,137 acres encompass some extremely rugged terrain, with elevations ranging from less than 2,000 feet to more than 8,000 feet. Many areas in this wilderness are characterized by slopes steeper than 45°.

Green ribbons of riparian vegetation cling to the narrow bottoms of the two principal drainages—Bear Creek and Devils Canyon—while dense chaparral forms an almost impenetrable cover on the lower canyon walls. Scattered big-cone Douglas-firs at lower elevations gradually give way to statuesque ponderosa, Jeffrey, Coulter, lodgepole, and sugar pines; incense cedars; and white firs on the higher slopes of Waterman Mountain and Twin Peaks.

This varied, rough, and remote habitat harbors mule deer, Nelson bighorn sheep, black bear, and mountain lions. You're most likely to see the former two, less likely to encounter bears (they love to hang around camp and picnic areas), and least likely to encounter a mountain lion. Grizzly bears, once a common hazard, were hunted to extinction here by about the turn of the 20th century.

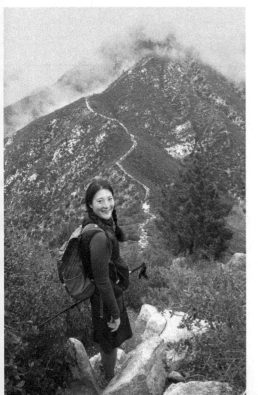

Although a transmountain Native American footpath once followed the length of Bear Creek, no such trails cross San Gabriel Wilderness today. The currently maintained hiking trails only graze the edges of the wilderness, leaving the interior (especially south of Twin Peaks) virtually unexplored in modern times.

You can easily enter San Gabriel Wilderness from any direction, as described in the trips listed below. Once inside the boundary the trails tend to fade, but the possibilities for further exploration (mostly of a very rugged kind) are almost endless. At present, you may enter San Gabriel Wilderness without having the usual wilderness permit that is required for most other wilderness areas around the state. This does not absolve you from obtaining a fire permit, if applicable. If you do plan

Descending Smith Mountain
(see Trip 27.4, page 358)

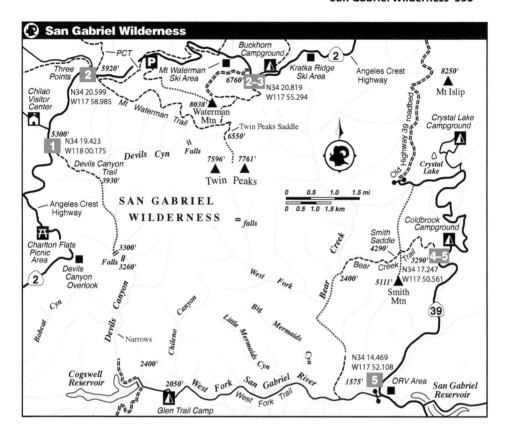

to venture well off the beaten track, then for your own safety it would be wise to consult with a ranger first.

The 2009 Station Fire in its closing stages burned into the west half of the San Gabriel Wilderness, affecting Devils Canyon and the western end of the Mount Waterman Trail in this chapter. The trails have reopened and you'll see the process of regeneration, with chaparral replacing many of the old trees.

trip 27.1   Upper Devils Canyon

Distance	6 miles (out-and-back)
Hiking Time	3.5 hours
Elevation Gain	1,600'
Difficulty	Moderately strenuous
Trail Use	Suitable for backpacking, dogs allowed
Best Times	October–June
Agency	Angeles National Forest
Optional Maps	Tom Harrison *Angeles Front Country* and *Angeles High Country* or Trails Illustrated *Angeles National Forest (811)*

DIRECTIONS Exit the 210 Freeway at Angeles Crest Highway (Highway 2) in La Cañada Flintridge. Drive 26 miles north and east to the Devils Canyon Trailhead, on the right at mile marker 2 LA 50.50, just south of the Chilao Visitor Center turnoff.

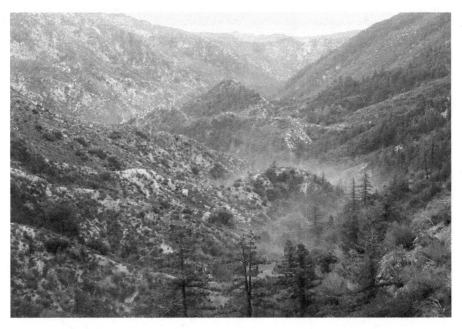

Thin morning fog adorns Devils Canyon.

If you stand at Devils Canyon Overlook (just below Charlton Flat on Angeles Crest Highway) on a warm spring day, a withering updraft fans your face like the hot breath of a furnace. There's no hint of the clear, cascading stream and the cool, shady microenvironment hidden in the deep crease of the canyon 2,000 feet below.

Getting down there isn't bad at all; most of the effort comes in getting back up. I'd recommend spending a full day (or parts of two days) exploring the canyon. You can splash around in some of the shallow pools (in May or June, when the water warms), watch ducks and water ouzels at work or play, fish for trout (you'll need a state license), and/or trek down to the upper of two waterfalls in the canyon. If the weather's warm, you should plan to wait until the sun sinks to the west before making the long climb back up the afternoon-shaded west canyon wall.

The trail starts at the Devils Canyon Trailhead, not the roadside Devils Canyon Overlook mentioned above. Your zigzagging descent on the trail quickly leaves the Coulter pines of the crest and takes you across slopes clothed alternately in chaparral and big-cone Douglas-fir–canyon live oak forest, occasionally mixed with incense cedar. Young men in the Civilian Conservation Corps cut this trail during the Great Depression. By 1.6 miles you reach a branch of what will soon become a trickling stream—one of the several tributaries that contribute to Devils Canyon's ample springtime flow. The deeply shaded trail leads to the main canyon (be sure to mark this spot or take note of surrounding landmarks so you can recognize this place when it's time to head back up the trail), at 2.8 miles, and then downstream a few hundred yards to the site of a former trail camp on a flat bench west of the Devils Canyon stream. In accordance with the philosophy of returning designated wilderness areas to as natural a condition as possible, this trail camp, as well as all others within the wilderness borders, have had their stoves and tables removed. However, the site remains large and well-used. Consider exploring downstream to look for pools, small cascades, and trout before returning the way you came.

VARIATION

It's possible to continue downstream for 2 miles to a 20-foot waterfall. Devils Canyon burned in the 2009 Station Fire, and the path downstream has not been maintained, so you're likely to encounter downed trees and bushwhacking. Along the way, watch for another two-tiered waterfall at the mouth of a side canyon on the east. The main waterfall effectively prevents farther descent without the use of technical gear; even with a rope, however, you'll have to return the way you came, because hiker access to the West Fork road is now blocked at Cogswell Reservoir.

---

trip 27.2   **Mount Waterman Trail**

Distance	8 miles (one-way)
Hiking Time	4.5 hours
Elevation Gain/Loss	1,400'/2,250'
Difficulty	Moderately strenuous
Trail Use	Suitable for backpacking, dogs allowed
Best Times	May–November
Agency	Angeles National Forest
Optional Map	Tom Harrison *Angeles High Country*

see map on p. 353

DIRECTIONS This trip requires a 5-mile car or bicycle shuttle. Leave your getaway vehicle at the Three Points Trailhead: From the 210 Freeway in La Cañada Flintridge, take the Angeles Crest Highway (Highway 2) 28 miles north and east to the signed Three Points Trailhead, at mile 52.8 by the intersection of Santa Clara Divide Road.
  To reach the start of the hike, continue 5.2 miles east on Highway 2 to the Buckhorn Trailhead, on the left at mile marker 2 LA 58.00.

The Mount Waterman Trail traverse across the north rim of San Gabriel Wilderness provides almost constant views of statuesque pines; yawning chasms; and distant, hazy ridges. You start near the entrance to Buckhorn Campground and end up half-circling broad-shouldered Waterman Mountain by the time you arrive at Three Points. Snow can linger on the easternmost mile of the trail until May, but it tends to disappear much earlier on the remaining (mostly south-facing) parts of the trail. The rugged topography of San Gabriel Wilderness below conceals the hangouts of herds of Nelson bighorn sheep. This area and another to the east, Sheep Mountain Wilderness, were classified as statutory wilderness areas in part to preserve the habitat of these magnificent animals. This is one of the most popular High Country summer hikes—heartily recommended for all but the warmest days. Robert Waterman was a forest ranger in the San Gabriel Mountains around 1904. His wife, Liz, was the first woman to cross the San Gabriel Mountains, taking a three-week backpacking trip with him in 1889. She built a cairn on the 8,038-foot summit, and the mountain was thus originally named Lady Waterman's Peak.

  If you plan to do a bicycle shuttle, it is more enjoyable to do the hike in reverse, leaving your bike at the Mount Waterman trailhead so that the shuttle is mostly downhill. This adds 850 feet of elevation gain to the trip.

  Pick up the Mount Waterman Trail on the south side of Angeles Crest Highway, opposite the Buckhorn Trailhead. Follow the well-graded foot trail—not the old road bed that parallels the trail at first—along a shady slope. After 1.1 miles of easy ascent through gorgeous mixed-conifer forest, you come to a saddle overlooking Bear Creek. The trail turns west, follows a scenic ridge, and then ascends on six long switchbacks to a trail junction

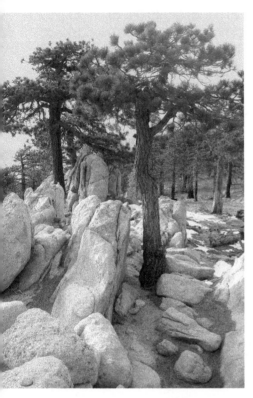

Granite boulders and Jeffrey pines congregate near Waterman Mountain's summit.

at 2.1 miles. A trail to Waterman Mountain's rounded 8,038-foot summit goes right (adding 0.7 mile and 400' of climbing one-way; see next trip), but you stay left and contour west about a half mile; then you zigzag south down to a second junction at 3.1 miles. Twin Peaks saddle, a spacious camping spot, lies below to the left. Wilbur Sturtevant (famed for Sturtevant Camp in Big Santa Anita Canyon) built a lean-to near a spring in the saddle in 1887 and regularly came here to escape the pressures of his business and family, prospect for gold, and drink.

If you're simply day-hiking this stretch, then stay right (west). The remaining 5 miles take you gradually downhill (steeper at the very end) along Waterman Mountain's south flank. You wind in and out of broad ravines, either shaded by huge incense cedars and vanilla-scented Jeffrey pines, or exposed to the warm sunshine on chaparral-covered slopes. The older cedar trees are gnarled veterans of past fires. Portions of this area burned again in the massive 2009 Station Fire, and the last 2 miles of the trail were severely affected. Near the end, you hook up briefly with the Pacific Crest Trail. On it you swing down to cross Angeles Crest Highway, and climb up to Three Points Trailhead.

VARIATION

Adventurous hikers can do this trip as an 11-mile loop with 2,600 feet of elevation gain from Three Points, ascending the trail and descending the west ridge of Mount Waterman. You'll find a use trail descending most of the west ridge, weaving through beautiful conifers and granite boulders, but route-finding occasionally becomes tricky around the rocks. A good map or GPS app and cross-country navigation skills are required.

---

trip 27.3	**Waterman Mountain & Twin Peaks**

see map on p. 353

Distance	12 miles (out-and-back)
Hiking Time	7.5 hours
Elevation Gain	4,000'
Difficulty	Strenuous
Trail Use	Suitable for backpacking, dogs allowed
Best Times	May–November
Agency	Angeles National Forest
Recommended Map	Tom Harrison *Angeles High Country*

DIRECTIONS Exit the 210 Freeway at Angeles Crest Highway (Highway 2) in La Cañada Flintridge. Drive 33 miles north and east to the Buckhorn Trailhead on the left, at mile 2 LA 58.00 on Angeles Crest Highway.

The top-of-the-world views from Waterman Mountain and especially the Twin Peaks ridge are among the best in the San Gabriel Mountains. This peak-bagging extravaganza visits both Waterman Mountain's summit and the east summit of Twin Peaks. You can, however, easily customize this hike to include less or more, to suit your ability and desire.

From the trailhead, start by crossing over to the south side of Angeles Crest Highway. Follow the well-graded Mount Waterman Trail—not the old road bed that parallels the trail at first—along a shady slope. After 1.1 miles of easy ascent through gorgeous mixed-conifer forest, you come to a saddle overlooking Bear Creek. The trail turns west, follows a viewful ridge, and then ascends on six long switchbacks to a trail junction, at 2.1 miles. A right turn here starts you on the way to the summit of Waterman Mountain, at 0.7 mile west. The trail itself swings around the north side of a lesser summit, crosses a saddle, and then bypasses, on the north, the true 8,038-foot summit. You leave the trail and walk about 200 yards up a sparsely treed slope to the summit plateau. A summit register has been in place here since 1924.

When you arrive back at the first trail junction, turn west and continue following the Mount Waterman Trail. You contour west for about a half mile, then start zigzagging down a forested south slope to a second trail junction. Make a hard left here and continue descending a more primitive trail to Twin Peak Saddle (6,550'), the lowest point on the divide separating upper Devil Canyon from upper Bear Creek. You could pitch a tent here, but there's much more room—and a better view—atop a 6,816-foot knob 0.3 mile southeast.

From Twin Peaks Saddle, the now-sketchy trail contours south to reach a second saddle (6,580') at the north base of Twin Peaks ridge. From there, you simply go straight up the slope, dodging boulders and trees, until you arrive on the ridgeline between the two peaks. Climb a short distance east to bag the 7,761-foot eastern peak. If you drop a short way down to rock outcrops south and east, just below the summit, you'll have a dizzying view of the secret, upper reaches of Bear Creek's West Fork. Serrated ridges of shattered diorite, a rock-climbers' nightmare, seem to tumble into the pit below. Quite often you can look out over a low-lying blanket of smog in the L.A. Basin and see Santa Catalina Island floating out at sea beyond the hazy dome of Palos Verdes. The Santa Anas, Palomar Mountain, the

Hikers celebrate a fun trek up Mount Waterman.

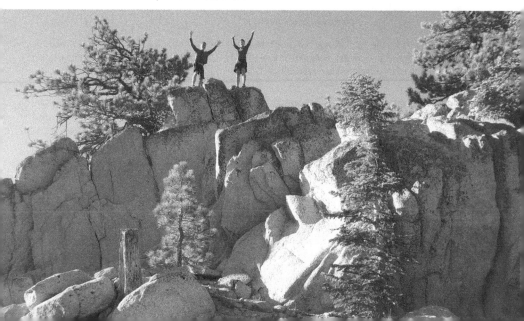

Santa Rosas, San Jacinto Peak and Old Baldy arc around the horizon from south to east. Also clearly in view, unfortunately, is the east wall of upper Bear Creek canyon, ripped apart during the grading for the now-closed upper segment of Highway 39.

Before returning to Buckhorn, consider visiting the 7,596-foot west summit of Twin Peaks. From there, the view south is even more vertiginous, and the ugly scars of Highway 39 are hidden by the slightly higher eastern peak. Just west of the west summit is a superbly situated small campsite—a flat, sandy hollow amid boulders and scattered pines. According to the summit registers on both peaks, more than 100 people climb the east peak every year, while only about a dozen make the west peak. Hikers signing in frequently report sightings of bighorn sheep.

VARIATIONS

Mount Waterman by itself is 5.5 miles with 1,300 feet of elevation gain. You can make it a loop by descending the ski area service road that starts just west of the peak. Twin Peaks by itself is 10 miles with 3,900 feet of elevation gain.

Mount Waterman can also be climbed cross-country from a turnout at mile marker 54.10 on the Angeles Crest Highway. Walk up the gated fire road, staying left at a fork in 0.1 mile onto an abandoned road/trail. When the road ends at a knoll in 1.2 miles, turn right and climb a steep use trail to gain the west ridge of Mount Waterman, then a faint climbers' trail along the ridge to the summit. This fun and scenic adventure is 6 miles round-trip with 1,800 feet of elevation gain.

---

trip 27.4   Smith Mountain

see map on p. 353

Distance	7 miles (out-and-back)
Hiking Time	4 hours
Elevation Gain	1,800'
Difficulty	Moderately strenuous
Trail Use	Dogs allowed
Best Times	October–April
Agency	Angeles National Forest
Recommended Map	Tom Harrison *Angeles High Country* or Trails Illustrated *Angeles National Forest (811)*

DIRECTIONS From the 210 Freeway in Azusa, take Exit 40 for northbound Azusa Avenue (Highway 39), which becomes San Gabriel Canyon Road. Continue 17 miles to the Bear Creek Trail parking area, on the left side of the road at mile marker 39 LA 32.14.

Smith Mountain (5,111') is a popular hike, especially on a winter day when the surrounding high peaks are blanketed in snow. An easy trail leads to Smith Saddle, beyond which you make a steep and strenuous but enjoyable scramble to the summit. Historians debate which Smith is the namesake of the mountain. Will Thrall argues for Eslies Smith, a Pasadena businessman who miraculously recovered from tuberculosis after staying a year at nearby Coldbrook Camp. John Robinson nominates Bogus Smith, a miner who worked the San Gabriel Canyon.

Wide and well graded, the Bear Creek Trail twists and turns up through sun-struck chaparral along Lost Canyon, gaining 1,000 feet in a moderately easy 3 miles to reach 4,290-foot Smith Saddle. Here at the boundary of the San Gabriel Wilderness, take the steep climbers' trail through scrub oak, manzanita, ceanothus, chamise, and granite boulders to the peak. From the top, you have unobstructed views of the central San Gabriel Mountains.

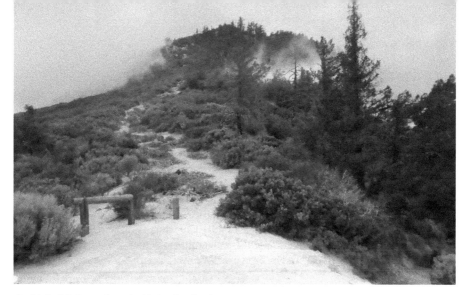

Smith Saddle is nearly socked in by the clouds.

VARIATION

Smith Mountain can be reached from the north in a more adventurous way along a steep firebreak from Highway 39. Park at a gate 0.2 mile beyond the Crystal Lake turnoff and follow the closed highway 0.9 mile to a gated firebreak on the left. Climb up to the ridge and follow the firebreak down to Smith Saddle where you join the regular route. This variation is also 7 miles, with 1,300 feet of elevation gain for a one-way trip ending at the Bear Creek Trail or 2,800 feet for an out-and-back.

trip 27.5 — Bear Creek Trail

see map on p. 353

Distance	11 miles (one-way)
Hiking Time	7 hours
Elevation Gain/Loss	1,100'/2,800'
Difficulty	Moderately strenuous
Trail Use	Suitable for backpacking, dogs allowed
Best Times	October–June
Agency	Angeles National Forest
Recommended Map	Tom Harrison *Angeles High Country* or Trails Illustrated *Angeles National Forest (811)*

DIRECTIONS This trip requires a 5-mile car or bicycle shuttle. From the 210 Freeway in Azusa, take Exit 40 for northbound Azusa Avenue (Highway 39), which becomes San Gabriel Canyon Road. In 12 miles you cross the West Fork San Gabriel River bridge; the spacious West Fork trailhead/staging area lies to the left at mile marker 39 LA 27.19. Leave one vehicle here; then continue north on Highway 39 another 5 miles to the start of the Bear Creek Trail, at the edge of a large roadside turnout at mile marker 39 LA 32.14.

Bear Creek and its myriad tributaries drain about half of San Gabriel Wilderness—roughly 25 square miles of steeply plunging ravines and canyons. Virtually none of this convoluted landscape ever experiences the tread of hiking boots except for the lower stretch of Bear Creek, reached by way of the Bear Creek Trail from Highway 39. The one-way route described here takes you into the heart of this wild area and includes almost 4 miles of boulder-hopping along perennially flowing Bear Creek. A short car shuttle along

Highway 39 can be used to connect the two ends of the hike. Wear long pants and sleeves to protect yourself from the encroaching brush. Beware of ticks, rattlesnakes, and poison oak in the Bear Creek drainage.

Wide and easy at first, the Bear Creek Trail twists and turns up through sun-struck chaparral, gaining 1,000 feet in a moderately easy 3 miles. The 4,290-foot Smith Saddle at the top of the grade marks the high point on the hike as well as the wilderness boundary. Down the other side you descend quickly on a narrower and rougher trail, and all vestiges of civilization (save an occasional passing aircraft) instantly disappear from view. Tall, nearly impenetrable chaparral on the steep north slopes keeps most of the sunlight away during the fall and winter months. Young men in the Civilian Conservation Corps hacked out this trail during the Great Depression, and persistent labor has been required ever since to prevent the chaparral from reclaiming the path. To the northwest, the Twin Peaks ridge soars impressively over the far wall of Bear Creek Canyon. Caution is in order in a couple of spots where the lightly maintained trail crosses perpetually eroding ravines.

The descent concludes with a zigzag passage down along a ridge between two steep ravines. You arrive at the small Upper Bear Creek Trail Camp on Bear Creek's east bank at 5.6 miles. (A spectacular narrow section of Bear Creek Canyon, with vertical granite walls, begins 0.3 mile upstream from this point—worth a look if you have time for the side trip.)

Little hint of any trail can be found in the next 4 miles as you follow the stream to its confluence with West Fork San Gabriel River. Narrow and vegetation-choked at first, the canyon becomes wider, flatter, and talus-filled as you press on ahead. Once the stream has room to meander across the canyon floor, it curves from wall to wall, forcing you to plunge into the streamside alders and boulder-hop or wade across the water. You'll repeat that process about 25 times.

Atop low, oak-shaded terraces at 6.9 miles (at the West Fork Bear Creek confluence) and at 8.6 miles (next to the remains of a stone cabin), you'll find plenty of room to set up a tent in a picturesque, shady setting. At 9.2 miles reach Lower Bear Camp, a long bench with room for several tents. Below the lower campsite, a well-beaten but intermittent path helps improve your speed for the last mile or so. At 10 miles you cross West Fork San Gabriel River and join the paved West Fork National Recreation Trail, which is the main access road to Cogswell Reservoir, doubling as a bike-and-hike trail. Turn left and walk a mile out to Highway 39 and your waiting vehicle.

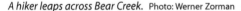

A hiker leaps across Bear Creek. Photo: Werner Zorman

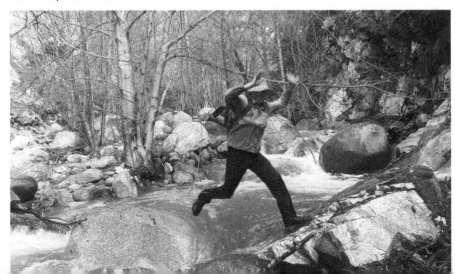

chapter 28

High Country & North Slope

North of Angeles Crest Highway and down the slopes toward Devil's Punchbowl country, the San Gabriel Mountains meld into desert in a most pleasant way. Timbered slopes dominate the cool crest, while on the warmer desert flats below, Joshua trees and high-desert scrub vegetation clearly hold sway. In between these two extremes there thrives an enigmatic mixture of oak and conifer forest, pinyon–juniper woodland, chaparral, and (in the bigger watercourses) riparian vegetation.

The trail system that runs through these parts is somewhat underutilized compared with trails farther west that are closer to the metropolis. The Pacific Crest Trail skims the crest of the range here, never straying too far from Angeles Crest Highway, while the High Desert National Recreation Trail probes the wild ridges and canyons of the slopes to the north. Not really a single trail, the High Desert Trail consists of several connected trails: Burkhart Trail, Punchbowl Trail, South Fork Trail, and Manzanita Trail. Serious backpackers could put together a marathon-length loop on the High Desert Trail by including the leg of the PCT that stretches from Vincent Gap to Islip Saddle (see Trip 33.33, page 444).

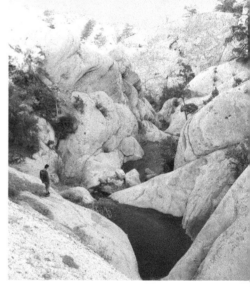

Lower Punchbowl Canyon's wild sandstone formations (see Trip 28.12, page 376)

In 2009, Congress designated the 26,839-acre Pleasant View Wilderness, the newest wilderness area in the San Gabriel Mountains. It encompasses most of the high country north of the Angeles Crest between Mount Hillyer and Mount Baden-Powell, including, of course, Pleasant View Ridge.

Roadside campgrounds in the area include Angeles Crest's seasonally open Buckhorn Campground, which was used as a high-country sportsman's camp long before Angeles Crest Highway permitted easy access to it. On the desert side, there are two campgrounds, Sycamore Flats and South Fork—both located in the Big Rock Creek drainage. These latter two are among the better sites for stargazing in the San Gabriels, as they're shielded by the mountains from much (but not all) of the L.A. Basin light pollution.

In winter, snow often closes the upper parts of Angeles Crest Highway (particularly east of Kratka Ridge Ski Area) and lesser roads in the area, so you'll want to check with the U.S. Forest Service before you head up there early in the season. If you're a cross-country skier, you'll want to take advantage of any and all unplowed roads while the snow is fresh.

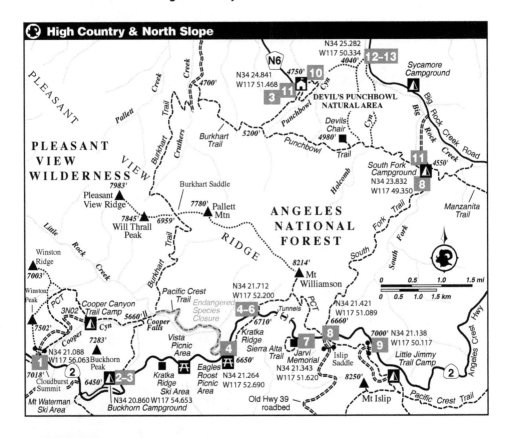

High Country & North Slope

trip 28.1   Winston Peak and Ridge

Distance	1.2 miles (out-and-back) or 4.4 miles (loop)
Hiking Time	1 hour or 3 hours
Elevation Gain	500' or 1,400'
Difficulty	Easy or moderate
Trail Use	Dogs allowed, good for kids
Best Times	May–October
Agency	Angeles National Forest
Optional Map	Tom Harrison *Angeles High Country* or Trails Illustrated *Angeles National Forest* (trail not shown)

DIRECTIONS Exit the 210 Freeway at Angeles Crest Highway (Highway 2) in La Cañada Flintridge. Drive 34 miles north and east to Cloudburst Summit at mile marker 2 LA 57.04. Park in a turnout on the north side of the road by Forest Service Road 3N02.

Winston Peak (7,502') is an appealing summit in the Pleasant View Wilderness accessible by an easy hike through an open forest of Jeffrey pines and white fir accented by lupine and other wildflowers. Although it lacks an official trail, hikers have worn a clear and straightforward path to the summit. If you're looking for a longer hike with more of the same fine scenery, you can continue on a climbers' trail down the far side and on to Winston Ridge, then loop back by way of the Pacific Crest Trail (PCT). The peak and ridge

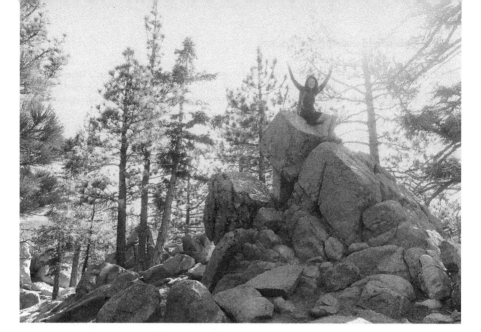

Granite summit boulders on Winston Peak

are named for L. C. Winston, a banker from Pasadena, who died here in 1900 when he was caught in a blizzard while hunting.

From the parking area, Forest Service Road 3N02 leads north past a gate and the PCT starts to the right, but we take an unsigned abandoned road that climbs steeply to the left instead. Within 0.1 mile join a climbers' trail on the left that shortcuts a bend in the road. Continue on this trail half a mile to the boulder pile on the summit of Winston Peak.

If you wish to continue to Winston Ridge, follow the climbers' trail down the steeper north side of Winston Peak to a saddle where you meet the PCT. Instead of taking the PCT, stay left onto another climbers' trail that circles around the west side of Peak 6903 to a second saddle. Continue along the climbers' trail to another boulder pile on the 7,003-foot high point of Winston Ridge.

When you are done, retrace your steps to the second saddle. For variety, stay left here and circle around the east side of Peak 6903 until you reach the PCT at a junction that is easily overlooked by PCT hikers. Turn right and follow the PCT back to the first saddle; then continue on the PCT as it contours across the east side of Winston Peak. When you reach a junction with FS 3N02, you can take either the PCT or the road to Cloudburst Summit. Enjoy the incense cedars and wildflowers along either path.

see map opposite

trip 28.2   Cooper Canyon Falls

Distance	3.2 miles (out-and-back)
Hiking Time	1.5 hours
Elevation Gain	800'
Difficulty	Moderate
Trail Use	Suitable for backpacking, dogs allowed, good for kids
Best Times	April–November
Agency	Angeles National Forest
Optional Map	Tom Harrison *Angeles High Country* or Trails Illustrated *Angeles National Forest (811)*

DIRECTIONS Exit the 210 Freeway at Angeles Crest Highway (Highway 2) in La Cañada Flintridge. Drive 34 miles north and east to the easily missed turnoff for Buckhorn Campground on the left, at mile 58.25 on Angeles Crest Highway. Drive all the way through the campground to the far (northeast) end, where a short stub of dirt road leads to a trailhead parking area.

Cooper Canyon Falls roars with the melting snows of early spring, then settles down to a quiet whisper by June or July. You can cool off in the spray of the 25-foot cascade, or at least sit on a water-smoothed log and soak your feet in the chilly, alder-shaded pool just below the base of the falls. In the right season (April or May most years) these falls are one of the best unheralded attractions of the San Gabriel Mountains. The trail takes you quickly to the falls, downhill all the way, and then uphill all the way back. The forest hereabouts is dense enough to give plenty of cool shade for most of the unrelenting climb back up. The canyon is named for brothers Ike and Tom Cooper, who hunted in the San Gabriel Mountains through the 1890s and favored this area.

From the trailhead, the Burkhart Trail takes off down along the western wall of an unnamed, usually wet canyon garnished by two waterfalls. The first, at 6,220 feet in the canyon bottom, is easy to reach by descending from the trail—this little gem of a cascade drops 10 feet into a rock grotto. The second, 30-foot-high falls, at 6,050 feet, is very hazardous to approach from above but is reachable from below by scrambling up the canyon bottom from Cooper Canyon.

At 1.2 miles the trail bends east to follow Cooper Canyon's south bank. Continue another 0.3 mile, down past the junction with the Pacific Crest Trail, which doubles back to follow the north bank upstream. Look or listen for water plunging over the rocky declivity to the left. A steep, rough, and potentially hazardous pathway leads down off the trail to the alder-fringed pool below.

VARIATION

With a car or bicycle shuttle or a risky 1.2-mile road walk along the Angeles Crest Highway, you can finish this trip at Cloudburst Summit via the Pacific Crest Trail, with a possible night at Cooper Canyon Trail Camp. This delightful one-way route is 5.5 miles.

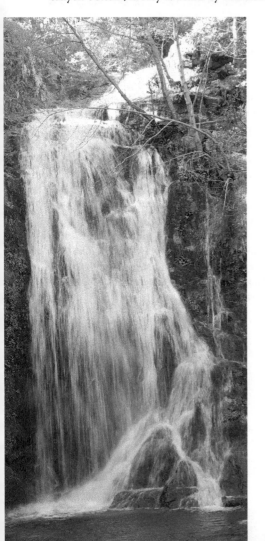

Cooper Canyon Falls can be exceptionally beautiful.

trip 28.3 **Burkhart Trail**

see map on p. 362

Distance	12 miles (one-way)
Hiking Time	7 hours
Elevation Gain/Loss	2,000'/3,700'
Difficulty	Moderately strenuous
Trail Use	Suitable for backpacking, dogs allowed
Best Times	April–November
Agency	Angeles National Forest
Optional Map	Tom Harrison *Angeles High Country* or Trails Illustrated *Angeles National Forest (811)*

DIRECTIONS This trip requires a 1.25-hour car shuttle. From the Antelope Valley Freeway (Highway 14) south of Palmdale, exit at Pearblossom Highway (Highway 138) and follow it for 14 miles to the small community of Pearblossom. At Pearblossom, turn right on Longview Road (County Road N6) at a sign for Devil's Punchbowl Natural Area. In 2.3 miles turn left on Fort Cajon Road. In 0.3 mile turn right to continue on N6 and, passing Pallett Creek Road, follow the twisting road 5.3 miles to its end at the Punchbowl—leave a shuttle vehicle here.

To reach the upper trailhead at Buckhorn Campground, return to Pallett Creek Road and turn right. In 2.2 miles turn right again onto Valyermo Road, which becomes Big Pines Road (County Road N4). When it ends at Highway 2, turn left and continue 21 miles to mile 58.25, where you turn right for Buckhorn Campground. Drive all the way through the campground to the far (northeast) end, where a short stub of dirt road leads to a trailhead parking area.

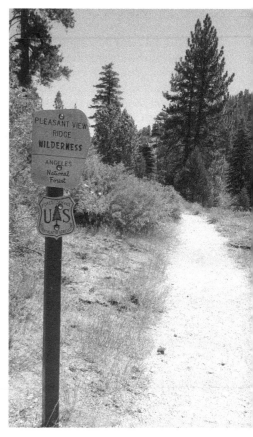

Established by Congress in 2009, Pleasant View Wilderness encompasses wild country on the north slope of the San Gabriel Mountains.

Far from the sights and sounds of the city, the Burkhart Trail blazes a lonely path over Pleasant View Ridge and down into the upper margins of the Mojave Desert. It is one of the few trails crossing the Pleasant View Wilderness. Here the natural landscape is not marred by canyon-carving highways and fire roads, not blemished by power lines, and mercifully free, for the most part, from the noxious clouds of air pollution that drift across the county. Here the clean, dry air bears the melded exudations of both pines and desert sage.

Although this is certainly one of the better hiking routes in the San Gabriels, relatively few hikers make the long climb, descent and traverse all the way to Devil's Punchbowl Natural Area. Of course, you'll need to solve some transportation problems first. At best, you can have someone drop you off at the start, Buckhorn Campground, and pick you up later at Devil's Punchbowl.

Start from Buckhorn Campground by descending to Cooper Canyon Falls, then descending farther to Little Rock Creek at 1.7 miles. After crossing the creek, bear left and commence a long climb to Burkhart Saddle, a gap on the high crest of Pleasant View Ridge. You wind steadily upward on sparsely forested slopes lacking underbrush, but resplendent (in springtime) with blue and white lupines, red and blue penstemons, sunflowers, and other wildflowers. Little Rock Creek lies below, its stream coursing through a thirsty-looking gorge.

Around 2.8 miles the trail crosses a perpetually sliding slope of sheared metamorphic rock, then gains better footing as it angles over to and finally crosses a tributary of Little Rock Creek. A series of long switchbacks takes you up the slope to the west, across the tributary once more, then up to Burkhart Saddle, 5.0 miles. There, a cool, dry breeze chills your sweat-soaked skin and clothing as you contemplate whether it's worth it to climb (as a side trip) either Pallett Mountain or Will Thrall Peak for a better view of what you can already see of the desert below.

Down the other side, conifer forest grades into chaparral as you drop north down along a canyon wall overlooking the upper gorge of Cruthers Creek. After a couple of zigzags near the bottom you join a ranch road (8.3 miles). Its crooked course takes you down along the creek, then east onto a gently sloping hillside. Look for the signed trail veering right toward Devil's Punchbowl Natural Area (the road itself continues north into the private Lewis Ranch).

You climb about 500 feet, then contour for almost 2 miles across the northern spurs of the San Gabriels, passing an odd but agreeable mix of beavertail cactus and sage; manzanita-rich chaparral; and scattered Coulter, pinyon, and Jeffrey pines. Views of the broad desert expanses below are frequent and inspiring. When you reach a dirt road at 11.1 miles where Punchbowl Trail keeps contouring ahead, bear left (northeast) on the road and walk down to a narrow trail continuing northeast along the rim of Punchbowl Canyon. The trail leads to the parking lot at Devil's Punchbowl Natural Area.

---

trip 28.4   **Kratka Ridge**

see map on p. 362

Distance	1.8 miles (out-and-back)
Hiking Time	1 hour
Elevation Gain	400'
Difficulty	Easy
Trail Use	Dogs allowed, good for kids
Best Times	May–October
Agency	Angeles National Forest
Optional Map	Tom Harrison *Angeles High Country* or Trails Illustrated *Angeles National Forest* (811)

DIRECTIONS Exit the 210 Freeway at Angeles Crest Highway (Highway 2) in La Cañada Flintridge. Drive 37 miles north and east to the Eagles Roost Picnic Area at mile marker 2 LA 61.65.

You won't find more outstanding views per step traveled along the Pacific Crest Trail (PCT) in the San Gabriel Mountains than you do on Kratka Ridge. This easy stretch of the trail is routed on the breathtaking ridge overlooking the upper reaches of Bear Creek in the San Gabriel Wilderness. The ridge is named for George and Walter Kratka of Pasadena. Don't confuse this hike with the nearby Kratka Ridge/Snowcrest ski area on Mount Waterman.

From the picnic area, follow the PCT northeast as it briefly parallels the highway before climbing onto Kratka Ridge. Look for Williamson Rock hulking across the canyon to the

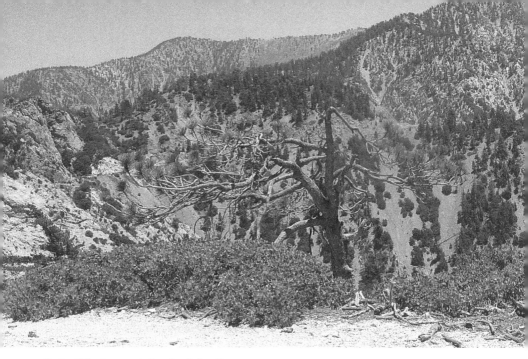

Kratka Ridge has great views in all directions.

north. The popular rock-climbing area and adjacent portion of the PCT have been closed by the U.S. Forest Service since 2005 to protect the endangered mountain yellow-legged frog.

The trail stays high for 0.9 mile before dropping to meet the highway again at mile 2 LA 62.50. If you left a bicycle shuttle here, you can pedal back. Otherwise, turn around and retrace your steps to enjoy the view in the opposite direction. Walking back on the shoulder of the busy highway is not recommended.

trip 28.5 Mount Williamson

see map on p. 362

Distance	4.2 miles (out-and-back)
Hiking Time	2.5 hours
Elevation Gain	1,500'
Difficulty	Moderately strenuous
Trail Use	Suitable for backpacking, dogs allowed
Best Times	April–November
Agency	Angeles National Forest
Optional Map	Tom Harrison *Angeles High Country* or Trails Illustrated *Angeles National Forest (811)*

DIRECTIONS Exit the 210 Freeway at Angeles Crest Highway (Highway 2) in La Cañada Flintridge. Drive 38 miles north and east to the large north-side turnout on Angeles Crest Highway at mile 2 LA 62.50.

Mount Williamson (8,244') isn't the highest peak on the San Gabriels' crest, but it hovers more closely over the desert than Mounts Islip, Hawkins, Baden-Powell, and others south of Angeles Crest Highway, and it is the highest mountain in the Pleasant View Wilderness. From the bare patch at the summit, you look down upon the obviously linear traces of the San Andreas and Punchbowl Faults, and often over thousands of square miles of

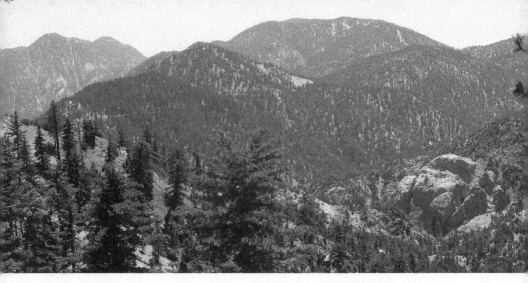

Williamson Rock with Twin Peaks and Waterman Mountain in the background

Mojave Desert. During the very best visibility, the southernmost Sierra Nevada can be seen, as well as Telescope Peak high on the west rim of Death Valley. The mountain is named for Lieutenant Robert Stockton Williamson, who conducted the Pacific Railroad Survey along the north side of the San Gabriel Mountains in 1853.

The hike to the top is short and sweet, but it involves steady elevation gain from a starting point at an elevation of nearly 7,000 feet. Follow the signed Pacific Crest Trail (PCT) east. That trail wastes no time in switchbacking up the steep, sparsely forested southwest flank of Mount Williamson. Behind you, from time to time, you can catch a great view of Bear Creek's V-shaped chasm and Twin Peaks to the south.

After only 1.3 miles (but 1,200 feet higher) you arrive at a trail junction on the south ridge of Mount Williamson. The PCT continues straight ahead, descending to Islip Saddle in 1.6 miles—that PCT segment can be used as an alternative route to or from Williamson. You then go left on the unmaintained but well-beaten path up the rocky ridge toward the summit.

In a cairn at the top you'll find a register, where you can dutifully add your name (and any comments) to the hundreds of other signatures recorded here annually. If you want to spend the night, there's plenty of room on the open summit to pitch a tent or lay out to watch the stars. If you do so, don't miss the spectacle of the sun rising as a fiery orange ball over the desert floor, May through August.

---

trip 28.6 Pleasant View Ridge

see map on p. 362

Distance	11 miles (out-and-back)
Hiking Time	8 hours
Elevation Gain	4,900'
Difficulty	Strenuous
Trail Use	Suitable for backpacking, dogs allowed
Best Times	May–November
Agency	Angeles National Forest
Recommended Map	Tom Harrison *Angeles High Country* or Trails Illustrated *Angeles National Forest* (811)

DIRECTIONS Exit the 210 Freeway at Angeles Crest Highway (Highway 2) in La Cañada Flintridge. Drive 38 miles north and east to the large, north-side turnout on Angeles Crest Highway at mile 2 LA 62.50.

From the conifer-clad heights of Pallett Mountain and Will Thrall Peak, Pleasant View Ridge delivers what its name promises. When north or northeast winds sweep smog and humid air away from Southern California, the ever-changing panoramas on this hike take in everything from sail-flecked Santa Monica Bay and the Channel Islands to the mind-stretching sweep of the Mojave Desert floor.

Earlier editions of this book described a one-way hike down from the high peaks of Williamson, Pallet, and Will Thrall to the Little Rock Recreation Area down near the desert floor. Due to a longtime closure of the recreation area for the purpose of protecting critical arroyo toad habitat, this hike has been revised here to include only the high part of the ridge. The elevation gains and losses are considerable on this all-day hike.

The hike begins as it does in Trip 28.5 previously: follow the signed Pacific Crest Trail (PCT) east. That trail wastes no time in switchbacking up the steep, sparsely forested southwest flank of Mount Williamson. After only 1.3 miles (but 1,200 feet higher) you arrive at a trail junction on the south ridge of Mount Williamson. The PCT continues straight ahead, and you go left on the unmaintained but well-beaten path up the rocky ridge toward the 8,214-foot Williamson summit, at 1.7 miles. There's a hikers' register on top.

Now you make your way northwest along the undulating spine of Pleasant View Ridge, following only hints of trail, heading northwest from Mount Williamson. You pass over two slightly higher but unnamed points—8,244 feet and 8,248 feet—at 2.0 and 2.3 miles, respectively, then begin the first of the many very sharp, rocky descents that characterize much of this trip. Over sparse pines and firs to the north, you'll look down upon some upthrust sandstone slabs known as sand rocks—a part of the same Punchbowl Formation that is abundantly exposed at Devil's Punchbowl Natural Area.

At around 2.7 miles, look for the glittering wreckage of a C-119 cargo plane caught near the top of a ridge 0.5 mile north in 1966. At 3.0 miles the Pleasant View ridgeline turns abruptly left (west) at a high point. (The wreckage lies about 0.2 mile northeast of here at **N34° 23.142' W117° 51.917'.**) You descend, then climb again, to Pallett Mountain (7,760+'), 4.0 miles from the start, where you'll find another summit register.

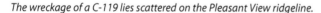

The wreckage of a C-119 lies scattered on the Pleasant View ridgeline.

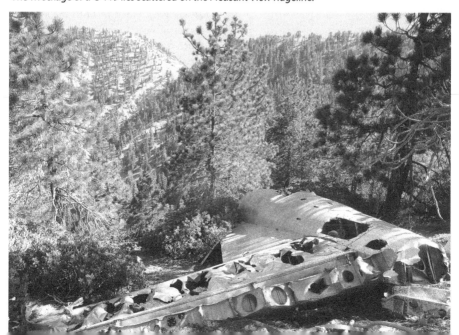

You then descend a well-worn climbers' path to Burkhart Saddle, cross the Burkhart Trail, and continue straight up the ridge west toward Will Thrall Peak (7,845'). The peak (5.1 miles), which offers the most pleasant view anywhere, also features a plaque honoring Will H. Thrall, editor of the Depression-era *Trails Magazine*. Thrall was an inveterate hiker of the San Gabriels from the 1920s through the 1950s.

There's a long, almost-never-visited segment of Pleasant View Ridge stretching northwest from Will Thrall Peak—a great area for some truly remote trail camping. The views, however, will not improve ahead, so Will Thrall Peak is the point for most hikers to turn around and return by way of the same demanding route. With a car or bicycle shuttle, you could take the Burkhart Trail south to Buckhorn Campground instead. Unfortunately, the PCT is closed between Cooper Canyon Falls and Eagles Roost, so you can't make a loop.

trip 28.7	**Sierra Alta Nature Trail**

see map on p. 362

Distance	0.2 mile (loop)
Hiking Time	1 hour
Elevation Gain	100'
Difficulty	Easy
Trail Use	Dogs allowed, good for kids
Best Times	April–November
Agency	Angeles National Forest
Optional Map	Tom Harrison *Angeles High Country* or Trails Illustrated *Angeles National Forest* (811)

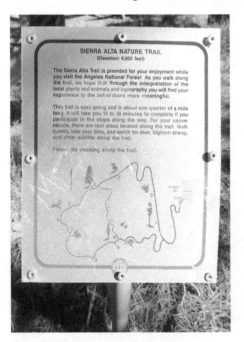

The short *Serra Alta Nature Trail* highlights some common trees in the high country.

DIRECTIONS Exit the 210 Freeway at Angeles Crest Highway (Highway 2) in La Cañada Flintridge. Drive 39 miles north and east to the Jarvi Memorial on the right, at mile 2 LA 63.50 on Angeles Crest Highway.

Jarvi Memorial Vista offers motorists great views of both the yawning gorges of Bear Creek to the south and a sheer, fractured slope to the north, punctured by two closely spaced tunnels on the highway. The memorial honors Sim Jarvi, a former Angeles National Forest supervisor, and also serves as a trailhead for the Sierra Alta Nature Trail. Jarvi died of a heart attack in 1964 while hiking Waterman Mountain.

The trail, strictly good for education, not exercise, features plaques highlighting some examples of ponderosa pine, Jeffrey pine, and canyon live oaks, as well as views in various directions. Clear-day vistas can include the ocean, as well as Santa Catalina and San Clemente islands.

trip 28.8   **South Fork Trail**

Distance	5 miles (one-way)
Hiking Time	2.5 hours
Elevation Gain/Loss	0'/2,100'
Difficulty	Moderate
Trail Use	Dogs allowed
Best Times	April–November
Agency	Angeles National Forest
Optional Map	Tom Harrison *Angeles High Country* or Trails Illustrated *Angeles National Forest (811)*

see map on p. 362

DIRECTIONS This trip requires a 1-hour car shuttle. Leave your getaway vehicle at South Fork Campground: From the Antelope Valley Freeway (Highway 14) south of Palmdale, exit at Pearblossom Highway (Highway 138) and follow it for 14 miles to the small community of Pearblossom. At Pearblossom, turn right on Longview Road (County N6). After 2.3 miles turn left (east) on Fort Tejon Road. Drive 2.3 miles to Pallett Creek Road, where you jog left and then promptly turn right onto Valyermo Road. Continue 2.9 miles and turn right on Big Rock Creek Road. In 2.4 miles turn right onto graded dirt Forest Service Road 4N11A, and proceed 0.9 mile to South Fork Campground. Just before the campground entrance, look for the signed Manzanita Trail on the left. Opposite this sign, take a short dirt spur on the right to the trailhead parking area, where you leave one vehicle.

To reach the upper trailhead at Islip Saddle, drive back down Big Rock Creek Road. At its junction with Valyermo Road, turn right instead onto Big Pines Road (County Road N4). When this road ends at Highway 2, turn left and continue 15 miles to mile marker 02 LA 64.00, where you find the large Islip Saddle Trailhead parking area on the right. If you have a high-clearance vehicle, you may be able to shortcut using the upper portion of Big Rock Creek Road, which climbs to Vincent Gap. Note that this road is only open seasonally, usually in the summer.

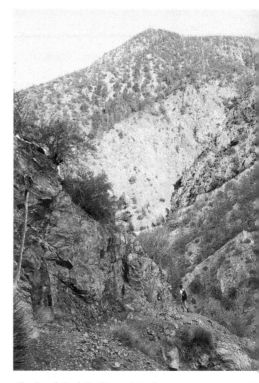

The South Fork Trail is cut into the crumbling mountainside.

The South Fork Trail descends the west wall of the dramatic V-shaped gorge cut by Big Rock Creek's South Fork through the Pleasant View Wilderness. It follows a natural, swaying contour as it curves around more than a dozen ravines indenting the canyon wall. South Fork creek murmurs far below (at least when swollen by melting snows), accompanied by the doleful trills of canyon wrens. Before construction of the Angeles Crest Highway, this trail was an important pack route into the high country. Now, because of the remote location and long car shuttle, you are likely to have the trail to yourself. In places, the narrow trail clings to the cliff above a drop-off. In other places, avalanches have covered the trail in scree. Thus this trail is not recommended for those who are afraid of heights. Shoes with good tread will be useful.

From Islip Saddle, take the poorly marked trail descending to the north from behind the picnic benches, not the sharply ascending Pacific Crest Trail, which climbs northwest toward Mount Williamson's summit. Traffic noises fade quickly as you enter a heterogeneous forest of Jeffrey pine, sugar pine, incense cedar, canyon live oak, and white fir. As you descend, the high-country forest thins; pinyon pine, big-cone Douglas-fir, manzanita, mountain mahogany, Whipple yucca, and blue- and white-blossoming ceanothus clothe the dry and rocky slopes.

In 1.1 miles pass seasonal Reed Spring, which trickles down a ravine beneath a canopy of alders. The trail loses elevation faster than the South Fork creek, so by 4.4 miles you'll be traversing a sheer slope only 200 feet above the stream. A couple of short switchbacks at 4.9 miles take you down to meet the alder- and sycamore-shaded creek. Cross over to the other side and follow the trail between the wash and South Fork Campground until you reach the trailhead parking area just below (north of) the campsites.

South Fork Campground is one of Angeles National Forest's more pleasant and secluded drive-in campgrounds. During April and May, flannel bush, or fremontia, blooms on the broad, alluvial terraces along the creek, opposite and downstream from the campground. Considered one of the showiest of California native plants, the fremontias here stand up to 15 feet high and bear thousands of large, waxy, yellow flowers.

If you have time for further exploration, climb southeast from the campground on the Manzanita Trail about 0.5 mile to some sandstone (Punchbowl Formation) outcrops. You'll get a great view of both the South Fork canyon and the main Big Rock Creek wash.

VARIATION

To avoid the long car shuttle, consider a 10-mile out-and-back from South Fork Campground.

---

trip 28.9   Mount Islip: North Approach

see map on p. 362

Distance	6 miles (out-and-back)
Hiking Time	3 hours
Elevation Gain	1,200'
Difficulty	Moderate
Trail Use	Suitable for backpacking, dogs allowed, good for kids
Best Times	May–November
Agency	Angeles National Forest
Optional Map	Tom Harrison *Angeles High Country*

DIRECTIONS Exit the 210 Freeway at Angeles Crest Highway (Highway 2) in La Cañada Flintridge. Drive 41 miles north and east to an unsigned gated service road on the right, at mile 65.3 on Angeles Crest Highway.

The ascent of Mount Islip from Crystal Lake to the south was described in Trips 26.2 and 26.4. The north approach described here—via an easier route—takes you through aromatic pine-and-fir forest most of the way. The gradual climb is well suited for children or anyone else who can handle moderate altitudes and hiking distances. If need be, you can shorten the hike by turning back at Little Jimmy Campground, 1.7 miles up the slope.

You begin on the shoulder of Angeles Crest Highway, opposite the site of the now-closed Pine Hollow Picnic Area shown on older maps. Walk up the pine cone–strewn gated road to where the Pacific Crest Trail (PCT) crosses it, 0.6 mile up and 350 feet higher. Both the road and the PCT go south and east to Little Jimmy Campground, but the trail is nicer.

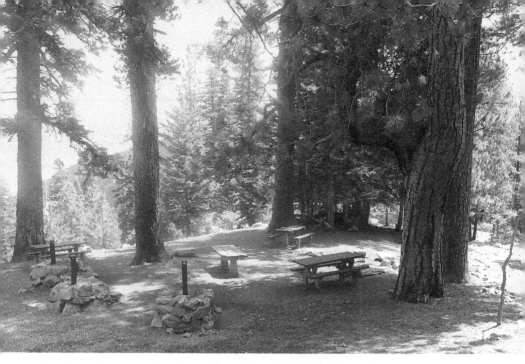

Little Jimmy Campground has the most basic of amenities: picnic tables and stone stoves.

Little Jimmy Campground, named for Jimmy Swinnerton, creator of the *Little Jimmy* comic strip, who summered here from 1890 to 1910, nestles comfortably in a little flat shaded by statuesque pines. Tables and stoves make this a convenient spot for a picnic or an overnight layover. If the main site is overrun by rambunctious Boy Scouts, you'll find more-private sites set farther back. Down the trail contouring south toward Windy Gap (below the trail a quarter mile away) is year-round Little Jimmy Spring.

Walk into the campground and pick up the signed Mount Islip Trail, which goes uphill (west at first) and continues looping upward to gain Mount Islip's east shoulder (stay right where a trail slants left and descends to meet the PCT). You ascend along this shoulder, swing around two switchbacks just below the summit, and arrive at the old hut and look-out site on top.

VARIATION

The section of Angeles Crest Highway between Islip Saddle and Vincent Gap may close for years at a time due to storm damage and landslides. If this is the case, you can begin your hike at Islip Saddle, following the PCT to Little Jimmy Campground. This variation adds about 1 mile and 400 feet of climbing round-trip.

---

trip 28.10   Devil's Punchbowl Loop Trail

see map on p. 362

Distance	1.0 mile (loop)
Hiking Time	30 minutes
Elevation Gain	300'
Difficulty	Easy
Trail Use	Dogs allowed, good for kids
Best Times	Year-round
Agency	Los Angeles County Parks & Recreation
Optional Map	Tom Harrison *Angeles High Country*

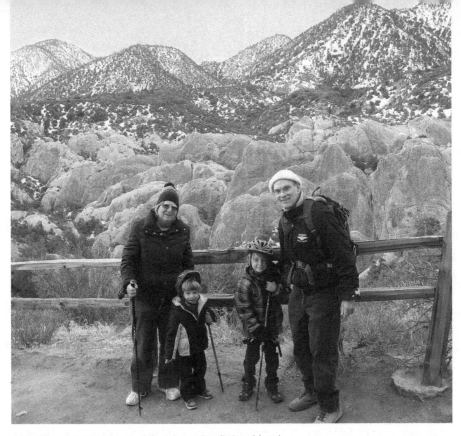

Little hikers join Grandma and Grandpa at Devil's Punchbowl.

DIRECTIONS From the Antelope Valley Freeway (Highway 14) south of Palmdale, exit at Pearblossom Highway (Highway 138) and follow it for 14 miles to the small community of Pearblossom. At Pearblossom, turn right on Longview Road (County Road N6) at a sign for Devil's Punchbowl. In 2.3 miles turn left on Fort Cajon Road. In 0.3 mile turn right to continue on N6, and follow the twisting road 5.3 miles to its end at the Punchbowl.

Tens of millions of years in the making, Devil's Punchbowl is L.A. County's most spectacular geological showplace. An observer looking down into this 300-foot-deep chasm immediately senses the enormity of the forces that produced the tilted and tangled collection of beige sandstone slabs.

The Punchbowl is caught between two active faults—the main San Andreas Fault and an offshoot, the Punchbowl Fault—along which old sedimentary formations have been pushed upward and crumpled downward, as well as transported horizontally. Erosion has put the final touches on the scene, roughing out the bowl-shaped gorge of Punchbowl Canyon and carving, in a host of unique ways, the rocks exposed at the surface.

Operated by the county as a special-use area under permit from Angeles National Forest, the 1,310-acre park consists of a superb nature center, a couple of short nature walks (including the loop trail described here), and the Punchbowl Trail—part of the High Desert National Recreation Trail. Devil's Punchbowl is open daily, sunrise–sunset, with no admission charge.

The Devil's Punchbowl Loop Trail is a perfect introduction to this fascinating area. It begins just behind the nature center, zigzags down off the rim to touch the seasonal creek in Punchbowl Canyon, and then climbs back out of the canyon opposite some of the tallest upright formations in the park. Near the start of the trail is a side path: the 0.3-mile Piñon Pathway, a self-guiding nature trail that loops through the piñon–juniper forest along the Punchbowl rim.

During winter, occasional snowfalls dust the 4,000-foot elevation of the Punchbowl itself and leave a lingering mantle of white on the pine-dotted slopes of the San Gabriel Mountains right above. During these episodes the trail can become muddy and slippery, and therefore probably unsuitable for small children.

trip 28.11   Devil's Chair

see map on p. 362

Distance	6 miles (one-way)
Hiking Time	3 hours
Elevation Gain/Loss	1,200'/1,500'
Difficulty	Moderate
Trail Use	Suitable for backpacking, dogs allowed
Best Times	September–June
Agency	Los Angeles County Parks & Recreation
Optional Map	Tom Harrison *Angeles High Country*

DIRECTIONS   This trip requires a 15-mile car shuttle. From the Antelope Valley Freeway (Highway 14) south of Palmdale, exit at Pearblossom Highway (Highway 138). Follow Pearblossom Highway for 14 miles to the small community of Pearblossom. At Pearblossom, turn right on Longview Road (County Road N6) at a sign for Devil's Punchbowl. In 2.3 miles turn left on Fort Cajon Road. In 0.3 mile pass a turn for southbound N6 on the right to which you will later return, but continue another 2.0 miles to Pallet Creek Road, where you jog left and then promptly turn right onto Valyermo Road. Continue 2.9 miles and turn right on Big Rock Creek Road. In 3.5 miles turn right onto a dirt road leading to South Fork Campground. In 0.9 mile, near the campground entrance, look for the signed Manzanita Trail on the left. Opposite this sign, take a short dirt spur on the right to the Punchbowl trailhead parking. Leave a vehicle here and return to Fort Cajon Road, where you turn south on N6 toward Devil's Punchbowl. Follow the twisting road 5.3 miles to its end at the Punchbowl.

The fenced viewpoint at Devil's Chair presides over what looks like frozen chaos— a vast assemblage of sandstone chunks and slabs tipped at odd angles, bent, seemingly pulled apart here, compressed there. This is really not so surprising when you realize that the Devil's Chair sits practically astride the "crush zone" of the Punchbowl Fault.

Devil's Chair can be reached with equal ease by starting either from Devil's Punchbowl Natural Area to the west or from South Fork Campground to the east. With a little help from a friend, perhaps, you can do the whole traverse from point to point, as we suggest here.; hiking from west to east gives you a slight downhill advantage. You'll need a permit, available free at Devil's Punchbowl Natural Area's nature center, if you plan to camp along the trail.

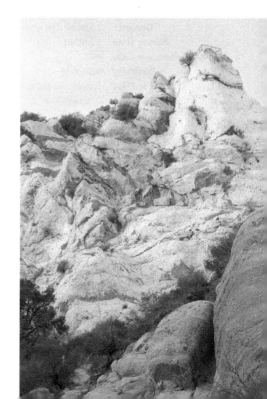

A fenced viewpoint perches atop this diabolically named rock formation.

If snow is present, check at the nature center to see if the route is safe. You should be aware that snow closes South Fork Campground, and that South Fork Big Rock Creek (next to the campground) could be difficult to ford after a storm.

From the south side of the Devil's Punchbowl parking lot, find and follow the signed Burkhart Trail as it climbs northwest along the rim of the punchbowl. You're actually following the upper (south) edge of a downward sloping terrace—part of an alluvial fan left high and dry when the Punchbowl creek began carving a new course northeast. You join an old road at 0.5 mile, pass a small reservoir at 0.7 mile, and arrive at a trail junction at 0.8 mile. Here, in a Coulter-pine grove, bear left on the Punchbowl Trail leading east. The delightful, contouring path takes you around several shady ravines, all draining into the Punchbowl. After some sharply descending switchbacks, you reach a trail junction (3.3 miles) from where a 0.1-mile spur goes west and then north over a narrow, rock-ribbed ridge to the high perch known as Devil's Chair. Protective fencing furnishes some psychological comfort for the nervous-making traverse.

East of the junction the trail keeps dropping, touches a saddle, descends crookedly past large manzanita shrubs, and crosses a small stream in the bottom of pine- and oak-shaded Holcomb Canyon beside a lovely campsite (3.8 miles).

Continue east up chaparral-smothered slopes to a saddle, then down the other side for a crooked mile to South Fork Campground.

VARIATION

To avoid the car shuttle, this trip can be done as an out-and-back from either trailhead. From the Devil's Punchbowl, it's 7 miles round-trip with 1,200 feet of elevation gain. From South Fork Campground, it's 5.4 miles with 1,300 feet of elevation gain.

---

trip 28.12   Lower Punchbowl Canyon

see map on p. 362

Distance	2.5 miles (out-and-back)
Hiking Time	1.5 hours
Elevation Gain	400'
Difficulty	Moderate
Trail Use	Suitable for backpacking, dogs allowed, good for kids
Best Times	October–June
Agency	Angeles National Forest
Optional Map	Tom Harrison *Angeles High Country*

DIRECTIONS From the Antelope Valley Freeway (Highway 14) south of Palmdale, exit at Pearblossom Highway (Highway 138) and follow it for 14 miles to the small community of Pearblossom. At Pearblossom, turn right on Longview Road (County Road N6). After 2.3 miles turn left (east) on Fort Tejon Road. Drive 2.3 miles to Pallet Creek Road, where you jog left and then promptly turn right onto Valyermo Road. Continue 2.9 miles and turn right on Big Rock Creek Road. After another 0.5 mile you pass the Angeles National Forest boundary (large sign). Go 0.2 mile farther to a parking turnout.

On this trip you enter Devil's Punchbowl by a little-known back way: the mouth of Punchbowl Canyon. Once above the lower canyon portals, you'll find yourself in a mazelike wonderland reminiscent of the slickrock country of southern Utah, save for the reddish hues. The hike is best done in winter or early spring, when snowmelt or runoff courses down the canyon and its tributaries.

Ford Big Rock Creek where you can, and start boulder-hopping up the narrow gorge to the west, Punchbowl Canyon. The canyon divides at 0.3 mile—stay right, in the main fork. Soon the familiar Punchbowl Formation rocks are all around you. The slabs of pebbly sandstone rise dramatically to the south—if you're game for it, scramble up for a great view of the brooding San Gabriels. Caution is in order when the rock is wet; it tends to disintegrate grain by grain much as Utah's slickrock does.

You may have to scramble up rocks or wade to bypass various obstacles. A narrow waterfall 1.2 miles up the meandering canyon blocks any farther easy walking. You can head back at this point, or you can find a way to scramble around it and reach the Devil's Punchbowl Loop Trail a short distance above.

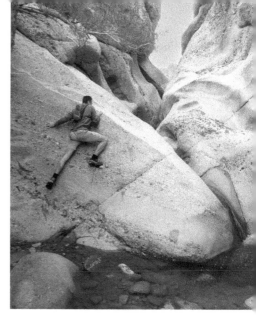

Playing on the rocks in Punchbowl Canyon

see map on p. 362

---

trip 28.13 **Holcomb Canyon**

Distance	4 miles (loop)
Hiking Time	3.5 hours
Elevation Gain	700'
Difficulty	Moderately strenuous
Trail Use	Suitable for backpacking, dogs allowed
Best Times	October–June
Agency	Los Angeles County Parks & Recreation
Recommended Map	Tom Harrison *Angeles High Country*

DIRECTIONS From the Antelope Valley Freeway (Highway 14) south of Palmdale, exit at Pearblossom Highway (Highway 138) and follow it for 14 miles to the small community of Pearblossom. At Pearblossom, turn right on Longview Road (County N6). After 2.3 miles turn left (east) on Fort Tejon Road. Drive 2.3 miles to Pallet Creek Road, where you jog left and then promptly turn right onto Valyermo Road. Continue 2.9 miles and turn right on Big Rock Creek Road. After another 0.5 mile you pass the Angeles National Forest boundary (large sign). Go 0.2 mile farther to a parking turnout.

Much of the fascination of the Devil's Punchbowl area lies in its trailless canyons, where the erosive forces of water have carved deep furrows in the soft sandstone. This beautiful loop trip, off-trail and requiring navigational skills almost the whole way, includes shady Holcomb Canyon as well as the large tributary of Punchbowl Canyon overlooked by the Devil's Chair. For adventurous hikers, it is the most interesting way to explore the heart of the Punchbowl. Several short scrambles and lots of rock-hopping is involved, so those uncertain of their footing will prefer a different trip.

Walk south along the shoulder of the road 0.3 mile to another turnout where the road turns sharply left, cross Big Rock Creek wherever most expedient, and stay right to start following the rocky banks of a tributary creek heading due south into Holcomb Canyon.

A mountain–desert mix of vegetation pervades the area: alder, willow, and sycamore along the creek banks; live-oak, incense cedar, big-cone Douglas-fir, and mountain mahogany higher on the banks; and pinyon pine dotting the dry slopes. The bedrock here is mostly the San Francisquito Formation—a marine sandstone formed about 60 million years ago. The Punchbowl Formation, which is a nonmarine sandstone only about 8 million years old, is seen briefly on the right (west) in the form of a blocky outcrop soaring over a pinched section of the canyon, 1.1 miles from the start. Soon you'll return to the Punchbowl Formation and stay in it for most of the remainder of the trip.

At 1.6 miles reach the crossing of the Punchbowl Trail a short distance ahead beside a gorgeous campsite. Use it to climb 0.3 mile west via switchbacks to a saddle. If you haven't been to visit the Devil's Chair, it's worth a short detour 0.25 mile west on the Punchbowl Trail to a signed spur leading out to the airy but fenced overlook, where you'll have wonderful views of the badlands you are about to explore.

Back at the saddle, leave the trail and descend cross-country, northwest through manzanita and scrub oak, into the head of a ravine. Proceed down the ravine to a three-way junction of ravines in a small flat just below the stony gaze of the Devil's Chair. From there on, you continue downcanyon (north), making two tricky drops, and eventually hook up with the lower end of Punchbowl Canyon. Turn right and go 0.3 mile to reach your car. Meanwhile, there are lots of interesting rock formations to explore along the way. Don't forget your camera!

Descending Holcomb Canyon

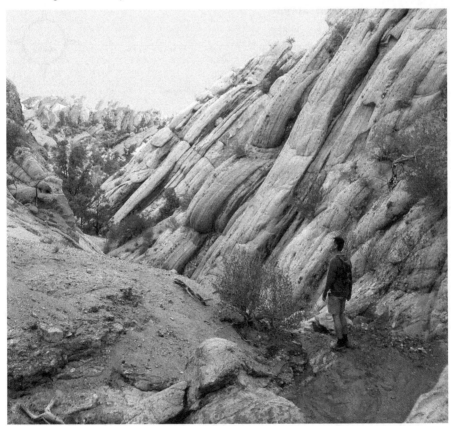

chapter 29

Big Pines &
Sheep Mountain Wilderness

On the eastern extremity of the Angeles Crest, quite removed from Los Angeles's often-smoggy blanket of air, lies Big Pines Recreation Area, set aside by the U.S. Forest Service specifically for year-round recreation. Perched high above the desert and blanketed by a heterogeneous mixture of pines, firs, and oaks, Big Pines boasts the clean, dry, evergreen-scented air and the crystalline blue skies that are characteristic of the melding of mountain and desert environments.

During the winter months, Big Pines' snow-play venues (Mountain High and Ski Sunrise) draw crowds of snow-starved skiers and snowboarders from the cities below who would rather not drive an extra 250 miles or more to reach the major-league Sierra Nevada ski resorts. In summer, several campgrounds, picnic areas, and interpretive trails serve the needs of visitors escaping the lowland heat. Ironically, relatively few people come up during seasons when the area is really most beautiful—spring and fall. Daytime temperatures are most pleasant then, and the colors of the foliage are bold and vibrant.

From most of the Los Angeles Basin, the most expedient way to get to the Big Pines area is by way of an eastern route: the 15 Freeway (I-15) and Highway 138 to Angeles Crest Highway, and then through Wrightwood. In the winter, Caltrans endeavors to plow the snow as far as Vincent Gap when possible, but the road beyond is closed frequently because of avalanches. The tedious west approach along Angeles Crest Highway from La Cañada Flintridge may involve winter closures due to snow cover, and sometimes long-term closures as a result of storm damage.

Big Pines and Wrightwood share the distinction of lying smack-dab on the San Andreas Fault. The crossroads of Big Pines itself (4 miles west of Wrightwood) marks the highest surface trace of the entire fault: 6,862 feet. Jackson Lake, a so-called sag pond in geologic parlance, fills a small, natural depression along the fault 2 miles northwest of Big Pines.

Wrightwood, one of the prettiest communities in L.A. County and the largest settlement in the San Gabriel Mountains, sprawls across another, much larger fault-caused depression known as Swarthout Valley. Unfortunately for

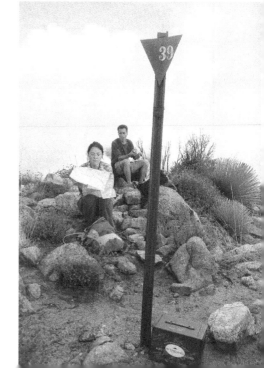

Hikers take a break on the summit of Rattlesnake Peak. (See Trip 29.2, page 383.)

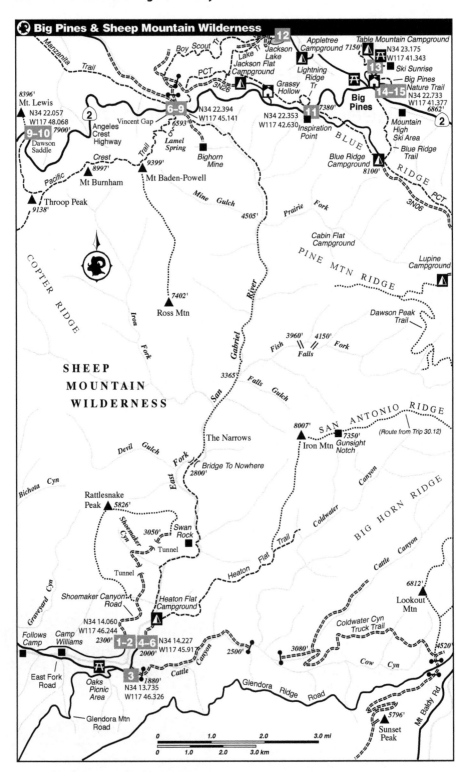

its roughly 5,000 summer residents, Wrightwood is acutely susceptible to destruction not only by Southern California's incipient Great Quake, likely to occur on this stretch of the San Andreas within a century, but also by fire, flooding, and mudslides.

At Big Pines you'll find the seldom-open Big Pines Information Station, housed in a corner of the former Swarthout Lodge. The lodge once served as headquarters for Big Pines County Park, which was open from 1923 to 1940. Unable to afford the cost of administering the park, Los Angeles County deeded the property to the U.S. Forest Service in 1940. The County had spent about $4 million creating a first-class recreational complex consisting of campgrounds, cabins, picnic areas, organizational camps, a swimming pool, an ice-skating rink, tennis courts, toboggan and ski runs, and more. An arched pedestrian overpass made of native stone was built over the access road, its twin towers containing barred holding cells for drunks and troublemakers. Only the north tower stands today near the visitor center. If you're looking for trail information, go to the Grassy Hollow Visitor Center instead.

After falling into disuse during and after World War II, Big Pines experienced a resurgence of attention in the 1950s. New facilities for campers and day users were constructed, and winter-sports areas were expanded and modernized. The use of snow-making machines today ensures that some of the ski slopes stay usable through much of the winter.

South of Big Pines, sprawling over some 44,000 acres, Sheep Mountain Wilderness is the largest and most recently (1984) designated federal wilderness in the San Gabriel Mountains. The name refers to the Nelson bighorn sheep, which are quite abundant throughout the area, and also to Iron Mountain—sometimes called Sheep Mountain—which lies near the geographic center of the wilderness.

The wilderness lies almost entirely in the grip of the many-branched, upper watershed of East Fork San Gabriel River. Rapid uplift and erosion have created topographical relief on a prodigious scale here. Boulder-strewn ridges dotted with sturdy conifers and clothed in tough blankets of chaparral fall thousands of feet to streams that tumble down V-shaped gorges. Elevations within the wilderness area range from 2,400 feet on the East Fork near Swan Rock to 10,064 feet at Old Baldy's summit, which lies on the east boundary.

From the 1850s until the early 1900s, gold mining was king on the East Fork, with important ore-producing prospects located high on the slopes of Mount Baden-Powell and Old Baldy and on some of the steep slopes overlooking the East Fork. On the banks of the East Fork itself, mountains of gold-bearing alluvium were literally washed away during a spate of hydraulic-mining activity in the 1870s. A fascinating history of East Fork's mining heyday is recounted in John Robinson's slender book *Mines of the East Fork*. Mining for gold and tungsten continues today at a number of sites within the wilderness; this is because certain mining claims were legally "grandfathered" when the area was declared a wilderness.

Most of the trails in Sheep Mountain Wilderness don't penetrate very far into its interior; cross-country hiking through the canyons and along many of the high ridges is possible, however. Three of the routes detailed in this chapter—Trips 29.5, 29.9, and 29.10—technically lie outside Sheep Mountain Wilderness but are included here because of their proximity to it.

It's not necessary to obtain a wilderness permit to enter Sheep Mountain Wilderness, *except* when you start from the end of East Fork Road. Pick up a self-issue permit at the East Fork Trailhead.

Even when a permit is not required, you should consult with an Angeles National Forest ranger to check on snow conditions, stream levels, and other possible hazards if you're planning a long trip to the interior of the wilderness. Also be aware that the Vincent Gap and Dawson Saddle Trailheads on Angeles Crest Highway can be unreachable by car for several months out of the year—and sometimes for a stretch of years—because of adverse weather conditions or storm damage.

see map on p. 380

trip 29.1 **Shoemaker Canyon Road**

Distance	5.5 miles (out-and-back)
Hiking Time	2.5 hours
Elevation Gain	800'
Difficulty	Moderate
Trail Use	Suitable for mountain biking, dogs allowed
Best Times	October–May
Agency	Angeles National Forest
Optional Map	Tom Harrison *Angeles High Country* or Trails Illustrated *Angeles National Forest (811)*

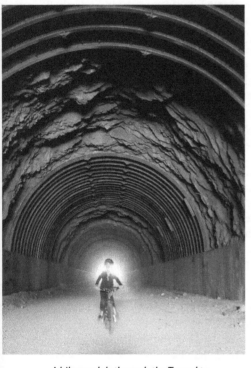

A biker pedals through the Tunnel to Nowhere on Shoemaker Canyon Road.

DIRECTIONS From the 210 Freeway in Azusa, take Exit 40 for northbound Azusa Avenue (Highway 39), and follow it into San Gabriel Canyon. In 11.9 miles turn right (east) on East Fork Road. Go 3.4 miles; then bear left on the paved, dead-end Shoemaker Canyon Road (Forest Service Road 2N11) at mile marker 3.39. Continue 1.9 miles to a vehicle gate and parking area.

Known colloquially as the Convict Road, Shoemaker Canyon Road should really be called the Road to Nowhere. The road was part of what was projected to be a 23-year effort to build a highway up along the East Fork canyon to Vincent Gap. (This project was not connected with an earlier road-building effort that included the construction of the famous, stranded Bridge to Nowhere; see Trip 29.4, page 385.)

During 1954–69, the county road department, using prison labor, managed to carve out and grade 4.5 miles of new roadway on the canyon wall opposite East Fork Station and Heaton Flat. The project was rendered moribund in 1969 in the face of rock slides, cost overruns, budget cuts, and opposition by conservationists. The creation of Sheep Mountain Wilderness in 1984 finally put to rest, probably once and for all, a project that would have irreparably scarred Southern California's deepest canyon: The Narrows of the East Fork. The enduring legacy of this misdirected road-building effort—massive cuts and fills—will probably be visible on the canyon walls for centuries to come.

Today you can drive the first 1.9 miles of Shoemaker Canyon Road on pavement, then walk the remaining graded-dirt section to reach a pair of tunnels. Beyond the second tunnel there's a great view of the East Fork gorge and its mile-high east wall culminating at 8,007-foot Iron Mountain.

From the trailhead, start walking up the unpaved road ahead. At 1.4 mile watch for an unsigned climbers' trail on the left heading up a gully to an old road cut and on to Rattlesnake Peak (see next trip). After 1.7 miles of walking, you reach the first tunnel, about 400 yards long, completed in 1961. Ahead lies a small abyss, Shoemaker Canyon. It was never bridged; instead, the road contours around it and continues northeast to a second tunnel, about 250 yards long, dated 1964. The canyon is named for Alonzo Shoemaker, a longtime miner who prospected here starting in 1855. On the far side of that tunnel, look over the edge for the best view of the East Fork gorge.

trip 29.2 — Rattlesnake Peak

Distance	9.5 miles (out-and-back)
Hiking Time	8 hours
Elevation Gain	4,200'
Difficulty	Strenuous
Trail Use	Dogs allowed
Best Times	October–April
Agency	Angeles National Forest
Recommended Map	Tom Harrison *Angeles High Country* or Trails Illustrated *Angeles National Forest (811)*

see map on p. 380

DIRECTIONS From the 210 Freeway in Azusa, take Exit 40 for northbound Azusa Avenue (Highway 39), and follow it into San Gabriel Canyon. In 11.9 miles turn right (east) on East Fork Road. Go 3.4 miles; then bear left on the paved, dead-end Shoemaker Canyon Road (Forest Service Road 2N11) at mile marker 3.39. Continue 1.9 miles to a vehicle gate and parking area.

Rattlesnake Peak (5,862') is the second most inaccessible major summit in the San Gabriels, after Iron Mountain. A steep climbers' trail ascends the south ridge from Shoemaker Canyon Road and descends the east ridge. The difficulty varies depending on how recently hikers and wildfires have beaten back the chaparral. The 2012 Williams Fire burned 4,192 acres, including most of Rattlesnake Peak; at the time of this writing, the brush has regrown but is not too bad along the route, and visitors have cut it back in places.

Picking a way up the south ridge of Rattlesnake Peak

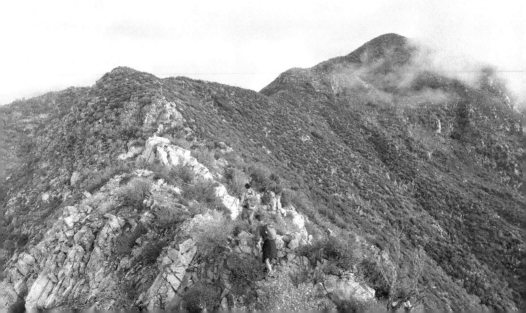

The U.S. Forest Service does not track information about this route, so your best bet is to search online for recent trip reports to make sure that other hikers are getting through before you venture up here. Long pants, long sleeves, boots with good tread, trekking poles, and gaiters will all be helpful. Go on a cool day. Rattlesnakes are no more common here than elsewhere at this altitude, but lizards are plentiful.

From the gate, hike up the so-called Road to Nowhere for 1.5 miles. Watch for mile markers placed by the overly optimistic roadbuilders. Just before a gully at mile marker 3.39, turn left off the road up a steep trail. You'll soon find yourself on traces of another abandoned road cut. In 0.2 mile leave the cut at a saddle and follow a climbers' trail steeply up the ridge, going west, then northwest, and then west again. Chamise, scrub oak, and buckwheat dominate the vegetation. Several ridges intersect at a bump just above 4,000'. Note this point carefully in case you need to retrace your path. Our ridge, rocky in places and steep in others, turns north and continues past some false summits to Rattlesnake Peak, 4.2 miles from the start. The summit benchmark is named Fang. Enjoy outstanding views in all directions, especially northeast toward Iron Mountain and Baldy.

You can return the way you came, but if the brush is not too bad, it is more fun to descend the east ridge. Carefully stay on the crest of the ridge, disregarding occasional animal paths that drop down the side, and quickly enter thick chaparral. Below 4,600 feet, the ridge steepens and at times you can boot-ski down the sandy parts. This is much better for descent than for climbing. At 3,650 feet, the climbers' trail abruptly turns right off the ridge and makes steep switchbacks southward. At 3,050 feet, you turn into a gully and join a good path contouring along the abandoned road cut. You soon reach the mouth of the northern tunnel and join the Shoemaker Canyon Road at 6.8 miles. From here, it's easy walking through a second tunnel back to the trailhead.

---

trip 29.3 Cattle Canyon

see map on p. 380

Distance	7.5 miles (out-and-back)
Hiking Time	3 hours
Elevation Gain	700'
Difficulty	Moderate
Trail Use	Suitable for backpacking, dogs allowed, good for kids
Best Times	September–June
Agency	Angeles National Forest
Optional Map	Tom Harrison *Angeles High Country* or Trails Illustrated *Angeles National Forest (811)*

DIRECTIONS From the 210 Freeway in Azusa, take Exit 40 for northbound Azusa Avenue (Highway 39), and follow it into San Gabriel Canyon. In 11.9 miles turn right (east) on East Fork Road. Go 5.2 miles to the intersection with Glendora Mountain Road. Park at this intersection, taking care to observe parking restrictions nearby.

From Coldwater Canyon to East Fork, Cattle Canyon carves a sinuous course through a gorge impressively flanked by walls abruptly soaring 1,000 feet or more. An old dirt road—now a pleasant hiking path—follows the canyon bottom, crossing the alder-lined stream about two dozen times. You can follow the gradually ascending trail through Cattle Canyon as far as 3.7 miles to a locked gate, posted NO ENTRY. Thompson Ranch and other private properties in Cattle and Coldwater Canyons lie beyond.

This is a great spring or early-summer trip. The stream flows clear and cool, but not normally so high as to create a hazard when you cross. Wear sandals or other shoes that you don't mind getting wet. Streamside vegetation flourishes, and wildflowers dot the sunny flats. The stream and its moist banks provide a perfect habitat for a variety of snakes, including rattlesnakes.

In May 1859, some prospectors found rich gold deposits in the East Fork and a gold rush began. Many of the miners settled on the flat at the mouth of Cattle Canyon, and the rowdy community soon became known as Eldoradoville. The miners built dams, waterwheels, pumps, and even railways to work their claims, but a heavy rainstorm in November of the same year washed away everything. The persistent men rebuilt and were back to full production by March. In January 1862 an even

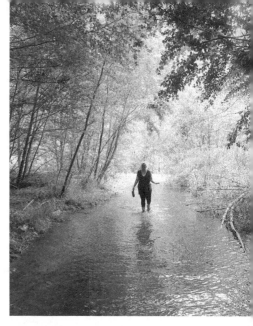

One of dozens of creek crossings in Cattle Canyon

larger storm flooded the canyon, washing away every trace of Eldoradoville along with all of the mine works. Finally discouraged, the miners dispersed. Unemployed men returned to this spot during the Great Depression and built another mining camp called Hooverville. A March 1938 storm swept away the town and mining works yet again, although recreational gold panning continues in the East Fork to this day. Flooding also continues to be a regular occurrence, as the builders of the Bridge to Nowhere and the Road to Nowhere eventually discovered.

From the parking at the intersection of East Fork Road and Glendora Mountain Road, continue up East Fork Road for 0.2 mile to the beginning of the gated dirt road at the south end of a bridge. Pass through the gate and follow the dirt road. You can go as far as you like, and turn back at any point short of Thompson Ranch.

trip 29.4 Bridge to Nowhere

Distance	9.5 miles (out-and-back)
Hiking Time	4.5 hours
Elevation Gain	1,000'
Difficulty	Moderately strenuous
Trail Use	Suitable for backpacking, dogs allowed
Best Times	October–June
Agency	Angeles National Forest
Optional Map	Tom Harrison *Angeles High Country*
Fees/Permits	Free self-issue wilderness permit required

see map on p. 380

DIRECTIONS From the 210 Freeway in Azusa, take Exit 40 for northbound Azusa Avenue (Highway 39), and follow it into San Gabriel Canyon. In 11.9 miles turn right (east) on East Fork Road. At a hairpin turn in 5.3 miles, stay straight (east) on a minor road that crosses a bridge and ends in 0.9 mile at a parking lot and closed gate. Get your free self-issue wilderness permit at a box near the entrance to the parking lot.

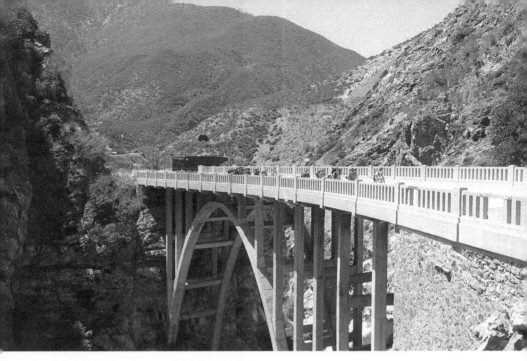

The Bridge to Nowhere is a reminder of man's hubris.

Born of snow-fed rivulets, the many tributaries of the East Fork gather together to form one of the liveliest mountain streams in the San Gabriels. At The Narrows of the East Fork, the water squeezes through the deepest gorge in Southern California. From the bottom of The Narrows, the east wall soars about 5,200 feet to Iron Mountain, and the west wall rises about 4,000 feet to the South Mount Hawkins divide.

During the 1930s, road-builders managed to push a highway up through the East Fork to as far as the lower portals of The Narrows. There, an arched, concrete bridge was constructed, similar in style to those that were built in the same era along Angeles Crest Highway. The bridge was to be a key link in a route that would one day carry traffic between the San Gabriel Valley and the desert near Wrightwood. But fate intervened. The great 1938 flood thoroughly demolished most of the road, leaving the bridge stranded far upstream. The next and last attempt to construct a road through the East Fork gorge utilized a high-line approach instead (see Trip 29.1, page 382), but that effort was ultimately abandoned as well.

The trek to the old bridge is in the same league as the climb of Old Baldy—an obligatory experience for L.A.-area hikers. On warm summer weekends, hundreds of people walk the trail going up from East Fork Station. A fraction venture as far as the bridge, a leisurely half-day's round-trip hike as long as the water flow in the East Fork isn't too great and swift. You'll find many places where you could spend a night, including near the river just beyond the bridge.

Over the last century or more, gold mining in the East Fork has evolved from a serious business to more of a recreational pastime. Today, claims are being worked around The Narrows area, but mostly it's the fun of playing around in the stream and catching a bit of color that keeps a number of recreational miners coming back year after year.

There are several creek crossings of ankle- to knee-depth, so wear shoes that you don't mind getting soaked. During parts of winter and spring, high water may render these crossings unsafe.

Follow the gated service road upstream, high along the right bank, to Heaton Flat Campground at 0.5 mile. Beyond Heaton Flat the road ends, but a well-traveled trail continues up the flood plain. At 2.5 miles you pass Swan Rock, a cliff-exposure of metamorphic rock branded with the light-colored imprint of a swan; you can see it best under flat lighting conditions. You're now entering Sheep Mountain Wilderness.

At 3.5 miles the trail swings abruptly right and climbs about 60 feet to meet a remnant of the old highway. The old road bed carves its way along the east canyon wall, high above what is now a wide, boulder-filled flood plain laced with the meandering, alder-lined stream. The Bridge to Nowhere appears at 4.8 miles, just as the canyon walls start to pinch in. The bridge appears remarkably undamaged after a half century of neglect, except for its crumbling concrete railings.

The bridge and the area just south of it lie within an island of posted private property. You're allowed passage across the bridge, but please don't stray from the road or the bridge when inside the posted area. From the north abutment of the bridge, a narrow trail contours above the stream, then drops into the lower part of The Narrows. Trip 29.6 (page 388) covers the upper portion of the canyon.

trip 29.5   Iron Mountain

see map on p. 380

Distance	13.5 miles (out-and-back)
Hiking Time	8 hours
Elevation Gain	6,200'
Difficulty	Strenuous
Trail Use	Dogs allowed
Best Times	October–November, April–May
Agency	Angeles National Forest
Recommended Map	Tom Harrison *Angeles High Country*
Fees/Permits	Free self-issue wilderness permit required

DIRECTIONS From the 210 Freeway in Azusa, take Exit 40 for northbound Azusa Avenue (Highway 39), and follow it into San Gabriel Canyon. In 12 miles turn right (east) on East Fork Road. At a hairpin turn in 5.3 miles, stay straight (east) on a minor road that crosses a bridge and ends in 0.9 mile at a parking lot and closed gate. Get a free self-issue wilderness permit at a box near the entrance to the lot.

Looking west from Iron Mountain over Rattlesnake Peak toward the San Gabriel Wilderness

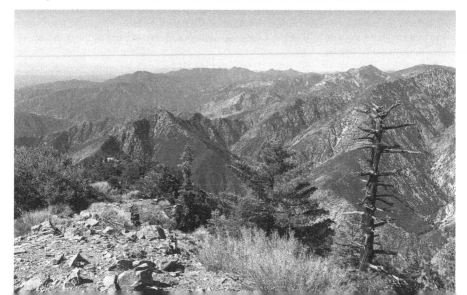

Big bad Iron Mountain stands west of Mount Baldy, towering over the headwaters of the San Gabriel River. It is the toughest single-peak hike in the San Gabriel Mountains. The hike begins near the river at 2,000 feet and climbs to the 8,007-foot summit. The first half is on a good trail to Heaton Saddle, but the second half follows a steep climbers' path up the interminable south ridge of Iron Mountain. The mountain is defended by sharp Whipple yuccas, so wear sturdy pants and gaiters. Most people will want at least 4 quarts of water on a cool day; don't even think about this shadeless climb on a hot day. This is also a popular conditioning hike and gets regular use by a number of hardy mountaineers. The route is south-facing and lower than many others in the region, so it can often be done in the winter months if snowfall has been light. The peak was originally named Sheep Mountain in 1890, but was renamed to Iron by 1907 because of the prominent outcrops of iron ore.

Hike north past the gate along the dirt road to Heaton Flat Campground. At a sign near the outhouse, turn right and follow the Heaton Flat Trail 3.9 miles to Allison Saddle. The maintained trail ends here, but a surprisingly good climbers' path leads up the crest of the south ridge for 2.5 intense miles with 3,500 feet of elevation gain. The route is distinct and straightforward to follow, even on a foggy day.

Return the way you came. Or, if you have plenty of time and are feeling extremely strong, follow the great San Antonio Ridge east to Mount Baldy (see Trip 30.12, page 419).

---

trip 29.6   Down the East Fork

see map on p. 380

Distance	15.5 miles (one-way)
Hiking Time	11 hours
Elevation Gain/Loss	200'/4,800'
Difficulty	Strenuous
Trail Use	Suitable for backpacking, dogs allowed
Best Times	April–November
Agency	Angeles National Forest
Recommended Map	Tom Harrison *Angeles High Country*
Fees/Permits	Free self-issue wilderness permit required only if hiking in reverse from the East Fork Trailhead

DIRECTIONS This trip requires a 1.5-hour, 81-mile car shuttle. Leave a getaway vehicle at the East Fork Trailhead: From the 210 Freeway in Azusa, take Exit 40 for northbound San Gabriel Canyon Road (Highway 39), and drive 12 miles to East Fork Road, on the right. Continue up East Fork Road 6 miles to a parking lot at the end. You can get a self-issue wilderness permit at a box by the outhouse.

   To reach the Vincent Gap Trailhead, return to the 210 Freeway and take it east to the 15 Freeway, then north to Highway 138. Drive west on Highway 138 for 8.6 miles; then turn left onto Angeles Crest Highway (Highway 2) and go 14 miles to the Vincent Gap Trailhead parking lot, at mile marker 74.88. Better yet, have somebody drop you off and then pick you up later.

Born from snow-fed rivulets, the many tributaries of the East Fork San Gabriel River gather together to form one of the liveliest and most remote streams in the San Gabriels. At The Narrows of the East Fork, the water squeezes through the deepest gorge in Southern California. From the bottom of The Narrows, the east wall soars about 5,200 feet to Iron Mountain, and the west wall rises about 4,000 feet to the South Mount Hawkins divide.

On this epic journey down the upper East Fork, you'll descend nearly a mile in elevation, travel from high-country pines and firs to sun-scorched chaparral, and cross three important geologic faults—the Punchbowl, Vincent Thrust, and San Gabriel faults. During the course of a single day you could experience a temperature increase of as much as 60°F.

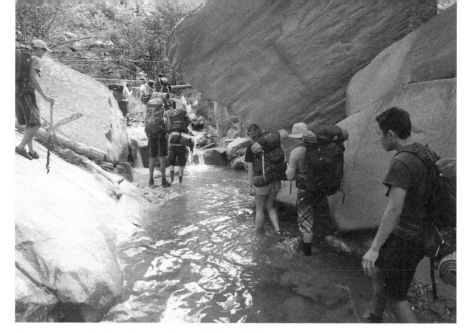

Backpackers wade through the unforgettable East Fork Narrows.

You can do this hike in one incredibly long day with an early start, or you can camp overnight on one of the shaded streamside terraces near the midpoint of the trek. The better camping sites include former trail camps at Fish and Iron forks, and the lower part of The Narrows. The route passes through the Sheep Mountain Wilderness, but a wilderness permit is required only if you start at East Fork, where a self-issue permit box is located in the parking area.

The upper part of the canyon receives few visitors and remains pristine, while the lower portion is heavily traveled by day hikers and "prospectors" panning for gold in the creek. If everyone hauls out a bit of the detritus left behind by thoughtless users, the canyon will become more attractive.

Except at the beginning, navigation on the trip is straightforward—you simply head downcanyon the whole way. Consult a detailed map often if you want to confirm exactly where you are. Heavy runoff after a storm or major snowmelt can create hazardous stream crossings, which is one of the reasons why this trip is only recommended for the late-spring through fall seasons. The other reason is the upper trailhead at Vincent Gap may be unreachable due to snow cover, although Highway 2 is often plowed to the gap. Check dot.ca.gov for road conditions; if Highway 2 is listed as closed 5 miles west of Big Pines, it's open to Vincent Gap.

The amount of time required to complete the trip can be highly variable due to problems with adverse weather or swift-flowing water, excessive bushwhacking along the banks of the upper river, how heavy your backpacks are, and the hiking ability of the slowest member of your party. This is not a trip for hikers without plenty of successful experience in off-trail wilderness travel.

From the parking area on the south side of Vincent Gap, walk down the gated road to the southeast. After only about 200 yards, a footpath veers left into Sheep Mountain Wilderness. Take it; the road itself continues toward the Bighorn Mine, an inholding of privately owned land inside the wilderness boundary.

Intermittently shaded by big-cone Douglas-firs, white firs, Jeffrey pines, and live oaks, the path descends along the south slope of Vincent Gulch. The gulch itself follows the Punchbowl Fault, a splinter of the San Andreas. At 0.7 mile, on a flat ridge spur, look for an indistinct path intersecting on the right. This leads about 100 yards, passing a tangle of downed trees, to an old cabin believed to have been the home of Charles Vincent. Vincent led the life of a hermit, prospector, and big-game hunter in the Baden-Powell–Old Baldy area from 1870 until his death in 1926.

After a few switchbacks, the primitive trail crosses Vincent Gulch (usually dry at this point, wet a short distance below) at 1.6 miles. Thereafter it stays on or above the east bank. Pass a tributary on the left in 0.4 mile and then a second one in another 0.5 mile. An unsigned trail leads to some fine campsites in the second tributary, but you should be careful to stay right and drop onto the floor of the main drainage.

The trail soon becomes indistinct and you must pick your own path down the rocky floor of Vincent Gulch. In 0.6 mile watch for the wreck of a Schweizer sailplane. In February 1974, the plane was caught in a downdraft on the flank of Mount Baden-Powell and became trapped in the canyon. The occupants walked away with minor injuries, but the plane was unsalvageable.

A sign marks the confluence of Prairie Fork, a wide drainage coming in from the east at 4.2 miles from the start. A trail once led up this canyon to Cabin Flat, but it was obliterated by the 1997 Beiderbach Fire and is now heavily overgrown with poison oak and stinging nettle. You veer right (west) down a gravelly wash, good for setting up a camp. In the summer, watch for brilliant yellow, five-petaled blazing star flowers in this area. Shortly after, at the Mine Gulch confluence, you bend left (south) into the wide bed of the upper East Fork. For several miles to come, there is essentially no trail. It may take several hours to traverse this stretch, depending on the energy and motivation of your group. Iron Mountain, the major summit to the south, often can be seen as an indicator of your progress.

Proceed down the rock-strewn flood plain, crossing the creek (and battling alder thickets) several times over the next mile. The canyon becomes narrow for a while starting at about 5.0 miles, and you must wade or hop from one slippery rock to another. Fish Fork, on the left at 7.3 miles from the start, is the first large stream below Prairie Fork. One of the best campsites along the canyon can be found here.

If you have the time for an intriguing side trip, Fish Fork canyon is well worth exploring. Chock-full of alder and bay, narrow with soaring walls, its clear stream tumbling over boulders, the canyon boasts one of the wildest and most beautiful settings in the San Gabriels. About 1.6 miles upstream lies a formidable impasse: There, the waters of Fish Fork drop 12 feet into an emerald-green pool set amid sheer rock walls. A bigger waterfall, inaccessible by means of this approach, lies farther upstream.

In another 0.3 mile, you may observe a thin column of water dropping over the cliff at the mouth of Falls Gulch on the left. In another mile you enter The Narrows. A rough trail, worn in by hikers, traverses this 1-mile-plus section of fast-moving water. You'll pass swimmable (if chilly) pools cupped in the granite and schist bedrock, and cross the stream when necessary. Listen and watch for water ouzels (dippers) by the edges of the pools. You might notice a travertine stalactite created by mineral-rich water seeping down the west wall. Old mining trails once threaded the canyon walls here and to the north, but all are virtually obliterated now.

At the lower portals of The Narrows (10.7 miles), you come upon the enigmatically named Bridge to Nowhere. During the 1930s, road-builders managed to push a highway up along the East Fork stream to just this far. The arched, concrete bridge, similar in style to those built along Angeles Crest Highway, was to be a key link in a route that would carry traffic between the San Gabriel Valley and the desert near Wrightwood. Fate intervened. A great flood in 1938 thoroughly demolished most of the road, leaving the bridge stranded.

Below the bridge, on remnants of the old road washed out in 1938, you'll run into more and more hikers, fishermen, and other travelers out for the day. A decent trail generally can be found on the east side of the canyon, occasionally becoming harder to find when it is forced over to the west side. At 12.7 miles Swan Rock—an outcrop of metamorphic rock branded with the light-colored imprint of a swan—comes into view on the right. At 15.0 miles you come upon Heaton Flat Campground. From there a final, easy 0.5-mile stroll takes you to the East Fork Station and trailhead at the end of East Fork Road.

---

trip 29.7   ## Big Horn Mine

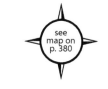

see map on p. 380

Distance	3.8 miles (out-and-back)
Hiking Time	2 hours
Elevation Gain	500'
Difficulty	Easy
Trail Use	Dogs
Best Times	March–November
Agency	Angeles National Forest
Recommended Map	Tom Harrison *Angeles High Country*

DIRECTIONS From I-15 north of San Bernardino, exit at Highway 138 and turn west. Drive 8.6 miles to Angeles Crest Highway (Highway 2), and turn left. Continue through Wrightwood and Big Pines on Angeles Crest Highway for 14 miles until you reach the large trailhead parking lot at Vincent Gap, at mile marker 2 LA 74.88.

Gold miners discovered placer gold in the East Fork of the San Gabriel river in the 1850s and amateurs still pan for flakes along its water course. Charles Tom Vincent, a hermit and mountain man who haunted the San Gabriel high country, discovered the mother lode high on the east flank of Mount Baden-Powell in 1895, and named it for the bighorn sheep he was hunting at the time. Lacking the capital to process or haul ore from such a remote location, he sold the mine. Twelve hundred feet of tunnels were laboriously hacked into the

Big Horn is the most impressive and best-preserved of the mines in the San Gabriel Mountains.

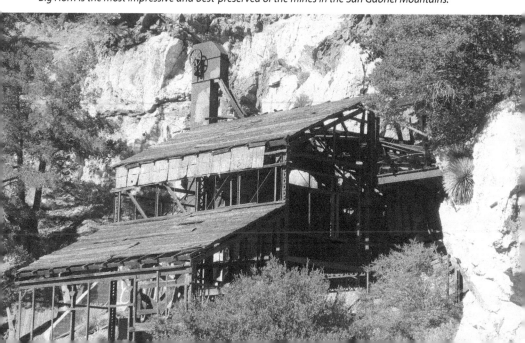

mountainside, and approximately $100,000 of gold was obtained, making Big Horn Mine the most famous of the many mines in the San Gabriel Mountains. On his deathbed, in 1926, Vincent confessed to his doctor that his true name was Charles Vincent Dougherty and that he was wanted for shooting three men who had been robbing his cabin at an Arizona mining claim. Various companies sporadically attempted to work the mine over the 20th century until the Wilderness Land Trust finally purchased the property in 2007 and bequeathed it to the U.S. Forest Service to become part of the Sheep Mountain Wilderness. The adits have been sealed with bat gates, but a large shed remains where the stamp mill once thundered. This is a good hike for those who enjoy mining history.

To visit the site, follow the gated wagon road left of the Mount Baden-Powell Trail. In 0.2 mile stay right at a signed junction where the Mine Gulch Trail descends into the canyon. In another 0.5 mile, pass above Vincent's well-preserved cabin, hidden in the woods (N34° 22.075' W117° 44.664').

Pass a partially flooded adit; then round the east ridge of Mount Baden-Powell, and reach the mill at the end of the trail. Use caution because the building could be unstable. Entering abandoned mines is never safe. A flat by the east ridge makes a good spot for lunch before you return.

VARIATION

One can climb Mount Baden-Powell via the east ridge. This 1.5-mile route with 2,400 feet of elevation gain tops out at the last switchback before the Pacific Crest Trail junction near the summit (see Trip 29.9, next page). No bushwhacking is necessary and you'll find a faint climbers' trail much of the way. It is usually easiest to stay near the crest of the ridge, until a thicket of chinquapin forces you off near the top. Limber pines (with small cones and bundles of five short needles) are found starting around 8,000 feet, unusually low in Southern California. They are propagated by the Clark's nutcracker, a bird that harvests the large pine nuts and hides them in the ground. Lodgepole pines join around 8,500 feet.

---

trip 29.8	**Ross Mountain**

see map on p. 380

Distance	14 miles (out-and-back)
Hiking Time	9 hours
Elevation Gain	5,500'
Difficulty	Strenuous
Trail Use	Suitable for backpacking
Best Times	May–November
Agency	Angeles National Forest
Recommended Map	Tom Harrison *Angeles High Country*

DIRECTIONS From I-15 north of San Bernardino, exit at Highway 138 and turn west. Drive 8.6 miles to Angeles Crest Highway (Highway 2), and turn left. Continue through Wrightwood and Big Pines on Angeles Crest Highway for 14 miles until you reach the large trailhead parking lot at Vincent Gap at mile marker 2 LA 74.88.

Isolated and difficult to reach, Ross Mountain (7,402') stands tall on the divide between the trenchlike East Fork San Gabriel River and a shallower but equally steep-walled tributary called Iron Fork. To get there you must first climb Mount Baden-Powell, and then descend 2,000 feet down a hardscrabble ridge. Weary peak-baggers have dubbed the mountain "Ross Pit"—you'll know why when it comes time to turn around and return the same way you came. Mr. Ross was an early homesteader in the area.

Starting from Vincent Gap, hike the 40 switchbacks of the Pacific Crest Trail to Mount Baden-Powell's summit (3.8 miles). Once you reach the top, you simply follow the rounded ridge leading south for another 3.0 miles to Ross Mountain's 7,402-foot high point.

From the Baden-Powell summit you swoop down along the eroding south rim of Mine Gulch and, 1 mile and 1,000 feet below, reach a flat area shaded by stately Jeffrey pines, suitable for camping. Ahead, there are fewer trees, and more chaparral. Short climbs alternate with long, steep, rocky downhill stretches.

According to the backcountry register kept on Ross Mountain, only a dozen or two climbers come this way every year. Die-hards have set speed records from Vincent Gap, while others have ascended the mountain by bushwhacking up the south slope from Iron Fork, a very impressive feat indeed.

A panoramic view of the canyons below Ross Mountain awaits if you walk 0.2 mile farther to the mountain's south brow. When

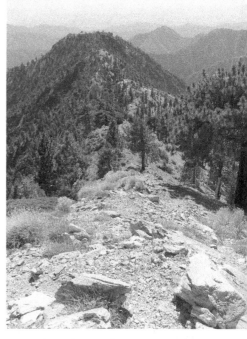

A view down the ridge from Baden-Powell to Ross Mountain

it's time to return, breathe a long sigh of regret and then tackle the job. The climb back up to Mount Baden-Powell is nearly always a sweaty affair, with a southern exposure all the way and very little shade.

trip 29.9 **Mount Baden-Powell Traverse**

see map on p. 380

Distance	8 miles (one-way)
Hiking Time	5.5 hours
Elevation Gain/Loss	2,100'/3,500'
Difficulty	Strenuous
Trail Use	Suitable for backpacking, dogs allowed
Best Times	May–November
Agency	Angeles National Forest
Recommended Map	Tom Harrison *Angeles High Country*

DIRECTIONS This trip requires a 5-mile car or bicycle shuttle. Leave your getaway vehicle at Vincent Gap: From I-15 north of San Bernardino, exit at Highway 138 and turn west. Drive 8.6 miles to Angeles Crest Highway (Highway 2), and turn left. Continue through Wrightwood and Big Pines on Angeles Crest Highway for 14 miles until you reach the large trailhead parking lot at Vincent Gap (mile marker 2 LA 74.88).

To reach the starting point, continue 5.3 miles west on Angeles Crest Highway to mile 69.6, just east of Dawson Saddle.

Named in honor of Lord Baden-Powell, the British Army officer who started the Boy Scout movement in 1907, massive Mount Baden-Powell stands higher than any other mountain in the San Gabriels—except the Mount San Antonio complex to the east. Many

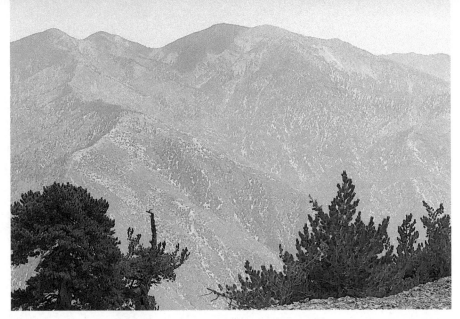

Mount Baldy's north backbone (left horizon; see Trip 30.13, page 420) from Mount Baden-Powell

thousands of hikers troop to Baden-Powell's summit yearly, mostly by way of Vincent Gap on Angeles Crest Highway.

Baden-Powell's summit is the last major milestone on the 52-mile trek from Chantry Flat to Vincent Gap known as the Silver Moccasin Trail (in this part of the range it coincides with the Pacific Crest Trail). The five-day-long Silver Moccasin backpack is a rite of passage for L.A.-area Scouts.

If you want to climb Mount Baden-Powell in a most interesting way, try this one-way hike from Dawson Saddle to Vincent Gap. The effort involved is only little more than what's involved in the usual round-trip from Vincent Gap, and you'll visit two other peaks as well. All three peaks offer their own unique and panoramic perspective of the rugged Sheep Mountain Wilderness below. The shuttle between ending and starting points (which can be done conveniently enough on a bicycle) is only 5 miles long. The following remarks assume that Angeles Crest Highway is open to vehicles west of Vincent Gap. Parts of this 5-mile stretch are notoriously susceptible to storm damage, and in the past landslides have closed the highway year-round.

Backpackers can find small, exposed campsites on the ridge between Throop and Baden-Powell. A medium-size site is available on the ridge south of the Baden-Powell summit. Sheltered sites are located in the forest along the switchbacks between Baden-Powell and Lamel Spring, including a large site three switchbacks above the spring.

Baden-Powell is also a popular winter ascent because Caltrans usually plows the road to Vincent Gap. The icy climb requires crampons, an ice ax, and suitable knowledge; unqualified mountaineers have repeatedly gotten in trouble here. Most winter climbers return the way they came.

Those planning a bicycle shuttle may prefer to do this hike in reverse so they can coast down the road on the bike.

Begin right at mile 69.6, just east of Dawson Saddle, where there's parking space on the north side of the highway. Cross the highway to get to the trail, which goes south along the top of a long, ascending ridge. You switchback up through pines and firs, heading toward the main crest of the San Gabriels at Throop Peak. An impressive 3,540 hours of volunteer labor by Boy Scouts were required to build this trail, which was completed in 1982.

At 1.8 miles, near the benchmark of 8,789 feet, you join the Pacific Crest Trail. Head southwest on the PCT; then climb cross-country about 300 yards to reach the summit of Throop Peak. Hikers' registers are found here, as well as on the other two peaks you'll be visiting.

Return to the Dawson Saddle Trail junction and continue northeast on the PCT, which follows the main ridgeline. You descend to a saddle and then ascend to Mount Burnham's north flank, where switchbacks take you over to Burnham's east shoulder. You can make an easy side trip to Burnham's summit from the east shoulder.

After bagging Burnham, continue east, climbing a breathless 400 feet more, to reach the impressive Boy Scout monument on Baden-Powell's 9,399-foot summit. Return by way of the trail descending Baden-Powell's northeast ridge. After 40 switchbacks and 3.8 miles of descent you'll reach the large Vincent Gap trailhead. About halfway down the trail, on the 25th switchback corner, a side trail leads about 200 yards east to a dribbling pipe at Lamel Spring. This spring occasionally dries up in drought years, so you're better off carrying your own water for the full day.

This is a great slope to observe the progression of conifers with altitude. The summit of Baden-Powell is covered in limber and lodgepole pines. Limber pines have 1.5- to 2.5-inch needles in tight bundles of five, medium cones, and famously flexible branches, while lodgepoles have short needles in bundles of two; round, golf ball–sized cones; and thin, flaky bark. The ancient limber pine grove is likely a remnant from the last ice age, during which the species was distributed more widely and at lower elevations. One of the most striking specimens is the signed Wally Waldron Tree, named for a longtime Scout leader who led the construction of the Mount Baden-Powell monument. Limber pines disappear below about 9,000 feet on your descent, although they persist down to 8,000 feet on the east ridge, their lowest elevation in Southern California.

By 8,650 feet, the beautiful pure stand of lodgepoles gives way to a mixed forest, including white fir and sugar pines. Fir has needles in rows rather than bundles, and the cones grow on the top of the trees and disintegrate in place rather than falling to the ground. Sugar pines have famously long cones, seasonally dripping with sap, and 2.5- to 4-inch needles in bundles of five. The lodgepoles become scarce below 8,100 feet. Jeffrey pines become common below 7,600 feet, with 5- to 10-inch needles in bundles of three and 4- to 8-inch oval cones. The sugar pines are scarce below 7,000 feet. Incense cedars, with bright green scales rather than needles, appear around 6,900 feet shortly before you reach the trailhead. Two stands of non-native giant sequoias were planted at Vincent Gap, recognizable by their awl-shaped leaves.

Backpackers will find room for at least two tents at each saddle on the Angeles Crest. These sites, as well as the north ridge of Baden-Powell, have tremendous views but are exposed to the wind. Larger sheltered sites are located along the trail 0.4 mile before the Throop Peak junction, on the northeast shoulder of Burnham, and about 0.5 mile above Lamel Spring.

---

trip 29.10 **Mount Lewis**

see map on p. 380

Distance	0.8 mile (out-and-back)
Hiking Time	1 hour
Elevation Gain	500'
Difficulty	Easy
Trail Use	Dogs allowed, good for kids
Best Times	May–November
Agency	Angeles National Forest
Optional Map	Tom Harrison *Angeles High Country*

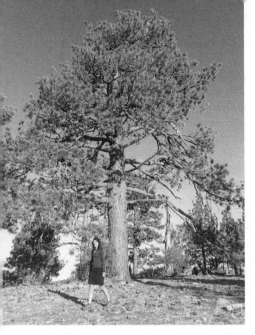

Jeffrey pine on the summit of Mount Lewis

DIRECTIONS From I-15 north of San Bernardino, exit at Highway 138 and turn west. Drive 8.6 miles to Angeles Crest Highway (Highway 2), and turn left. Continue through Wrightwood and Big Pines on Angeles Crest Highway for 19 miles until you reach Dawson Saddle, at mile 69.5. Park in the turnout beside a maintenance shed.

Mount Lewis (8,396') is a short but steep ascent from Dawson Saddle through a fine forest of Jeffrey pine and white fir on the edge of the Pleasant View Wilderness. While it might be a long drive for a short hike, Lewis is an enjoyable excursion if you find yourself on the Angeles Crest for a picnic or another hike and have a bit of extra time. The peak is named for Washington Bartlett "Dusty" Lewis, who surveyed the San Gabriels before becoming the first Superintendent of Yosemite National Park from 1917 to 1928.

The peak has no official trail, but a surprisingly good use path starts just left of the maintenance shed and makes a no-nonsense climb. It ends at a grizzled old Jeffrey pine on the high point. Explore a little farther north for great views of the Antelope Valley.

trip 29.11 Lightning Ridge Nature Trail

see map on p. 380

Distance	0.6 mile (loop)
Hiking Time	30 minutes
Elevation Gain	200'
Difficulty	Easy
Trail Use	Dogs allowed, good for kids
Best Times	April–November
Agency	Angeles National Forest
Optional Map	Tom Harrison *Angeles High Country*

DIRECTIONS From I-15 north of San Bernardino, exit at Highway 138 and turn west. Drive 8.6 miles to Angeles Crest Highway (Highway 2), and turn left. Continue through Wrightwood and Big Pines on Angeles Crest Highway for 11 miles until you reach the trailhead parking area on the right at mile marker 2 LA 78.00 (across from Inspiration Point, which is on the left).

The Lightning Ridge Nature Trail contours through the cool precincts of a wooded northeast-facing slope, then switchbacks upward to meet the Pacific Crest Trail (PCT) on a windblown crest. You'll see Jeffrey pines, sugar pines, and white firs, and pass right through a beautiful glade of black oaks called Oak Dell—very nice in October, when the leaves turn crispy gold and acorns fall. Near the crest are a number of stunted and distorted trees battered by winds and flattened by snowdrifts that can pile up to 10 feet high.

The signed PCT starts beside a corral. At the very start, the easily overlooked Lightning Ridge Nature Trail splits off to the right. It wiggles across the hillside and through Oak Dell, eventually climbing to rejoin the PCT at an unsigned junction on the ridge near a bench.

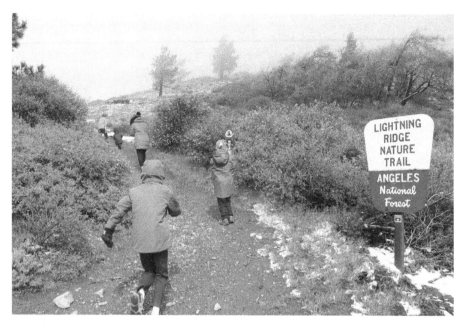

Lightning Ridge after a chilly spring storm

The view from there is similar to that from Inspiration Point below, only a bit more panoramic. Old Baldy and Mount Baden-Powell rise like massive sentinels, bracketing the rugged slopes and canyons of Sheep Mountain Wilderness. To the south you look straight down the V-shaped, linear gorge of East Fork San Gabriel River. Turn left and descend the PCT to the trailhead.

trip 29.12   Jackson Lake Loop

Distance	7 miles (loop)
Hiking Time	4 hours
Elevation Gain	1,300'
Difficulty	Easy
Trail Use	Suitable for mountain biking, dogs allowed
Best Times	April–November
Agency	Angeles National Forest
Optional Map	Tom Harrison *Angeles High Country*

see map on p. 380

DIRECTIONS From I-15 north of San Bernardino, exit at Highway 138 and turn west. Drive 8.6 miles to Angeles Crest Highway (Highway 2), and turn left. Continue through Wrightwood on Angeles Crest Highway for 9 miles; then, at mile marker 2 LA 80.00, turn right on Big Pines Highway (County Road N4) and proceed 3.0 miles to signed Jackson Lake, on the left. Continue 0.2 mile to the parking lot by the lake.

The oak and pine–forested slopes between Jackson Lake and Vincent Gap are just as lovely as the Blue Ridge above Wrightwood. In the spring, chickadees sing and lupine, paintbrush, and wallflower lend color to the woods. Visitors are lured by a chain of fine campgrounds and picnic areas along Big Pines Highway. Jackson Lake, a natural sag pond

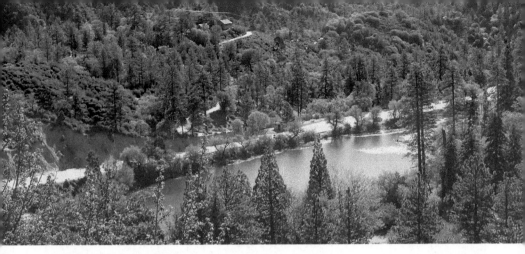

The Jackson Lake area is laced with a maze of interesting trails.

on the San Andreas Fault, is stocked with fish and well-used by anglers and picnickers. Those looking to stretch their legs will enjoy this hike, climbing up on the Jackson Lake Trail, then following the Pacific Crest Trail (PCT) and a segment of dirt road before descending the Boy Scout Trail back to the lake. The trails are in good condition but are oddly not shown on U.S. Forest Service maps.

From the west end of the parking area, take the signed Jackson Lake Trail, which climbs steeply for 0.1 mile to a dirt Forest Service road. Turn left and follow the road, passing above a campfire circle for a youth camp. In 0.6 mile veer left at a fork. Pass the signed Boy Scout Trail on the right, by which you will return; then soon reach the signed Jackson Lake Trail on the right in 0.1 mile. Follow this scenic trail as it climbs 1.3 miles to meet the PCT.

Turn right (west) on the PCT. Immediately pass a fork on the left leading a few yards up to Forest Service Road 3N26. Take the trail or road west until they rejoin. This is 0.6 mile by the road or 0.8 mile by the more scenic trail; cyclists are prohibited on the PCT and must choose the road.

From the second junction, continue west on FS 3N26 for 0.7 mile, passing a locked gate. Veer right at a hairpin turn onto the signed Boy Scout Trail, which descends 2.5 miles back to the dirt road near where your trip began. Turn left and promptly reach the fork in the road.

You could turn right and return the way you came, but, for a change of scenery, turn left instead and continue 0.2 mile on the rough road. Watch for the unsigned Serra Trail on the right, descending a draw just beyond a sharp bend in the road. Take this trail, which eventually widens to become an abandoned dirt road. In 0.5 mile stay right at a fork in a large clearing, and soon reach the short trail down to Jackson Lake.

VARIATION

If you're short on time, turn around at the PCT and return on the Jackson Lake Trail the way you came. This option is 4.2 miles with 1,300 feet of elevation gain.

---

trip 29.13   **Table Mountain Nature Trail**

Distance	1.0 mile or 2.7 miles (loops)
Hiking Time	30 minutes
Elevation Gain	200'/500'
Difficulty	Easy

see map on p. 380

Trail Use	Dogs allowed, good for kids
Best Times	April–November
Agency	Angeles National Forest
Optional Map	Tom Harrison *Angeles High Country*

DIRECTIONS From I-15 north of San Bernardino, exit at Highway 138 and turn west. Drive 8.6 miles to Angeles Crest Highway (Highway 2), and turn left. Continue through Wrightwood for 9 miles until you reach the crossroads of Big Pines at mile marker 2 LA 80.00. As you pass the Big Pines Information Station, turn right on Table Mountain Road and drive uphill 1 mile to Table Mountain Campground. If you aren't staying in the campground, park outside at the large lot just up the road.

The Table Mountain Nature Trail is primarily of interest to campers staying at the Table Mountain Campground. You'll be introduced to Jeffrey pines, canyon live oaks, black oaks, and several other plants and trees that grow in the immediate area. Numbered posts correspond to the entries on a long-lost self-guiding leaflet. You can do a short loop from the campground entrance and back on the campground road, or a longer loop circumnavigating the entire campground.

The signed trail begins near the campground entrance. As you descend the south-facing slope traveled by the trail, you'll spot Mount Baden-Powell rising impressively in the west, and Blue Ridge, complete with the scars of ski runs, in the southeast. Blue Ridge was logged many decades ago, accounting for the even-aged appearance of the trees on its slopes.

When the trail passes near campsite 49, you can turn right and follow the paved campground road back to the entrance to make the short loop. Or continue on the trail around the campground for the longer loop.

---

trip 29.14 Big Pines Nature Trail

Distance	0.5 mile (loop)
Hiking Time	30 minutes
Elevation Gain	100'
Difficulty	Easy
Trail Use	Dogs allowed, good for kids
Best Times	Year-round
Agency	Angeles National Forest
Optional Map	Tom Harrison *Angeles High Country*

see map on p. 380

DIRECTIONS From I-15, north of San Bernardino, exit at Highway 138 and turn west. Drive 8.6 miles to Angeles Crest Highway (Highway 2), and turn left. Continue through Wrightwood; stay on Angeles Crest Highway for 9 miles until you the Big Pines Information Station at mile marker 02 LA 80.00.

The short, easy, self-guiding Big Pines Nature Trail highlights many of the native trees and shrubs of the Big Pines area. The trail originates behind the Big Pines Information Station and starts by winding up through a sparse grove of centuries-old Jeffrey pines. If you aren't, as yet, familiar with the local flora, this is a good trail to further your education.

Along the way, you'll be introduced to the canyon live oak and black oak; four kinds of pines; and shrubs such as ceanothus (mountain lilac), manzanita, yerba santa, flannel bush, serviceberry, and mountain mahogany. Interpretive plaques cover some of the uses of these native plants by the Gabrielino, Serrano, and Cahuilla Indians.

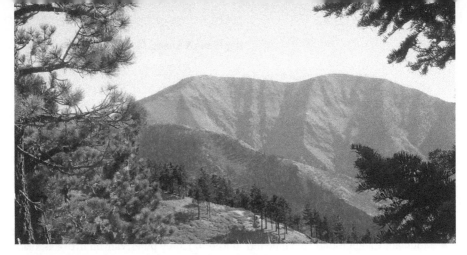

Mount Baldy dominates the eastern skyline from Blue Ridge.

see map on p. 380

trip 29.15 Blue Ridge Trail

Distance	5 miles (out-and-back)
Hiking Time	2.5 hours
Elevation Gain	1,300'
Difficulty	Moderate
Trail Use	Dogs allowed, good for kids
Best Times	May–November
Agency	Angeles National Forest
Optional Map	Tom Harrison *Angeles High Country*

DIRECTIONS From I-15 north of San Bernardino, exit at Highway 138 and turn west. Drive 8.6 miles to Angeles Crest Highway (Highway 2), and turn left. Continue through Wrightwood on Angeles Crest Highway for 9 miles until you reach the Big Pines Information Station at mile marker 02 LA 80.00.

Tall, aromatic pines and firs plus thin air (elevation averages 7,500') lend a High Sierra feel to the north slope of Blue Ridge. The well-maintained Blue Ridge Trail climbs about 1,100 feet up this slope to meet the Pacific Crest Trail (PCT) just outside Blue Ridge Campground. From there you can climb a bit farther for a panoramic view of Mount San Antonio, Mount Baden-Powell, and other giants on the roofline of Angeles National Forest.

You have a lot of flexibility on this hike: From the campground you can return the way you came, walk down the PCT to Angeles Crest Highway, or descend with a prearranged bicycle or car (assuming the road is snow-free and open to traffic).

The Blue Ridge Trail starts near the restrooms opposite the Information Station. It briefly descends to a lower trailhead and then begins climbing to the south through a forest of black oak, Jeffrey pines, and white fir. About halfway up the slope (1.1 mile), the trail crosses an old road bed and continues climbing. To the north, on Table Mountain, you'll spot the white domes of the Table Mountain and Smithsonian observatories. After several switchbacks, you meet the Blue Ridge road at Blue Ridge Campground. The PCT swings around the far side of the campground; you can join it (easy to miss) by walking southeast about a hundred yards up the road. Head southeast on the PCT, uphill along a ski run for another quarter mile. Then veer right to the top of a sage-covered rise dotted in spring and early summer with paintbrush and wallflower blossoms. Here you'll have a panoramic view of Old Baldy's north slope—streaked with snow and often wreathed in cottony clouds in springtime.

This a good spot to turn around and go back the way you came. Or, with a car or bicycle shuttle, you could descend Blue Ridge to Inspiration Point.

chapter 30

San Antonio Canyon & Old Baldy

Best beloved of all the [San Gabriel] peaks is San Antonio, whose ample crown, in shape somewhat like an inverted dish, is the dominating feature of the range. It is the one mountain whose elevation—10,080 feet above the sea—is sufficient to support a snow-cap throughout the winter, and from December to June in ordinary seasons, the white summit against the blue makes from the valley a sight of chaste loveliness, which becomes still lovelier when the setting sun entenders it to color of rose. . . . It looks an easy enough back to climb, and, if you have anything of the Californian in you, you mark it for the objective of an outing sometime.

—Charles Francis Saunders, The Southern Sierras of California, *1923*

San Antonio Canyon, a yawning gap in the fortresslike south front of the San Gabriels, also serves as the main gateway to the third-highest mountain mass in Southern California—Mount San Antonio, or Old Baldy. At 10,064 feet, Baldy's summit looms large over the eastern Los Angeles Basin, the Inland Empire communities of Riverside and San Bernardino, and the western Mojave Desert. It can be seen as far north as the southern Sierra Nevada, and as far south as the Mexican border adjoining San Diego County.

Both San Antonio Canyon and Old Baldy lie astride the Los Angeles–San Bernardino County line. Old Baldy's summit is a county-line benchmark, making it the highest point in Los Angeles County but not in San Bernardino County. Our coverage of the trails in this chapter includes some that are outside the L.A. County boundary, but we don't include

Southern Californians can enjoy snowcapped Mount Baldy and then head to the beach the same day.

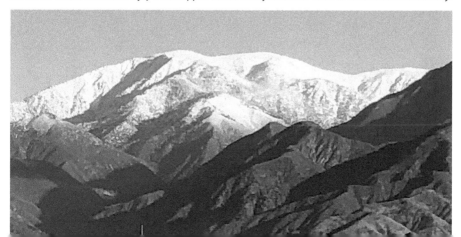

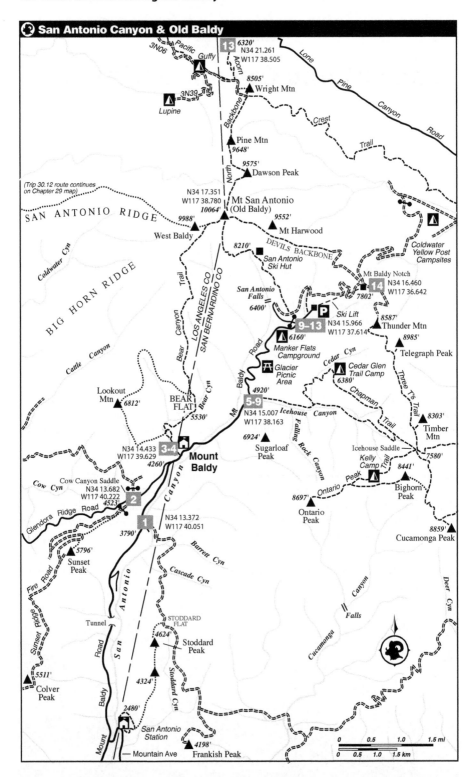

San Antonio Canyon & Old Baldy

3N06 Pacific Guffy 3N39 Lupine

13 6320' N34 21.261 W117 38.505

Lone Pine Canyon Road

8505' Wright Mtn

Backbone North Crest Trail

Pine Mtn 9648'

9575' Dawson Peak

(Trip 30.12 route continues on Chapter 29 map)

N34 17.351 W117 38.780 Mt San Antonio 10064' (Old Baldy)

SAN ANTONIO RIDGE

9988' West Baldy

9552' Mt Harwood

DEVILS BACKBONE

8210' San Antonio Ski Hut

Coldwater Yellow Post Campsites

Coldwater Cyn

BIG HORN RIDGE

Cattle Canyon

San Antonio Falls 6400'

Mt Baldy Notch **14** N34 16.460 W117 36.642 7802'

San Antonio Falls

Bear Canyon Trail

LOS ANGELES CO SAN BERNARDINO CO

9-13 N34 15.966 W117 37.614' Ski Lift 6160' Manker Flats Campground

8587' Thunder Mtn

8985' Telegraph Peak

Cedar Cyn Cedar Glen Trail Camp 6380'

Three T's Trail

Glacier Picnic Area 4920'

Baldy Road

Lookout Mtn 6812'

BEAR FLAT 5530' Bear Cyn

5-9 N34 15.007 W117 38.163 Icehouse Canyon

Chapman Trail

8303' Timber Mtn

Falling Rock Canyon

N34 14.433 W117 39.629 **3-4** Mount Baldy 4260'

6924' Sugarloaf Peak

Icehouse Saddle 7580'

Kelly Camp 8441'

Cow Cyn Cow Canyon Saddle N34 13.682 W117 40.222 4523' **2**

Glendora Ridge Road

N34 13.372 W117 40.051 **1** 3790'

8697' Ontario Peak

Ontario Peak

Bighorn Peak

8859' Cucamonga Peak

5796' Sunset Peak

Barrett Cyn Cascade Cyn

San Antonio

Canyon Falls Deer Cyn

Fire Road Sunset Ridge

Tunnel STODDARD FLAT 4624' Stoddard Peak

Cucamonga Canyon

5511' Colver Peak

Road Baldy 4324' Stoddard Cyn 2480'

San Antonio Station

Mount Mountain Ave Frankish Peak 4198'

| 0 | 0.5 | 1.0 | 1.5 mi |
| 0 | 0.5 | 1.0 | 1.5 km |

anything east of the divide defined by Cucamonga Peak, the so-called Three Ts, and Mount Baldy Notch. See *Afoot & Afield Inland Empire* for more on the Lytle Creek area, which is a part of San Bernardino County's share of the San Gabriel Mountains.

The San Gabriel Mountains, and Mount San Antonio in particular, were spiritually important to the Serrano and Gabrielino peoples. According to one creation legend, the Land God angered the Sea God by creating humans. The Sea God sent huge waves, but the Land God raised the hills and mountains to protect himself and his people. The Land God stands atop his highest mountain, San Antonio.

The first recorded ascent of Mount San Antonio was made by the Wheeler Survey party in 1875. Louis Nell, chief topographer, climbed San Antonio, while Lieutenant Bergland and others climbed Cucamonga Peak. Two soldiers from Bergland's group got lost and nearly died of thirst before being rescued.

Prospectors began working the slopes of Mount Baldy in the 1860s and organized the San Antonio Mining District by 1872. By the 1880s and 1890s, they had built the Hocumac Mine cabin community just below Baldy Notch, and ran a pipeline from San Antonio Creek. They sprayed the high-pressure water through a nozzle to wash away the dirt and collect gold-bearing gravel. This hydraulic mining sent floods of muddy red water pouring into San Antonio Creek and fouling the water supply in the Pomona Valley. The San Antonio Water Company got an injunction against the miners in 1895 and eventually bought out the mine and demolished the pipeline. In California, water is more valuable than gold. Other well-known mines in the area included the Gold Ridge Mine, near the present site of the Sierra Club ski hut, and John Kelly's mine at the present site of Kelly's Camp on Ontario Peak.

The opening of San Antonio Canyon to automobiles, starting in 1908, helped facilitate the rapid development of cabins and resorts in the area. Several hundred cabins dotted the main canyon and its tributaries by the mid 1930s. Camp Baldy—the site of today's Mount Baldy Village—grew to become one of the most popular mountain retreats in Southern California. The great flood of 1938, which tore up the whole front face of the San Gabriels, washed away most of Camp Baldy, as well as scores of other cabins that were sited too close to the streams.

The resort era is long-forgotten today, but Mount Baldy (or Baldy Village, as it's known to many residents) remains a thriving cabin community. The greater Mount Baldy area, with a population of about 1,000, is the second-largest community in the San Gabriels after Wrightwood.

San Antonio Canyon gets a big influx of skiers and snow seekers during the winter, while a less hectic crowd of hikers and sightseers makes use of the area during the warmer months. In Mount Baldy you can stop by the U.S. Forest Service (USFS) visitor center (open Saturday and Sunday, 7 a.m.–3:30 p.m.) for the latest information on trail conditions; you can also obtain free self-issue Cucamonga Wilderness permits here even if the visitor center is closed.

The upper end of San Antonio Canyon is home to the USFS's Manker Flats Campground and Glacier Picnic Area, as well as a large parking lot for the privately operated ski lift. Backpackers can camp just about anywhere on Forest Service land, subject to the regulations for remote camping.

One of the best-known hikers in the canyon was Seuk Doo "Sam" Kim, a 78-year-old South Korean who climbed Mount Baldy more than 700 times before slipping to his death off the icy summit in April 2017. Four other hikers died on the Devils Backbone in the winters of 2016 and 2017. Many other highly experienced hikers have been killed or injured on the seemingly innocuous mountain in icy conditions. Ali Aminian, former president of the California Mountaineering Club, died after slipping off icy Bear Ridge in 2004, and R. J. Secor, author of the leading guidebook on the Sierra Nevada Mountains, took a near-fatal head injury when his glissade down the Baldy Bowl got out of control in 2005.

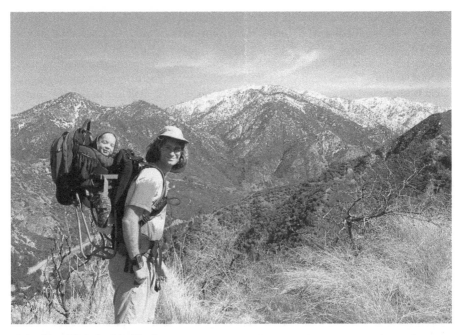

Going for a ride to Stoddard Peak

trip 30.1   **Stoddard Peak**

see
map on
p. 402

Distance	6 miles (out-and-back)
Hiking Time	3 hours
Elevation Gain	1,100'
Difficulty	Moderate
Trail Use	Dogs allowed
Best Times	October–May
Agency	Angeles National Forest
Recommended Map	Tom Harrison *Angeles High Country* or Trails Illustrated *Angeles National Forest (811)*

DIRECTIONS From the 210 Freeway in Claremont, take Exit 52 for Base Line Road. Go west on Base Line for 0.2 mile; then turn right (north) on Padua Avenue. In 1.8 miles turn right onto Mount Baldy Road. In 6.4 miles, just after passing over the dirt hogback blocking San Antonio Canyon, turn right onto Barrett–Stoddard Road and park in the small lot before crossing the bridge.

Stoddard Peak's 4,624-foot height places it above most of the shaggy, chaparral-covered foothill country but well below the stony gaze of the western ramparts of the Cucamonga Wilderness. When dusted or spotted with snow, the peak becomes a dichotomous perch between the white-mantled world above and sun-warmed slopes and canyons below. The hike to the top involves mostly road walking, with a short, rugged stretch near the peak itself. The peak and nearby canyon were named for William Stoddard, who settled here in 1880, and around 1886 founded the first of many mountain resorts in San Antonio Canyon. These resorts were immensely popular before the development of air-conditioning. Ranchers sent their families up into the high country to escape the oppressive heat that blankets the Inland Empire during the summer months.

From the trailhead, hike east down the road, and cross the bridge over San Antonio Creek. On the west side of the creek, you can see traces of the old Mount Baldy Road that once ran along the creek before being washed out one too many times. Follow Barrett–Stoddard Road past some private residences near Barrett Canyon and in 0.8 mile pass a gate. Continue, generally southward, past the mouth of Cascade Canyon and above the flat-topped Spring Hill, where traces of an old farm can still be seen. In another 1.7 miles, cross a saddle to reach Stoddard Flat. Look to the right (west) for a trail chopped through the chaparral. Follow it up the hill, then along the rocky crest of a ridge. Hike 0.4 mile, passing two false summits before reaching the true summit of Stoddard Peak at the south end of the ridge.

The ridge falls sharply beyond Stoddard Peak, so there's no need to go on—the view is the best from here. Looking down into San Antonio Canyon, you can see disconnected segments of the old canyon-bottom road, pummeled in the past by floods and slides. Old Baldy, its snowcap gleaming in winter, dominates the view to the north. To the south, beyond San Antonio Dam (and its usually dry flood-control reservoir), spread the Pomona valley and the Chino Hills. If it's clear enough to see the ocean horizon, you can often see sprawling Santa Catalina Island, plus the low dome of San Clemente Island a little to the left.

ALTERNATIVE FINISH

Follow the Cucamonga Truck Trail south from Stoddard Flat 5.6 miles to Cucamonga Canyon and out to the top of Skyline Drive in Alta Loma. At the time of this writing, some sections have been obliterated by flooding. Beware of poison oak. Another option with a shuttle is to descend 2.2 miles cross-country along Stoddard's south ridge over Peak 4324 to the Lower San Antonio Fire Station, on Mountain Avenue beside San Antonio Creek.

---

trip 30.2   Sunset Peak

see map on p. 402

Distance	6 miles (out-and-back)
Hiking Time	3 hours
Elevation Gain	1,200'
Difficulty	Moderate
Trail Use	Suitable for backpacking, suitable for mountain biking, dogs allowed
Best Times	October–May
Agency	Angeles National Forest
Optional Map	Tom Harrison *Angeles High Country* or Trails Illustrated *Angeles National Forest (811)*

DIRECTIONS From the 210 Freeway in Claremont, take Exit 52 for Base Line Road. Go west on Base Line for 0.2 mile; then turn right (north) on Padua Avenue. In 1.8 miles turn right onto Mount Baldy Road. Follow it 7.1 miles to Mount Baldy Village. Just as you approach the village, turn left on Glendora Ridge Road and go 0.8 mile to Cow Canyon Saddle, where parking is available on the shoulder (be aware of signed parking restrictions). If the gate at the bottom of Glendora Ridge Road is closed, park outside the gate and hike the road.

The hike to Sunset Peak from Cow Canyon Saddle offers up fine views of the archipelago of high peaks stretching from San Gabriel Wilderness in the west to Cucamonga Wilderness in the east. Mount San Antonio rises from center stage in the north, its bald summit sometimes accented by a brilliant snowcap.

From the parking area at Cow Canyon Saddle, start hiking up the gated fire road on the south side of the road. You gain elevation steadily, accompanied by a mixture of tall chaparral, live oaks, big-cone Douglas-firs, and big-leaf maples. You reverse direction at

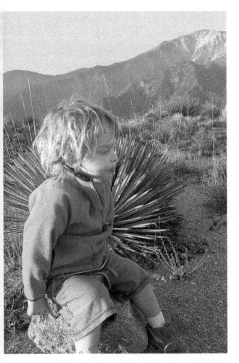

First lesson for little hikers: don't get stuck-a by yucca.

1.9 miles, and again at 2.5 miles. Just after the latter switchback, bear left on an old firebreak, and head southwest straight to the summit (2.9 miles). This worthwhile and enjoyable shortcut, with some easy rock scrambling at the top, saves time and distance over the alternative—a mile of tedious road walking.

Sunset Peak's flat, barren summit makes a fine (but dry) campsite. A fire lookout stood here from the 1920s to the 1970s; you'll notice the building's foundation and also the remains of a rainwater-collection system.

Much of what lies in view to the south is a large, closed-to-the-public parcel of the Angeles National Forest called the San Dimas Experimental Forest. Much of our current knowledge about fire ecology and erosion in the chaparral plant community has been gained from carefully controlled experiments performed in this outdoor laboratory over the past seven or eight decades.

VARIATION

For a shorter but steeper climb (1.5 miles one-way), you can take the steep firebreak all the way from Cow Canyon Saddle. For a great loop, go up the firebreak, enjoy a picnic at sunset, and then descend the dirt road by headlamp.

VARIATION

The Sunset Ridge Fire Road continues all the way to San Dimas Canyon Road, at mile marker 1.32 near the top of San Dimas Dam. This excursion is 15 miles, with 1,500 feet of elevation gain and 4,700 feet of knee-pounding elevation loss. Keen-eyed hikers will notice paths along firebreaks dropping off Sunset Ridge Fire Road to Evey Canyon, the Claremont Hills Wilderness Park, and Marshall Canyon.

---

trip 30.3   Bear Flat

Distance	4.0 miles (out-and-back)
Hiking Time	2 hours
Elevation Gain	1,300'
Difficulty	Moderate
Trail Use	Dogs allowed, good for kids
Best Times	Year-round
Agency	Angeles National Forest
Optional Map	Tom Harrison *Angeles High Country*

see map on p. 402

DIRECTIONS From the 210 Freeway in Claremont, take Exit 52 for Base Line Road. Go west on Base Line for 0.2 mile; then turn right (north) on Padua Avenue. In 1.8 miles turn right onto Mount Baldy Road. Follow it 7.6 miles to the Mount Baldy Trout Ponds, where you'll find plenty of parking across the road above Mount Baldy Village.

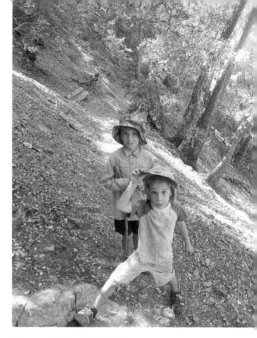

Barely a mile's walk from the busy little community of Mount Baldy, you can be sitting on a rock, communing with nature, feet dangling in the sun-and-shade-dappled, crystalline stream of Bear Canyon. With a bit more time and energy, you can climb to Bear Flat, where a binocular sweep of the surrounding hillsides often nets sightings of bighorn sheep.

Walk back down Mount Baldy Road 0.3 mile and turn right onto Bear Canyon Road just below the visitor center. Hiker parking is not permitted along this road. Walk up Bear Canyon Road past numerous cabins. When the road ends in 0.4 mile, turn right onto the Bear Canyon Trail (7W12). Switchback up through the canyon live oaks and big-cone Douglas-firs, then across a sunbaked slope and back into the canyon to reach Bear Flat.

Fun on the Bear Flat Trail

Bear Flat is the bracken-fern-filled, sloping meadow just above a creek crossing. This is the place to sniff a few spring wildflowers, look for bighorn sheep tracks, and then think about turning back. Beyond this, the Bear Canyon Trail switchbacks up to the south ridge of Mount San Antonio and relentlessly continues all the way to the summit, almost 5 miles away, 4,500 feet higher than Bear Flat (see next trip).

trip 30.4   Mount Baldy via Bear Ridge

see map on p. 402

Distance	13 miles (out-and-back)
Hiking Time	7 hours
Elevation Gain	5,800'
Difficulty	Strenuous
Trail Use	Suitable for backpacking, dogs allowed
Best Times	June–October
Agency	Angeles National Forest
Recommended Map	Tom Harrison *Angeles High Country* or Trails Illustrated *Angeles National Forest (811)*

DIRECTIONS From the 210 Freeway in Claremont, take Exit 52 for Base Line Road. Go west on Base Line for 0.2 mile; then turn right (north) on Padua Avenue. In 1.8 miles turn right onto Mount Baldy Road. Follow it 7.6 miles to the Mount Baldy Trout Ponds, where you'll find plenty of parking across the road above Mount Baldy Village.

The great south ridge of Mount Baldy rises directly from Mount Baldy Village to the summit, and climbs nearly 6,000 feet in 3.5 horizontal miles. The trail offers the greatest sustained elevation gain of any in the San Gabriel Mountains. According to the Winter 1934 issue of *Trails Magazine*, "This is a hard one-day trip, but is often done." Nowadays you will avoid the usual Baldy crowds until reaching the summit. Start early in summer because the switchbacks above Bear Flat are long and shadeless.

This trail was built in the summer of 1889 by Fred Dell and his crew. Dell was the owner of Dell's Camp, a resort in San Antonio Canyon. The trail, passable by horses, cut about 4 miles off the previous approach of taking a miner's trail to Baldy Notch and then hiking the backbone. The work was financed by Dr. B. H. Fairchild of Claremont, who hoped to persuade Harvard to place an observatory on the summit. A November blizzard discouraged the Harvard astronomers, and the observatory stayed on Mount Wilson, but hikers still enjoy the trail. From 1910 to 1913, William Dewey used the trail to operate the Baldy Summit Inn, six tent cabins on the mountaintop. The venture ended when the tents burned in a cooking fire.

Walk back down Mount Baldy Road 0.3 mile and turn right onto Bear Canyon Road just below the visitor center. Hiker parking is not permitted along this road. Walk up Bear Canyon Road past numerous cabins. When the road ends in 0.4 mile, turn right onto the Bear Canyon Trail (7W12). Switchback up through the canyon live oaks and big-cone Douglas-firs, then across a sunbaked slope and back into the canyon to reach Bear Flat.

The 2008 Bighorn Fire burned from Bear Flat up to the ridge. The trail makes 16 long, steep switchbacks through the burn zone before reaching the first intact Jeffrey pines. Enjoy views of Icehouse Canyon and the surrounding peaks. Another 20 or so shorter switchbacks bring you to Bear Ridge, the halfway point on the trip and 1,800 feet up from Bear Flat.

Hike up the ridge, enjoying more great views. In another 1,000 feet of climbing, near the 8,400-foot contour, the ridge merges with a second ridge to the east, rising from Lookout Mountain, and dramatic views open into Cattle Canyon. In another 600 feet of climbing, cross a section known as the Narrows where the ridge drops steeply on both sides.

The last 1.6 miles are gentler, climbing the upper ridge and traversing across the southeast side of West Baldy to reach the high point of the San Gabriel Mountains. The forest gives way to lodgepole pines, which become ever more stunted by wind and ice as you climb until they vanish entirely on the bald summit. This is a good place to watch for elusive desert bighorn sheep. The trail passes close by West Baldy before reaching the true summit. Return the way you came.

ALTERNATIVE FINISH

If you left a vehicle at Manker Flats, descend the Devils Backbone or Baldy Bowl Trail (see Trip 30.11, page 417). These options are highly recommended because they are spectacular, you avoid retracing your steps, and you save your knees from the brutal descent.

Upper Bear Ridge from the south

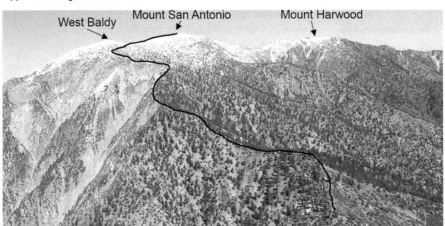

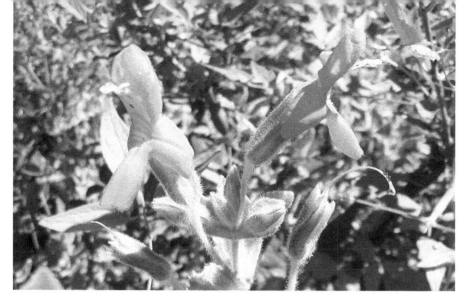

Striking scarlet monkey flower (Mimulus cardinalis) prefers moist areas such as Icehouse Canyon.

trip 30.5 Icehouse Canyon

see map on p. 402

Distance	7 miles (out-and-back)
Hiking Time	4 hours
Elevation Gain	2,600'
Difficulty	Strenuous
Trail Use	Dogs allowed
Best Times	May–November
Agency	Angeles National Forest
Optional Map	Tom Harrison *Angeles High Country*
Fees/Permits	Cucamonga Wilderness Permit required (self-issue at trailhead)

DIRECTIONS From the 210 Freeway in Claremont, take Exit 52 for Base Line Road. Go west on Base Line for 0.2 mile; then turn right (north) on Padua Avenue. In 1.8 miles turn right onto Mount Baldy Road. Follow it 9.0 miles to Ice House Canyon Road on the right, where you'll reach a large trailhead parking area that can fill early on the weekends. You may find overflow parking on the shoulder of Mount Baldy Road.

Icehouse Canyon is the most accessible hike in the beautiful Cucamonga Wilderness. The canyon was formed by earthquake fault activity. It is part of a larger system of east-to-west-running canyons that stretches along the southern San Gabriel Mountains out to the west fork of the San Gabriel River. This trip climbs through the forest to the saddle at the head of the canyon. A five-way junction on the saddle tempts the ambitious hiker with numerous ways to continue exploring (see Trips 30.7–30.9, pages 412, 413, and 415).

Old newspaper reports suggest that an ice-packing operation existed in or near Icehouse Canyon during the late 1850s. The ice was hauled down San Antonio Canyon on mules to a point accessible to wagons (below the Hogback), whereupon it was carted, as quickly as possible, to Los Angeles for use in making ice cream and for chilling beverages. Whether ice was actually quarried in this canyon or in another, Icehouse Canyon's name is apt enough: cold-air drainage produces refrigerator-like temperatures on many a summer morning, and deep-freeze temperatures in winter.

Hike east along the popular Icehouse Canyon Trail past numerous cabins along the north side of the creek. Icehouse Canyon had its heyday during the great age of hiking and mountain resorts in the 1920s and 1930s. The devastating floods of 1938 wiped out many cabins. Fires and avalanches have also taken their toll.

In the summer and fall, the rabbitbrush and boulders alongside the stream are sometimes clothed with swarms of ladybugs, more formally known as convergent lady beetles or *Hippodamia convergens*. Their antifreeze-like blood enables them to survive the winter buried by snow, and their bright-red coloration indicates "toxic and distasteful" to would-be predators.

In 1.0 mile pass an intersection with the Chapman Trail to the left (see next trip). As you ascend, the canyon bottom becomes dry. Pass the wilderness boundary, and then watch for Columbine Spring on the downhill side of the trail, 2.4 miles from the start. The spring is located immediately before a series of switchbacks and is often surrounded by a patch of columbine in the summer. In 0.5 mile of serious climbing, pass the second junction with the Chapman Trail, and then saunter up the last 0.6 mile to Icehouse Saddle.

trip 30.6	**Cedar Glen**

see map on p. 402

Distance	4.5 miles (out-and-back), or 7.5 miles (loop)
Hiking Time	2.5–4 hours
Elevation Gain	1,300' or 2,200'
Difficulty	Moderate
Trail Use	Suitable for backpacking, dogs allowed
Best Times	May–November
Agency	Angeles National Forest
Optional Map	Tom Harrison *Angeles High Country*
Fees/Permits	Cucamonga Wilderness Permit required (self-issue at trailhead)

DIRECTIONS From the 210 Freeway in Claremont, take Exit 52 for Base Line Road. Go west on Base Line for 0.2 mile; then turn right (north) on Padua Avenue. In 1.8 miles turn right onto Mount Baldy Road. Follow it 9.0 miles to Ice House Canyon Road on the right, where you'll reach a large trailhead parking area that can fill early on the weekends. You may find overflow parking on the shoulder of Mount Baldy Road.

Cedar Glen Trail Camp is perched on a bench overlooking Icehouse Canyon. This beautiful trip up to the glen follows the shady Icehouse Canyon Trail to the Chapman Trail, and then climbs the wall of the canyon, alongside Cedar Creek, passing chaparral and wildflowers. Cedar Glen has one of the most diverse conifer groves in Southern California, with most of the local species growing together. This trip can be done as a short out-and-back jaunt or, better yet, as a loop continuing on to rejoin Icehouse Canyon and returning via the canyon floor. It is also an enjoyable destination for a short backpacking trip. The climb to Cedar Glen is steep and shadeless. If you are going in the summer, start in the morning before it gets too hot.

From the popular Icehouse Canyon Trailhead, hike east up the canyon past cabins. The dirt road soon narrows to a trail and continues along the north bank of the rushing creek beneath oaks, incense cedars, and broad-leaf trees. In the summer, expect to pass a field of fragile red- and yellow-flowered columbines growing along the trail.

In 1 mile reach a trail junction with the Chapman Trail; at the time of this writing, the sign was damaged. Turn sharply left and follow the Chapman Trail up the north slope of the canyon along Cedar Creek. This slope is exposed to the searing sun and is covered with yuccas, buckthorns, manzanitas, and other chaparral adapted to the harsh conditions. Watch for rattlesnakes, especially in the summer. The trail crosses to the west side of Cedar Creek, then crosses back east again in a lush field of vines and wildflowers. This is the best place to get water if you are camping. Follow one more switchback and arrive at Cedar Glen, 1.3 miles up from Icehouse Canyon.

The small grove on the bench includes Jeffrey, ponderosa, and sugar pines; big-cone Douglas-firs; white firs; and, of course, incense cedars. It's a great place to study the trees and learn to identify the different species. Incense cedars have distinctive scalelike leaves instead of needles. White firs and big-cone Douglas-firs have short needles, which grow individually rather than in bundles. White fir cones are rarely seen at the base of the tree; the barrel-shaped cones grow near the top of the tree and decompose on the branch rather than falling. Big-cone Douglas-fir, also called big-cone spruce, is neither a fir nor a spruce. Its cones grow up to 7 inches long. Pines have longer needles growing in bundles. Sugar pines have bundles of five needles, about 4 inches long, and are easily recognized by their long, skinny cones; sugar pine cones are the world's longest, often exceeding 12 inches. Jeffrey and ponderosa have long needles in bundles of three and are much more difficult to distinguish. The size of the cones is your best clue: Jeffrey pine cones grow up to 10 inches, while ponderosa pine cones are 3–5 inches long.

Return the way you came.

ALTERNATIVE FINISH

You can make a wonderful 7.5-mile loop by continuing 2.2 miles up the Chapman Trail to where it rejoins the Icehouse Canyon Trail. This stretch offers fantastic views of the north wall of Ontario Peak across the canyon, and out to Sunset Peak and Bear Ridge to the west. Reach the Icehouse Canyon Trail at a switchback beneath some sugar pines. It's possible to head uphill 0.6 mile to Icehouse Saddle, and then on to any of several terrific peaks (see Trips 30.7–30.9, pages 412, 413, and 415). But for now, turn right and follow the switchbacks downhill 0.6 mile. At the base of the last switchback is Columbine Spring, whose clear, cold waters gush forth beneath the trail in a patch of columbine and scarlet monkey flower. Continue down the trail past the wilderness boundary into a talus field, and soon reach the stone foundations of old cabins. Icehouse Creek begins flowing strongly again. In 1.3 miles from Columbine Spring, reach the lower junction with the Chapman Trail; then hike the final mile down to the trailhead.

Admiring the view from the Chapman Trail above Cedar Glen

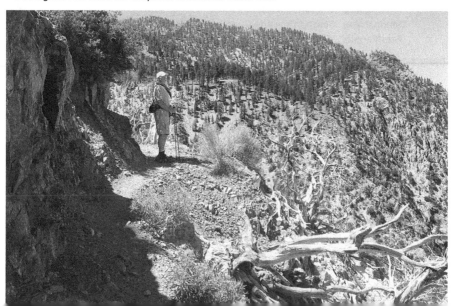

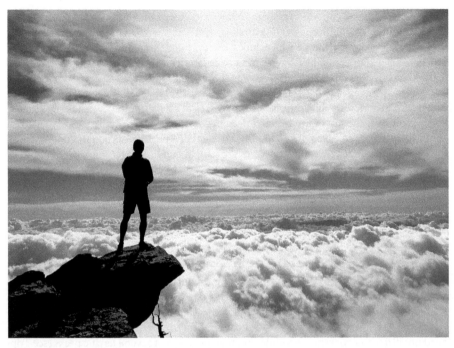

Cucamonga Peak often floats above the clouds.

trip 30.7   Cucamonga Peak

see
map on
p. 402

Distance	12 miles (out-and-back)
Hiking Time	7 hours
Elevation Gain	3,800'
Difficulty	Strenuous
Trail Use	Suitable for backpacking, dogs allowed
Best Times	May–November
Agency	Angeles National Forest
Optional Map	Tom Harrison Angeles High Country
Fees/Permits	Cucamonga Wilderness Permit required (self-issue at trailhead)

DIRECTIONS From the 210 Freeway in Claremont, take Exit 52 for Base Line Road. Go west on Base Line for 0.2 mile; then turn right (north) on Padua Avenue. In 1.8 miles turn right onto Mount Baldy Road. Follow it 9.0 miles to Ice House Canyon Road on the right, where you'll reach a large trailhead parking area that can fill early on the weekends. You may find overflow parking on the shoulder of Mount Baldy Road.

Cucamonga Peak's south and east slopes feature some of the most dramatic relief in the San Gabriel range. At 8,859 feet, the peak stands sentinel-like only 4 miles from the edge of the broad inland valley region known as the Inland Empire. Go all the way to the top for the view, but don't be too disappointed in case there's nothing below but haze and smog. So much beautiful high country can be seen along the way that reaching the top is just icing on the cake. The peak is named for Rancho Cucamonga; Cucamonga, in turn, is a Shoshonean place-name. The portion above Icehouse Saddle was built by young men in the Civilian Conservation Corps during the Great Depression.

Most of the hike lies within Cucamonga Wilderness, requiring a permit for both day and overnight use. Near Cucamonga's summit you'll tackle a steep, north-facing gully that can retain snow into May. Check for possible snow and ice early or late in the season.

From the trailhead, walk along the path that follows the alder-shaded stream. The first couple of miles along the canyon are a fitting introduction to a phase of Southern California scenery not familiar to a lot of visitors and newcomers. Huge big-cone Douglas-fir, incense cedar, and live oak trees cluster on the banks of the stream, which dances over boulders and fallen logs. Moisture-loving, flowering plants like columbine sway in the breeze. Some old cabins along the lower canyon still survive, while others, destroyed by flood or fire, have left evidence in the form of foundations or rock walls.

The Chapman Trail intersects on the left at 1.0 mile. It goes up Icehouse Canyon's north wall, passes Cedar Glen Trail Camp, and contours over to meet the older, canyon-bottom trail (see previous trip). Stay on the latter (Icehouse Canyon) trail; it's about 1.7 miles shorter, it's cooler, and it offers better scenery. At Columbine Spring (2.4 miles, last water during the warmer months), the trail starts switchbacking up the north wall. After passing the upper intersection of the Chapman Trail at 2.9 miles, you continue to pine-shaded Icehouse Saddle, at 3.5 miles, where trails converge from five directions. The signed trail to Cucamonga's summit contours southeast, descends moderately near an abandoned mine shaft, and climbs to a 7,654-foot saddle (4.4 miles) between Bighorn and Cucamonga Peaks. Thereafter, it switchbacks up a steep slope dotted with sugar pines and white firs, which give way to lodgepole pines near the summit.

At 5.8 miles the trail crosses a shady draw 200 feet below and northwest of the summit. The trail continues east toward Etiwanda Peak, while a spur on the right goes straight up to the summit, 6.0 miles from your starting point in Icehouse Canyon. You can camp on the summit, where you'll have incredible views of the night lights of the Inland Empire, or in a more sheltered grove a few hundred yards east along the Etiwanda Peak Trail. Return the same way, or take the alternate route, the Chapman Trail, if you'd like a longer but more scenic descent from Icehouse Saddle.

VARIATION

Etiwanda Peak is east of Cucamonga, along a good but lightly maintained trail. A round-trip to visit the summit is 2.2 miles with 600 feet of elevation gain. See *Afoot & Afield Inland Empire* for details.

---

trip 30.8   **Ontario Peak**

see map on p. 402

Distance	12 miles (out-and-back)
Hiking Time	7 hours
Elevation Gain	3,600'
Difficulty	Strenuous
Trail Use	Suitable for backpacking, dogs allowed
Best Times	June–October
Agency	Angeles National Forest
Recommended Map	Tom Harrison *Angeles High Country*
Fees/Permits	Cucamonga Wilderness Permit required (self-issue at trailhead)

DIRECTIONS From the 210 Freeway in Claremont, take Exit 52 for Base Line Road. Go west on Base Line for 0.2 mile; then turn right (north) on Padua Avenue. In 1.8 miles turn right onto Mount Baldy Road. Follow it 9.0 miles to Ice House Canyon Road on the right, where you'll reach a large trailhead parking area that can fill early on the weekends. You may find overflow parking on the shoulder of Mount Baldy Road.

Ontario and Cucamonga Peaks form an imposing wall overlooking the western end of the Inland Empire. They rise more than a vertical mile from the endless subdivisions at the 2,000-foot base to the summits at almost 9,000 feet. Ontario Peak is one of the classic climbs of Southern California. It is named for the town of Ontario, which in turn was named by the founding Chaffey brothers for their home province of Ontario, Canada. The easiest way to the summit is to ascend the Icehouse Canyon Trail; then turn southwest and hike up past Kelly Camp, along the long ridge to the summit. The north side of the ridge can be deceptively icy in early summer and after the first storms of the fall.

Follow the Icehouse Canyon Trail 3.5 miles to the signed five-way junction at Icehouse Saddle (see Trip 30.5, page 409). Turn sharply right and take the Ontario Peak Trail 0.9 mile to Kelly Camp. John Kelly began prospecting here in 1905 and Henry Delker turned the site into a backcountry resort in 1922. It is now a simple trail camp and an excellent place to stay if you are backpacking. In the early summer, you may find water trickling from a small spring by the camp. It is always prudent to treat water before drinking.

Beyond Kelly Camp, continue 0.4 mile to the ridge, where there are breathtaking views down into Cucamonga Canyon and out over the Inland Empire. Continue west along the undulating ridge. This area is in a burn zone, but the annoying deadfalls that once blocked the trail have been cleared by enterprising Boy Scouts. In a seemingly endless 1.2 miles, reach the 8,693-foot summit, which is readily recognizable by a granite spire. You'll find an exposed but spectacular tent site near the peak.

ALTERNATIVE FINISH

Most parties descend the way they came. It's also possible to take cross-country routes down Falling Rock Canyon or Shortcut Ridge, but these routes are recommended only for experienced cross-country travelers. Yet another option is to follow the ridge east over Bighorn Peak, then down and up to Cucamonga Peak (see previous trip).

Falling Rock Canyon is accessed from the broad bowl beneath the trail 0.3 mile east of Ontario Peak. Pick a way down to the north through the fallen timber. The canyon steepens and passes a small saddle next to Sugarloaf Peak. It then veers right and descends through talus fields before reaching the bottom of Icehouse Canyon 0.5 mile east of the trailhead. This route saves substantial distance but not much time because of the difficult terrain. Be careful not to be lured down the wrong canyon because some of the canyons have cliff bands of decomposing rock.

On the summit rocks of Ontario Peak, with the Inland Empire spread out below

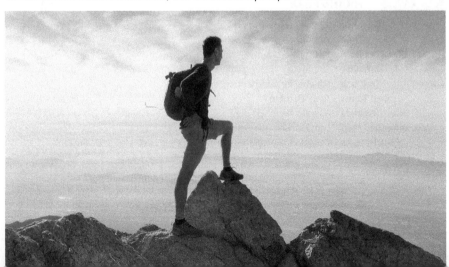

Shortcut Ridge descends from Kelly Camp and reaches Icehouse Canyon 0.1 mile east of the wilderness-boundary sign. It is flanked by Delker Canyon to the east and Lost Creek Canyon to the west. Descending the ridge on the return from Ontario Peak saves distance but likely increases time and effort. The upper part of the ridge is brushy in places, while the lower section involves easy scrambling on loose metamorphic rock.

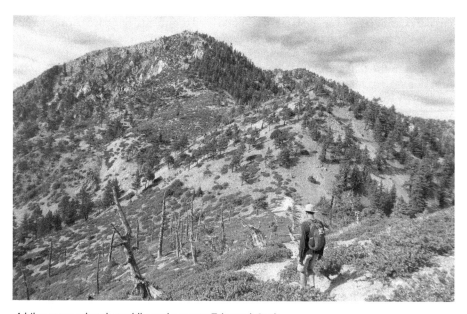

A hiker approaches the saddle on the way to Telegraph Peak.

trip 30.9 The Three Ts

see map on p. 402

Distance	13 miles (one-way with short shuttle)
Hiking Time	8 hours
Elevation Gain	5,000'
Difficulty	Strenuous
Trail Use	Suitable for backpacking, dogs allowed
Best Times	June–October
Agency	Angeles National Forest
Recommended Map	Tom Harrison *Angeles High Country*
Fees/Permits	Cucamonga Wilderness Permit required (self-issue at Icehouse Canyon Trailhead)

DIRECTIONS This trip requires a short car or bicycle shuttle. From the 210 Freeway in Claremont, take Exit 52 for Base Line Road. Go west on Base Line for 0.2 mile; then turn right (north) on Padua Avenue. In 1.8 miles turn right onto Mount Baldy Road. Follow it 11.7 miles to Manker Flats, where you leave one vehicle. Drive or pedal 2.7 miles down the hairpin turns and turn left into Icehouse Canyon; then park at the trailhead on the left.

Timber, Telegraph, and Thunder Mountains form the undulating northeast wall of San Antonio Canyon. This superb romp over the Three Ts begins up Icehouse Canyon and descends through the ski resort at Baldy Notch. For an easier hike with only 9.5 miles of distance and 2,100 feet of elevation gain, take the ski lift from the top of Mount Baldy Road up to the notch and do the trip in reverse.

Follow the Icehouse Canyon Trail 3.5 miles to the signed five-way junction at Icehouse Saddle (see Trip 30.5, page 409). Turn left and climb north 0.7 mile toward Timber Mountain. The trail curves around the west side, so you will have to make a 0.2-mile detour to reach the true summit. You can find sheltered camping in the trees near the summit.

Follow the trail 2 miles down to a saddle and steeply up to Telegraph Peak. The origin of this peak's name is obscure and is probably not related to an actual telegraph. Again, make a short detour on a use trail to the northeast to reach the summit, which is the highest point of the trip. You can find exposed camping just south of the start of the use trail.

Return to the trail and drop steeply to a third saddle, and then climb back up to the final summit, reaching Thunder Mountain in 1.2 miles. The mountain was once known as Mount Harwood in honor of Aurelia Harwood, the first female Sierra Club president. It was renamed over the Club's protests by Herb Leffler and Jim Chafee, who wanted a more exciting name and alliteration with the other Ts when they built the ski area at Baldy Notch in 1952. Harwood's name was transferred to the rounded summit near Mount Baldy.

From Thunder Mountain, the Gold Ridge ski road leads 1.5 miles back down to Mount Baldy Notch. Continue down the service road 3.2 miles to Manker Flats. Alternatively, the ski lift runs on weekends and is a tempting way to save the wear and tear on your knees.

trip 30.10   San Antonio Falls

Distance	1.2 miles (out-and-back)
Hiking Time	1 hour
Elevation Gain	200'
Difficulty	Easy
Trail Use	Suitable for mountain biking, dogs allowed, good for kids
Best Times	April–July
Agency	Angeles National Forest
Optional Map	Tom Harrison *Angeles High Country*

see map on p. 402

DIRECTIONS From the 210 Freeway in Claremont, take Exit 52 for Base Line Road. Go west on Base Line for 0.2 mile; then turn right (north) on Padua Avenue. In 1.8 miles turn right onto Mount Baldy Road. Follow it 11.7 miles to Manker Flats, where you can park alongside the road.

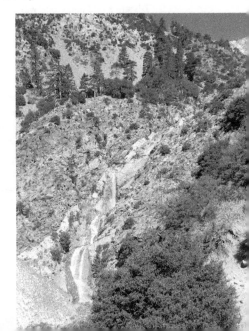

At San Antonio Falls, San Antonio Canyon's fledgling stream shoots down a broken rock face, falling a total of about 100 feet in three tiers. With a drainage area of only a few hundred acres, the falls puts on a decent show only after a rather big storm or when the snow above is melting at a rapid

San Antonio Falls drops in several tiers.

rate. Three springs in the headwaters of the canyon help keep the falls alive, at a greatly subdued level, after all the snow has melted.

The easy hike to the base of the falls begins on the gated fire road just above Manker Flats Campground. The road, which is closed to all but ski-lift-maintenance vehicles, is thinly paved for the first 0.6 mile. That's just enough to reach a hairpin curve with a good glimpse of the falls to the left.

From the curve, a short but slightly precarious trail contours to the base of the falls, where the plummeting water hits not a pool but a streambed of broken rock and gravel. If you have small kids, watch them carefully on this trail and near the base of the falls to ensure their safety.

VARIATION

You could follow San Antonio Creek up the falls all the way to the Sierra Club ski hut. Stay left of the first waterfall and then right of the next ones; many parties will want a rope for this Class 4 stretch. The walking then eases until you reach the abandoned Agamemnon and Penelope Mines (now sometimes called Gold Ridge) and another waterfall just below the ski hut. Climb loose rock on the left side or bushwhack up the steep slope farther left.

---

trip 30.11 Baldy Loop

Distance	10.5 miles (loop)	
Hiking Time	6 hours	
Elevation Gain	3,900'	
Difficulty	Strenuous	
Trail Use	Suitable for backpacking, dogs allowed	
Best Times	June–October	
Agency	Angeles National Forest	
Recommended Map	Tom Harrison *Angeles High Country*	

see map on p. 402

DIRECTIONS From the 210 Freeway in Claremont, take Exit 52 for Base Line Road. Go west on Base Line for 0.2 mile; then turn right (north) on Padua Avenue. In 1.8 miles turn right onto Mount Baldy Road. Follow it 11.7 miles to Manker Flats, where you can park alongside the road.

Mount Baldy is one of the most popular hikes in Southern California. Its summit, the highest in the San Gabriel Mountains and Los Angeles County, offers breathtaking views, yet the route is straightforward for a hiker of average ability. There are many routes on the mountain, but this one is especially enjoyable because it makes a loop up past the Baldy Bowl and down along the stunning Devils Backbone to the ski area at the Baldy Notch. From here, one can follow a dirt service road back to Manker Flats. This is a deceptively dangerous route when icy, and only experienced mountaineers with ice ax, crampons, and sufficient knowledge should attempt it under winter or spring conditions.

From Manker Flats, walk west through a gate and up a service road. In 0.5 mile the road makes a hairpin turn, and you have an excellent view of San Antonio Falls (see previous trip). At 0.9 mile look for the Baldy Bowl Trail switchbacking up the slope to the left. It is easy to miss; if you get to a point directly overlooking Manker Flats, you have gone too far.

Follow the trail up through an open forest up to a Sierra Club ski hut, built by volunteers in 1937, located off the right side of the trail (2.4 miles). Use of the hut is by reservation only, through the Angeles Chapter of the Sierra Club. Trail campers without reservations are invited to camp in the so-called Rock Garden about 200 yards southwest of the hut.

The ski hut marks the halfway point of the ascent in distance and elevation gain. Just beyond, cross the head of San Antonio Creek beneath the scree-filled Baldy Bowl. This area

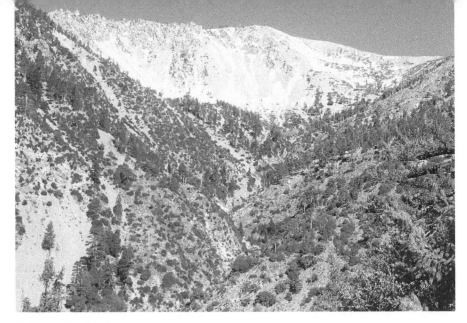

Baldy Bowl is a favorite among hikers.

is a backcountry skier's paradise in the winter and early spring. On a rare quiet day, it is also a good place to look for bighorn sheep.

The trail continues around the southwest edge of Baldy Bowl, crossing a field of talus and switchbacking up to the ridge, 3.1 miles. Shady spots along this part of the trail remain icy long after most of the mountain has melted out. Expert mountaineers have had serious and fatal slips on this seemingly innocuous stretch of trail.

Now follow the ridge north. At 3.5 miles, at a sign labeled BALDY BOWL TRAIL, look for a use trail dropping into the canyon. On October 5, 1945, a Curtiss C-46 Commando grazed the cloud-socked ridge of Mount Baldy and tumbled down the canyon. You can find wreckage strewn down the gully, with the largest wing section 0.1 mile below the trail. Our trip, however, climbs on to the windswept summit above tree line, at 4.1 miles. Rock rings provide partial shelter while you picnic. Camping can be magnificent on a calm day, or an ordeal in adverse weather.

After taking in the magnificent scenery, descend east along the Devils Backbone Trail. Beware that five trails depart the summit ridge and that many hikers have headed the wrong way, especially when visibility is poor. This spectacular trail passes along the south side of Mount Harwood, and then follows a knife-edge ridge down to the ski area at Baldy Notch. Again, be especially careful in icy conditions because a slip down one of the steep chutes has repeatedly proven fatal.

From the lodge at Baldy Notch (7.2 miles, 7,800'), follow the service road descending to the southwest. Pass the original junction with the Baldy Bowl Trail before reaching Manker Flats.

VARIATION

Baldy Bowl is a popular winter snow climb and ski descent. The couloirs at the top reach an angle of 35–40° and can be icy, so bring crampons and an ice ax. Sierra Club members and the general public can stay at the ski hut. See angeles.sierraclub.org/san_antonio_ski_hut for details and reservations.

VARIATION

With a car shuttle, you could descend the spectacular but foot-punishing Bear Ridge Trail, which loses 5,800 feet in 6.4 miles, ending at Mount Baldy Village (see Trip 30.4, page 407).

trip 30.12 ## San Antonio Ridge

Distance	16 miles (one-way)
Hiking Time	14 hours
Elevation Gain/Loss	6,000'/10,200'
Difficulty	Very strenuous
Trail Use	Suitable for backpacking
Best Times	May–November
Agency	Angeles National Forest
Recommended Map	Tom Harrison *Angeles High Country*
Fees/Permits	Self-issue permit required only if hiking in reverse from the East Fork Trailhead

see map on p. 402

DIRECTIONS This trip requires a 1-hour car shuttle. Leave a getaway vehicle at the East Fork Trailhead: From the 210 Freeway in Azusa, take Exit 40 north on the San Gabriel Canyon Road, Highway 39, for 11 miles to East Fork Road, on the right. Continue up East Fork Road 6 miles to a parking lot at the end. You can get a self-issue wilderness permit at a box by the outhouse.

Return to the 210 Freeway and go east; then take Exit 52 for Base Line Road. Go west on Base Line for 0.2 mile; then turn right (north) on Padua Avenue. In 1.8 miles turn right onto Mount Baldy Road. Follow it 11.7 miles to Manker Flats, where you can park alongside the road.

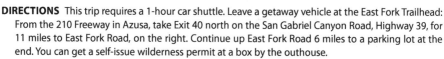

Get set for a spectacular and extremely challenging traverse along the spine of the San Gabriel Mountains. From the top of Old Baldy, you descend a net elevation of 8,000 feet to East Fork San Gabriel River by way of San Antonio Ridge and Iron Mountain. Done in the manner described here (net downhill), the trip is certainly the most tortuous hike of all those included in this book.

The authors did the trip in reverse, from East Fork to Baldy, an option open to you if you're a real glutton for punishment. One of Jerry's rewards, besides the aerial-like views, was the sighting of a large herd of bighorn sheep. Some 25 sheep scooted over a rocky saddle on San Antonio Ridge as he watched in amazement from a hundred yards away.

It's prudent to know the area well before attempting this trip. Climb Baldy (see previous trip) and Iron Mountain (see Trip 29.5, page 387) on their own, and be sure neither feels overly demanding. You'll be glad to wear boots, long pants, and gaiters, and trekking poles can be helpful for the long, steep, loose descents. Some hikers who are uncomfortable on loose Class 3 rock will find a rope helpful. Although it is possible to camp on the summit of Baldy or Iron, or on flat spots along San Antonio Ridge, you may need to haul 10 quarts or more of water for such an arduous backpacking trip.

You begin with the standard approach to Old Baldy's summit from the Manker Flat Trailhead by way of the ski-hut trail (see previous trip) at 4 miles. You might be tempted to take the ski lift, but check the current schedule because it may not be running at the early hour you'll need to start this trip.

From Old Baldy's summit, proceed west to 9,988-foot West Baldy (4.3 miles). From there you can visually trace the rounded San Antonio Ridge in the distance as it curves gradually left and finally becomes a serrated spine leading to Iron Mountain's summit. Based on what you can see, estimate how long it will take you to walk over to Iron Mountain—then multiply that figure by at least two.

From West Baldy, you descend through talus and timberline krummholz (stunted, almost prostrate trees) and then through taller trees to the first saddle in the ridge (7,772'). On the undulating ridge ahead, you travel through sparse groves of timber and thickets of snowbrush, a low-growing but very thorny variety of ceanothus. The USGS topo map

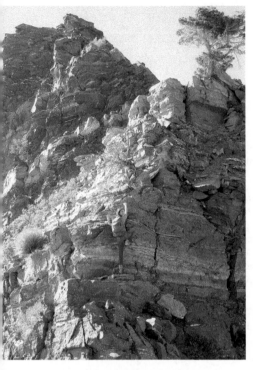

Scrambling up the shattered rock out of Gunsight Notch

shows trails connecting several old mines in the upper Coldwater Canyon drainage to the south, but mines and trails alike have been unused for decades.

The crux of the trip begins at Gunsight Notch, the lowest point along the ridge (7.7 miles, 7,350'). Work your way over and around pinnacles of shattered metamorphic rock on the arête, mostly a slow process of stepping over or bashing through low chaparral. Bighorn sheep tracks may guide you. Take great care not to pull on or otherwise dislodge blocks of rock; many seem to be delicately balanced and poised to tumble. Also make sure that no two climbers are in the same fall line—some parties who are uncomfortable on loose Class 3 rock may find a rope helpful. While you're on this tense stretch, try to relax occasionally and enjoy the dizzying vistas into the precipitous Fish Fork canyon on the north and the more gentle Coldwater Canyon drainage on the south.

When you finally reach Iron Mountain's 8,007-foot summit (8.6 miles), you'll find a register in a red can appropriately labeled BIG BAD IRON. In it, a scribe has written, "Through bad chaparral and stinging nettle; to do Big Iron you need pants of metal." Take a long breather on top and revel in the view. Some nice camp or picnic sites can be found amid the scattered pines just below the summit.

When it's time to leave, head down the south ridge on a rather-well-beaten but occasionally very steep climbers' path. Huge yuccas, some with a thousand slender daggers, grow uncomfortably close to the path. Keep your speed down lest you slide into one of them. A couple of pine- and-fir dotted flat areas on the way down offer a chance to rest and cool off. At the 4,582-foot Allison Saddle (11.1 miles), you come upon the comparatively well-maintained Heaton Flat Trail, which zigzags southeast up a hill, gaining about 150 feet, then descends, more or less steadily to Heaton Flat. From there, walk out on the service road to the East Fork Trailhead.

trip 30.13 Baldy North Backbone Traverse

Distance	11.5 miles (one-way)
Hiking Time	7 hours
Elevation Gain	5,100'
Difficulty	Strenuous
Trail Use	Suitable for backpacking, dogs allowed
Best Times	June–October
Agency	Angeles National Forest
Recommended Map	Tom Harrison *Angeles High Country*

see map on p. 402

DIRECTIONS This trip requires a 75-minute car shuttle. From I-15 south of the Cajon Pass, drive northwest on Highway 138 for 8.8 miles and then west on Highway 2 for 5.3 miles to Wrightwood. At mile marker 2 SBD 1.00, turn left onto Spruce Street, then immediately right onto Apple Avenue, and then immediately left again onto Acorn Drive. Follow Acorn Drive 0.6 mile to where it becomes a private road, and park off the pavement.

Drive the other car back down to I-15, and then south to the 210 Freeway and west to Exit 54 for Mountain Avenue in Upland. Take Mountain north and stay on it as it turns right, then back left (west), passes San Antonio Dam and Fire Station, and eventually reaches a T-junction with Mount Baldy Road in 4.2 miles. Turn right and drive 9 miles up to the Manker Flat Trailhead parking area.

This trip traverses the San Gabriel Mountains from south to north, climbing over Mount Baldy and following its rugged north backbone over Dawson Peak and Pine Mountain down to Wrightwood. It features grand views from the rarely visited north face of Baldy down into the remote Fish Fork of the San Gabriel River. The long drive is justified by the fantastic scenery and seclusion of Sheep Mountain Wilderness. With an early start, you can reach Wrightwood in time for lunch with a friend who picks you up. Alternatively, you could spend the night on any of the summits. Beware: these north slopes hold snow and ice in the spring long after the south face snow has completely melted.

Follow the Baldy Bowl Trail 5 miles to the summit of Mount Baldy (see Trip 30.11, page 417). Descend the steep North Backbone Trail on the north side to a saddle of 8,800 feet; then follow the trail that climbs steeply up to 9,575-foot Dawson Peak, 1.5 miles from Baldy. Dawson Peak was named for Ernest Dawson, who served as the Sierra Club Angeles Chapter outings chair from 1916 to 1927 and as president from 1935 to 1937. His son Glen was a pioneering rock climber of the Sierra Nevada, establishing the first route up the East Face of Mount Whitney in 1931.

Descend the far ridge 0.5 mile past a junction with the unmaintained Dawson Peak Trail, which soon fades to oblivion as it drops westward into Fish Fork Canyon. Stay north on the Backbone Trail over 9,648-foot Pine Mountain; a 100-foot detour is necessary to reach the true summit. Then drop back down to a saddle and up to an unmarked trailhead on Forest Route 3N06.

Follow a use path up to the Pacific Crest Trail on the north side of the road, and continue west as it contours around Wright Mountain. In 0.8 mile turn north onto the Acorn Trail, and follow it 2.1 miles down to the top of Acorn Drive. Continue 0.2 mile to a gate, then another 0.4 mile down the paved private road to your vehicle.

Baldy's North Backbone is especially pretty (but potentially treacherous) in spring snow.

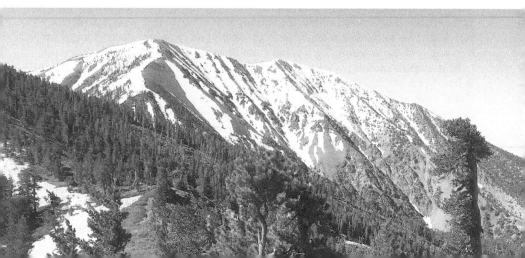

ALTERNATIVE FINISH

It's possible to end the at Forest Service Road 3N06, which is reached from Inspiration Point on Highway 2 by driving 7.2 miles east on fair dirt Blue Ridge Road (labeled FS 3N26 at the start but soon becoming FS 3N06) to the point above the prominent saddle between Pine and Wright Mountains. The driving time may exceed the time you save hiking, but the views of the North Backbone, Iron Mountain, the San Antonio Ridge, and the San Gabriel River Canyon are breathtaking.

VARIATION

Peak baggers may choose to make a short excursion to the 8,505-foot summit of Wright Mountain. From FS 3N06, cross the road and continue, very steeply for the first few yards, straight up the toe of the ridge. Soon, cross the PCT and look for traces of an old jeep trail. In 0.1 mile the slope levels out under the Jeffrey pines and white firs. In another 0.2 mile, the jeep trail dips and climbs back up to reach a T-junction on top of the ridge. Turn left and walk 100 yards to a yellow triangular sign. Look for a faint climbers' trail on the right leading north 100 feet to the indistinct summit, which is marked with a large cairn. Then continue west on the jeep trail to rejoin the PCT. This option adds 200 feet of climbing and negligible distance.

---

trip 30.14   Baldy Devils Backbone

see map on p. 402

Distance	6 miles (out-and-back)
Hiking Time	3.5 hours
Elevation Gain	2,300'
Difficulty	Moderately strenuous
Trail Use	Suitable for backpacking, dogs allowed
Best Times	May–November
Agency	Angeles National Forest
Optional Map	Tom Harrison *Angeles High Country*

DIRECTIONS From the 210 Freeway in Claremont, take Exit 52 for Base Line Road. Go west on Base Line for 0.2 mile; then turn right (north) on Padua Avenue. In 1.8 miles turn right onto Mount Baldy Road. Follow it 12 miles to the end at the Mount Baldy Ski Lift.

N o Southland hiker's repertoire of experiences is complete without at least one ascent of Mount San Antonio—Old Baldy. The east approach is the least taxing of the several routes to the summit, but it's by no means a picnic. You start at 7,800 feet, with virtually no altitude acclimatization, and climb expeditiously to over 10,000 feet. With ready access, it's beguilingly easy to come unprepared for high winds or bad weather, which although fairly rare, may come up suddenly. Ice, if present, can be a serious hazard as well.

By mechanical means (a car) you can get to the upper terminus of Mount Baldy Road in less than a half hour from the valley flatlands below. Further mechanical means—the Mount Baldy ski lift—carries you to an elevation of 7,800 feet at Mount Baldy Notch, where you begin hiking. Although the ski lift caters mostly to skiers (seven days a week during the winter season), it remains open during the summer season on weekends and holidays (8 a.m.–5 p.m.) for the benefit of sightseers and hikers. Call Mount Baldy Resort at 909-982-0800 for more information.

If it's a weekday, or you don't like being dangled over an abyss, you can always walk up the ski-lift-maintenance road starting from Manker Flats. That option adds 3.2 miles and an elevation change of about 1,600 feet both on the way up and on the way down. A lodge at the upper terminus of the lift offers food and beverages. From Mount Baldy Notch, technically the spot about 200 yards northeast of the top of the ski lift, take the maintenance road to the northwest that climbs moderately, then more steeply through groves of Jeffrey pine and incense cedar. After a couple of bends, you come to the road's end (1.3 miles) and the beginning of the trail along the Devils Backbone ridge.

The stretch ahead, once a hair-raiser, lost most of its terror when the Civilian Conservation Corps constructed a wider and safer trail, complete with guard rails, in 1935–36. The guard rails are gone now, but there's plenty of room to maneuver, unless there are problems with strong winds and/or ice. Devils Backbone offers grand vistas of both the Lytle Creek drainage on the north and east and San Antonio Canyon on the south.

The backbone section ends at about 2.0 miles as you start traversing the broad south flank of Mount Harwood. Scattered lodgepole pines now predominate. At 2.6 miles you arrive at the saddle between Harwood and Old Baldy, where backpackers sometimes set up camp (no water, no facilities here). Continue climbing up the rocky ridge to the west, past stunted, wind-battered lodgepole pines barely clinging to survival in the face of yearly onslaughts by cold winter winds. You reach the summit after a total of 3.1 miles.

On the rocky summit, barren of trees, you'll find a rock-walled enclosure. Most days you can easily make out the other two members of the triad of Southern California giants—San Gorgonio Mountain and San Jacinto Peak—about 50 miles east and southeast, respectively. On days of crystalline clarity, the Old Baldy panorama includes 90° of ocean horizon, a 120° slice of the tawny desert floor, and the far-off ramparts of the southern Sierra Nevada and Panamint ranges, as much as 160 miles away.

Aerial view of the Devils Backbone from the east, looking toward the summit of Mount Baldy at the top right

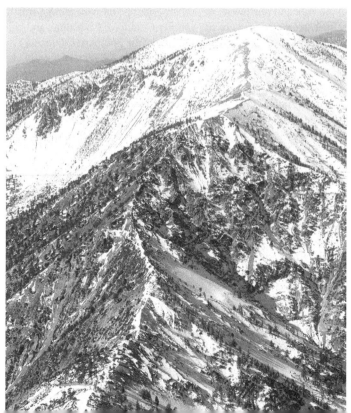

chapter 31

Santa Catalina Island: Avalon

From high points on the mainland, Santa Catalina Island is often seen either floating over a blanket of fog like a mirage, or rising boldly from the surface of the sea. The island, third largest of the several Channel Islands strung along the Southern California coast, lies only 19 miles at its closest point from the Palos Verdes Peninsula. It's the only Channel Island with a town of any real size, and the only one catering to large numbers of tourists.

The island has been inhabited by the Gabrielino-Tongva people and their ancestors since about 7000 B.C. The Tongva called the island Pimu or Pimugna. Juan Rodríguez Cabrillo was the first European visitor, claiming the island for Spain in 1542 and naming it San Salvador after his ship. Another Spanish explorer, Sebastian Vizcaino, rediscovered the island on the night before Saint Catherine's Day 1602 and renamed the island Catalina, Spanish for "Catherine."

Catalina stretches 21 miles in length and up to 8 miles at its maximum width. A half-mile-wide isthmus called Two Harbors separates the 6-mile-long northwestern end of the island (called the West End) from the larger southeastern part. The town of Avalon and Avalon Bay snuggle into an eastern corner of the island, protected from the prevailing winds, which come out of the west and northwest. Avalon experiences the same almost-frost-free climate as the most even-tempered areas of the Southern California coastline, and enjoys what is probably the cleanest air of any populated area near the Southern California coastline.

For most of this century, Catalina was owned by the Wrigley family (of chewing-gum and Chicago Cubs fame), whose interest in developing the island as a vacation destination was mostly limited to the Avalon area. Catalina's interior remained largely off-limits to tourists until the creation of the Catalina Island Conservancy in 1972, whose function is to preserve and protect the wild landscape and biological diversity of the island. Today 88% of the island is owned by the Conservancy and is open to light recreational use.

The languid pace of life on Catalina Island reflects its aloofness from the often-frantic business of living on the Southern California mainland. A weekend visit here is truly relaxing, whether you choose to lodge in Avalon or prefer to rough it at one of the several campgrounds spread around the island's coast and interior.

So why is Catalina included in this book on Los Angeles County hikes? Because it lies within the county's jurisdictional boundary, and because many L.A.-area residents vacation there. Of the million or so visitors to the island per year, many engage in hiking and mountain biking. To do that, you need to obtain a free permit for hiking (or a $35 Freewheeler permit for mountain biking) from The Trailhead visitor center in Avalon (at the corner of Crescent Avenue and Pebbly Beach Road as you walk toward town from the Catalina Express terminal) or online.

Ferries to Catalina depart from terminals at Dana Point, San Pedro, Long Beach, and Newport Beach. The *Catalina Express* ferry departs from terminals at San Pedro, Long Beach, and Dana Point; the *Catalina Flyer* departs from Newport Beach. The trip takes

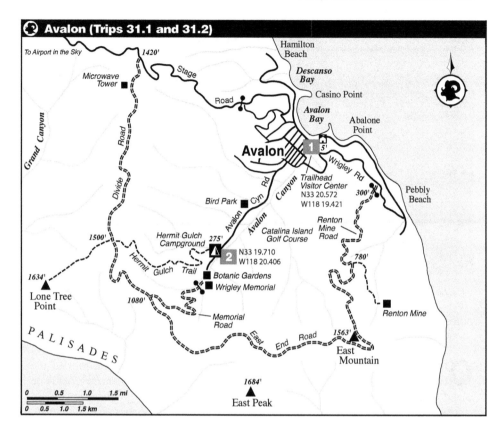

Avalon (Trips 31.1 and 31.2)

about an hour and costs about $70 per round-trip. Helicopter flights are available from Long Beach and San Pedro. Lodging in Avalon ranges from $75-per-night cottages to $400-plus bed-and-breakfasts.

For information, contact Catalina Island Conservancy, 310-510-2595, catalinaconservancy .org. Book campsites at 310-510-4205 or the Wildlands Express Shuttle at 310-510-0143.

In this chapter and the next, we profile some of the best hikes on Catalina—in this chapter near the Avalon area and in the next chapter originating from Two Harbors. See Trip 33.5 (page 457) for the popular Trans-Catalina Trail.

trip 31.1   East Mountain

Distance	10 miles (loop)
Hiking Time	5 hours
Elevation Gain	2,000'
Difficulty	Moderately strenuous
Trail Use	Dogs allowed
Best Times	October–June
Agency	Catalina Island Conservancy
Recommended Map	Free *Catalina Island Trail Map*
Fees/Permits	Free permit required, available online or at The Trailhead visitor center

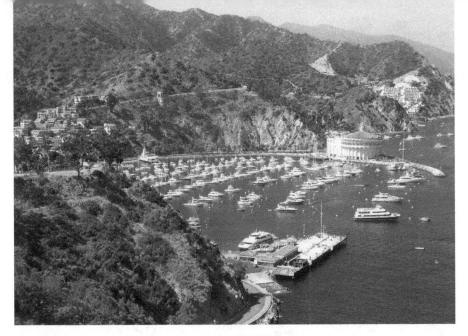
Most hikers on Catalina start with a ferry ride to Avalon Harbor.

DIRECTIONS Pick up your free permit at The Trailhead visitor center, at the corner of Crescent Avenue and Pebbly Beach Road, which you'll pass as you walk from the Catalina Express terminal toward town.

On certain crystal-clear days (generally November–March), this grand tour of the island's eastern end affords an ever-changing panorama of blue ocean, San Clemente Island to the south, and the snowcapped summits of the San Gabriels on the mainland.

The route takes you up along moderately graded paved and dirt roads to East Mountain, a broad summit area marking the last gasp of the island spine before it falls eastward into the ocean. No matter what the time of year, beware of the sun. You'll be climbing along the lee side of the island, fully exposed to morning and midday temperatures easily 20° higher than along the immediate coastline. Bring lots of water, and don't forget your shade hat.

Mountain bikers, who are allowed only on the island's primary road system, can make a longer loop variation on the hikers route described here. They are allowed to use Renton Mine Road, East End Road, Divide Road, and Stage Road.

From The Trailhead visitor center, walk along the waterfront toward the green pleasure pier, but make an immediate left onto Clarissa Avenue. Walk two blocks on Clarissa, left on Beacon Street, immediately right on Clemente Avenue, and then immediately left onto Wrigley Road. Climbing paved Wrigley Road, swing around the high ridge overlooking Avalon Bay, enjoying picture-postcard views of boats at anchor and of the famous round Casino building on the bay's far side. The distinguished edifice on the right at 0.5 mile is The Inn on Mount Ada, formerly the Wrigley family home. The home was designed to take advantage of the sunrises and sunsets visible from its commanding perch.

Go right at 1.3 miles past a gate onto Renton Mine Road; the paved road descends left toward a power plant at Pebbly Beach. A gradual ascent takes you to another junction, at 2.7 miles, where you make another right on East End Road. On the slopes hereabouts, notice the St. Catherine's lace, a type of buckwheat endemic to the dry slopes of the island. The flower clusters on this large (up to several feet high) shrub can spread as wide as a foot, with a creamy white color fading to rust in the fall.

After curling around East Mountain, East End Road proceeds due west along the ridge-crest, with spectacular views north down to Avalon Bay and south over the sparkling waters to San Clemente Island. Thick accumulations of chaparral coat the north-facing slopes, while the sunnier, south-facing slopes are much more parched and brown. Drought-resistant prickly-pear cacti grow abundantly on the ridgecrest and down along the drier slopes.

At 7 miles you'll veer sharply right on Memorial Road. Some easy walking down this dirt road takes you along a cool, north-facing slope covered with scrub oak, manzanita, and toyon. At the bottom of the hill you come upon the 130-foot-tall Wrigley Memorial, built in honor of chewing-gum magnate William Wrigley Jr., who purchased the island in 1918.

The botanic gardens started by Wrigley's wife, Ada, in the 1920s lie just below the monument. Distinguished by a virtually frost-free Mediterranean climate, they're home to an array of native Southern California plants plus exotics from around the world. Beyond the garden gates, 1.4 miles of road-walking down Avalon Canyon will take you back to Avalon.

trip 31.2　Lone Tree Point

Distance	6 miles (loop)
Hiking Time	3 hours
Elevation Gain	1,800'
Difficulty	Moderately strenuous
Trail Use	Dogs allowed, good for kids
Best Times	October–June
Agency	Catalina Island Conservancy
Recommended Map	*Catalina Island Trail Map*
Fees/Permits	Free permit required, available online or at The Trailhead visitor center

see map on p. 425

DIRECTIONS Pick up your free permit at The Trailhead visitor center, at the corner of Crescent Avenue and Pebbly Beach Road, which you'll pass as you walk from the Catalina Express terminal toward town.

    The hike starts at Hermit Gulch Campground. The easiest access is via the Garibaldi City Bus, which makes a loop around town. For schedules, check at The Trailhead or cityofavalon.com /transit. Get off at Stop 13. If you prefer to walk, take any street leading away from the waterfront, jog right on Tremont Street and then left onto Avalon Canyon Road, and follow it 1.5 miles to the campground.

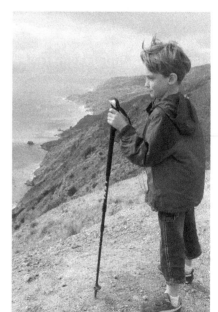

This popular springtime hike starts from Hermit Gulch Campground and loops over the main divide of the island overlooking Avalon. The highlight is a side trip over to Lone Tree Point, which commands an unparalleled view of the clifflike Palisades falling sheer to the ocean. You'll encounter a couple of very steep grades on the old firebreak leading to Lone Tree Point, so be sure to wear running shoes or boots with good tread. Small children would need some assistance

Lone Tree Point has incredible ocean views, provided that the fog hasn't rolled in.

on that stretch. The hike is especially enjoyable during the spring wildflower season or on a crisp fall or winter day.

Bison, boar, deer, and goats have all been introduced on the island at one time or another. Efforts to eradicate feral goats and pigs, whose impacts on vegetation were extreme in some areas, have been successful. On this hike and across the island today, you may see deer. Also keep an eye on the sky for bald eagles: the Catalina Island Conservancy, in partnership with the Institute for Wildlife Studies, has restored the eagles to the skies above Catalina after their populations suffered DDT contamination.

From the top end of Hermit Gulch Campground, follow the signed Hermit Gulch Trail up the ravine to the west. This is also the start of the Trans-Catalina Trail, which leads 38.5 miles across the island (see Trip 33.5, page 457). Before long you leave the stream in the canyon bottom and begin ascending along a shaggy slope. Red monkey flower, shooting star, paintbrush, and lupine dot the trailside in spring during a good rain year. Also watch for Saint Catherine's lace, a gigantic species of buckwheat endemic to the Channel Islands.

After a 1,200-foot gain (1.7 miles) you meet Divide Road, a fire road following the eastern spine of the island. Most of the elevation gain for the hike is now behind you.

Turn right, walk 0.1 mile to a stone restroom, and then turn left onto a steep fire road signed LONE TREE TRAIL. Continue for 1.0 mile over several rounded barren hills, to the peaklet designated Lone Tree. Continue to the end of the firebreak, where you'll find the best view of the ocean and shoreline. Sometimes you can gaze south over the shore-hugging fog and spy the low dome of San Clemente Island, some 40 miles across the glistening Pacific. During the best visibility you can trace the mainland shoreline down as far as San Diego, and also spy the long crest of the Peninsular Ranges.

After taking in the visual feast, backtrack to Divide Road. From there you can loop back to the starting point via a somewhat longer but more gradually descending route. Head south down Divide Road for 0.8 mile; then veer left on Memorial Road. Easy walking down this dirt road takes you down to Wrigley Memorial, through the botanic gardens, and finally to Hermit Gulch Campground, a short distance down Avalon Canyon Road.

trip 31.3 Airport Loop Trail

see map opposite

Distance	2.3 miles (loop)
Hiking Time	1 hour
Elevation Gain	400'
Difficulty	Easy
Trail Use	Dogs allowed, good for kids
Best Times	October–June
Agency	Catalina Island Conservancy
Recommended Map	*Catalina Island Trail Map*
Fees/Permits	Free permit required, available online or at the airport office

DIRECTIONS This trip starts at the Airport in the Sky, a popular destination for private pilots. If you aren't flying in, you can take the Safari Bus from Island Plaza in Avalon or the Wildlands Express Shuttle from The Trailhead visitor center. Reservations are required for both; for schedules and booking information, call 310-510-4205 or go to tinyurl.com/safaribus, or call 310-510-0143 or go to tinyurl .com/wildlandsexpress.

Airport in the Sky is located on a mesa in the center of Catalina Island. A trail circumnavigating the airport gives you a chance to stretch your legs and enjoy the views. The trail

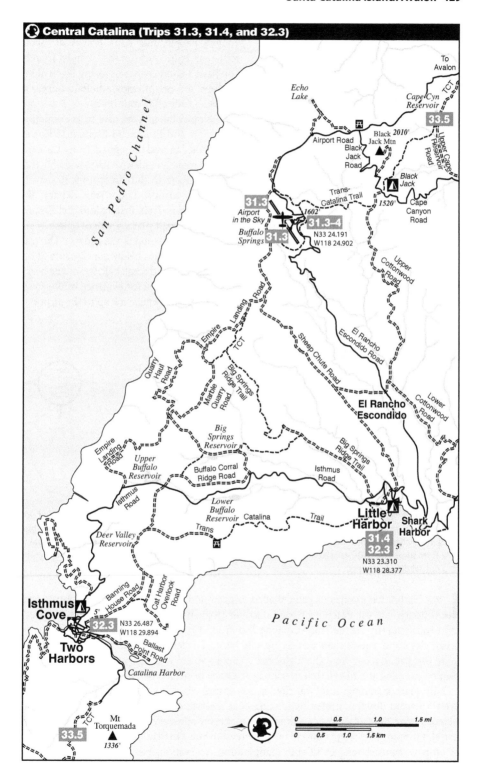

Central Catalina (Trips 31.3, 31.4, and 32.3)

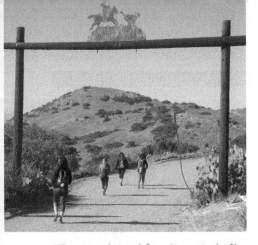

Hikers start their trek from Airport in the Sky.

passes a soapstone quarry used by the native Tongva people and visits groves of island scrub oak found only on the Channel Islands. You have a good chance of seeing bison along the way. You might enjoy a buffalo burger at the DC-3 Café after your hike.

Walk out the airport gate to the junction of Airport and El Rancho Escondido Roads, where you can find the signed Trans-Catalina Trail. To make a clockwise loop, take this trail west and north to Buffalo Springs Reservoir, where our Airport Loop Trail departs the Trans-Catalina Trail. Briefly join dirt Empire Landing Road; then continue along a trail paralleling the road past a grove of oaks.

Rejoin the road again as it curves around a bluff at the north end of the runway. The trail resumes at a sign on the right, cuts across Airport Road, and dips below the east side of the airport. Here is some of the most lush vegetation, including island scrub oak, lemonade berry, toyon, and prickly pear cactus. Watch for signs of bison and look for evidence of the soapstone quarry. Stay right to rejoin the Trans-Catalina Trail and switchback up to the airport.

trip 31.4   Airport in the Sky to Little Harbor

Distance	12 miles (loop)
Hiking Time	6 hours
Elevation Gain	2,000'
Difficulty	Strenuous
Trail Use	Suitable for backpacking, dogs allowed
Best Times	October–May
Agency	Catalina Island Conservancy
Recommended Map	*Catalina Island Trail Map*
Fees/Permits	Free permit required, available online or at the airport office

DIRECTIONS This trip starts at the Airport in the Sky, a popular destination for private pilots. If you aren't flying in, you can take the Safari Bus from Island Plaza in Avalon or the Wildlands Express Shuttle from The Trailhead visitor center. Reservations are required for both; for schedules and booking information, call 310-510-4205 or go to tinyurl.com/safaribus, or call 310-510-0143 or go to tinyurl.com/wildlandsexpress.

Little Harbor has a gorgeous palm-shaded campground and picnic area beside a sandy cove. Although you can reach it by the Safari Bus from Avalon or Two Harbors, it is a much more satisfying trip via the Trans-Catalina Trail from Airport in the Sky. The hike offers great ocean views and a good chance of seeing wild bison. The ferry schedule makes it impractical to do this trip in a day from the mainland, so unless you're coming by private plane or boat, plan on camping at Little Harbor or staying at a hotel in Avalon or Two Harbors.

Little Harbor Campground was cited in *Sunset* magazine's list of Best Campgrounds in the West, so avoid disappointment by making your reservation well in advance at visitcatalinaisland.com or 877-778-1487 (minimum two-night stay on weekends and three nights on holidays). Camping fuel is not allowed on the ferry, but you can arrange for firewood, charcoal, or propane canisters as part of your campground reservation. You can also make advance reservations for sea kayaks through Wet Spot Rentals (310-510-2229, wetspotrentals.com). You'll find tap water and restrooms at the campground for campers or picnickers.

Walk out the main gate from Airport in the Sky to the signed Trans-Catalina Trail and take it toward Little Harbor. Your route is initially a dirt road, but it soon veers right onto a trail that circles around the west side of the airport before reaching the dirt Empire Landing Road near the Buffalo Springs pond, at 1.0 miles. Continue west on this road, which is still part of the Trans-Catalina Trail. At 1.9 miles leave the Trans-Catalina Trail/Empire Landing Road, and turn left onto Sheep Chute Road, which is rough and steep in places but offers great ocean views. At 5.0 miles join a better road, turn right, and make your way down to Little Harbor, 5.3 miles.

Stingrays frequent the waters in Little Harbor. They don't want to sting humans but will do so if stepped upon. If you wish to venture into the water, shuffle your feet to alert them of your presence and don't tread upon one accidentally.

When you're ready to loop back, your first challenge is to find your way back to the Trans-Catalina Trail up Big Springs Ridge. Either wander a maze of faint paths northeast (uphill) from the campground until you reach the signed Trans-Catalina Trail, departing a good road, or follow the campground road north until you can turn hard right and follow another good road south to the same trail junction. The broad Trans-Catalina Trail climbs a steep northeast-trending ridge. Pass a signed connector trail on the left to Big Springs Reservoir at 6.9 miles. Shortly beyond the trail narrows, curves left, and switchbacks to gain another ridge, then follows this ridge over several false summits to a trail junction. Stay right and descend to join the Empire Landing Road at 9.4 miles. Take this to the right, and pass Sheep Chute Road at 9.8 miles; then retrace your path back to the airport, where you might get a buffalo burger at the café while waiting for your transportation back to civilization.

You'll likely see bison when you hike in the Catalina backcountry. They're large and wild, and they must be accorded respect.

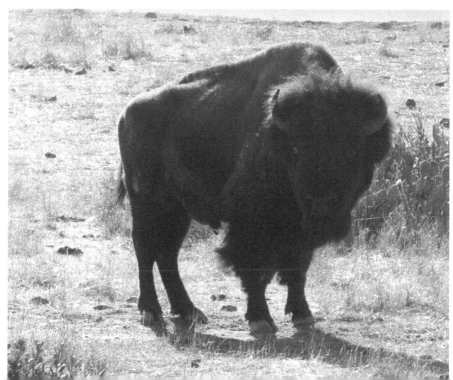

chapter 32

Santa Catalina Island: Two Harbors

If the popular Avalon area is too crowded for you, try Two Harbors, a quintessential sleepy village. Camping, hiking, backpacking, water sports, and wildlife-watching are the norms here.

In addition to a small lodge and cabins in tiny Two Harbors itself, hillside campsites abound at Two Harbors Campground just east of town. The more remote Parsons Landing Campground is accessible by way of a 7-mile road walk (see Trip 32.1, below).

Two Harbors is served by ferry from San Pedro and by helicopter from Long Beach and San Pedro. For information, contact Catalina Island Conservancy, 310-510-2595, catalina conservancy.org. Book campsites at 310-510-4205 or the Wildlands Express Shuttle at 310-510-0143.

If you're camping and plan to cook your own meals, be sure to ask at the Island Company visitor center in Two Harbors about the availability of firewood, charcoal, or stoves at either campground. (Stove fuel is not allowed on the ferry boats that serve the island.) Note that camping and transportation on Catalina are expensive.

---

trip 32.1   Parsons Landing

see map on next page

Distance	14 miles (loop)
Hiking Time	7 hours
Elevation Gain	2,300'
Difficulty	Moderately strenuous
Trail Use	Suitable for backpacking, dogs allowed
Best Times	Year-round
Agency	Catalina Island Conservancy
Recommended Map	*Catalina Island Trail Map*
Fees/Permits	Free permit required, available online or at the Two Harbors Visitor Center

DIRECTIONS The hike begins at the small community of Two Harbors, accessible by *Catalina Express* ferry from San Pedro.

Parsons Landing is not only the site of a small beach and a spacious camping area; it is also the home of one of the best examples of native Southern California grassland. Gray-green after winter rains, bleached gray during drought, the perennial grasses here have found the right combination of fine-grained soil, soaking winter rains, and desiccating summer drought.

The native grasslands of Parsons Landing are only one example of the botanical richness and diversity of the north slope of Catalina's West End. The chaparral and oak-woodland habitats here look healthy. On the sheltered north-facing slopes (especially at Cherry Valley), you'll find plenty of the native Catalina cherry, a large shrub or tree (up to 45 feet

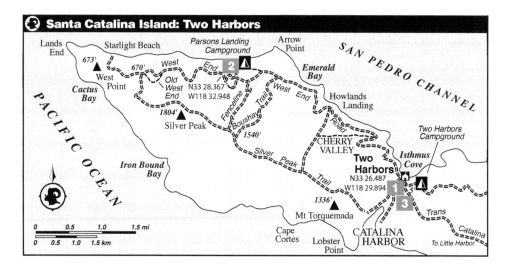

tall) displaying spike-shaped clusters of white flowers during the spring. Its dark, red fruits resemble large black cherries.

This route follows the western end of the Trans-Catalina Trail, looping west from Two Harbors along a scenic ridge on the Silver Peak Trail, then returning on the West End Road that hugs the coast, swinging around every ravine and canyon along the way.

The trip is most rewarding, and not at all exhausting, if you can spend a night at Parsons Landing Campground. Considering the ferry schedule, you are likely to be spending a night on the island in any event, and it's hard to find a better site than Parsons. From there, if you're ambitious, you can loop around the island's west end—see the next trip.

Stop by the Two Harbors Visitor Services office if you need to pick up a hiking or camping permit. The office will also arrange water and firewood for you at Parsons Landing for a fee. You can pick up camping-fuel canisters at the General Store.

Parsons Landing offers incredible, secluded beach camping, with amazing views of the lights of Palos Verdes across the channel.

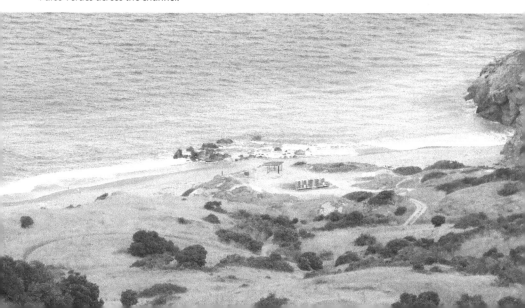

Walk south to the Isthmus Yacht Club. Jog right and then turn left again toward Catalina Harbor, following signs for the Trans-Catalina Trail. Soon, pass through a gate onto a dirt road called the Silver Peak Trail. Your strenuous climb onto the ridge is rewarded with outstanding views over the coastline and east toward Black Jack Mountain.

Pass Water Tank Road and Boushay Canyon Road on the right before reaching Fenceline Road, where the Trans-Catalina Trail turns right and descends toward Parsons Landing. Follow signs for Trans-Catalina/Parsons Landing as you pass two junctions on your way down.

Parsons Landing is one of the finest campsites in Southern California, especially on a weeknight when you have it mostly to yourself. You can camp on the sand beside huge boulders and listen to the sea lions frolicking in the water through the night. The sunsets can be spectacular, and you'll have a great view across the channel to the lights of Los Angeles.

Return on the West End Road segment of the Trans-Catalina Trail. This sinuous route takes 7.5 air miles to cover 3.5 miles as the crow files, weaving in and out of every cove but scarcely gaining any elevation. You'll pass Boy Scout camps at Emerald Bay and Cherry Valley, and a private camp at Howlands Landing. Watch for dolphins off the coast.

trip 32.2	**Silver Peak & Starlight Beach**

Distance	11 miles (loop)
Hiking Time	5.5 hours
Elevation Gain	3,100'
Difficulty	Moderately strenuous
Trail Use	Dogs allowed
Best Times	October–June
Agency	Catalina Island Conservancy
Recommended Map	*Catalina Island Trail Map*
Fees/Permits	Free permit required, available online or at the Two Harbors Visitor Center

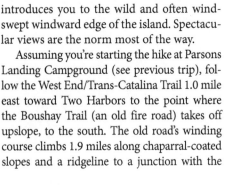

see map on previous page

DIRECTIONS The hike begins at Parsons Landing Campground, which can be reached from Two Harbors by hiking the previous trip for Parsons Landing or by kayaking up the coast.

This hike to the highest point on the west end of Catalina, 1,804-foot Silver Peak, introduces you to the wild and often wind-swept windward edge of the island. Spectacular views are the norm most of the way.

Assuming you're starting the hike at Parsons Landing Campground (see previous trip), follow the West End/Trans-Catalina Trail 1.0 mile east toward Two Harbors to the point where the Boushay Trail (an old fire road) takes off upslope, to the south. The old road's winding course climbs 1.9 miles along chaparral-coated slopes and a ridgeline to a junction with the

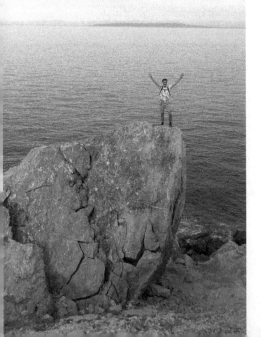

Starlight Beach is about as remote as you can get by trail on Catalina.

Silver Peak Trail—a fire road traversing the spine of the island's west end. Here, amid brick-red soils and rock outcrops, you get your first glimpses of the west end's dry and heavily eroded south-facing slopes falling precipitously to the blue and emerald ocean below.

In 1.2 miles Silver Peak Road passes about 100 feet below Silver Peak's nearly barren summit. You can scramble up near a sparse grove of Catalina ironwood trees and reach the top for an all-inclusive panorama. San Nicolas and Santa Barbara islands can be seen to the west on many days. Very rarely, Anacapa, Santa Cruz, and Santa Rosa Islands off the coast of Santa Barbara, as well as the mainland shoreline west of Ventura, can be seen in the northwest. Quite often, especially in spring and summer, there's nothing to see at all, as you may be wreathed in low clouds scudding over the island's spine.

Past Silver Peak, the fire road swings sharply downhill, beginning a sometimes very sheer descent down the wind-buffeted ridgeline to the west. After descending a total of about 1,100 feet, you reach a T-intersection. You'll return to Parson's Landing on the road to the right. But first make the side trip left down to Starlight Beach, one of the most isolated and wild stretches of Catalina's coastline. (This excursion is 1.1 miles each way, with 800 feet of elevation loss and gain; if you are pressed for time, you could shorten the trip by omitting it.) You'll have to scramble a bit in the end to reach the rocky shore, where the ebb and flow of the waves dance over rock-dimpled sand. On clear days you can see the low dome of the Palos Verdes Peninsula some 20 miles across the San Pedro Channel, and it's hard to believe such a serene and beautiful place as Catalina's northwest shore can exist so close to the L.A. metropolis.

Climb back up to the T-intersection and return to Parsons Landing on the road that contours and lazily drops across steep, north-facing slopes. At a signed fork, stay right on the Old West End Road, now faded to a trail in places, which is shorter and avoids the gratuitous dips and climbs found on the vehicular West End Road. It rejoins the main road in 0.8 mile. Each ravine you cross harbors a mini-forest of tangled oaks and chaparral. By the late afternoon, the often-misty atmosphere of the morning may have turned transparent, rendering the waters of the San Pedro Channel down below a deep azure.

trip 32.3   Harbor to Harbor

see
maps on
pgs. 429
& 433

Distance	5.5 miles (one-way)
Hiking Time	3 hours
Elevation Gain	1,500'
Difficulty	Moderate
Trail Use	Suitable for backpacking, dogs allowed
Best Times	October–June
Agency	Catalina Island Conservancy
Recommended Map	*Catalina Island Trail Map*
Fees/Permits	Free permit required, available online or at the Two Harbors Visitor Center

DIRECTIONS The hike begins at the small community of Two Harbors, accessible by *Catalina Express* ferry from San Pedro. If you don't wish to retrace your steps, arrange a shuttle in advance from Little Harbor to Two Harbors with the Safari Bus (for fares and schedules, call 310-510-4205 or go to tinyurl .com/safaribus). The bus runs frequently in the summer but only once a day in the winter.

Perhaps the most scenic hike on Catalina Island, this trip follows the Trans-Catalina Trail from Two Harbors up a steep hill and along a narrow ridge with views of dramatic sea cliffs, then brings you to a marvelous beach and campground at Little Harbor. Consider

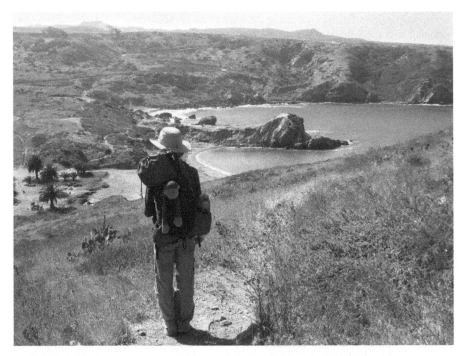

A boy and his stuffed monkey approach Little Harbor on the Trans-Catalina Trail.

making a reservation to enjoy the night at the Little Harbor Campground: 877-778-1487, tinyurl.com/littleharborcampground. Contact Wet Spot Rentals (310-510-2229, wetspot rentals.com) to arrange kayak rentals at Little Harbor.

From the Visitor Center in Two Harbors, walk south along the main road to a T-junction at the Isthmus Yacht Club. Turn left and follow the Trans-Catalina Trail as it ascends a steep dirt road. Pass the Banning House, originally constructed in 1910 by the Banning brothers as a summer home, and now operated as a bed and breakfast. Stay straight at various junctions, pass through a gate (closing it behind you to keep the bison out of town), and reach a crest at 1.8 miles.

Continue on the Trans-Catalina Trail as it departs Banning House Road. At 2.6 miles reach a picnic shelter with tremendous views of the sea cliffs to the west. Now on narrow trail, descend the steep ridge to Little Harbor.

The trail ends at the Little Harbor Campground, where you'll find tap water and restrooms. The Safari Bus stop is near the ranger station, 150 yards south along the main road. The adjacent bay contains both Little Harbor and Shark Harbor, split by an outcrop known as the Whales Tail. If you venture into the water, shuffle your feet to avoid surprising the stingrays that frequent the area.

chapter 33

Long-Distance Trails

Los Angeles County is fortunate to have the most interesting and diverse long distance trails in California south of the Sierra Nevada. The Pacific Crest Trail (PCT) is the granddaddy of them all, running 2,650 miles from Mexico to Canada including a magnificent stretch through the San Gabriel Mountains, but this trail is already the topic of many books (including *Pacific Crest Trail: Southern California* and *Day & Section Hikes Pacific Crest Trail: Southern California,* both by Wilderness Press). This chapter covers a diverse set of long trails in the San Gabriel Mountains, the Santa Monica Mountains, Santa Catalina Island, and across the Los Angeles basin.

Most of the trips in this chapter are best done as backpacking trips. There are two schools of thought about backpacking. Old-school backpackers find the biggest pack they can buy and fill it up with a heavy tent, a heavy sleeping bag, all the luxuries one might want in camp, and maybe even a cast-iron Dutch oven. Sometimes they must carry gallons of water because reliable water sources are two days apart. They lumber up the mountain for 8 to 10 miles in heavy boots, then set up camp at a heavily used site, switch into the spare shoes they've been hauling, and rest their aching backs and feet. At night, they fend off the bears that prowl the campsite.

Modern backpacking has been pioneered by thru-hikers on the PCT and other long treks. They ruthlessly strip their packs down to the essentials. Anyone can get their summer pack base weight (excluding consumables such as food, water, and fuel) below 20 pounds with a bit of thought, and 12 pounds is readily achievable without any loss of safety, if one invests in a lightweight (less than 2 pounds) sleeping bag, pack, and shelter.

Compared with old-school backpackers, ultralight hikers almost float up the trail. They're walking by sunrise to enjoy the cool temperatures and splendid lighting of the early morning. At a moderate 2-mph pace with plenty of breaks, practiced hikers can readily cover 20 miles or more before sunset. At this pace, they carry fewer days of food, and rarely travel a day without reliable water. They may cook near a water source, then continue on to camp at a secluded clearing where they won't be bothered by animals or noisy campers. While they carry a shelter if there is any chance of rain, they often "cowboy camp" under the stars on pleasant nights.

The suggested itineraries in this chapter generally average about 10 miles per day and are suited to youth groups and old-school backpackers, but ultralight hikers will readily shorten the trips.

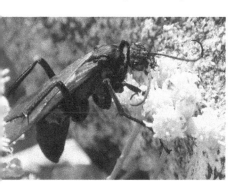

The tarantula hawk wasp (Pepsis formosa) is a striking sight with its orange wings and blue-black body that's up to 2 inches long.

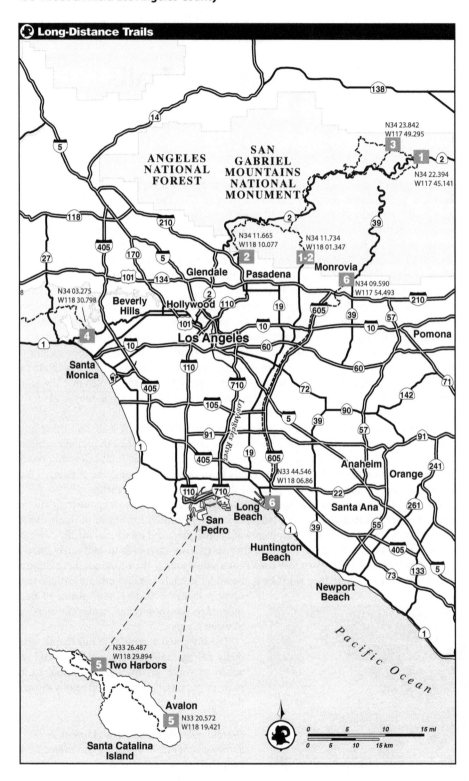

Long-Distance Trails

trip 33.1   Silver Moccasin Trail

Distance	52 miles (one-way)
Hiking Time	3–7 days
Elevation Gain/Loss	14,600'/10,200'
Difficulty	Strenuous
Trail Use	Suitable for backpacking, equestrians, dogs allowed; Three Points to Chantry Flat suitable for mountain biking
Best Times	May–November
Agency	Angeles National Forest
Recommended Map	Tom Harrison *Angeles High Country* and *Angeles Front Country*

DIRECTIONS This hike begins at Chantry Flat and ends at Vincent Gap on the Angeles Crest. The 71-mile shuttle between the trailheads takes about 1.5 hours without traffic. To leave a vehicle at Vincent Gap, take I-15 north to Highway 138 west to Highway 2 west to the gap at mile marker 2 LA 74.8.

To reach Chantry Flat, return to I-15, and take it south to the 210 Freeway. Go west to Exit 32 for Santa Anita Avenue in Arcadia. Drive north 5 miles to the parking lots at Chantry Flat, passing a vehicle gate that's open 6 a.m.–8 p.m. The lot fills early on weekends, so you may have to backtrack and park along the shoulder of the road.

The Silver Moccasin National Recreation Trail (11W06) runs the length of the San Gabriel Mountains. Starting through chaparral and woods and past a waterfall in Big Santa Anita Canyon, it visits the secluded West Fork San Gabriel River, Chilao's peaceful forest, Cooper Canyon Falls, and the Angeles Crest, culminating on the summit of Mount Baden-Powell. The trail was named by the Boy Scouts, and is a rite of passage for thousands of boys seeking the coveted 50 Miler or Silver Moccasin badge, but the path has been used for centuries by Native Americans and Anglo settlers for hunting and trade before becoming formalized in the 1930s. The Silver Moccasin Trail coincides with the Gabrielino Trail from Chantry Flats to West Fork Campground, with the Pacific Crest Trail (PCT) from Three Points to Vincent Gap, and with the Angeles Crest 100 ultramarathon route. The trip is long enough for you to adapt to the rhythm of trail life and lose track of time and civilization. You won't find a better trip of this length in Southern California.

There is no good group camping between West Fork and Chilao or between Cooper Canyon and Little Jimmy, so you'll have some strenuous hiking days even if you allocate a week for the trip. In the winter and spring, the ridge near Mount Baden-Powell is icy and requires an ice ax and crampons and suitable experience; unprepared hikers have died here. By late spring, water can be unreliable for 34 miles between West Fork and Little Jimmy. Check with the U.S. Forest Service before your trip, and cache water jugs near the Angeles Crest Highway crossings if necessary (but be sure to carry out the jugs when you collect them). You can find information about water at Cooper Canyon, Buckhorn Campground, and Lamel Spring at the Pacific Crest Trail Water Report at pctwater.com (click "Part Two, Idyllwild to Agua Dulce"). The PCT is indefinitely closed between the Buckhorn Trail and Eagles Roost to protect the endangered yellow-legged mountain frog, so this trip involves a potentially dangerous walk along the shoulder of the Angeles Crest Highway to bypass the closure. Be careful of poison oak along the trail.

The PCT segment from Vincent Gap to Three Points is closed to mountain bikers, but the Silver Moccasin segment from Three Points to West Fork is considered one of the best rides in the range for advanced cyclists.

From the Chantry Flat Trailhead, start down the Gabrielino Trail, which begins as a gated paved road descending into Big Santa Anita Canyon. The pavement ends at 0.6 mile as you bridge Winter Creek and hike up alder-lined Big Santa Anita Canyon on a roadbed that passes some cabins and soon narrows to a foot trail.

At 1.4 miles come to a four-way junction in a tranquil oak woodland. The right branch goes to Sturtevant Falls, which is a worthy 0.3-mile detour if the creek is flowing well, but generally not impressive in the summer. The left branch is recommended for equestrians or hikers who dislike heights. The middle branch is the most scenic, traversing the face above the waterfall and then following the fern-lined creek past cascades and pools. The left and middle trails reconverge at 2.2 miles.

Continuing up the canyon, reach Cascade Picnic Area at 2.7 miles, where you'll find picnic tables and restrooms near the stream. You'll see many check dams built from concrete blocks resembling Lincoln logs. These dams were installed in the 1960s by the U.S. Forest Service and the Los Angeles County Flood Control District in an effort to reduce the flow of rock and sand into the Big Santa Anita Reservoir. It is hard to imagine that a road once ran through here to bring cement mixers and cranes up the canyon, or that forest managers once believed that pouring cement on a pristine creekbed was a good idea. There's something in nature that doesn't love a dam, and floods and vegetation are gradually restoring the canyon to its original character.

At 3.3 miles reach Spruce Grove Trail Camp, which has water seasonally. (*Spruce* is an older name for the big-cone Douglas-firs that thrive on this side of Mount Wilson.) At 3.5 miles the signed Sturtevant Trail veers left to reach Sturtevant Camp in 0.1 mile. This historic camp was established in 1893 and now has four cabins that you could rent with advanced reservations at sturtevantcamp.com. In a pinch, you could also get water there. However, we stay on the Gabrielino Trail, which steepens as it climbs through chaparral to Newcomb Pass at 5.7 miles.

Switchback down the north side of the pass, crossing the often-closed Rincon–Red Box jeep road, to DeVore Trail Camp on the West Fork of the San Gabriel River at 7.1 miles.

Follow the trail west (upstream) to West Fork Trail Camp at 8.2 miles. Both of these fine trail camps have a remote feel as well as reliable water from the river—this may be the last dependable water for a long time. The Gabrielino Trail continues west, but you'll stay on the Silver Moccasin Trail, which veers north into Shortcut Canyon and then climbs to Shortcut Saddle at mile marker 2 LA 43.30 on the Angeles Crest Highway (Highway 2) at 11.8 miles.

Descend to cross seasonal Big Tujunga Creek at 12.8 miles; then begin a hot climb through chaparral recovering from the 2009 Station Fire. At 14.5 miles pull over a low saddle to cross a service road by a picnic table. At 14.7 miles cross another paved road near the Charlton Flats picnic grounds. The trail curves around the hillside, passing a spur to Vetter Mountain at 15.3 miles; then it meets paved Forest Service Road 3N16B in the picnic grounds at 15.5 miles. Hike north through a gate; then leave

The Silver Moccasin and Gabrielino National Recreation Trails are both memorable backpacking trips.

the road at a hairpin turn and continue north along the East Fork of Alder Creek. Eventually, the trail climbs out to meet FS 3N21 near the Chilao Campground Little Pines Loop, just north of the Angeles Crest Highway at mile marker 2 LA 49.69 17.6 miles. The first-come, first-served campground sometimes has piped water.

Continue on the Silver Moccasin Trail through a pine forest, over a low ridge, and down to the edge of the Upper Chilao Picnic Area at 18.2 miles, where you might again find a faucet. At 18.6 miles recross FS 3N21 at the Chilao Trailhead. Pass Horse Flats Campground (no water) at 19.7 miles and then the Bandido Group Camp (also no water) at 20.1 miles. The trail now turns east and parallels the paved Santa Clara Divide Road to its junction with the Angeles Crest Highway at Three Points (mile marker 2 LA 52.85), where you'll find trailhead parking and an outhouse, 22.2 miles.

Your route now coincides with the PCT and exits the Station Fire burn area. Climb near the Angeles Crest Highway, crossing it three times to reach Cloudburst Summit at 27.0 miles by mile marker 2 LA 57.04. Follow the circuitous trail down (or short cut down the dirt service road) into Cooper Canyon to find a spacious and scenic trail camp shaded by pines at 29.7 miles. Seasonal water flows in the nearby creek. At 31.0 miles reach a junction with the Buckhorn Trail. Cooper Canyon Falls is just to the east and is well worth a visit if the creek is flowing. The PCT is closed ahead indefinitely to protect habitat of the endangered yellow-legged mountain frog. Unless the closure has been lifted, our route turns right and climbs the Burkhart Trail, passing two waterfalls, to reach Buckhorn Campground at 32.6 miles. You may find working water spigots at the campground.

Walk up through the campground and find the paved exit road leading east to meet the Angeles Crest Highway at mile 2 LA 59.05, 33.4 miles. You now face a dull and dangerous walk along the shoulder of the highway to Eagles Roost picnic area at 2 LA 61.65, 36.1 miles. The PCT resumes along Kratka Ridge, a low ridge with stunning views, then crosses back to the north side of the highway at 2 LA 62.50, 37 miles. It then climbs high onto the shoulder of Mount Williamson, passes a spur leading to Williamson's summit, and drops back to cross the highway once more at Islip Saddle, 2 LA 64.0, 39.9 miles.

Beyond the saddle, begin a long gradual climb toward Mount Baden-Powell. Watch for red currants, which ripen by late summer. At 42.2 miles reach the spacious Little Jimmy Trail Camp, named for cartoonist Jimmy Swinnerton, who drew the *Little Jimmy* comic strip and spent his summers here from 1890 to 1910. The camp has picnic benches and stone ovens. If the sites near the trail are full or noisy, look farther back for more-private spots. Less than a quarter mile beyond the camp, you'll find reliable Little Jimmy Spring beside two huge incense cedars and many wildflowers.

Continuing on the PCT, reach aptly named Windy Gap at 42.5 miles. Pressure differences between the desert and valley air masses funnel air through this low point in the Angeles Crest. A web of trails radiates from the gap; be sure to continue east on the PCT. At 42.9 miles pass an undeveloped large campsite at the edge of the burn zone from the 2002 Curve Fire. Continue past climbers' trails leading to Middle Hawkins, Mount Hawkins, and Throop Peak to reach a signed junction with the Dawson Saddle Trail at 45.5 miles.

The next section of the trail, along the Angeles Crest, is perhaps the best part of the whole trip. You'll find a small exposed tent site with amazing views here, and at each saddle between Throop and Baden-Powell. At 46.6 miles bypass Mount Burnham on the north side. You'll find another campsite large enough for a troop of Scouts on the northwest slope of the mountain. Major Fredrick Burnham was a cofounder of the Boy Scout movement. At 47.9 miles reach a short trail on the right leading to the 9,399-foot summit of Mount Baden-Powell. A monument here celebrates Lord Robert Baden-Powell (1857–1941), who founded the Boy Scouts in 1907. You can find more exposed camping on the ridge south of the peak. The only trees growing this high are lodgepole and limber pines, which favor the tallest mountains in Southern California. Lodgepole pines have needles in bundles of two and round, golf ball–size cones, while limber pines have needles in bundles of five and longer, 4- to 6-inch cones on their flexible branches. The Wally Waldron Tree at the junction below the summit is a twisted limber pine believed to be 1,500 years old.

The trip concludes with 40 knee-jarring switchbacks descending to Vincent Gap. Halfway down, you'll pass three undeveloped campsites and then a signed spur at a switchback that leads 100 yards to seasonal Lamel Spring, in a ravine.

POSSIBLE ITINERARY			
DAY	CAMP	MILES	ELEVATION GAIN
1	West Fork	8.2	2,700'
2	Chilao	9.4	3,400'
3	Cooper Canyon	12.1	2,600'
4	Little Jimmy	12.5	3,600'
5	(exit)	9.5	2,300'

trip 33.2   Gabrielino Trail

see map on p. 438

Distance	28 miles (one-way)
Hiking Time	2–4 days
Elevation Gain	4,900'
Difficulty	Strenuous
Trail Use	Suitable for backpacking, mountain biking, dogs allowed
Best Times	Year-round (hot in summer)
Agency	Angeles National Forest
Recommended Map	Tom Harrison *Angeles Front Country*

DIRECTIONS This hike begins at Chantry Flat and ends at Arroyo Seco, requiring a 16-mile shuttle. To reach Arroyo Seco from the 210 Freeway in Pasadena, take Exit 22B for Windsor Avenue. Go north 0.8 mile to the parking area at the corner of Ventura Street—leave a shuttle vehicle here.

To reach Chantry Flat, return to the 210 Freeway eastbound and take Exit 32 for Santa Anita Avenue in Arcadia. Drive north 5 miles to the parking lots at Chantry Flat, passing a vehicle gate that's open 6 a.m.–8 p.m. The lot fills early on weekends, so you may have to backtrack and park along the shoulder of the road.

The Gabrielino National Recreation Trail from Chantry Flat to Arroyo Seco was designated in 1970. It follows historic Native American hunting and trading paths across three major watersheds: Big Santa Anita, West Fork San Gabriel, and Arroyo Seco. The trail offers diverse scenery and gorgeous wild streams. The portion from Chantry Flat to West Fork coincides with the southern end of the Silver Moccasin Trail. Most hikers just use small segments of the trail (see Chapters 23 and 24), but those seeking a longer trip can walk the entire Gabrielino Trail, either in one very long day or a backpacking trip enjoying the fine remote trail camps along the way. Water may be seasonal in Big Santa Anita Canyon but is reliable beyond; be sure to treat before using. Trail junctions are well signed, but some of the mileages are remarkably inaccurate. Finally, watch out for poison oak along the trail.

From the Chantry Flat Trailhead, start down the Gabrielino Trail, which begins as a gated paved road descending into Big Santa Anita Canyon. The pavement ends at 0.6 mile as you bridge Winter Creek and hike up alder-lined Big Santa Anita Canyon on a roadbed that passes some cabins and soon narrows to a foot trail.

At 1.4 miles come to a four-way junction in a tranquil oak woodland. The right branch goes to Sturtevant Falls, which is a worthy 0.3-mile detour if the creek is flowing well, but generally not impressive in the summer. The left branch is recommended for equestrians or hikers who dislike heights. The middle branch is the most scenic, traversing the face above the waterfall and then following the fern-lined creek past cascades and pools. The left and middle trails reconverge at 2.2 miles.

Continuing up the canyon, reach Cascade Picnic Area at 2.7 miles, where you'll find picnic tables and restrooms near the stream. You'll see many check dams built from concrete blocks resembling Lincoln logs. These dams were installed in the 1960s by the U.S. Forest Service and Los Angeles County Flood Control District in an effort to reduce the flow of rock and sand into the Big Santa Anita Reservoir. It is hard to imagine that a road once ran through here to bring cement mixers and cranes up the canyon, or that forest managers once believed that pouring cement on a pristine creekbed was a good idea. There's something in nature that doesn't love a dam, and floods and vegetation are gradually restoring the canyon to its original character.

At 3.3 miles reach Spruce Grove Trail Camp, which has water seasonally. (*Spruce* is an older misnomer for the big-cone Douglas-firs that thrive on this side of Mount Wilson.) At 3.5 miles the signed Sturtevant Trail veers left to reach Sturtevant Camp in 0.1 mile. This historic camp was established in 1893 and now has four cabins that you could rent with advanced reservations at sturtevantcamp.com. In a pinch, you could also get water there. However, we stay on the Gabrielino Trail, which steepens as it climbs through chaparral to Newcomb Pass at 5.7 miles.

Switchback down the north side of the pass, crossing the often-closed Rincon–Red Box jeep road, to DeVore Trail Camp on the West Fork of the San Gabriel River at 7.2 miles. Follow the trail west (upstream) to West Fork Trail Camp at 8.3 miles, fording the river 10 times en route—note that the crossings could be difficult in times of high water. Both of these fine trail camps have a remote feel as well as reliable water from the river.

The Gabrielino Trail runs above Arroyo Seco to avoid the Royal Gorge.

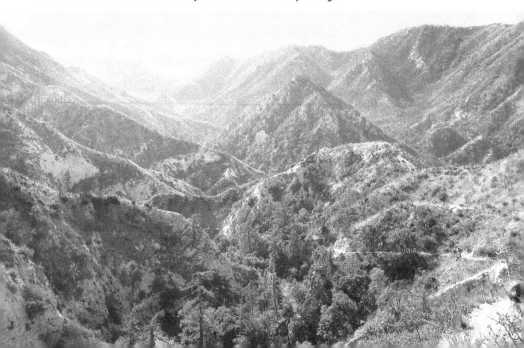

Your route departs the Silver Moccasin Trail here and continues paralleling the West Fork upstream. At 9.8 miles pass the Kenyon DeVore Trail, which climbs to Mount Wilson. At 11.2 miles pass the Valley Forge Trail, which climbs to Eaton Saddle. Shortly beyond, you'll reach a spur to Valley Forge Campground. Staying on the main trail, pass some cabins; then top out at Red Box Saddle (4,666') at 13.3 miles, named for a box of firefighting tools that were stationed here in the 19th century. Here, you'll find a ranger station, toilets, and trailhead parking.

From here, your trip is nearly all downhill. A unremarkable stretch parallels the Angeles Crest Highway along a hillside that burned in the 2009 Station Fire. The scenery and tree cover improve when you reach the Switzer Picnic Area at 17.6 miles. The remainder of your hike follows Trip 23.2 (see page 283) down the Arroyo Seco under a delightful canopy of live oak, sycamore, bay, alder, and maple. Spring wildflowers can be outstanding.

Follow the shady creek to the site of the historic Switzer resort at 18.7 miles, where you'll find stone stoves (day use only). Beware that the water here is heavily polluted by the hordes of day users in the drainage. Pass above Switzer Falls (difficult to see from the trail), and come to a fork at 18.9 miles—the left branch, Bear Canyon Trail, descends to the base of the falls, a short and worthy side trip if the water is flowing well. Dispersed camping is possible out of sight of the trail. Our trail stays high to bypass the rugged Royal Gorge before descending Long Canyon to rejoin the Arroyo Seco at 21.5 miles.

The trail is cut into the steep east wall of the canyon. At 22.5 miles pass the Ken Burton Trail, which ascends toward Brown Mountain. Now you follow the floor of the canyon, repeatedly crossing the creek. You can count on wet feet in the spring.

Oakwilde Campground just beyond was obliterated by the Station Fire. At 23.2 miles make a short but steep climb onto the canyon wall to bypass the Brown Canyon Debris Dam, reaching the Paul Little Memorial Picnic Area near the foot of the dam.

You have now have an easy downhill journey back to civilization. You'll see foundations, bits of eroded asphalt, and eight bridges left from the resort developments that were repeatedly wiped out by fire and flood. Pass the Nino Picnic Area; then come to busy Gould Mesa Campground at 25.3 miles. Then you'll pass Teddy's Outpost Picnic Area and some U.S. Forest Service residences before joining the final paved section of the trail.

POSSIBLE ITINERARY			
DAY	CAMP	MILES	ELEVATION GAIN
1	West Fork	8.3	2,700'
2	Bear Canyon Trail junction	10.6	1,900'
3	(exit)	9.2	300'

trip 33.3 High Desert Loop

Distance	41 miles (loop)
Hiking Time	2–5 days
Elevation Gain	10,000'
Difficulty	Strenuous
Trail Use	Suitable for backpacking, dogs allowed
Best Times	May–November
Agency	Angeles National Forest
Recommended Map	Tom Harrison *Angeles High Country*

see map on p. 438

DIRECTIONS From Highway 138, 26.5 miles northwest of I-15 or 16.7 miles east of Highway 14, turn south on 165th Street. Follow the meandering road 6.4 miles as it changes name to Bob's Gap Road.

Turn left on Highway N4 (Big Pines Highway), go 0.3 mile; then turn right on Big Rock Creek Road and go 2.4 miles. Turn right onto graded Forest Service Road 4N11A and proceed 0.9 mile to South Fork Campground. Just before the campground entrance, look for the signed Manzanita Trail on the left. Opposite this sign, take a short dirt spur on the right to the trailhead parking.

The High Desert National Recreation Trail is the name given in 1981 to the Burkhart, Devil's Punchbowl, Manzanita, and South Fork Trails that climb the northern flank of the San Gabriel Mountains between the Mojave Desert and the Pacific Crest Trail (PCT). In combination with the Pacific Crest Trail, these trails form a splendid loop touring many ecological zones as you climb from the desert to the highest ridges. Peak baggers will enjoy short detours to climb to 10 named peaks along the Angeles Crest. If you do this hike in the summer, get an early start to climb out of the desert before the heat of the day. You may wish to cache water in the fall because natural sources are scarce. The Angeles Crest can be icy December–April. The trip can be shortened to 23 miles with 5,500 feet of elevation gain by descending the South Fork Trail from Islip Saddle.

This loop has an unsurpassed diversity of conifers along any trail in Southern California. Big-cone Douglas-firs predominate along the lower Manzanita Trail. As you approach Vincent Gap, white fir, sugar pine, Jeffrey pine, and incense cedar join the mix. A grove of non-native giant sequoias shades the picnic benches at Vincent Gap. The Mount Baden-Powell climbs into a forest of pure lodgepole pines, eventually joined by gnarled limber pines at the highest elevations. A smattering of ponderosa pines can be found along the South Fork Trail just below Reed Spring. Coulter and pinyon pines grow on the desert slopes near the Devil's Punchbowl.

Water may be a concern on this trail. Little Jimmy Spring is the only reliable year-round source. Lamel Spring and Cooper Canyon may have water earlier in the season. Look for recent water reports at pctwater.com; click "Part Two, Idyllwild to Agua Dulce," and scroll down to mile 375.9 for Lamel Spring and 395.2 for Cooper Canyon. In a dry year, you might cache water at Vincent Gap, Islip Saddle, and Buckhorn Campground on Angeles Crest Highway (Highway 2), especially if you're leading a youth group that can't haul too much water.

Start your trip on the signed Manzanita Trail back on the campground road. This attractive but poorly named trail leads through shrub oak and birch-leaf mountain mahogany but passes very little manzanita in its entire length. The trail makes four switchbacks to climb around a sandstone outcrop. At the first switchback you'll encounter a stand of trees, mostly big-cone Douglas-fir and canyon live oak, which are codominant for the next 3 miles.

Big-cone Douglas-fir is a conifer with rows of needles on all sides of the twigs. The cones are generally 4–6 inches long, big compared only with the ordinary Douglas-firs that grow in the Sierra and northward. Nearly all of the oaks along the trail are canyon live oaks, with large acorns, flat elliptical leaves that remain on the tree year-round, and, often, many trunks from a common root. The acorns were favored by American Indians, who harvested up to 400 pounds per tree, soaked the kernels in water to leach out the bitter tannins, ground them into flour using bedrock mortars called metates, and cooked them into soup, mush, biscuits, or bread. This forest community is also associated with gnats, which don't bite but love to swarm in hikers' faces.

At 0.8 mile pass a short spur to the sandstone outcrop. It's worth walking 100 yards out to the rocks to take in the view. From here, the trail climbs at a steady grade. At 1.8 miles pass another trail descending to Paradise Springs, a private camp. Continue over a small saddle and across often-dry Big Rock Creek in Dorr Canyon. After another small saddle, pass a smaller but more reliable creek decorated with wildflowers including scarlet monkey flower and columbine. The trail follows the linear Punchbowl Fault line, and the saddles are created by the fault.

Soon you'll catch the sights and sounds of the Angeles Crest Highway bridging the canyon above, and should watch for the striking yellow blazing star flower, which is uncommon in Southern California. Observe the forest transition to white fir, Jeffrey pine, sugar pine, and incense cedar before you reach Dawson Saddle at 5.7 miles. White fir has individual needles in rows. The green cones grow upright at the tops of the trees and rarely are seen on the ground. Mistletoe infests many of the white firs in this area. Jeffrey pine has long needles in bundles of three and shapely 4- to 8-inch cones. Sugar pines have short needles in bundles of five and skinny cones of 12 inches or more in length; they often drip with sugary sap. Incense cedar has bright green scales rather than needles, ropy bark, and small seed pods rather than pine cones.

Cross the Angeles Crest Highway to a large and popular parking area at mile marker 2 LA 74.88. A picnic bench is shaded by a grove of nonnative sequoias. Several trails depart Dawson Saddle; be sure you take the PCT toward Mount Baden-Powell. This trail makes 40 switchbacks on its way up the mountain. Mount Baden-Powell is named for Lord Robert Baden-Powell, the British lieutenant-general who founded the Boy Scouts Association in 1910. At the 14th switchback (7.3 miles), a signed spur leads to Lamel Spring in a ravine, but don't rely on water here unless you have recent reports that it is running.

The switchbacks become longer. Watch for three undeveloped campsites near the 17th and 20th switchbacks. By the 17th switchback, the forest becomes almost a pure stand of lodgepole pines. These pines, which have thin, flaky bark, needles in bundles of two, and round, golf ball–size cones, are found only at high elevations in Southern California. At the 21st switchback, you'll meet two gnarled limber pines beside the trail. These pines have short needles in bundles of 5 on flexible twigs resembling bottlebrushes. The cones are longer, 3–6 inches, and resemble small sugar pine cones. The bark is thicker and the trees, which live for over 1,000 years, are often twisted by wind and ice into fantastic shapes. Limber pines, found only on the highest summits in Southern California, mingle with the lodgepoles the rest of the way up the mountain.

The switchbacks abruptly tighten, until they stop after number 38 and you get great views along the upper ridge. Reach a trail junction beside the Wally Waldron Tree, a 1,500-year-old limber pine named for a Boy Scout leader.

From the junction, stay left and continue 0.1 mile up two final switchbacks to the summit of Mount Baden-Powell (9,399', 9.6 miles). From here, you'll have exquisite views east toward Mount Baldy above the East Fork of the San Gabriel River, south over the Los Angeles Basin (as far as Catalina Island on a clear day), north over the Mojave Desert, and west over the San Gabriel Mountains where you are soon to travel. This marks the end of your long climb from the desert. You can find unsheltered campsites with breathtaking views on the ridge just south of the summit.

Return to the trail junction and turn west on the PCT. The next leg of this trip stays on or near the crest and is mostly downhill and unusually straight, so you'll cover territory quickly. At each saddle between here and Throop Peak, you'll find room for one to three tents. On a clear calm evening, these are unbeatable camping sites with the city lights far below. The trail circles the north side of Mount Burnham (8,997'), named for Lord Baden-Powell's friend and mentor who helped found the Scouting movement. On the northeast side of the mountain, at 11.1 miles, you'll find a sheltered campsite large enough for a troop of Scouts.

At 12.2 miles pass the signed Dawson Saddle Trail leading down to the saddle, where you could bail out in case of bad weather. Pass Throop Peak (9,138'), named for Amos Throop, who founded Throop University in Pasadena, which eventually became the California Institute of Technology. Next up is Mount Hawkins (8,850'), accessed by a 0.1-mile

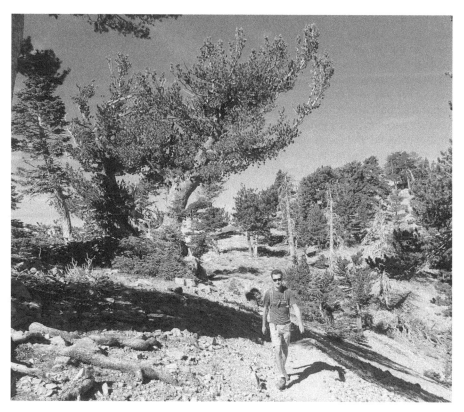

On the Pacific Crest Trail above Windy Gap

climbers' trail. At 13.7 miles pass the signed Hawkins Ridge Trail leading 0.4 mile to Middle Hawkins (8,505'); then enter a zone burned in the 2002 Curve Fire. At 14.7 miles you'll find another large campsite sheltered at the edge of the burn zone.

Descend to Windy Gap at 15.1 miles. This aptly named saddle is the lowest point in this part of the San Gabriel Mountains, and it funnels masses of air moving between the desert and Los Angeles basins. Several trails radiate from the gap. Peak-baggers could follow the 1.1-mile trail up to Mount Islip (8,250'), but this trip stays on the PCT. At 15.3 miles, a signed trail on the right leads down to Little Jimmy Spring. This reliable spring near two huge incense cedars is surrounded by wildflowers and has log benches where you can rest your legs for a bit. A trail continues from the spring and promptly rejoins the PCT, which reaches Little Jimmy Campground at 15.5 miles. The excellent campground has many large sites with picnic tables and stone fireplaces. If the sites near the trail are crowded or noisy, walk farther back to find some more secluded elevated sites. The camp and spring are named for the *Little Jimmy* comic strip, which ran in Hearst newspapers from 1904 to 1958. The cartoonist, Jimmy Swinnerton, spent summers drawing here from 1890 to 1910.

The PCT descends to Islip Saddle at 17.6 miles, where you'll cross the Angeles Crest Highway to reach another parking area and outhouse. The South Fork Trail descends the canyon on the right (a shortcut back to your vehicle, if you wish to abbreviate the loop), but this trip continues on the PCT up the shoulder of Mount Williamson. At 19.2 miles pass a trail on the right continuing 0.7 mile up to the 8,244-foot summit, but stay on the PCT, which switchbacks down to the Angeles Crest Highway at 20.7 miles.

Cross the highway and climb onto the Kratka Ridge, where you'll enjoy incredible views over the San Gabriel Wilderness and pass over the 7,515-foot high point. At 21.6 miles meet the highway yet again at Eagles Roost.

At the time of this writing, the next segment of the PCT is closed to protect habitat for the endangered mountain yellow-legged frog along Little Rock Creek. The U.S. Forest Service has proposed building a bridge to separate hikers from frogs, but if that hasn't yet happened, you'll need to carefully walk west along the shoulder of the highway to the access road for Buckhorn Campground (24.3 miles). You'll sometimes find the spigot running in the campground, and you could camp here if you don't mind the company of cars and RVs.

Follow the road to the bottom end of the campground (25.0 miles) where the Buckhorn Trail starts. Descend the unnamed creek (listen for two waterfalls) to a junction where the Burkhart Trail merges with the PCT at 26.5 miles. Turn right (east) and pass marvelous Cooper Canyon Falls; then reach a trail junction at Little Rock Creek at 26.7 miles. If the PCT has reopened, you can reach this point from Eagles Roost in only 3.3 miles.

Leave the PCT and take the northern segment of the Burkhart Trail. This area is resplendent in spring with lupine and penstemon. Make the long, hot climb to Burkhart Saddle (6,950'), at 29.8 miles, the low point on Pleasant View Ridge. If you have energy to spare, you could make a steep half-mile climb on use trails to Will Thrall Peak (7,845') or Pallett Mountain (7,760'+) for a dry camp with great views. Will Thrall is the patron saint of Southern California guidebook writers.

The conifers give way to chaparral and then desert scrub as you descend the northern slope of the San Gabriel Mountains. At 33.2 miles cross seasonal Cruthers Creek and join a ranch road; then depart on a signed trail on the right leading to Devil's Punchbowl. Climb out of the Cruthers drainage and traverse the desert slopes, watching for Jeffrey, Coulter, and pinyon pines over the beavertail cactus, sage, and manzanita. Coulters are easily recognized by their gigantic "widowmaker" cones, and also have long needles in bundles of three like the Jeffrey. Scraggly pinyon pines have single needles (not bundled) and a tennis ball–size cone with delicious pine nuts in October or November. At 35.9 miles reach a road on the left descending to Devil's Punchbowl Natural Area headquarters.

This trip stays right on the Punchbowl Trail, promptly crossing usually dry Punchbowl Creek. At 38.4 miles pass a signed trail on the left for the Devil's Chair. The short excursion to this viewpoint on an airy ridge is well worth the effort for its splendid views into the heart of the Punchbowl, where layers of sedimentary rocks have been stirred into otherworldly forms by the Punchbowl and San Andreas faults.

Continue east on the Punchbowl down to seasonal Holcomb Creek (39.1 miles), where you'll find a peaceful unimproved campsite in the woods. Then climb again to a saddle at 40.1 miles. A few switchbacks and then a straightaway take you down to the South Fork of Big Rock Creek, where you pick a path north across the wash to the trailhead parking where you began.

POSSIBLE ITINERARY			
DAY	CAMP	MILES	ELEVATION GAIN
1	Camp above Lamel Spring	8.0	3,800'
2	Little Jimmy Campground	7.5	1,800'
3	Buckhorn Campground	8.8	1,800'
4	Cruthers Creek	8.9	1,400'
5	(exit)	8.1	1,200'

trip 33.4 Santa Monica Mountains Backbone Trail

see map on p. 438

Distance	67 miles (one-way)
Elevation Gain	13,300'
Difficulty	Strenuous
Trail Use	Equestrians; certain sections are suitable for backpacking, biking, and dogs
Best Times	February–May
Agency	National Park Service
Recommended Maps	Trails Illustrated *Santa Monica Mountains National Recreation Area (253)* or Tom Harrison *Point Mugu State Park, Zuma–Trancas Canyons, Malibu Creek State Park,* and *Topanga State Park*

The Santa Monica Mountains Backbone Trail stretches 67 miles from Point Mugu State Park to Will Rogers State Park by way of Malibu Creek State Park; Topanga State Park; and land administered by the National Park Service (NPS), including Circle X Ranch, Zuma and Trancas Canyons, and Upper Solstice Canyon.

More than 50 years in the making, the last segment of this National Recreation Trail was completed in 2016. The trail visits much of the best scenery in the Santa Monica Mountains, including the highest peaks, ocean views, rocky outcrops, wooded canyons with hidden creeks, and miles of chaparral-blanketed mountains.

The trail is constantly climbing or descending as it hugs the undulating spine of the range, so even though the highest point is only 3,111 feet at Sandstone Peak, the elevation change per mile is much higher than that of other long-distance trails.

At present, the Backbone Trail is more practical for day hikes than thru-hiking because long stretches lack legal campsites or overnight trailhead parking, although the NPS is planning to open more camping facilities. Thus, this trip description is divided into multiple segments between roads.

The hike can be done in either direction but is described from west to east. Although it can be done any time of year, the summer can be unpleasantly hot. February–May offers the most wildflowers and greenery. Dogs are prohibited in the state park sections, and cyclists are prohibited on certain parts.

DIRECTIONS

Ray Miller Trailhead From Highway 1 at mile marker 001 VEN 5.9, turn north into Point Mugu State Park. Parking fee ($12).

Mishe Mokwa Trailhead From Highway 1 at mile marker 001 VEN 1.00, turn north onto Yerba Buena Road and proceed 6.4 miles to the Mishe Mokwa Trailhead.

Encinal Trailhead From Highway 1, 0.5 mile west of mile marker 001 LA 59.00, turn north onto Encinal Canyon Road. Proceed 9 miles to the Backbone crossing near mile 2.45.

Kanan Trailhead From Highway 1 at mile marker 001 LA 54.00, turn north onto Kanan Dume Road and proceed 4.5 miles to the trailhead at mile marker 9.62.

Latigo Trailhead From Highway 1 just east of mile marker 001 LA 51.00, turn north onto Latigo Canyon Road and proceed 7.3 miles to the dirt parking area on the right.

Corral Canyon Trailhead From Highway 1 just west of mile marker 001 LA 50.0, turn north onto Corral Canyon Road and proceed 5.4 miles to the trailhead parking area just after the road turns to dirt.

Tapia Trailhead From Highway 1 at mile 48.17, turn north onto Malibu Canyon Road and proceed 4.1 miles to the trailhead. Parking fee ($12).

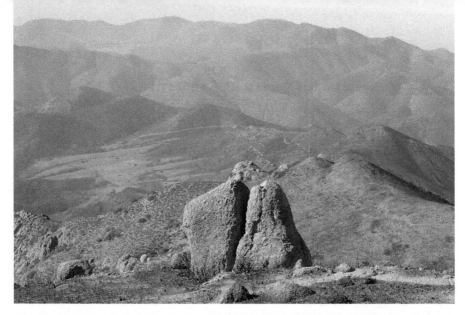

Chamberlain Rock stands out from the bare earth after the Woolsey Fire burned away the chaparral.

Lois Ewen Overlook From Highway 1 near mile marker 001 LA 44.0, turn north onto Los Flores Canyon Road. In 3.5 miles turn right on Rambla Pacifico Street. In 0.6 mile turn right on Schueren Road. In 1.8 miles reach the overlook parking area on the crest.

Dead Horse Trailhead From Highway 1 at mile 40.77, turn north onto Topanga Canyon Boulevard. Proceed 4.8 miles to a parking area on the wide shoulder at mile marker 4.80 opposite Greenleaf Canyon Road. If there is no space here, you can go 0.1 mile up Entrada Road to the official Dead Horse Trailhead lot with pay parking ($10).

Will Rogers Trailhead From Highway 1 a third of a mile west of mile marker 001 LA 39.0, turn east onto Sunset Boulevard and proceed 3.8 miles to Will Rogers State Park. Parking fee ($12).

| **trip 33.4** | **SEGMENT A: Ray Miller Trailhead to Mishe Mokwa Trailhead** |

see map on p. 438

Distance	16.1 miles (one-way)
Elevation Gain/Loss	4,300'/2,100'
Trail Use	Suitable for backpacking, equestrians

This is the longest roadless stretch of the Backbone Trail. Start eastbound on the Ray Miller Trail, which winds up onto a ridge. This area burned in the 2013 Spring Fire. (Ray Miller was California's first official state campground host, serving here from 1979 until his death in 1989.) On the crest, stay left onto the Overlook Fire Road, which leads north. Turn right onto Wood Canyon Vista Trail and descend into Big Sycamore Canyon. Follow the fire road up the canyon. For some reason, the official Backbone route bypasses the more-direct Old Boney Trail and continues north to Danielson Ranch Group Campground, 7.7 miles from the start. If this segment is too long to do in a day, you may be able to stay at the campground with advance permission from the park ranger; call 818-880-0363.

The biggest climb of the Backbone Trail begins here. Ascend Blue Canyon to reach the edge of the 2018 Woolsey Fire burn area, near another junction with the Old Boney Trail. Where the Old Boney Trail turns west, go east on the Chamberlain Trail. When you finally reach the top in the Boney Mountain area, stay right at two junctions with the Tri-Peaks Trail loop. Pass Sandstone Peak, the high point of the Santa Monica Mountains and a worthy short detour if you have the energy. Pass a trail on the right down to the Sandstone Peak Trailhead. Most parties will get off the Backbone Trail here to detour to the Circle X Group Campground, west of the trailhead via Yerba Buena Road. Otherwise, stay left on the Backbone Trail, which continues to the Mishe Mokwa Trailhead on Yerba Buena Road.

trip 33.4   SEGMENT B: **Mishe Mokwa Trailhead to Encinal Trailhead**

see map on p. 438

Distance	10.1 miles (one-way)
Elevation Gain/Loss	1,000'/1,300'
Trail Use	Suitable for mountain biking, equestrians, dogs permitted

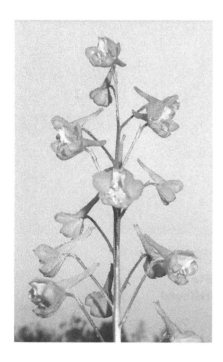

This stretch is noteworthy for its expansive views down the Arroyo Sequit Watershed. The 4.1-mile Triunfo Pass segment was the last stretch of the trail to be completed, when the land was acquired in 2016. The Backbone Trail initially parallels Yerba Buena Road on the south side, then crosses to the north side to join the old dirt Etz Meloy Motorway, named for an early homesteader. Watch for redshank, a tall, peeling, red-barked chaparral shrub that is found only in this area and along the Peninsular Ranges. It switchbacks down to cross Mulholland Highway at 8.9 miles (poor parking). Pay attention to stay on the Backbone Trail as it passes some spurs before reaching the Encinal Trailhead.

The Trans-Catalina Trail has exceptional spring wildflowers, such as this scarlet larkspur (Delphinium cardinale).

trip 33.4   SEGMENT C: **Encinal Trailhead to Kanan Trailhead**

see map on p. 438

Distance	4.9 miles (one-way)
Elevation Gain/Loss	1,100'/1,100'
Trail Use	Suitable for mountain biking, equestrians, dogs permitted

This stretch includes another of the final segments to be completed, following a donation of a 40-acre parcel in Zuma Canyon by fitness expert Betty Weider and former governor Arnold Schwarzenegger in 2016. It features lovely oak woodlands, chaparral, and seasonal waterfalls in Zuma and Trancas Canyons (*Zuma* is the Chumash word for "abundance"). Saddle Rock is the prominent landmark north of Mulholland Highway.

trip 33.4 SEGMENT D: **Kanan Trailhead to Latigo Trailhead**

see map on p. 438

Distance	2.2 miles (one-way)
Elevation Gain/Loss	700'/200'
Trail Use	Suitable for mountain biking, equestrians, dogs permitted

This short segment climbs through coast live oak, overlooking Newton Canyon and vineyards. The high point to the east with antennas is Castro Peak (2,624'), the high point of the central Santa Monica Mountains. During the Woolsey Fire, a Los Angeles Fire Department helicopter made a daring rescue of three people and two dogs from the burning peak.

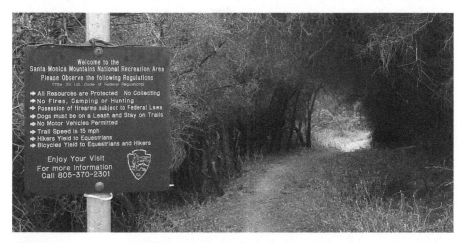

Maintaining the Backbone Trail through fast-growing chaparral is a major effort.

trip 33.4 SEGMENT E: **Latigo Trailhead to Corral Canyon Trailhead**

see map on p. 438

Distance	4.0 miles (one-way)
Elevation Gain/Loss	800'/800'
Trail Use	Suitable for mountain biking, equestrians, dogs permitted

This segment traverses south of Castro Crest, visiting two canyons with riparian woodlands. The spring wildflowers, particularly sticky monkey flower, can be remarkable. This area was hit particularly hard by the Woolsey Fire and will take time to recover. The top of the mountain is on private property and closed to visitors. Cyclists should use caution toward other travelers on the steep mountainside.

trip 33.4 SEGMENT F: **Corral Canyon Trailhead to Tapia Trailhead**

see map on p. 438

Distance	5.4 miles (one-way)
Elevation Gain/Loss	600'/2,100'
Trail Use	Suitable for mountain biking, equestrians

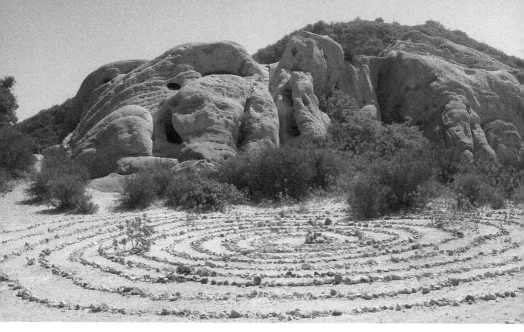

Somebody put a lot of work into this spiral labyrinth near Corral Canyon.

This segment starts with one of the most scenic parts of the trail, following a narrow ridge studded with fascinating sandstone fins (cyclists and equestrians must bypass this portion on the road below). The well-known Corral Canyon Cave on the north slope is presently closed due to graffiti vandalism, but it is still enjoyable to scramble on other rocks if you have the time. The trail then joins Mesa Peak Motorway on the long backbone ridge with terrific ocean views to the south. Look north into Malibu Creek State Park's Udell Gorge by the Goat Buttes. The 1930s *Tarzan* movies and *Planet of the Apes* were filmed here, while *M*A*S*H* was filmed just west of the buttes. Watch for fossils from an ancient seabed in the sandstone. Pass a 2,049-foot hill topped with a distinctive sandstone boulder. In 2015, the hill was renamed McAuley Peak in honor of Milt McAuley, a longtime Santa Monica Mountains guidebook author and trails advocate. Just beyond, come to a hairpin turn by a spur road to Mesa Peak just before switchbacking down to the Tapa Trailhead on Malibu Canyon Road.

This marks the end of your time in the Woolsey Fire burn area. If you're looking for a place to sleep, you can follow Malibu Canyon Road or a confusing trail west of the road north to Malibu Creek State Park, where you'll find a large (and expensive) campground.

---

trip 33.4   SEGMENT G: **Tapia Trailhead to Lois Ewen Overlook**

see map on p. 438

Distance   7.1 miles (one-way)
Elevation Gain/Loss   2,500'/600'
Trail Use   Suitable for equestrians (some sections are narrow)

This section features a demanding climb up Saddle Peak through intriguing sandstone formations. The first challenge is to get established on the trail. From the Tapia Trailhead, the official but vague trail wanders north through the brush west of Malibu Canyon Road. It fords Malibu Creek (sometimes impassible during high water) and crosses under the road before turning east along the south side of Piuma Road. If you can't find the route

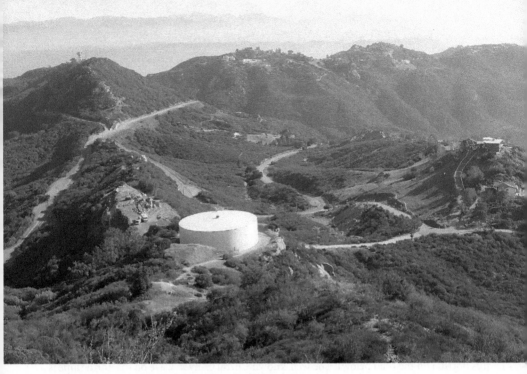

A view east from Saddle Peak toward Lois Ewen Overlook

or ford the creek, you can take your chances walking north on the shoulder of fast-moving Malibu Canyon Road and crossing at the Piuma Road traffic signal.

The trail closely parallels Piuma Road for some time before veering away and passing the California Wildlife Center and a residential area. At 2.1 miles cross Piuma Road at a hairpin turn. Limited parking can be found nearby. Be sure to stay on the Backbone Trail as you pass some unauthorized trails coming up from the houses of Monte Nido. Enjoy a brief foray through Dark Canyon along a creek and through riparian woods before embarking on countless switchbacks up Saddle Peak through chaparral and weathered sandstone. This beautiful and timeless section of trail was built in 1990 by the California Conservation Corps. At 1,975 feet, pass a short connecting trail on the left to a trailhead on Stunt Road.

The Backbone Trail soon turns south and passes Gateway Rock and the Rock Garden and an elfin forest of manzanita. You can take a 0.2-mile detour on the Summit Spur Trail to the 2,700-foot East Summit of Saddle Peak, the easternmost high summit in the Santa Monica Mountains. Back at the spur intersection, the Backbone Trail descends east to the Lois Ewen Overlook at the three-way junction of Schueren, Stunt, and Saddle Peak Roads. Mayor Lois Ewen was a founding board member of the Mountains Restoration Trust that has acquired and protected land in the Santa Monica Mountains since 1981.

trip 33.4 SEGMENT H: Lois Ewen Overlook to Dead Horse Trailhead

Distance	4.9 miles (one-way)
Elevation Gain/Loss	400'/2,000'
Trail Use	Suitable for equestrians

see map on p. 438

This section features a gorgeous descent of Hondo Canyon. It begins on the Fossil Ridge Trail paralleling Saddle Peak Road. The 30- to 40-million-year-old Sespe Formation sandstone holds marine fossils including pectin shells, though you'll need a keen eye to spot them from the trail. You're more likely to see graffiti that mars the abandoned microwave tower and rocks near the trail.

The trail then veers away from the road and begins a switchbacking descent through Hondo Canyon. (*Hondo* is Spanish for "deep," a fitting name for this area.) Oak-and-bay forest mixes with chaparral-clad slopes and trickling streams. At the bottom of the canyon, ford Old Topanga Canyon Creek and cross the road (parking available). Climb onto low Henry Ridge, where you meet Topanga School Road/Henry Ridge Motorway by a water tank. Turn left onto the road, go 0.1 mile, and then turn right where the Backbone Trail resumes.

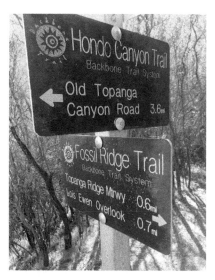

The National Park Service signage along the Backbone Trail is much better than you'll find elsewhere in Southern California.

The next portion above the school has a poorly marked maze of trails. Immediately pass a trail on the left climbing Henry Ridge, then two trails on the right to Topanga School. Descend to Green Leaf Canyon Road, where you turn right. Promptly reach and cross busy Topanga Canyon Road. You'll find trailhead parking here on the shoulder or the Dead Horse parking lot 0.1 mile up Entrada Road.

trip 33.4   SEGMENT I: **Dead Horse Trailhead to Will Rogers Trailhead**

see map on p. 438

Distance	12.2 miles (one-way)
Elevation Gain/Loss	1,900'/2,300'
Trail Use	Suitable for backpacking, equestrians

This long but mellow easternmost stretch of the Backbone follows trails and fire roads through Topanga and Will Rogers State Parks. Highlights include Eagle Rock, Chicken Ridge Bridge, and the Will Rogers mansion. The trail portion west of Eagle Junction is closed to mountain bikers, but cyclists can park at Trippet Ranch, then ride the Eagle Springs Fire Road to Eagle Junction and join the Backbone Trail the rest of the way to Will Rogers.

From the shoulder of Topanga Canyon Boulevard, follow the Backbone Trail as it climbs 0.1 mile to the Dead Horse parking area. Beware of spur trails leading to nearby neighborhoods. Cross an unusual band of black basalt rock, pass a house close by the trail, and cross a bridge over Trippet Creek. Pass the signed 92 Trail on the right and come to a junction with a narrow paved road just north of the Trippet Ranch Visitor Center at the Topanga State Park headquarters. Judge Oscar Trippet acquired this cattle ranch in 1917, and the state bought the land in the 1960s to preserve it for recreation and open space.

Turn left (north) on the paved road and follow it briefly before veering off to the right onto Musch Trail. Go about 2 miles and reach Musch Camp, which has toilets and running water. Continue to four-way Eagle Junction, where you turn sharply left up the Eagle Springs

Fire Road that passes next to Eagle Rock (consider a short detour to the summit). Next is Hub Junction, another four-way intersection. Stay right, pass Cathedral Rock, and come to a junction by Temescal Peak (2,126'). The summit is a short detour, but the views are scarcely better than from the trail.

Leave the Temescal Ridge Road and turn left to stay on the Backbone, which loops north and east before turning south down a long ridge. The monotony is broken by Lone Oak, a massive coast live oak offering shade and a good rest spot. Watch for a trail on the left into Rustic Canyon; then come to Chicken Ridge, a narrow fin separating Rivas and Rustic Canyons. Will Rogers must have had an exciting time riding his horse along this crest, but it is now spanned by Chicken Ridge Bridge, complete with guard rails.

You soon reach a T-junction with a road by Inspiration Point at the top of Will Rogers State Park. Consider a brief detour to the crowded lookout point; then take the west road. Midway down, watch for the Lower Betty Rogers Trail, which shortcuts a long bend in the road. Emerge at the lawn just above the house where the Backbone Trail concludes.

THRU-HIKING ITINERARY

The Backbone Trail is short of adequate camping, and camping is prohibited outside of designated sites. The following west–east itinerary is a legal route, but it involves some long days and one hotel stay.

Circle X Ranch (12896 Yerba Buena Road; 877-444-6777, 805-370-2301, recreation.gov /camping/campgrounds/233381) is a group campground 1.7 miles off the Backbone Trail. Contact the campground regarding your thru-hiking intentions, and request a waiver to reserve a single site.

From the Kanan Trailhead, you may be able to hail a ride to a hotel where you've previously made a room reservation. **Calamigos Ranch** (327 Latigo Canyon Road; 818-889-6280,

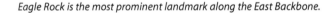

Eagle Rock is the most prominent landmark along the East Backbone.

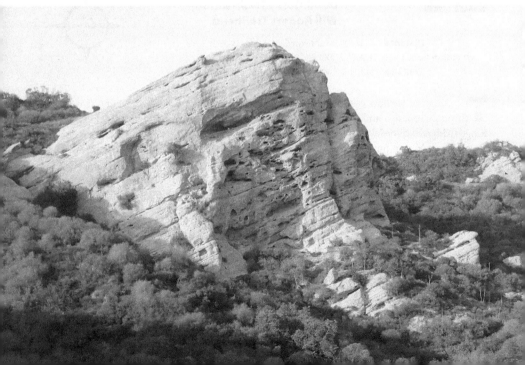

calamigos.com) has high-end accommodations just 1.4 miles north of the trail. **Homewood Suites by Hilton Agoura Hills** (28901 Canwood St.; 818-865-1000, tinyurl.com/homewood suitesagoura) is more reasonably priced. Or perhaps a friend could give you a ride home and back to the trail the next day.

Malibu Creek State Park Campground is 1.5 miles north of the Backbone Trail; for reservations, go to reservecalifornia.com. **Topanga State Park's Musch Trail Camp** has eight sites directly on the trail (no vehicle access), but they're first come, first served only.

The + numbers in the mileages below indicate extra walking to and from campgrounds off the Backbone Trail.

SUGGESTED ITINERARY			
DAY	CAMP	MILES	ELEVATION GAIN
1	Circle X Ranch Group Campground	16.1 + 1.7	4,300'
2	Kanan Trailhead (drive to hotel)	1.7 + 15.2	2,100'
3	Malibu Creek State Park Campground	11.6 + 1.5	2,100'
4	Musch Trail Camp	1.5 + 13.4	3,300'
5	(exit)	10.8	1,500'

trip 33.5   Trans-Catalina Trail

see map on p. 438

Distance   38.5 miles (one-way)
Hiking Time   4–5 days
Elevation Gain 8,000'
Difficulty   Strenuous
Trail Use   Suitable for backpacking
Best Times   October–May, closed during and after rainstorms
Agency   Catalina Island Conservancy
Recommended Map *Catalina Island Trail Map*
Fees/Permits   Free permit and camping reservations required; both are available at The Trailhead visitor center

DIRECTIONS This trip requires a 75-minute ferry ride from San Pedro to Avalon and a return ferry from Two Harbors. The *Catalina Express* ferry schedule changes seasonally and on weekends—in winter, there may be only one ferry a day from Two Harbors and none at all on Tuesdays and Thursdays. The fare is presently $37.25 each way; check current schedules at catalinaexpress.com.

Catalina Express parking is located at Berth 95 in San Pedro. From the 110 Freeway, take Exit 1A for Highway 47. Take an immediate exit onto Harbor Boulevard, and then continue straight on Swinford Street to the ferry terminal. Camping fuel is prohibited on the ferry, but you can purchase all kinds of fuel at Chet's Hardware in Avalon or the General Store in Two Harbors.

The Trans-Catalina Trail is an increasingly popular backpacking trip across the length of California's most visited Channel island. It traverses diverse scenery, from view-rich ridges to secluded coves to intimate woodlands. You'll likely encounter bison and deer along the trail (give them plenty of space!), and you might see the Catalina Island fox and other endemic species. The campgrounds along the trail are some of the most memorable (and expensive) in California. This trip is far more than the sum of its parts. While portions involve walking dusty fire roads or traversing weedy hillsides, the experience of hiking the entire island and seeing it from so many perspective is unforgettable.

Go during cool weather; the beaches are appealing in the summer, but the interior is too hot for enjoyable hiking. Carry at least 3 quarts of water between campgrounds, or more

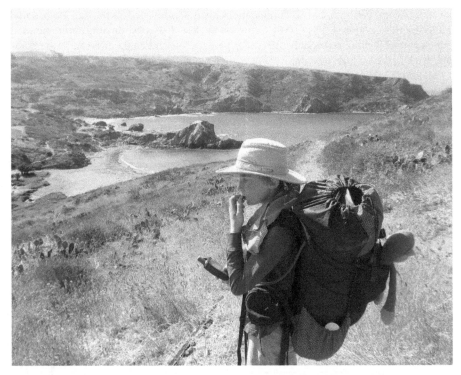

Little Harbor is a delightful respite after the dry grasslands of the Trans-Catalina Trail.

on a hot day. Some portions of the trail are very steep, and trekking poles may be useful. Hiking at night is prohibited.

A free hiking permit is required and can be obtained online at the Catalina Island Conservancy website or at the visitor centers. Expensive camping permits are required in advance for each campsite and are obtained by calling Two Harbors Visitor Services (310-510-4205). Some campgrounds have two-night minimum stays, but these are waived for Trans-Catalina hikers. Campsites fill up, so make your reservation well in advance. Parsons Landing lacks tap water, but you can request a water jug and/or firewood for a fee as part of your camping reservation.

Start at The Trailhead, the Catalina Conservancy's visitor center, near the boat landing in Avalon. Here you can pick up your permit, buy a map, or inquire about current conditions.

The first leg of the trip follows paved Avalon Canyon Road from the back of town to Hermit's Gulch Campground, at 1.5 miles. You can walk the road or take the Avalon Transit Garibaldi Bus, which loops through town. If you arrive on the afternoon ferry, you might want to spend the first night at Hermits Gulch and make a side trip to the Wrigley Memorial and Botanic Garden.

From the top of the campground, follow the Hermit Gulch Trail as it switchbacks up through chaparral and wildflowers. At 3.2 miles reach Divide Road, where you turn right (north). Enjoy excellent views of Avalon Bay from the ridge. At 5.0 miles veer left onto a trail that leads to the small Haypress Reservoir. Circle around the north side of the lake to Haypress Recreation Area at 5.6 miles, where you'll find tap water, restrooms, and picnic tables beside a playground. Be sure you have plenty of water because the stretch ahead can be hot.

The trail briefly follows the reservoir before turning north and rejoining Airport Road at 6 miles. At 6.5 miles, near a viewpoint, turn left onto singletrack. The next stretch of undulating but scenic trail crosses three lightly used roads and the Skull Ridge Trail before reaching Black Jack Campground at 10.5 miles. Here you'll find tap water, restrooms, and a cold shower at the large campsite nestled in a pleasant grove of oaks and conifers.

Follow trail signs carefully as you climb through a maze of roads between Black Jack Mountain (2,010') and Mount Orizaba (2,102'). Orizaba, the highest point on the island, is easily recognized from afar by its flat summit, bulldozed to hold a white bowling pin-shaped aircraft radio beacon. At 11.5 miles, beyond the saddle, the route leaves Upper Cottonwood Road and becomes a steep but scenic singletrack dropping north into Cottonwood Canyon and climbing back toward a mesa where Airport in the Sky is situated. Turn left near the old soapstone quarry and meet Airport Road just outside the airport, at 12.8 miles. Consider stopping at the DC3 Grill at the airport for their famous buffalo burger or just to refill your water bottle.

Pass under a decorative Western arch and join the trail that circles the west end of the airport. At 13.7 miles join Empire Landing Road near Buffalo Springs Reservoir. Turn left and head west on this dull and dusty road. At 15.0 miles be sure to pick up the singletrack on the left descending Big Springs Ridge. Your long descent is rewarded by reaching Little Harbor, one of the most scenic parts of the island. At the bottom of the trail, jog right on Isthmus Road, then left on the trail to reach the corner of the Little Harbor Campground, at 19.0 miles. This jewel of a campground fronting a sandy beach is shaded by palms and has water, restrooms, and cold showers. Beware that sting rays frequent the harbor; if you go in the water, shuffle your feet to warn them you are coming and avoid stepping on one. With (expensive) advance reservations through Wet Spot Rentals (310-510-2229, wetspotrentals .com), you can rent kayaks here and explore the windward side of the island on a layover day.

The signed Trans-Catalina Trail switchbacks up to the northeast above the campground. The first several hundred yards have some of the best photo opportunities on the whole trail. Send your photographer ahead to capture the rest of the group hiking up a switchback with Little Harbor in the background. The trail is steep and rough in places as it climbs

The higher peaks of Catalina often rise out of the marine layer blanketing the Pacific Ocean.

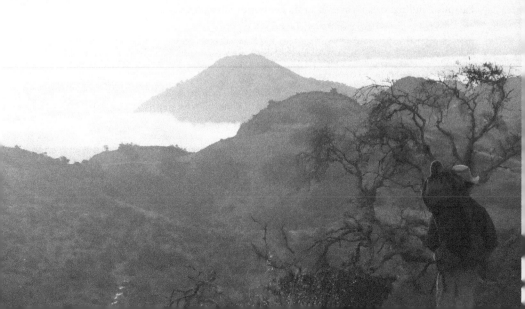

to a high ridge, where you may appreciate a shade structure at a vista point at 21.7 miles. Now continuing on a dirt road, follow the ridge north to meet Banning House Road at 22.4 miles. Turn left and descend the steep road to the small town of Two Harbors (24.2 miles), on a narrow bridge of land between Isthmus Cove and Catalina Harbor.

In Two Harbors, you could enjoy a hot meal at one of several restaurants, resupply on groceries or hiking gear at the General Store, lounge on the beach, or spend a night at the Two Harbors Campground or at the historic Banning House Lodge bed-and-breakfast. The Visitor Services office at the foot of the pier is staffed by knowledgeable rangers who can help with last-minute permits (if available) or answer questions about the sights you've seen. If you want to shorten your trip, you can catch the ferry back to San Pedro from here.

Otherwise, complete the Trans-Catalina Trail around the west end of the island on fire roads by way of Parsons Landing campsite. Return to the south end of town where the signed Trans-Catalina Trail resumes, following the west shore of Catalina Harbor before climbing steeply onto the ridge. At 28.7 miles reach a road junction. If you're looking for a side trip, you could continue west on Silver Peak Road for 1.0 mile to Silver Peak, which, at 1,804 feet, is the highest point on the west end of the island. From here, you could continue 2.8 miles farther to Starlight Beach on the rocky, lonely coast near the extreme west end. The Trans-Catalina Trail, however, turns north and descends Fenceline Road.

At 30.0 miles turn left; then, at 30.4 miles, turn right and descend to Parsons Landing, at 30.8 miles. This spectacular campground is right on the sandy beach. You'll hear the sea lions barking in the surf and will have spectacular sunsets followed by million-dollar views of the Palos Verdes lights across the channel. There is no tap water, but you may request as part of your reservation that the rangers leave a water jug for you in the locker. With a layover day here, you could enjoy the ocean or hike out to Starlight Beach.

When you're ready to loop back to Two Harbors, find the signed Trans-Catalina Trail leading east. At 31.3 miles it joins West End Road. Follow this road east as it contours 100–200 feet above the ocean, dipping in and out of coves and ravines and passing several youth camps. Watch for dolphins playing off the coast. The last stretch has great views of Isthmus Cove. Follow the trail into town, where your journey is complete at 38.5 miles. You may have time to stop at a restaurant or relax on the beach before your ferry back to San Pedro.

If you have more time, you can add a day at Two Harbors between Little Harbor and Parsons Landing, or a layover at Little Harbor or Parsons Landing.

POSSIBLE FOUR-DAY ITINERARY			
DAY	CAMP	MILES	ELEVATION GAIN
1	Blackjack	10.7	3,000'
2	Little Harbor	8.2	1,000'
3	Parsons Landing	11.9	3,600'
4	Two Harbors	7.7	400'

POSSIBLE FIVE-DAY ITINERARY			
DAY	CAMP	MILES	ELEVATION GAIN
1	Blackjack	10.7	3,000'
2	Little Harbor	8.2	1,000'
3	Two Harbors	5.3	1,600'
4	Parsons Landing	6.6	2,000'
5	Two Harbors	7.7	400'

trip 33.6   San Gabriel River Trail

Distance	38 miles
Elevation Loss	700'
Difficulty	Strenuous
Trail Use	Suitable for mountain biking, equestrians, dogs allowed
Best Times	October–June
Agency	Los Angeles County Parks & Recreation
Maps	Interactive trail map at tinyurl.com/sgrtmap

see map on p. 438

DIRECTIONS This trail starts at the San Gabriel Canyon Gateway Center on Highway 39 in Azusa and ends at First Street in Seal Beach; the locations of trailheads along the path are provided in the description.

The smoothly paved San Gabriel River Trail runs 38 miles from the mouth of the San Gabriel River canyon in Azusa to the Pacific Ocean in Seal Beach. This popular trail attracts legions of road bikers, along with joggers, equestrians, and families. It traverses a fascinating cross-section of Los Angeles County, from sage scrub at the foothills to stables, backyards, industrial zones, manicured parks, busy freeways, wilderness areas, and homeless encampments. The upper river runs free until the massive flood-control basin behind the Santa Fe Dam. Most of the river then runs underground beneath a concrete channel that is designed to take floodwaters to the sea. The river emerges again near the ocean, and you might see green sea turtles plying the waters. While the concrete river channel is often dry, it deserves a healthy respect when it's flowing strong. The trail closes during storms.

The San Gabriel River Trail is part of the Emerald Necklace Regional Park Network. The Emerald Necklace aims to preserve and restore the Los Angeles and San Gabriel watersheds, rivers, and tributaries for recreation, habitat, conservation, and education.

Cyclists often ride the entire way, while joggers and equestrians are more likely to pick a shorter segment. The trail has very few street crossings, so cyclists can maintain their speed. Fit road bikers may ride the distance in 2 hours, while occasional riders might wish to plan 4–5 hours, with breaks in the parks along the way. Southbound riders usually face a headwind from the on-shore breeze, while northbound riders have 500 feet of elevation gain to reach Azusa. The fittest riders go out and back in a day, but you can also set up

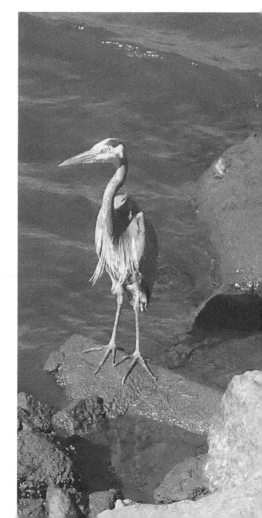

A California brown pelican chills out at the mouth of the San Gabriel River.

a car shuttle or spend 3–4 hours on public transit to close the loop: take the bus to Long Beach, the Metro Blue Line to downtown Los Angeles, the Red Line (or bike) past City Hall to Union Station, the Gold Line to the Azusa Downtown Station, and finally bike back to your starting point.

The waypoints below include many parks and access points so that you could go the whole distance or plan a shorter trip along any segment of the trail. Numbers painted on the pavement will help you track your progress.

MILE	NOTES
37.7	**SAN GABRIEL CANYON GATEWAY CENTER** 1960 San Gabriel Canyon Road (Highway 39), Azusa. Restrooms, limited parking, friendly volunteer rangers. The Azusa BikeTrail forks left near here. It's possible to follow the San Gabriel River Trail upstream 0.7 mile to a dead end with no parking, but this trip starts downstream.
37.4	**AZUSA BIKETRAIL TRAILHEAD PARKING LOT** San Gabriel Canyon Road (Highway 39) at Ranch Road, Azusa. More parking 0.1 mile southwest of San Gabriel Canyon Gateway Center (see above). Backtrack north on the Azusa BikeTrail to join the San Gabriel River Trail opposite Gateway Center.
35.6	**ENCHANTO PARK TRAILHEAD** 777 Enchanto Parkway, Duarte. Take the 1907 Puente Largo Bridge across the river to park on the street near Enchanto Park and the Duarte Historical Society.
35.3	**LARIO PARK STAGING AREA** 3089 E. Huntington Drive, Irwindale
34.5	**210 FREEWAY UNDERPASS**
33.3	**SANTA FE DAM NATURE CENTER** 15501 E. Arrow Highway, Irwindale. Nature trail nearby.
32.4	**SANTA FE DAM RECREATIONAL AREA ENTRY STATION** 15501 E. Arrow Highway, Irwindale. $10 entry fee for cars; swimming beach, playground, picnic area, restrooms.
30.2	**EMERALD NECKLACE BIKE TRAIL** This 1.1-mile trail leads from Arrow Highway to City of Hope hospital and the Duarte Gold Line Metro station.
29.8	**SANTA FE DAM PARKING** 1636 Arrow Highway, Irwindale. Look for street parking below dam near a pocket park on the San Gabriel River Trail.
28.8	**605 FREEWAY UNDERPASS**
25.7	**10 FREEWAY UNDERPASS**
23.0	**60 FREEWAY UNDERPASS**
22.5	**WHITTIER NARROWS NATURE CENTER TRAIL** 1000 N. Durfee Ave., El Monte. This spur trail leads to the nature center.
21.5	**RIO HONDO TRAIL CONNECTOR** Access this signed spur to the Rio Hondo Trail just before the trail crosses the Whittier Narrows Dam.
20.9	**PICO RIVERA BIKE STOP** Pico Rivera Golf Club, 3260 Fairway Drive, Pico Rivera. Water, tools, and a snack bar are available at this biker-friendly golf course.
20.5	**CROSS TO EAST SIDE** At San Gabriel River Parkway, turn left and follow the road bridge over the river; the San Gabriel River Trail resumes on the east side.
19.7	**WHITTIER GREENWAY TRAIL** A signed trail on the left leads 4.5 miles along an abandoned Union Pacific Railroad right-of-way.
15.5	**SANTA FE SPRINGS PARK** 10068 Cedardale Drive, Santa Fe Springs
15.3	**5 FREEWAY UNDERPASS**
14.7	**WILDERNESS PARK** 10999 Little Lake Road, Downey
13.0	**105 FREEWAY UNDERPASS**
10.3	**91 FREEWAY UNDERPASS**
8.8	**LIBERTY PARK** 19211 Studebaker Road, Cerritos
7.3	**RYNERSON PARK** 20711 Studebaker Road, Lakewood
5.8	**EL DORADO EAST REGIONAL PARK** 7550 E. Spring St., Long Beach. Entry fee for cars (varies; check tinyurl.com/eldoradoeast for details).
4.1	**COYOTE CREEK TRAIL JUNCTION** A signed trail on the left leads about 10 miles to Santa Fe Springs.
3.5	**405 FREEWAY UNDERPASS**
2.6	**22 FREEWAY UNDERPASS**
0.0	**FIRST STREET PARKING LOT** 95 First St., Seal Beach

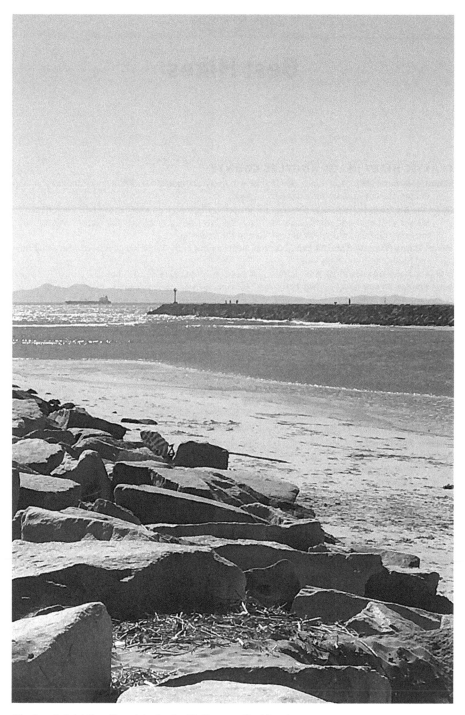

The San Gabriel River flows into the Pacific Ocean at Seal Beach.

Best Hikes

CLASSIC HIKES IN LOS ANGELES COUNTY

Mount Hollywood (Trip 14.3) Enjoy views of the HOLLYWOOD sign and Griffith Observatory as you loop through the city's largest and most famous park.

Down the Arroyo Seco (Trip 23.2) Descend the historic trail through an iconic canyon. In the spring, enjoy the waterfall and wildflowers. In the fall, brightly colored sycamores and maples contrast with the somber browns and greens of the oaks and the chaparral.

Mount Wilson (Trips 24.8 and 24.13) This prominent summit of the Front Range is laced with delightful and historic trails on every side.

Bridge to Nowhere (Trip 29.4) A beautiful canyon walk to a testament of man's hubris.

Mount Baden-Powell Traverse (Trip 29.9) The 360° view encompasses mountains, deserts, and the ocean.

Cucamonga Peak (Trip 30.7) From shady brook to high mountain crest, Cucamonga offers a complete mountain experience.

The Three Ts (Trip 30.9) Three alliterating peaks with great views over the high country.

Baldy Loop (Trip 30.11) An obligatory climb, 10,064-foot Old Baldy is the highest point in the San Gabriel Mountains as well as in Los Angeles County.

BEST BEACH HIKE

Point Dume to Paradise Cove (Trip 1.1) During the lowest of low tides, the Point Dume coastline offers up the finest array of tide-pool life in the county.

BEST SUBURBAN HIKES

Paradise Falls (Trip 3.2) A glorious waterfall hidden in an intimate little gorge.

Los Padres Loop (Trip 3.3) A popular loop with oaks and views.

Santa Clarita Woodlands (Trips 5.11–5.13) Lush woods and trickling streams just beyond the San Fernando Valley.

Will Rogers Park (Trip 10.7) Ocean and city lie at your feet on this island of open space on L.A.'s West Side.

Placerita Canyon (Trip 12.3) This quiet, woodsy retreat is only a few minutes away from the San Fernando Valley.

Ben Overturff Trail (Trip 18.2) Serene and pristine canyon country, just uphill from the San Gabriel Valley.

Upper Marshall Canyon (Trip 19.3) Hike through two of the best-preserved canyons of the San Gabriel foothills.

Millard Canyon (Trips 23.15 and 23.16) A deep, shady cleft graced by a small stream and a 50-foot waterfall, barely 10 minutes by car from the edge of Pasadena and other suburbs nearby.

BEST MOUNTAIN HIKES

Strawberry Peak (Trip 23.8) A fun and airy climb up the west ridge.

Mount Hillyer (Trip 25.3) A mellow climb through pines and granite boulders reminiscent of the Sierra Nevada Mountains.

Mount Islip (Trips 26.2 and 26.4) Great views and a good workout on a fun mountain.

Mount Hawkins Loop (Trip 26.5) Ever-changing scenery above the Crystal Lake Basin.

Mount Waterman (Trip 27.2) A very popular rocky summit with a scenic trail through the conifers.

Winston Peak and Ridge (Trip 28.1) An easy introduction to mountain climbing. Woods, wildflowers, and interesting boulders.

Ontario Peak (Trip 30.8) Strenuous and popular trail to unsurpassed views of the Inland Empire.

BEST CANYON HIKES
The Grotto (Trip 7.4) Here, the primeval mountain and canyon country of the Santa Monica Mountains survives intact.
Zuma Canyon (Trips 8.1 and 8.2) Big-scale canyon country within a small-scale mountain range.
Lower Solstice Canyon (Trip 9.2) Alongside a trickling stream, enjoy some of the county's finest oak woodlands.
Hoegees Loop (Trip 24.10) The riparian splendor of the San Gabriels' Front Range at its best.
East Fork San Gabriel River (Trip 29.6) The East Fork has carved out the granddaddy of Southern California canyons, a mile deep as measured from the top of the east wall.
Icehouse Canyon (Trip 30.5) An easy mile or two up the tumbling Icehouse stream takes you to tall-timbered canyon recesses.

BEST WATERFALLS
Escondido Falls (Trip 9.1) By far the best waterfall in the Santa Monica Mountains.
Monrovia Canyon Falls (Trip 18.1) Easy hike along a shaded canyon stream, ending at a 40-foot cascade.
Fish Canyon Falls (Trip 18.3) A real payoff in the end when you discover a magnificent 100-foot cascade.
Trail Canyon Falls (Trip 22.2) A beautiful and unexpected find tucked amid the chaparral country of lower Big Tujunga Canyon.
Sturtevant Falls (Trip 24.11) A scenic attraction for more than a century, it's popular and easy to reach.
Cooper Canyon Falls (Trip 28.2) A small but beautiful cascade in a sublime High Country setting.
San Antonio Falls (Trip 30.10) Dependably impressive when swollen with snowmelt during spring and early summer. A very easy walk to the base.

BEST VIEW HIKES
Top of the Peninsula (Trip 2.1) Features a stunning panorama of ocean and islands on clear, winter days.
Sandstone Peak (Trip 7.5) This volcanic outcrop crowning the Santa Monica Mountains overlooks the ocean, the Channel Islands, and much of Los Angeles and Ventura Counties.
Topanga Overlook (Trip 10.4) Unbelievably spacious views of Santa Monica Bay and the ocean.
La Tuna Loop (Trip 13.4) Spectacular vistas of San Fernando Valley and all the basin-bordering mountain ranges.
Cahuenga Peak (Trip 14.1) A top-of-the-city view in every direction from over the HOLLYWOOD sign.
Inspiration Point (Trip 23.13) Summon the energy to go an extra mile to Panorama Point, where there's an even better perspective of the L.A. megalopolis below.
Echo Mountain (Trip 23.19) A quick climb to the site of historic White City overlooking coastal and urban L.A.
Twin Peaks (Trip 27.3) Some of Southern California's most wild and inaccessible terrain lies directly below these crags.
Kratka Ridge (Trip 28.4) A short ridge run that packs quite a punch, with airy views of the San Gabriel Wilderness and the basin beyond.
Lone Tree Point (Trip 31.2) The pseudo-Hawaiian vista atop Catalina's east end includes eroded palisades and the green- and blue-tinted ocean.

BEST BACKPACKING TRIPS
Silver Moccasin Trail (Trip 33.1) Classic traverse of the San Gabriel Mountains from the High Country to the Los Angeles Basin. Overlaps with Southern California's best segment of the Pacific Crest Trail. A rite of passage for thousands of Boy Scouts.
Santa Monica Mountains Backbone Trail (Trip 33.4) Recently completed trail across the length of the Santa Monica Mountains. Varied scenery including wildflowers, oaks, rock formations, ocean views, chaparral. Logistics of backpacking are difficult until more trail camps get built.
Trans-Catalina Trail (Trip 33.5) Grand tour of Southern California's most famous island. Word has gotten out, and this unique trail is drawing visitors from around the world.

BEST HISTORICAL WALKS
Old Stagecoach Road (Trip 5.5) Trace the notorious Devil's Slide segment of a 19th-century stage road linking Northern California with Southern California.
Pico Canyon (Trip 5.14) Roll the clock back a century and appreciate Southern California's early oil-drilling industry.

Mount Lowe Railway (Trip 23.20) Follow the path of more than 3 million passengers who rode rails into the sky.

BEST WILDFLOWERS

La Jolla Valley & Mugu Peak (Trip 6.3) The giant coreopsis in La Jolla Canyon are especially noteworthy.

Charmlee Wilderness Park (7.7) Wildflowers here are characteristic of grassland, chaparral, and oak-woodland habitats.

Lookout Loop (Trip 9.8) Good displays of meadow wildflowers.

Eagle Rock Loop (Trip 10.1) A broad range of wildflowers characteristic of the Santa Monica Mountains is represented here.

Antelope Valley Poppy Reserve (Trip 11.2) Iconic desert bloom in March or April after a wet winter.

Vasquez Rocks Natural Area (Trip 12.6) A convergence of three plant communities here yields a plethora of blooms during wet years.

Devil's Punchbowl (Trips 28.10–28.12) Flora from both mountain and high desert areas are represented on this trek.

BEST AUTUMN COLORS

Serrano & Big Sycamore Loop (Trip 6.5) Big Sycamore Canyon is touted as the finest example of sycamore savanna in the California State Park system.

Placerita Canyon (Trip 12.3) Willow, sycamore, cottonwood, big-leaf maple, and California walnut trees contribute various shades of yellow and rust.

Liebre Mountain (Trip 21.1) The golden leaves of the black oak, a common tree in these northern reaches of L.A. County, put on a fine autumnal show.

Bear Canyon (Trip 23.14) Alders, sycamores, and maples line the narrow canyon floor.

BEST BIRD- AND WILDLIFE-WATCHING

Cheeseboro Canyon (Trip 4.6) At dawn and at dusk, deer, bobcats, and coyotes roam the oak-dotted hills and canyon floor. Birds of prey patrol the skies.

Lost Cabin Trail (Trip 9.10) The trail probes an area set aside for special protection within Malibu Creek State Park.

Vetter Mountain (Trip 25.1) Birds and animals typical of yellow-pine forests are found here.

Santa Catalina Island (Chapters 31 and 32) Wildlife on the island includes deer, fox, and bison.

BEST MOUNTAIN BIKING

Cheeseboro and Palo Comado Canyons (Trip 4.6) Old ranch roads and an open oak forest. Cyclists stay on the doubletrack sections.

Hummingbird and Chumash Trails (Trips 5.1 and 5.2) Varied route with tough climbs, technical sections, fast portions, and intriguing rocks.

Point Mugu State Park, Sycamore Canyon (Chapter 6) Popular ride on fire road in the canyon. Gentle except for the steep stretch up to Satwiwa at the north end.

New Millennium Loop (Trip 9.14) Fun, flowing singletrack with some very tight switchbacks and intriguing views into a community of ostentatious mansions.

Mount Wilson Toll Road (Trip 24.2) Historic dirt road with great views. Good downhill ride for kids.

Blue Ridge Trail (Trip 29.15) Fast and sometimes technical descent through the pines. Make a loop by climbing the Angeles Crest Highway to Inspiration Point and then Blue Ridge Road to the top of the trail.

Gabrielino Trail (Trip 33.2) Long and challenging backcountry route, reopened after the Station Fire of 2009, thanks to great effort by mountain bike clubs.

Santa Monica Mountains Backbone Trail (Trip 33.4) Portions are open to mountain biking. The portion from Newton Canyon (Kanan Dume Road) to Corral Canyon is particularly interesting, with great views and rock formations.

BEST EPIC HIKES

Piru Creek (Trip 20.3) A demanding journey down the county's only designated Wild & Scenic River. Your trip may involve wading, swimming, and dodging rattlesnakes, poison oak, and thorn bushes as you trek to the waterfall and narrows in remote Piru Gorge.

San Antonio Ridge (Trip 30.12) L.A. County's hardest test piece, running the ridge from the county's highest peak to its most inaccessible summit, by way of airy Gunsight Notch. Tremendous views reward those who endure the journey.

Recommended Reading

Los Angeles–Area Outdoor Guidebooks

California Coastal Commission. *California Coastal Access Guide.* 7th ed. Berkeley: University of California Press, 2014.

Chamberlin, Doug and Caroline. *The Complete Hiker's Guide to the Backbone Trail.* Glendale, CA: Riviera Books, 2017.

Harris, David. *Afoot & Afield Inland Empire.* Birmingham, AL: Wilderness Press, 2018.

Harris, David. *Day & Section Hikes Pacific Crest Trail: Southern California.* Birmingham, AL: Wilderness Press, 2012.

McAuley, Milt. *Hiking Trails of the Santa Monica Mountains,* 6th ed. Los Angeles: Canyon Publishing Company, 1998.

McKinney, John. *John McKinney's New Day Hiker's Guide to Southern California.* Santa Barbara, CA: Olympus Press, 2004.

Randall, Laura, et al. *Pacific Crest Trail: Southern California.* 7th ed. Birmingham, AL: Wilderness Press, 2019.

Randall, Laura. *60 Hikes Within 60 Miles: Los Angeles.* 3rd ed. Birmingham, AL: Menasha Ridge Press, 2016.

Robinson, John W., and Doug Christiansen. *Trails of the Angeles: 100 Hikes in the San Gabriels.* 9th ed. Birmingham, AL: Wilderness Press, 2013.

Schad, Jerry, and David Harris. *101 Hikes in Southern California.* 3rd ed. Birmingham, AL: Wilderness Press, 2013.

Schad, Jerry. *Top Trails Los Angeles.* Birmingham, AL: Wilderness Press, 2010.

Schreiner, Casey. *Dayhiking Los Angeles.* Seattle: Mountaineers Books, 2016.

Stone, Robert. *Day Hikes Around Los Angeles.* 6th ed. Red Lodge, MT: Day Hike Books, 2015.

———. *Day Hikes in the Santa Monica Mountains.* Red Lodge, MT: Day Hike Books, 2012.

Ward, Sam. *Trans-Catalina and Backbone Trails.* San Diego: Sandiburg Press, 2017.

History and Natural History

Bakker, Elna S. *An Island Called California.* Berkeley: University of California Press, 1984.

Bailey, H. P. *The Climate of Southern California.* Berkeley: University of California Press, 1966.

Belzer, Thomas J. *Roadside Plants of Southern California.* Missoula, MT: Mountain Press Publishing Company, 1986.

Bortugno, E. J., and T. E. Spittler. *Geologic Map of the San Bernardino Quadrangle.* Sacramento: California Division of Mines and Geology, 1986.

Hall, Clarence A. *Introduction to the Geology of Southern California and Its Native Plants.* Berkeley: University of California Press, 2007.

Hanna, W. F., et al. *Bouguer Gravity Map of California: Los Angeles Sheet.* Sacramento: California Division of Mines and Geology, 1975.

Keator, Glenn. *Pacific Coast Fern Finder.* Birmingham, AL: Nature Study Guild Publishers, 1981.

Lederer, Roger J. *Pacific Coast Bird Finder.* Birmingham, AL: Nature Study Guild Publishers, 1977.

Mackay, Pam, and Tim Thomas. *Southern California Mountain Wildflowers.* Guilford, CT: FalconGuides, 2017.

McPhee, John. *The Control of Nature.* New York: Farrar, Straus and Giroux, 1990.

Munz, Philip A., and Dianne Lake. *Introduction to California Spring Wildflowers of the Foothills, Valleys, and Coast.* Berkeley: University of California Press, 2004.

Munz, Philip A., et. al. *Introduction to California Mountain Wildflowers, Revised Edition.* Berkeley: University of California Press, 2003.

Peterson, P. Victor. *Native Trees of Southern California.* Berkeley: University of California Press, 1966.

continued on next page

Raven, Peter H. *Native Shrubs of Southern California*. Berkeley: University of California Press, 1966.

Robinson, John W. *Mines of the East Fork*. Glendale, CA: La Siesta Press, 1980.

———. *Mines of the San Gabriels*. Glendale, CA: La Siesta Press, 1973.

———. *The San Gabriels*. Arcadia, CA: Big Santa Anita Historical Society, 1991.

Rundel, Philip W., and John Robert Gustafson. *Introduction to the Plant Life of Southern California*. Berkeley: University of California Press, 2005.

Russo, Ron, and Pam Olhausen. *Pacific Coast Mammals*. Birmingham, AL: Nature Study Guild Publishers, 1987.

Saunders, Charles F. *The Southern Sierras of California: A Complete New Edition of the 1923 Classic*. Pasadena, CA: Many Moons Press, 2014.

Schoenherr, Allan A. *A Natural History of California*. Berkeley: University of California Press, 1995.

Sharp, Robert P. *Coastal Southern California*. Dubuque, IA: Kendall/Hunt Publishing Company, 1978.

———. *Geology Field Guide to Southern California*. Dubuque, IA: William C. Brown Company, 1972.

Sharp, Robert P., and Allen F. Glazner. *Geology Underfoot in Southern California*. Missoula, MT: Mountain Press Publishing Company, 1993.

Thrall, Will, ed. *Trails Magazine*. 6 vols. Los Angeles: Los Angeles County Department of Recreation, Camps, and Playgrounds, 1934–39.

———. *Trails Magazine* (reestablished). 1 vol. Los Angeles: Southern California Outdoor Federation, 1941.

Watts, Tom. *Pacific Coast Tree Finder*. 2nd ed. Birmingham, AL: Nature Study Guild Publishers, 2004.

appendix c

Local Organizations

The three largest private environmental organizations in Los Angeles County are listed below. Scores of other organizations and outdoor groups can be found at websites such as Meetup.com.

LOS ANGELES AUDUBON SOCIETY For general information about L.A. Audubon programs and events, call 323-876-0202 or visit laaudubon.org. The **Audubon Center at Debs Park** is located at 4700 N. Griffith Ave. The visitor center is open Wednesday–Saturday, 9 a.m.–5 p.m. April–October and 8 a.m.–4 p.m. November–March; trails are open daily, sunrise–sunset; pets are prohibited. For more information, call 323-221-2255 or visit debspark.audubon.org.

THE NATURE CONSERVANCY IN CALIFORNIA For more information on the conservancy's programs and preserves in the state and L.A. County in particular, call 213-327-0104 or visit tinyurl.com /tnc-california.

SIERRA CLUB The **Angeles Chapter,** with nearly 60,000 members, has 13 regional groups, numerous standing committees, and several special activities sections. Its outings program offers more than 4,000 hikes and backpack trips each year, the majority of them in Los Angeles County. All outings are published in a three-times-yearly schedule distributed free to members and also available for purchase at outdoor-equipment stores. For more information, call 213-387-4287 or visit angeles.sierraclub.org.

Agencies & Information Sources

See trip profiles for information about fees and permits where they apply. Check the agency websites for information about parks and preserves not specifically listed here.

CALIFORNIA STATE PARKS

parks.ca.gov
Note: For camping reservations, call 800-444-7275 or visit reservecalifornia.com. Hours for the following parks are daily, 8 a.m.–sunset except as noted. Dogs are prohibited on trails except at Kenneth Hahn State Recreation Area and Santa Susana Pass and Will Rogers State Historic Parks, where they are permitted on leash.

Antelope Valley California Poppy Reserve

15101 Lancaster Road
Lancaster, CA 93536
661-724-1180, parks.ca.gov/?page_id=627
Hours: Daily, sunrise–sunset

Arthur B. Ripley Desert Woodland State Park

Lancaster Road at 205th Street West
Lancaster, CA 93536
661-946-6092, parks.ca.gov/?page_id=634
Hours: Daily, sunrise–sunset

Baldwin Hills Scenic Overlook

6300 Hetzler Road
Culver City, CA 90232
310-558-5547, parks.ca.gov/?page_id=22790
Hours: Daily, sunrise–sunset

Kenneth Hahn State Recreation Area

4100 S. La Cienega Blvd.
Los Angeles, CA 90056
323-298-3660, parks.ca.gov/?page_id=612
Hours: Daily, sunrise–sunset

Leo Carrillo State Park

35000 W. Pacific Coast Highway
Malibu, CA 90265
310-457-8143
parks.ca.gov/leocarrillo
Hours: Daily, 8 a.m.–10 p.m.

Malibu Creek State Park

1925 Las Virgenes Road
Calabasas, CA 91302
818-880-0367; parks.ca.gov/malibucreek
Hours: Daily, 8 a.m.–10 p.m.

Point Mugu State Park

9000 W. Pacific Coast Highway
Malibu, CA 90265; 310-457-8143
parks.ca.gov/pointmugu

Santa Susana Pass State Historic Park

10200 block of Larwin Avenue
Chatsworth, CA 91311
818-784-4849
parks.ca.gov/santasusana

Saddleback Butte State Park

43230 172nd St.
East Lancaster, CA 93534; 661-946-6092
parks.ca.gov/page_id=618
Hours: Daily, sunrise–sunset

Topanga State Park

20828 Entrada Road
Topanga, CA 90290; 310-455-2465
parks.ca.gov/topanga

Will Rogers State Historic Park

1501 Will Rogers State Park Road
Pacific Palisades, CA 90272; 310-230-2017
parks.ca.gov/willrogers

NATIONAL PARK SERVICE

nps.gov

Santa Monica Mountains National Recreation Area

26876 Mulholland Highway
Calabasas, CA 91302; 805-370-2300
nps.gov/samo
Hours: Visitor center open daily, 9 a.m.–5 p.m., except January 1, Thanksgiving Day, December 25, and other federal holidays; parking areas open daily, 8 a.m.–sunset except as noted above; trails open daily, 24/7. For pet policies, see nps.gov/samo/planyourvisit/pets.htm.

U.S. FOREST SERVICE
fs.usda.gov

Angeles National Forest
fs.usda.gov/angeles

HEADQUARTERS
701 N. Santa Anita Ave.
Arcadia, CA 91006
626-574-1613
Hours: Monday–Friday, 8 a.m.–4:30 p.m.

Chilao Visitor Center
Angeles Crest Highway (CA 2)
La Cañada Flintridge, CA 91011
626-796-5541
Hours: Saturday–Sunday, 9 a.m.–4 p.m.

Grassy Hollow Visitor Center
Angeles Crest Highway (CA 2)
Wrightwood, CA 92397
626-821-6737
Hours: Saturday–Sunday, 10 a.m.–4 p.m.

Mount Baldy Visitor Center
Mount Baldy Road
Mount Baldy, CA 91759
909-982-2829
Hours: Saturday–Sunday, 7 a.m.–3:30 p.m.

LOS ANGELES GATEWAY RANGER DISTRICT
12371 N. Little Tujunga Canyon Road
San Fernando, CA 91342
818-889-1900
Hours: Monday–Friday, 8 a.m.–4:30 p.m.

SAN GABRIEL MOUNTAINS NATIONAL MONUMENT
110 N. Wabash Ave.
Glendora, CA 91741
626-335-1251
Hours: Monday–Friday, 8 a.m.–4:30 p.m.

SANTA CLARITA/MOJAVE RIVERS RANGER DISTRICT
33708 Crown Valley Road
Acton, CA 93510
661-269-2808
Hours: Monday–Friday, 8 a.m.–4:30 p.m.

Los Padres National Forest
fs.usda.gov/lpnf

HEADQUARTERS
6750 Navigator Way
Goleta, CA 93117
805-968-6640
Hours: Monday–Friday, 8 a.m.–4:30 p.m.

OJAI RANGER DISTRICT
1190 E. Ojai Ave.
Ojai, CA 93023
805-646-4348
Hours: Monday–Friday, 8 a.m.–4:30 p.m.

L.A.-AREA PARK DISTRICTS, LAND-MANAGEMENT AGENCIES, AND CONSERVANCIES

Catalina Island Conservancy
310-510-1445, catalinaconservancy.org

City of Burbank Parks and Recreation
818-238-5300
burbankca.gov/departments/parks-and-recreation

WILDWOOD CANYON PARK
1701 Wildwood Canyon Road
Burbank, CA 91501
818-238-5440, tinyurl.com/wildwoodcanyon
Hours: Daily, sunrise–sunset; dogs must be leashed

City of Claremont Human Services Department, City Parks
909-399-5490, tinyurl.com/claremontparks

CLAREMONT HILLS WILDERNESS PARK
North Mills Avenue
Claremont, CA 91711
909-399-5460, tinyurl.com/claremonthills
Hours: Seasonal (see website for details); dogs must be leashed

City of Glendora Parks and Recreation
626-914-8228, tinyurl.com/glendoraparksandrec

City of Malibu Community Services
310-456-2489
malibucity.org/335/community-services

CHARMLEE WILDERNESS PARK
2577 S. Encinal Canyon Road
Malibu, CA 90265
323-221-9944, tinyurl.com/charmleewildernesspark
Note: Closed at press time due to damage from the 2018 Woolsey Fire; contact the park for updates.

City of Monrovia Parks
626-932-5550
cityofmonrovia.org/your-government/parks

MONROVIA CANYON PARK
1200 N. Canyon Blvd.
Monrovia, CA 91016
626-256-8282, tinyurl.com/monroviacanyon
Hours: Open to vehicles Monday, Wednesday, Thursday, and Friday, 8 a.m.–5 p.m., Saturday–Sunday, 7 a.m.–5 p.m.; pedestrians permitted daily, sunrise–10 p.m.; dogs must be leashed

City of Palos Verdes Estates
310-378-0383, pvestates.org

PALOS VERDES ESTATES SHORELINE PRESERVE
Along Paseo del Mar from Bluff Cove to
    Lunada Bay
Palos Verdes Estates, CA 90274
Hours: Daily, sunrise–sunset; leashed dogs permitted on trails but prohibited on beach

City of Santa Clarita Open Space Preservation District
hikesantaclarita.com

City of Rancho Palos Verdes Department of Recreation, Parks, and Open Space
310-544-5260, rpvca.gov

PALOS VERDES NATURE PRESERVE
Comprises 11 parks along/above the Palos Verdes shoreline
Rancho Palos Verdes, CA 90275
310-544-5200
rpvca.gov/998/palos-verdes-nature-preserve
Hours: Daily, 1 hour before sunrise–1 hour after sunset; leashed dogs permitted on trails but prohibited on beach

City of Sierra Madre
626-355-7135, cityofsierramadre.com

Conejo Open Space Conservation Agency
805-495-6471, conejo-openspace.org

Conejo Recreation & Park District
805-495-6471, crpd.org

Glendale Community Services & Parks
818-548-2000, parksonline.glendaleca.gov

Los Angeles Department of Recreation and Parks
213-202-2700, laparks.org

GRIFFITH PARK
4730 Crystal Springs Drive
Los Angeles, CA 90027
323-644-2050, laparks.org/griffithpark
Hours: Daily, 5 a.m.–10:30 p.m.; dogs must be leashed

Los Angeles County Parks & Recreation
626-588-5364, parks.lacounty.gov

DEVIL'S PUNCHBOWL NATURAL AREA
28000 Devil's Punchbowl Road
Valyermo, CA 93563
661-944-2743, tinyurl.com/devilspunchbowlnaturalarea
Hours: Daily, sunrise–sunset; dogs must be leashed

EATON CANYON NATURAL AREA AND NATURE CENTER
1750 N. Altadena Drive
Pasadena, CA 91107
626-398-5420, tinyurl.com/eatoncanyonnaturalarea
Hours: Nature center open Tuesday–Sunday, 9 a.m.–5 p.m.; trails open daily, 7:30 a.m.–7 p.m.; closed December 25 and January 1; dogs must be leashed

PLACERITA CANYON NATURAL AREA
19152 Placerita Canyon Road
Newhall, CA 91321
661-259-7721, placerita.org
Hours: Nature center open Tuesday–Sunday, 9 a.m.–5 p.m.; park open daily, sunrise–sunset; dogs must be leashed

VASQUEZ ROCKS NATURAL AREA
10700 Escondido Canyon Road
Santa Clarita, CA 91390
661-268-0840, tinyurl.com/vasquezrocksnaturalarea
Hours: Daily, sunrise–sunset; dogs must be leashed

Los Angeles County Department of Beaches & Harbors
424-526-7777, beaches.lacounty.gov

WHITE POINT/ROYAL PALMS BEACH
1799 Paseo del Mar
San Pedro, CA 90732
310-305-9546
beaches.lacounty.gov/white-point-royal-palms-beach
Hours: Daily, sunrise–sunset; dogs prohibited

Los Angeles County Fire Department, Forestry Division
fire.lacounty.gov/forestry-division

HENNINGER FLATS FORESTRY UNIT
Visitor Information Center
2260 Pinecrest Drive
Altadena, CA 91001-2123
626-794-0675

Mountains Recreation & Conservation Authority
323-221-9944, mrca.ca.gov

Puente Hills Landfill Habitat Preservation Authority
562-945-9003, habitatauthority.org

Rancho Simi Recreation and Park District
818-584-4400, rsrpd.org

Santa Monica Mountains Conservancy
310-858-7272, smmc.ca.gov

United Water Conservation District
805-525-4431, unitedwater.org

LAKE PIRU RECREATION AREA
4780 Piru Canyon Road
Piru, CA 93040
805-521-1500, camplakepiru.com
Hours: Vary seasonally; check before you go for the latest information. Dogs must be leashed.

Maps

The following maps are available in digital and hard-copy formats, some at no cost. Most can be obtained directly from the publishers; many are also sold at ranger stations as well as outdoors stores such as REI. Beware of relying on your phone for navigation—if your battery dies, you'll have not only no maps but no way to call for help.

For **Angeles National Forest** maps and brochures, see fs.usda.gov/main/angeles/maps-pubs. For an interactive map showing fee-charging and free-access areas of the forest, see tinyurl.com/anfrecreation.

The **Catalina Island Conservancy** has free downloadable maps at its website. See tinyurl.com/catalinamaps.

Free relief-shaded maps of the trails in **Griffith Park** are available on-site and online. See tinyurl.com/griffithparkmap1 and tinyurl.com/griffithparkmap2.

National Geographic **Trails Illustrated** maps (natgeomaps.com) covering trips in this book are *Angeles National Forest (811)* ($11.95) and *Santa Monica Mountains National Recreation Area (253)* ($14.95).

The **Santa Monica Mountains Conservancy**'s free *Map of the Conservancy Zone: Santa Monica Mountains and Rim of the Valley Corridor* is available for download at smmc.ca.gov/about.html.

Tom Harrison Maps (tomharrisonmaps.com) sells waterproof topographic maps of hiking locales throughout Angeles National Forest and the Santa Monica Mountains. Click "Southern CA Maps" on the homepage for details. You can also buy these maps in handy digital format through the **Avenza Maps app.**

Finally, **U.S. Geological Survey (USGS)** 7.5-minute topographic maps are sold at store.usgs.gov but are widely available elsewhere online. For example, *National Geographic* **Maps** (see above) offers free PDFs of all USGS topo maps covering the continental United States; see natgeomaps.com/trail-maps/pdf-quads. You can access these maps through various apps (I presently prefer Gaia GPS).

Index

About the Authors

Jerry Schad (1949–2011) was Southern California's leading outdoors writer. His 16 guidebooks, including those in Wilderness Press's popular and comprehensive Afoot & Afield series, along with his "Roam-O-Rama" column in the *San Diego Reader,* helped thousands of hikers discover the region's diverse wild places. Jerry ran or hiked many thousands of miles of distinct trails throughout California, in the Southwest, and in Mexico. He was a sub-24-hour finisher of Northern California's 100-mile Western States Endurance Run, and served in a leadership capacity for outdoor excursions around the world. He taught astronomy and physical science at San Diego Mesa College and chaired its physical sciences department from 1999 until 2011. His sudden, untimely death from kidney cancer shocked and saddened the hiking community.

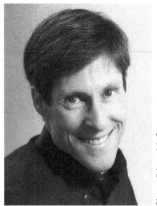

Photo: Edward A. Brown

David Harris is a professor of engineering at Harvey Mudd College. He is the author or coauthor of seven hiking guidebooks and five engineering textbooks. David grew up rambling about the Desolation Wilderness as a toddler in his father's pack and later roamed the High Sierra as a Boy Scout. As a Sierra Club trip leader, he organized mountaineering trips throughout the Sierra Nevada. Since 1999, he has been exploring the mountains and deserts of Southern California. David is the father of three sons, with whom he loves sharing the outdoors.

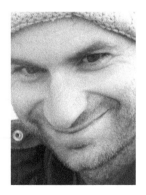

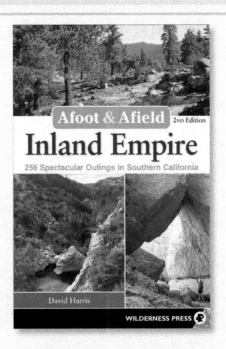

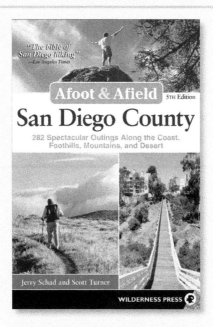
 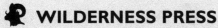

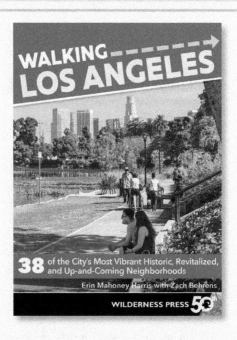
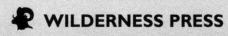

Ingram Content Group UK Ltd.
Milton Keynes UK
UKHW021256170323
418744UK00006B/45

9 781643 590417